Instructor's Resource Manual for

Community Health Nursing
Advocacy for Population Health

FIFTH EDITION

Mary Jo Clark
RN, MSN, PhD, PHN
Professor
Hahn School of Nursing and Health Science
University of San Diego
San Diego, California

Denise A. Smart, BSN, MPH, DrPH
Washington State University/Intercollegiate College of Nursing
Spokane, Washington

D1065736

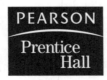

Upper Saddle River, New Jersey 07458

Notice: Care has been taken to confirm the accuracy of information presented in this book. The authors, editors, and the publisher, however, cannot accept any responsibility for errors or omissions or for consequences from application of the information in this book and make no warranty, express or implied, with respect to its contents.

The authors and publisher have exerted every effort to ensure that drug selections and dosages set forth in this text are in accord with current recommendations and practice at time of publication. However, in view of ongoing research, changes in government regulations, and the constant flow of information relating to drug therapy and reactions, the reader is urged to check the package inserts of all drugs for any change in indications or dosage and for added warning and precautions. This is particularly important when the recommended agent is a new and/or infrequently employed drug.

Publisher: Julie Levin Alexander
Assistant to Publisher: Regina Bruno
Editor-in-Chief: Maura Connor
Executive Acquisitions Editor: Pamela Lappies
Associate Editor: Michael Giacobbe
Development Editor: Elizabeth Tinsley
Managing Editor, Development: Marilyn Meserve
Editorial Art Manager: Patrick Watson
Media Product Manager: John J. Jordan
Director of Marketing: Karen Allman
Senior Marketing Manager: Francisco del Castillo
Marketing Coordinator: Michel Sirinides
Managing Editor, Production: Patrick Walsh
Production Liaison: Anne Garcia
Media Project Manager: Stephen Hartner
Manufacturing Manager: Ilene Sanford
Manufacturing Buyer: Pat Brown
Senior Design Coordinator: Mary Siener
Printer/Binder: Bind-Rite Graphics/Robbinsville
Composition: GGS Book Services
Interior Design: Janice Bielawa
Cover Design: Robert Aleman
Cover Illustration: Top, Corbis, Melanie Burford, *Dallas Morning News;*
Middle, George Dodson; Bottom, Photodisk; Background, Jupiter Images, Biran Haglwara
Cover Printer: Phoenix Color

Pearson Prentice Hall™ is a trademark of Pearson Education, Inc.
Pearson® is a registered trademark of Pearson plc
Pearson Hall® is a registered trademark of Pearson Education, Inc.

Pearson Education LTD.
Pearson Education Australia PTY, Limited
Pearson Education Singapore, Pte. Ltd
Pearson Education North Asia Ltd
Pearson Education Canada, Ltd.

Pearson Educación de Mexico, S.A. de C.V.
Pearson Education—Japan
Pearson Education Malaysia, Pte. Ltd
Pearson Education, Upper Saddle River, New Jersey

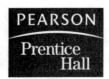

10 9 8 7 6 5 4 3 2 1
ISBN-13: 978-0-13-613556-2
ISBN: 0-13-613556-0

CONTENTS

PREFACE

Community health nurses must have the depth and breadth of knowledge that allows them to work independently and in conjunction with clients and others to improve the health of the world's populations. In part, this improvement occurs through care provided to individuals and families, but it must also occur on a larger scale through care provided to communities and population groups. *Community Health Nursing: Advocacy for Population Health,* Fifth Edition provides community health nurses with the knowledge needed to intervene at these levels. This accompanying *Instructor's Resource Manual* is designed to support your teaching in this stepped-up environment, and to reduce your preparation time for class. It will help you provide an optimal learning experience for your students and their many learning needs.

Each chapter in the Instructor's Resource Manual is thoroughly integrated with the corresponding chapter in the textbook *Community Health Nursing,* Fifth Edition. Chapters are organized by learning outcomes, and the teaching unit flows from these outcomes. You will find the following features to support the objectives:

- The Concepts for Lecture in this manual may be used in their entirety for class presentation or they may be merged with the classroom activities for a mixture of teaching styles that will meet the needs of students with various learning styles.
- The Lecture Outlines can be found on your Instructor's Resource DVD-ROM in PowerPoint. The number in the slide icon ▣ refers to the Concept for Lecture to which the slide correlates. Some lecture concepts have more than one slide, in which cases the slide icon will contain a letter after the Concept for Lecture number.
- Suggestions for Classroom and Clinical Experiences attempt to go beyond the traditional activities that have been the mainstay of nursing education for many years.
- The Resource Library identifies for you—the instructor—all the specific media resources and activities available for that chapter on the Companion Website and Instructor's Resource DVD-ROM. Chapter by chapter, the Resource Library helps you decide what resources from the Companion Website and Instructor's Resource DVD-ROM to use to enhance your course and your students' ability to apply concepts from the book into practice.

This IRM also contains a brand new "Strategies for Success" module written by Sandra DeYoung. Included within are Learning Theories, Planning for Instruction, How to Use Effective Pedagogies, Assessing Learning, and more! There is also a guide on "Teaching Nursing to Students who Speak English as a Non-Native Language." This tool is intended to guide you in reaching across cultural barriers to train nurses.

Finally, the following additional resources are also available to accompany this textbook. For more information or sample copies, please contact your Prentice Hall Sales Representative:

- **Companion Website www.prenhall.com/clark** This on-line study guide is designed to help students apply the concepts presented in the book. Each chapter-specific module features Learning Outcomes, Exam Review Questions with rationales, Chapter Outlines for lecture notes, Case Studies, Advocacy Interviews, Challenge Your Knowledge, Update *Healthy People 2010*, answers to textbook case studies, MediaLink Applications, WebLinks, Audio Glossary, and more.
- **Community Assessment Reference Guide (ISBN 0-13-240400-1)** This valuable collection of 38 tools is intended for students and community health nurses to use in providing outstanding care to individuals, families, and population groups. Two types of tools are included: assessment tools and inventories. Assessment tools provide guidance for assessing the health status of individual clients or population groups and provide space for recording data collected. These tools also provide direction for the development of nursing diagnoses, planning interventions, and evaluating the outcomes of care. Inventories are checklists of client/population-specific interventions or risk factors for selected community health problems.
- **Instructor's Resource DVD-ROM (ISBN 0-13-170987-9)** This cross-platform DVD-ROM provides text slides and illustrations in PowerPoint for use in classroom lectures. It also contains an electronic test bank and slides for use in Classroom Response Systems. This supplement is available to faculty upon adoption of the textbook. *Note: Instructor's Resource CD-ROM also available upon request.*

It is our hope that the information provided in this manual will decrease the time it takes you to prepare for class and will optimize the learning experience for your students.

Teaching Nursing to Students who Speak English as a Non-native Language

We are fortunate to have so many multi-national and multi-lingual nursing students in the US in the 21st century. As our classrooms become more diverse, there are additional challenges to communication, but we in the nursing education community are ready. Our goal is to educate competent and caring nurses to serve the health needs of our diverse communities.

We know that ENNL students experience higher attrition rates than their native English-speaking counterparts. This is a complex problem. However, there are teaching strategies that have helped many students be successful.

The first step toward developing success strategies is understanding language proficiency. Language proficiency has four interdependent components. Each component is pertinent to nursing education. *Reading* is the first aspect of language. Any nursing student will tell you that there are volumes to read in nursing education. Even native speakers of English find the reading load heavy. People tend to read more slowly in their non-native language. They also tend to recall less. Non-native speakers often spend inordinate amounts of time on reading assignments. These students also tend to take longer to process exam questions.

Listening is the second component of language. Learning from lectures can be challenging. Some students are more proficient at reading English than at listening to it. It is not uncommon for ENNL students to understand medical terminology, but to become confused by social references, slang, or idiomatic expressions used in class. The spoken language of the teacher may be different in accent or even vocabulary from that experienced by immigrant students in their language education. ENNL students may not even hear certain sounds that are not present in their native languages. Amoxicillin and Ampicillin may sound the same. Asian languages do not have gender-specific personal pronouns (he, she, him, her, etc.). Asian students may become confused when the teacher is describing a case study involving people of different genders.

Speaking is the third component of language proficiency. People who speak with an accent are often self-conscious about it. They may hesitate to voice their questions or to engage in discussion. Vicious cycles of self-defeating behavior can occur in which a student hesitates to speak, resulting in decreased speaking skills, which results in more hesitation to speak. Students may develop sufficient anxiety about speaking that their academic outcomes are affected. Students tend to form study groups with others who have common first languages. Opportunities to practice English are therefore reduced, and communication errors are perpetuated. When the teacher divides students into small groups for projects, ENNL students often do not participate as much as others.

If these students are anxious about speaking, they may withdraw from classroom participation. ENNL students may feel rejected by other students in a small group situation when their input is not sought or understood.

The fourth aspect of language is *writing*. Spelling and syntax errors are common when writing a non-native language. Teachers often respond to student writing assignments with feedback that is too vague to provide a basis for correction or improvement by ENNL students. When it comes to writing lecture notes, these students are at risk of missing important details because they may not pick up the teacher's cues about what is important. They might miss information when they spend extra time translating a word or concept to understand it, or they might just take more time to write what is being said.

Another major issue faced by ENNL nursing students is the culture of the learning environment. International students were often educated in settings where students took a passive role in the classroom. They may have learned that faculty are to be respected, not questioned. Memorization of facts may have been emphasized. It may be a shock to them when the nursing faculty expect assertive students who ask questions and think critically. These expectations cannot be achieved unless students understand them.

Finally, the European-American culture, which forms the context for nursing practice, creates challenges. Because they are immersed in Euro-American culture and the culture of nursing, faculty may not see the potential sources of misunderstanding. For example, if a teacher writes a test question about what foods are allowed on a soft diet, a student who understands therapeutic diets may miss the question if s/he does not recognize the names of the food choices. Nursing issues with especially high culture connection are: food, behavior, law, ethics, parenting, games, or choosing the right thing to say. These topics are well represented in psychiatric nursing, which makes it a difficult subject for ENNL students.

Minimizing Culture Bias on Nursing Exams

Our goal is not really to eliminate culture from nursing or from nursing education. Nursing exists in a culture-dependent context. Our goal is to practice transcultural nursing and to teach nursing without undue culture bias.

Sometimes our nursing exam questions will relate to culture-based expectations for nursing action. The way to make these questions fair is to teach transcultural nursing and to clarify the cultural expectations of a nursing student in the Euro-American-dominated health care system. Students must learn the cultural aspects of the profession before they can practice appropriately within it. Like other cultures, the professional culture of nursing has its own language (medical terminology and nursing diagnosis, of course). We have our own accepted way of dress, our own implements, skills, taboos, celebrations, and behavior. The values accepted by our culture are delineated in the ANA Code of Ethics, and are passed down to our young during nursing education.

It is usually clear to nursing educators that students are not initially aware of all the aspects of the professional culture, and that these must be taught. The social context of nursing seems more obvious to educators, and is often overlooked in nursing education. Some aspects of the social context of nursing were mentioned above (food, games, social activities, relationships, behavior, what to say in certain situations). Students must also learn these social behaviors and attitudes if they are to function fully in nursing. If they do not already know about American hospital foods, what to say when someone dies, how to communicate with an authority figure, or what game to play with a 5-year-old child, they must learn these things in nursing school.

Try for yourself the following test. It was written without teaching you the cultural expectations first.

CULTURE BIASED TEST

1. Following radiation therapy, an African American client has been told to avoid using her usual hair care product due to its petroleum content. Which product should the nurse recommend that she use instead?
   A. Royal Crown hair treatment
   B. Dax Wave and Curl
   C. Long Aid Curl Activator Gel
   D. Wave Pomade
2. A Jewish client is hospitalized for Pregnancy Induced Hypertension during Yom Kippur. How should the nurse help this client meet her religious needs based on the tradition of this holy day?
   A. Order meals without meat-milk combinations
   B. Ask a family member to bring a serving of *Marror* for the client
   C. Encourage her to fast from sunrise to sunset
   D. Remind her that she is exempt from fasting
3. Based on the Puerto Rican concept of *compadrazco*, who is considered part of the immediate family and responsible for care of children?
   A. Parents, grandparents, aunts, uncles, cousins, and godparents
   B. Mother and father, older siblings
   C. Mother, father, any blood relative
   D. Parents and chosen friends *(compadres)* who are given the honor of childcare responsibility
4. A 60-year-old Vietnamese immigrant client on a general diet is awake at 11 PM on a summer night. What is the best choice of food for the nurse to offer to this client?
   A. warm milk
   B. hot tea
   C. ice cream
   D. iced tea

5. Which of the following positions is contraindicated for a client recovering from a total hip replacement?
   A. Side-lying using an abductor pillow
   B. Standing
   C. Walking to the restroom using a walker
   D. Sitting in a low recliner

When you took this test, did it seem unfair? It was intended to test nursing behaviors that were based on culture-specific situations. Your immigrant and ENNL students are likely to face questions like these on every exam.

Item #1 is about hair care products for black hair. Option C is the only one that does not contain petroleum products. Students could know this, if they were given the information before the exam. Otherwise the item is culture-biased.

Item #2 is about the Jewish holiday Yom Kippur. To celebrate this holiday, it is customary to fast from sunrise to sunset, but people who are sick, such as the client in the question, are exempted from fasting. This is only unfair if students did not have access to the information.

Item #3 expects you to know about *compadrazco*, in which parents, grandparents, aunts, uncles, cousins, and godparents are all considered immediate family. This can be an important point if you are responsible for visiting policies in a pediatrics unit.

Item #4 tests knowledge about the preferred drink for an immigrant Vietnamese client. Many people in Asia feel comforted by hot drinks and find cold drinks to be unsettling.

Item #5 does not seem so biased. If you understand total hip precautions, it is a pretty simple question, unless you have never heard of a "low recliner." An ENNL student who missed this question, said, "I saw the chairs in clinical called 'geri chairs' and I know that the client cannot bend more than 90 degrees, but 'low recliner' was confusing to me. I imagined someone lying down (reclining) and I think this would not dislocate the prosthesis."

The best way to avoid culture bias on exams is to know what you are testing. It is acceptable to test about hip precautions, but not really fair to test about the names of furniture. The same is true of foods. Test about therapeutic diets, but not about the recipes (an African immigrant student advised us to say "egg-based food" instead of custard).

Behavior in social and professional situations is especially culture-bound. Behavior-based questions are common on nursing exams. Make behavior expectations explicit. Especially when a student is expected to act in a way that would be inappropriate in his or her social culture, these are very difficult questions. For example, we expect nurses to act assertively with physicians and clients. It is inappropriate for many Asian students to question their elders. When a client is their elder, these students will choose the option that preserves respect for the client over one that provides teaching. We must make our expectations very clear.

Finally, talk with your ENNL and immigrant students after your exams. They can provide a wealth of information about what confused them or what was ambiguous. Discuss your findings with your colleagues and improve your exams. Ultimately your exams will be clearer and more valid.

SUCCESS STRATEGIES

The following strategies were developed originally to help ENNL students. An interesting revelation is that they also help native English speakers who have learning styles that are not conducive to learning by lecture, or who read slowly, or have learning disabilities or other academic challenges.

STRATEGIES FOR PROMOTING ENNL STUDENT SUCCESS

1. You cannot decrease the reading assignment because some students read slowly, but you can help students prioritize the most important areas.
2. Allow adequate time for testing. The NCLEX is not a 1-minute-per-question test anymore. Usually 1.5 hours is adequate for a 50 item multiple-choice exam.
3. Allow students to tape lectures if they want to. You might have lectures audio-taped and put in the library for student access.
4. Speak clearly. Mumbling and rapid anxious speech are difficult to understand. If you have a problem with clarity, provide handouts containing the critical points. Provide the handouts anyway. You want to teach and test nursing knowledge, not note-taking skills.
5. Avoid slang and idiomatic expressions. This is harder than heck to do, but you can do it with practice. When you do use slang, explain it. This is especially important on exams. When in doubt about whether a word is confusing, think about what the dictionary definition would be, if there are two meanings, use another word.
6. Allow the use of translation dictionaries on exams. You can say that students must tell you what they are looking up, so they cannot find medical terminology that is part of the test.
7. Be aware of cultural issues when you are writing exams. Of course you will test on culture-specific issues, but be sure you are testing what you want to test (the student's knowledge of diets, not of recipes).
8. Feel free to use medical terminology, after all this is nursing school. However, when you use an important new term, write it on the board so students can spell it correctly in their notes.
9. In clinical, make the implied explicit. It seems obvious that safety is the priority, but if a student thinks the priority is respecting her elders, when a client with a new hip replacement demands to get out of bed there could be a disaster.
10. Hire a student who takes clear and accurate lecture notes to post his/her notes for use by ENNL and other students. The students will still attend class and take their own notes, but will have this resource to fill in the details that they miss.
11. SOA (spell out abbreviations).
12. Many international students learned to speak English in the British style. If something would be confusing to a British person, they will find it confusing.
13. Provide opportunities for students to discuss what they are learning with other students and faculty. A faculty member might hold a weekly discussion group where students bring questions. It can be interesting to find a student having no trouble tracing the path of a red cell from the heart to the portal vein, but having difficulty understanding what cream of wheat is ("I thought it was a stalk of grain in a bowl with cream poured on it").
14. Make it clear that questions are encouraged. When a student is not asking, and you think they may not understand, ask the student after class if s/he has questions. Make it easier for students to approach you by being approachable. Learn their names, and learn to pronounce them correctly. Hearing you try to pronounce their name might be humorous for them, and it will validate how difficult it is to speak other languages.
15. Take another look at basing grades on class participation. You may be putting inordinate demands on the ENNL students. Of course nurses must learn to work with others, but the nurse who talks most is not necessarily the best.
16. Be a role model for communication skills. You might even say in class when you talk about communication that if you respect a person who is trying to communicate with you, you will persist until you understand the message. Say, "Please repeat that," or "I think you said to put a chicken on my head, is that correct?" or "You want me to do what with the textbook?" It may be considered socially rude to ask people to repeat themselves repeatedly. Make it clear that this is not a social situation. In the professional role, we are responsible for effective communication. We cannot get away with smiling and nodding our heads.
17. In clinical, if a student has an accent that is difficult for the staff to understand, discuss clarification techniques (#16 above) to the student and staff member. Make it explicit that it is acceptable for the student to ask questions and for the staff to ask for clarification.
18. If your college has a writing center where students can receive feedback on grammar and style before submitting papers, have students use it. If you are not so fortunate, view papers as a rough draft instead of a final product. Give specific feedback about what to correct and allow students to resubmit them.

19. Make any services available to ENNL students available to all students (such as group discussions and notes). These services may meet the learning needs of many students while preventing the attitude that "they are different and they get something I don't."

20. Faculty attitudes are the most important determinant of a successful program to promote the success of ENNL nursing students. Talk with other faculty about the controversial issues. Create an organized program with a consistent approach among the faculty. The rewards will be well worth the work.

STRATEGIES FOR SUCCESS

Sandra De Young, Ed. D., R.N.
William Paterson University
Wayne, New Jersey

IMPROVING OUR TEACHING

Every faculty member wants to be a good teacher, and every teacher wants the students to learn. In particular, we want to achieve the student learning outcomes that our educational institutions say we must achieve. How can we best meet both goals? We cannot just teach as we were taught. We have to learn a variety of teaching methods and investigate best practices in pedagogy. We also have to learn how to measure student learning outcomes in practical and efficient ways. The next few pages will introduce you to principles of good teaching and ways to evaluate learning. Keep in mind that this is only an introduction. For a more extensive study of these principles and pedagogies, you might consult the resources listed at the end of this introduction.

LEARNING THEORY

In order to improve our teaching, we must have some familiarity with learning theory. Nurses who come into educational roles without psychology of learning courses in their background should read at least an introductory-level book on learning theories. You should, for example, know something about stages and types of learning, how information is stored in memory and how it is retrieved, and how knowledge is transferred from one situation to another.

BEHAVIORIST THEORIES

Behaviorist theories are not in as much favor today as they were 25 years ago, but they still help to explain simple learning. Conditioning and reinforcement are concepts with which most educators are familiar. Conditioning explains how we learn some simple movements and behaviors that result in desired outcomes, such as a nurse responding when an alarm sounds on a ventilator. Reinforcement refers to the fact that behavior which is rewarded or reinforced tends to reoccur. Therefore, reinforcement is a powerful tool in the hands of an educator.

COGNITIVE LEARNING THEORIES

Cognitive learning theories are much more sophisticated. They deal with how we process information by perceiving, remembering, and storing information. All of these processes are a part of learning. One of the most useful concepts in cognitive theory is that of mental schemata.

Schemata (plural) are units of knowledge that are stored in memory. For example, nurses must develop a schema related to aseptic technique. Once a schema is stored in memory, related information can be built on it.

For instance, changing a dressing is easier to learn if the learner already has a schema for asepsis.

Metacognition is another concept identified in cognitive theories. This concept refers to thinking about one's thinking. To help learners who are having difficulty mastering certain material, you might ask them to think about how they learn best and help them evaluate whether they really understand the material.

Transfer of learning occurs when a learner takes information from the situation in which it is learned and applies it to a new situation. Transfer is most likely to occur if the information was learned well in the first place, if it can be retrieved from memory, and if the new situation is similar to the original learning situation. Educators can teach for transfer by pointing out to students how a concept is applied in several situations so that learners know the concept is not an isolated one, and the students begin to look for similar patterns in new situations.

ADULT LEARNING THEORIES

Adult learning theories help to explain how learning takes place differently for adults than for children. Adults usually need to know the practical applications for the information they are given. They also want to see how it fits with their life experiences. When teaching adults, nurse educators need to keep in mind adult motivation for learning.

LEARNING STYLE THEORIES

Learning style theories abound. Research has shown that some learners are visually oriented, some are more auditory or tactile learners, some are individualistic and learn best alone, others learn best by collaboration, some deal well with abstract concepts, and others learn better with concrete information. Measurement instruments that can determine preferred learning styles are readily available. Although not many educators actually measure their students' learning styles, they should keep learning styles in mind when they plan their instruction.

PLANNING FOR INSTRUCTION

With some background knowledge of how students learn, the nurse educator can begin to plan the learning experiences. Planning includes developing objectives, selecting content, choosing pedagogies, selecting assignments, and planning for assessment of learning. All nurse educators come to the teaching process already knowing how to write objectives. Objectives can be written in the cognitive, psychomotor, and affective domains of learning. In the cognitive domain, they can be written at the knowledge, comprehension, application, analysis, and synthesis levels of complexity. The critical aspect of objectives is to keep referring to them as you plan your lesson or course. They will help you focus on the "need to know" versus the "nice to know" material. They will help you decide which assignments will be most suitable, and they will guide your development of evaluation tools.

SELECTING ASSIGNMENTS

Selecting and developing out-of-class assignments calls for creativity. You may use instructor's manuals such as this for ideas for assignments or you may also develop your own. To encourage learning through writing, you can assign short analysis papers, position papers, or clinical journals, all of which promote critical thinking. Nursing care plans of various lengths and complexity may be assigned. You may create reading guides with questions to help students read their textbooks analytically. You might also ask students to interview or observe people to achieve various objectives.

USING EFFECTIVE PEDAGOGIES

Selecting teaching methods or pedagogies takes considerable time. You must consider what you are trying to achieve. To teach facts, you may choose to lecture or assign a computer tutorial. To change attitudes or motivate learners, you may use discussion, role-playing, or gaming. Developing critical thinking may be done effectively using critical-thinking exercises, concept maps, group projects, or problem-based learning. There are traditional pedagogies, activity-based pedagogies, and technology-based pedagogies.

TRADITIONAL PEDAGOGIES

Traditional pedagogies include lecture, discussion, and questioning. Lecturing is an efficient way to convey a great deal of information to large groups of people. However, the lecture creates passive learning. Learners just sit and listen (or not) and do not interact with the information or the lecturer. Research has shown that students learn more from active learning techniques (i.e., from being able to talk about, manipulate, deduce, or synthesize information). If you are going to lecture, it would be wise to intersperse lecture with discussion and questioning.

Discussion gives students an opportunity to analyze and think critically about information that they have read or were given in a lecture. By discussing key concepts and issues, they can learn the applicability of the concepts and see how they can transfer to varied situations. Discussions can be formal or informal, but they generally work best if they are planned. For a formal discussion, students must be held accountable for preparing for it. The teacher becomes a facilitator by giving an opening statement or question, guiding the discussion to keep it focused, giving everyone a chance to participate, and summarizing at the end.

Questioning is a skill that develops over time. The first principle to learn is that you have to give students time to answer. Most teachers wait only 1 second before either repeating the question or answering it themselves. You should wait at least 3 to 5 seconds before doing anything, to allow students time to think and prepare a thoughtful answer. Research has revealed that most instructor-posed questions are at a very low level (lower-order), eliciting recall of facts. But questioning can be used to develop critical thinking if it is planned. Higher-order questions are those that require students to interpret information, to apply it to different situations, to think about relationships between concepts, or to assess a situation. If you ask higher-order questions during your classes or clinical experiences, students will rise to the occasion and will be challenged to provide thoughtful answers.

ACTIVITY-BASED PEDAGOGIES

Activity-based teaching strategies include cooperative learning, simulations, games, problem-based learning, and self-learning modules, among others. Cooperative learning is an old pedagogy that has received more research support than any other method. This approach involves learners working together and being responsible for the learning of group members as well as their own learning. Cooperative learning groups can be informal, such as out-of-class study groups, or they can be formally structured in-class groups. The groups may serve to solve problems, develop projects, or discuss previously taught content.

Simulations are exercises that can help students to learn in an environment that is low risk or risk-free. Students can learn decision making, for example, in a setting where no one is hurt if the decision is the wrong one. Simulations in skill laboratories are frequently used to teach psychomotor skills. Simulations can be written (case studies), acted out (role-playing), computer-based (clinical decision-making scenarios), or complex technology-based (active simulation manikins).

Games can help motivate people to learn. Factual content that requires memorization (such as medical terminology) can be turned into word games such as crossword puzzles or word searches. More complex games can teach problem solving or can apply previously learned information. Board games or simulation games can be used for these purposes.

Problem-based learning (PBL) provides students with real-life problems that they must research and analyze and then develop possible solutions. PBL is a group activity. The instructor presents the students with a brief problem statement. The student group makes lists of what they know and don't know about the problem. They decide what information they must collect in order to further understand the problem. As they collect the information and analyze it, they further refine the problem and begin to investigate possible solutions. The educator serves as a facilitator and resource during the learning process and helps keep the group focused.

Self-learning modules are a means of self-paced learning. They can be used to teach segments of a course or an entire course or curriculum. Modules should be built around a single concept. For example, you might design a module for a skill lab based on aseptic technique, or you could develop a module for a classroom course around the concept of airway impairment. Each module contains components such as an introduction, instructions on how to use the module, objectives, a pretest, learning activities, and a posttest. Learning activities within a module should address various learning styles. For example, you should try to include activities that appeal to visual learners and tactile learners, conceptual learners and abstract learners, and individual learners and collaborative learners. Those activities could be readings, audiovisuals, computer programs, group discussion, or skills practice. The educator develops and tests the module and then acts as facilitator and evaluator as learners work through the module.

TECHNOLOGY-BASED PEDAGOGIES

Technology-based pedagogies include computer simulations and tutorials, Internet use, and distance learning applications. Computer simulations include decision-making software in which a clinical situation is enacted and students are asked to work through the nursing process to solve problems and achieve positive outcomes. They also include simulation games such as SimCity, which can be a useful tool in teaching community health principles. Computer tutorials are useful for individual remedial work such as medication calculations or practice in answering multiple-choice test questions.

The Internet is a rich resource for classroom use and for out-of-class assignments. There are hundreds of websites that can be accessed for health-related information. Students need to be taught how to evaluate the worth of these websites. The criteria they should apply to this evaluation include identifying the intended audience, the currency of the information, the author's credentials or the affiliated organization, and content accuracy. Students may not know how to identify online journal sources compared to other websites. It is worth spending time, therefore, teaching students how to use the Internet before giving them such assignments. If your classroom is Internet access enabled, you can visually demonstrate how to identify and use appropriate websites. For example, if you want students to find relevant information for diabetic teaching, you can show them the differing value of information from official diabetes associations versus pharmaceutical sites versus chat rooms or public forums.

You may be using this instructor's manual in a distance learning course. Distance learning takes the forms of interactive television classes, webcasting, or online courses. In any form of distance learning, students are learning via the technology, but they are also learning about technology and becoming familiar with several computer applications. Those applications may include synchronous and asynchronous applications, streaming video, and multimedia functions.

ASSESSING LEARNING

You can assess or evaluate learning in a number of ways. Your first decision is whether you are just trying to get informal, ungraded feedback on how well students are learning in your class, or whether you are evaluating the students for the purpose of assigning a grade. Following are a number of techniques that can be used for one or both purposes.

CLASSROOM ASSESSMENT TECHNIQUES

Classroom assessment techniques (CATs) are short, quick, ungraded, in-class assessments used to gauge students' learning during or at the end of class. Getting frequent feedback on students' understanding helps educators to know if they are on the right track and if students are benefiting from the planned instruction. If you wait until you give a formal quiz or examination, you may have waited too long to help some students who are struggling with the material. The most popular CAT is probably the minute paper. This technique involves asking students to write down, in 1 or 2 minutes, usually at the end of class, what was the most important thing they learned that day or what points remain unclear. A related technique is the muddiest point, in which you ask the class to write down what the "muddiest" part of the class was for them. In nursing, application cards can be especially useful. After teaching about a particular concept or body of knowledge, and before you talk about the applications of the information, ask the students to fill out an index card with one possible clinical application of the information. This technique fosters application and critical thinking. Always leave class time during the following session to give feedback on the CAT results.

Another means of doing a quick assessment of learning in the classroom is the use of a classroom (or student) response system, sometimes called clicker technology. By the use of radio frequency technology, a laptop computer, a projector, and student remote controls (the clickers), an instructor can pose a written question on the screen and ask students to use their clickers to select the correct answer. The answers are then tallied and can be projected as a graph of results on the screen. This technology permits quick assessment of student understanding of critical information and keeps students active during a lecture. Classroom response systems are often made available by publishers in conjunction with their textbooks.

TESTS AND EXAMINATIONS

Tests and examinations are also used to assess or evaluate learning. Tests should be planned carefully to measure whether learning objectives have been met. You should form a test plan in which you decide the number of test items to include for each objective as well as the complexity of the items. Just as objectives can be written at the knowledge through synthesis levels of knowing, test items can be written at each level, too. Some types of items lend themselves to the lower levels of knowing, such as true-false and matching items, while multiple-choice and essay questions can be used to test higher levels.

TRUE-FALSE QUESTIONS

True-false questions are used simply to determine if the student can identify the correctness of a fact or principle. This type of question should be used sparingly, because the student has a 50% chance of guessing the correct answer. Well-written true-false questions are clear and unambiguous. The entire statement should be totally true or totally false. An example of a question that is ambiguous is:

(T F) A routine urinalysis specimen must be collected with clean technique and contain at least 100 mL.

The answer to this question is false because the specimen does not require 100 mL of volume. However, the clean technique part of the question is true. Because part of the statement is true and part is false, the question is misleading. A better question is:

(T F) A routine urinalysis specimen must be collected with clean technique.

True-false questions can be made more difficult by requiring the student to explain why the statement is true or false.

MATCHING QUESTIONS

Matching questions also test a low level of learning-that of knowledge. They are most useful for determining if students have learned definitions or equivalents of some type. They should be formatted in two columns, with the premise words or statements on the left and the definitions or responses on the right. You should have more responses than premises so that matching cannot be done simply by process of elimination. Instructions should be given that indicate if responses can be used more than once or even not used at all. An example of a matching question is:

Match the definition on the right with the suffix on the left. Definitions can be used only once or not at all.

_____ 1. -itis	a. presence of
_____ 2. -stalsis	b. abnormal flow
_____ 3. -rrhage	c. inflammation
_____ 4. -iasis	d. discharge or flow
_____ 5. -ectomy	e. contraction
	f. surgical removal of

MULTIPLE-CHOICE QUESTIONS

application through evaluation. At these higher levels they can test critical thinking. A multiple-choice question has two parts. The first part, the question, is also called the stem. The possible answers are called options. Among the options, the correct one is called the answer, while the incorrect options are termed *distractors*. You can word stems as questions or as incomplete statements that are completed by the options. For example, an item written as a question is:

WHAT IS A QUICK WAY TO ASSESS THE APPROXIMATE LITERACY LEVEL OF A PATIENT?

a. Pay attention to her vocabulary as she speaks.

b. Give her an instruction sheet to read.

c. Administer a literacy test.

d. Ask her whether she graduated from high school.

The same knowledge can be tested by a stem written as an incomplete statement:

A QUICK WAY TO ASSESS THE APPROXIMATE LITERACY LEVEL OF A PATIENT IS TO

a. pay attention to her vocabulary as she speaks.

b. give her an instruction sheet to read.

c. administer a literacy test.

d. ask her whether she graduated from high school.

Notice the differing formats of each item. When the stem is a question it is also a complete sentence, so each option should be capitalized because each is also a complete sentence and each ends with a period. When the stem is an incomplete statement, it does not end with a period, so the options that complete the statement do not begin with a capital letter but do end with a period. Stems should be kept as brief as possible to minimize reading time. Avoid negatively stated stems. For example, a poor stem would be:

WHICH OF THE FOLLOWING IS NOT A GOOD WAY TO ASSESS A PATIENT'S LITERACY LEVEL?

It is too easy for readers to miss the word not and therefore answer incorrectly. If you feel compelled to write negative stems occasionally, be sure to capitalize or underline the word *not,* or use the word *except* as in the following example:

ALL OF THE FOLLOWING ARE GOOD WAYS TO ASSESS A PATIENT'S LITERACY LEVEL EXCEPT

In this case, the reader is less likely to miss the negative word because of the sentence structure and also because the word except is capitalized.

Options usually vary from three to five in number. The more options you have, the more difficult the item. However, it is often difficult to write good distractors. Be sure that your options are grammatically consistent with the stem. Next is a test item in which all of the options do not fit grammatically with the stem:

The lecture method of teaching is best suited to

a. when the audience already knows a lot about the topic.

b. large audiences.

c. times when you are in a hurry to cover your material and don't want to be interrupted.

d. young children.

Not only are the options grammatically inconsistent, they are also of varied lengths. Attempt to keep the options about the same length. The following restatement of the item corrects the problems with grammar and with length:

The lecture method of teaching is best suited to

a. an audience that already knows the topic.

b. an audience that is very large.

c. times when you must cover your material quickly.

d. an audience of young children.

Distractors that make no sense should never be used. Instead, try to develop distractors that reflect incorrect ideas that some students might hold about a topic.

ESSAY QUESTIONS

Essay-type questions include short answer (restricted-response questions) and full essays (extended-response questions). These types of items can be used to test higher-order thinking. Extended-response essays are especially suited to testing analysis, synthesis, and evaluation levels of thinking. An example of an essay that might test these higher-order levels of thinking is:

Explain how exogenous cortisone products mimic a person's normal cortisol functions and why long-term cortisone administration leads to complications. Also explain how nursing assessment and intervention can help to reduce those complications.

The educator must plan how the essay is going to be graded before the test is given. An outline of required facts and concepts can be developed and points given to each. Then a decision must be made as to whether it is appropriate to give points for writing style, grammar, spelling, and so on.

TEST ITEM ANALYSIS

After a test is given, an analysis of objective items can be conducted. Two common analyses are item difficulty and item discrimination. Most instructors want to develop questions that are of moderate difficulty, with around half of the students selecting the correct answer. A mixture of fairly easy, moderate, and difficult questions can be used. The difficulty index can be calculated by dividing the number of students who answered the question correctly by the total number of students answering the question. The resulting fraction, converted to a percentage, gives an estimate of the difficulty, with lower percentages reflecting more difficult questions.

Item discrimination is an estimate of how well a particular item differentiates between students who generally know the material and those that don't. In other words, a discriminating item is one that most of the students who got high scores on the rest of the examination got right and most of the students who got low scores got wrong. The discrimination index can be calculated by computer software or by hand using a formula that can be found in tests and measurement textbooks.

HELPFUL RESOURCES

These few pages are but an introduction to teaching techniques. To be fully prepared for the educator role, you will need to enroll in formal courses on curriculum and teaching or do more self-learning on educational topics. For more information, you might consult the following print and Web-based resources:

DeYoung, S. (2003). Teaching Strategies for Nurse Educators, Upper Saddle River, NJ: Prentice Hall.

Web sites:

www.crlt.umich.edu/tstrategies/teachings.html

www.gmu.edu/facstaff/part-time/strategy.html

www.ic.arizona.edu/ic/edtech/strategy.html

Community Health Nursing as Advocacy

RESOURCE LIBRARY

COMPANION WEBSITE

Audio Glossary
Appendix A: Quad Council PHN Competencies
Exam Review Questions
Case Study: Empowerment Through Literacy
MediaLink Applications: Lillian Wald, Nurse Advocate
  (Video)

Media Links
Challenge Your Knowledge
Advocacy Interviews

IMAGE LIBRARY

Figure 1-1 Problem Solving in Community Health Nursing

Table 1-1 Client-Oriented Community Health Nursing Roles and Related Functions

Table 1-2 Delivery-Oriented Community Health Nursing Roles and Related Functions

Table 1-3 Population-Oriented Community Health Nursing Roles and Related Functions

LEARNING OBJECTIVE 1

Define community health nursing.

CONCEPTS FOR LECTURE

1. Definitions of community health nursing incorporate the use of the nursing process and concepts of public health with a primary focus on population health.
2. Public health nursing has historical roots imbedded in environmental sanitation and control of communicable diseases. More recently, community health nursing has been associated with health education and individual behavior change. Today, community health nursing incorporates actions to change a broad range of factors that influence health.

POWERPOINT LECTURE SLIDES

NOTE: The number on each PPT Lecture Slide directly corresponds with the Concepts for Lecture.

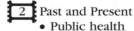 Definition of Community Health Nursing
- Science and practice of public health
- Systematic use of nursing process
- Promotes health and prevents illness
- Focuses on population groups

Past and Present
- Public health
  - Environmental sanitation
  - Control of communicable diseases
- Community health
  - Health education
  - Individual behavior change
  - Actions to change factors that influence health

SUGGESTIONS FOR CLASSROOM ACTIVITIES

What's in a name? Have the class divide into two groups: public health and community health. Ask each group to review the Principles of Public Health Nursing, the Standards of Public Health Nursing Practice, and Tables 1–1 through 1–3, pertaining to community health nursing. Next, have each group present an argument for their specific specialty title.

SUGGESTIONS FOR CLINICAL ACTIVITIES

Invite a community health nurse to discuss the various programs offered at the local health department. Clarify and discuss the relationship between the local, regional, and state health departments.

LEARNING OBJECTIVE 2

Distinguish among community-based, community-focused, and community-driven nursing and describe their relationship to community health nursing.

CONCEPTS FOR LECTURE

1. Community-based nursing provides care to individuals in community settings. Often these individuals require care for a specific illness.
2. Community-focused nursing brings nursing knowledge and expertise to the community.
3. Community-driven nursing focuses on the needs of the community as a whole and emphasizes community participation in determining those needs.
4. Community health nurses focus on the health of population groups. They may provide aggregate care for a population with a common characteristic or for an entire population. The mission of community health nursing is to improve the overall health of a population through health promotion, illness prevention, and protection from biological, behavioral, social, and environmental threats. The goal is to promote health by preventing illness and injury. Community health nursing's overall expectation is that improving population health benefits the individuals of that population.

POWERPOINT LECTURE SLIDES

NOTE: The number on each PPT Lecture Slide directly corresponds with the Concepts for Lecture.

1 Community-Based Nursing
- Provides care to individuals (often to those who are ill)
- Delivers care in a community setting

2 Community-Focused Nursing
- Brings nursing knowledge and expertise to community

3 Community-Driven Nursing
- Focuses on whole community needs as identified by community members
- Emphasizes community participation to determine needs

4 Community Health Nursing
- Mission, goals, and expectations
  - Promote and improve health
  - Prevent illness and injury
  - Protect from threats
    - Biological
    - Behavioral
    - Social
    - Environmental

SUGGESTIONS FOR CLASSROOM ACTIVITIES

1. Use the Internet to locate various local and state health department goals and objectives.
2. Invite local community health nurse to discuss specific populations that receive care or services.

SUGGESTIONS FOR CLINICAL ACTIVITIES

Have students research biological, behavioral, social, and environmental threats to population groups after Hurricane Katrina. Present findings to classmates.

LEARNING OBJECTIVE 3

Differentiate between district and program-focused community health nursing.

CONCEPTS FOR LECTURE

1. Aspects of program-focused community health nursing and district nursing can be differentiated from the literature. Program-focused community health nursing is a service delivery system designed to address specific health problems or the needs of specific target populations. District nursing originated in England and emphasizes community health nurses' responsibility for addressing all the health needs of a specific geographical segment of the population.

POWERPOINT LECTURE SLIDES

NOTE: The number on each PPT Lecture Slide directly corresponds with the Concepts for Lecture.

1 Program-focused
- Service delivery system
- Specific health problems
- Specific target populations
- Specialist practice
- Focus on a specific set of services
- More focus on services to groups

1a District Nursing
- Originated in England
- Addresses health needs of given geographic segment of the population
- Broad spectrum of services
- Generalist practice
- More services to individuals

SUGGESTIONS FOR CLASSROOM ACTIVITIES

Divide students into two groups: a program-focused group and a district nursing group. Ask each group to describe and to distinguish how they would meet the population health needs for a specific target group or geographical segment.

SUGGESTIONS FOR CLINICAL ACTIVITIES

1. Provide an opportunity for students to research specific health problems identified in the local community using Internet resources and other published data for the community.
2. Invite a community health practitioner to discuss specific health problems, target populations, and services provided in the local community.

LEARNING OBJECTIVE 4

Identify at least five attributes of community health nursing.

CONCEPTS FOR LECTURE

1. The eight unique attributes for community health nursing include population consciousness, orientation to health, autonomy, creativity, continuity, collaboration, intimacy, and variability.

POWERPOINT LECTURE SLIDES

NOTE: The number on each PPT Lecture Slide directly corresponds with the Concepts for Lecture.

1 Eight Unique Attributes of Community Health Nurses
- Population consciousness
- Orientation to health
- Autonomy
- Creativity

1a Eight Unique Attributes of Community Health Nurses (continued)
- Continuity
- Collaboration
- Intimacy
- Variability

 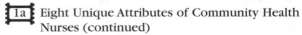

1. Have students identify how the eight attributes apply to community health nursing in their community. Compare and contrast hospital, clinic, and community nursing attributes.
2. Have students identify examples of the attributes as they have seen them in their own clinical practice.
3. Share community resources and types of group meetings that community health nurses may attend. Discuss how community health nurses exemplify specific attributes such as collaboration, autonomy, and creativity when they organize community forums and specific community committee meetings.

Have students select a community support group, meeting, or educational class from the list of community resources. Have students research their community assignment prior to scheduling clinical experience. Ask them to develop a list of questions for the group leader that emphasize the attributes described in this section.

LEARNING OBJECTIVE 5

Describe the process of advocacy as enacted by community health nurses.

CONCEPTS FOR LECTURE

1. Advocacy is defined as the act of pleading or arguing in favor of a cause, idea, or policy on someone else's behalf. Nursing advocacy extends the concept of protecting clients against harm through such activities as informing clients, protecting client rights, mediating between clients and health care providers, and supporting client autonomy.
2. Community health nursing advocacy is defined as action taken on behalf of, or in concert with, individuals, families, or populations to create or support an environment that promotes health.
3. Advocacy models include guardian of legal rights, preservation of patient values, champion of social justice and access to care, and client empowerment. Advocacy for social justice is an essential aspect of the core mission of community health nursing.
4. The advocacy process involves three essential categories of participants: a recipient of the advocacy, an advocate, and an adversary, and a consequence for all the participants in the process. Within this process are three factors that influence participants in an advocacy situation: knowledge, conviction, and emotion.
5. Approaches to effective advocacy involve the advocate taking action that is situation- and client-specific, using a collaborative and cooperative approach with the adversary, educating the advocacy recipient or adversary, confronting the adversary, requesting a change, explaining, and enlisting the aid of others.
6. Community health nurses serve in an advocacy role when they engage in several activities: determining the need for advocacy, determining the point at which advocacy is most effective, collecting facts

POWERPOINT LECTURE SLIDES

NOTE: The number on each PPT Lecture Slide directly corresponds with the Concepts for Lecture.

1 Advocacy
- Definition
- Nursing advocacy

2 Community Health Nursing Advocacy
- Definition

3 Advocacy Models
- Guardian of legal rights
- Preservation of patient values
- Champion of social justice and access to care
- Client empowerment

4 Advocacy Process
- A recipient of the advocacy
- An advocate
- An adversary
- A consequence for all the participants in the process

4a Advocacy Process (continued)
- Factors that influence participants in an advocacy situation
  - Knowledge
  - Conviction
  - Emotion

5 Approaches to Effective Advocacy
- Advocate takes action that is situation- and client-specific
- Use a collaborative and cooperative approach with the adversary

CONCEPTS FOR LECTURE continued

surrounding the problem, presenting the client's case to the appropriate decision makers, and preparing clients to speak for themselves.

- Educate the advocacy recipient or adversary
- Confront the adversary
- Request a change
- Explain
- Enlist the aid of others

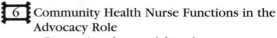 Community Health Nurse Functions in the Advocacy Role
- Determine the need for advocacy
- Determine the point at which advocacy is most effective
- Collect facts surrounding the problem
- Present the client's case to the appropriate decision makers
- Prepare clients to speak for themselves

SUGGESTIONS FOR CLASSROOM ACTIVITIES

Divide students into three groups: recipient of advocacy, the advocate, and the adversary. Provide students with a case scenario of a family with a medically fragile child in need of specialized care not provided in the local community. Ask groups to role play their position using knowledge, conviction, and emotion as influencing factors.

SUGGESTIONS FOR CLINICAL ACTIVITIES

Have students identify situations or examples of advocacy in action in their clinical practice setting. During post conference, ask students to discuss their examples from all three perspectives: recipient, advocate, and adversary.

LEARNING OBJECTIVE 6

Summarize the standards for community health nursing practice.

CONCEPTS FOR LECTURE

1. The key concept is that standards of practice are essential to a profession.
2. The American Nurses Association delineates standards that incorporate a framework for the community health nursing process and core functions of public health.
3. Professional standards address expected levels of professional performance, quality of practice, education, practice evaluation, collegiality, ethics, collaboration, research, resource utilization, leadership, and advocacy.

POWERPOINT LECTURE SLIDES

NOTE: The number on each PPT Lecture Slide directly corresponds with the Concepts for Lecture.

1 Standards of Practice
- Essential to a profession

2 Developed by Quad Council of Public Health Nursing Organizations
- Apply nursing process to community/public health nursing practice
- Incorporate core functions of public health

3 Professional Standards
- Expected levels of professional performance
- Quality of practice
- Education
- Practice evaluation
- Collegiality

3a Professional Standards (continued)
- Ethics
- Collaboration
- Research
- Resource utilization
- Leadership
- Advocacy

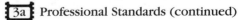

SUGGESTIONS FOR CLASSROOM ACTIVITIES

Have the class search the Web for practice standards for different nursing specialties. Have students develop a diagram that explains the benefits of practice standards for the nurse, client, and community.

SUGGESTIONS FOR CLINICAL ACTIVITIES

Assign students one standard to focus on as they begin their clinical experience Ask students to discuss their standard in their journal writing for that week.

LEARNING OBJECTIVE 7

Identify the eight domains of competency for community health nursing.

CONCEPTS FOR LECTURE

1. The eight domains of community health nursing practice include the following: analytic assessment, policy development and program planning, communication, cultural competence, community dimensions of practice, basic public health practice, financial planning and measurement, and leadership and systems thinking.

POWERPOINT LECTURE SLIDES

NOTE: The number on each PPT Lecture Slide directly corresponds with the Concepts for Lecture.

1 Eight Domains of Competency
- Analytic assessment
- Policy development and program planning
- Communication
- Cultural competence

1a Eight Domains of Competency (continued)
- Community dimensions of practice
- Basic public health practice
- Financial planning and measurement
- Leadership and systems thinking

SUGGESTIONS FOR CLASSROOM ACTIVITIES

Assign students to groups to prepare examples of how these eight domains are applied at the two levels of community health nursing practice.

SUGGESTIONS FOR CLINICAL ACTIVITIES

1. Contact the health department for a schedule of local and community meetings in which community health nurses are chairing, co-chairing or otherwise responsible for the overall direction of the meeting (such as a disaster-preparedness meeting, a pandemic influenza committee meeting, or a community needs assessment meeting. Assign students to attend and report to class how the eight domains of competency were evidenced at the various meetings.
2. Have students examine the practice of community health nurses in their clinical practice setting and identify activities that exemplify the PHN competencies. Have them distinguish between activities that exemplify generalist- and specialist-level competencies.

LEARNING OBJECTIVE 8

Distinguish among client-oriented, delivery-oriented, and population-oriented community health nursing roles.

CONCEPTS FOR LECTURE

1. Client-oriented, delivery-oriented, and population-oriented roles vary based on the focus of activity.
2. Client-oriented roles apply to the care of specific individuals or families. Delivery-oriented roles focus on the mechanisms by which care is delivered.

POWERPOINT LECTURE SLIDES

NOTE: The number on each PPT Lecture Slide directly corresponds with the Concepts for Lecture.

1 Community Health Nursing Roles
- Vary based on specific practice setting

CONCEPTS FOR LECTURE continued

population-oriented roles are organized around the care of communities or populations.

3. The types of and emphasis placed on specific roles will vary by practice setting.

POWERPOINT LECTURE SLIDES continued

- Focus of activity
  - Client-oriented roles
  - Delivery-oriented roles
  - Population-oriented roles

 Focus of Services
- Types and emphasis placed on specific roles vary by practice setting
- Client-oriented roles
  - Emphasize direct care of specific individuals or families
- Delivery-oriented roles
  - Focus on mechanisms of care delivery
  - Primarily address care delivery to individuals and families
- Population-oriented roles
  - Care of communities or populations

SUGGESTIONS FOR CLASSROOM ACTIVITIES

Have students research, summarize, and present to the class articles in public health and community health nursing journals that address the three specific roles. Discuss key words to use for their literature search.

SUGGESTIONS FOR CLINICAL ACTIVITIES

Invite a guest speaker from the local community health department to share how the nurse prepares for each of these roles. Discuss various programs at local, state, and national level that emphasize these three roles.

LEARNING OBJECTIVE 9

Describe at least five client-oriented roles performed by community health nurses.

CONCEPTS FOR LECTURE

1. The key objectives for a client-oriented role are to the nursing process to clients at any level. The functions for these roles are assessing client needs, developing nursing diagnoses, planning nursing interventions, and evaluating nursing care and its outcomes.

2. Client-oriented roles include, but are not limited to, caregiver, educator, counselor, referral resource, role model, primary care provider, and case manager.

3. The community health nurse as a caregiver provides primary care and delegated care for individuals, families, groups, and communities with a focus on health promotion and illness prevention interventions such as routine prenatal assessments, well-child care, and immunizations. The caregiver role may also encompass care to ill individuals.

4. As an educator, the community health nurse facilitates learning with a focus on positive health behaviors through the development of population-based health education programs.

5. Counseling focuses on choosing viable solutions to health problems by assisting clients to identify and clarify their health problem, identifying alternative solutions, assisting clients in developing criteria for acceptable solutions to their problem, and assisting in the evaluation of alternative solutions and problem-solving processes.

POWERPOINT LECTURE SLIDES

NOTE: The number on each PPT Lecture Slide directly corresponds with the Concepts for Lecture.

1. Client-Oriented Objectives
- Apply the nursing process
- Assess client needs
- Develop nursing diagnoses
- Plan nursing interventions
- Evaluate nursing care and outcomes

2. Client-Oriented Roles
- Caregiver
- Educator
- Counselor
- Referral resource
- Role model
- Primary care provider
- Case manager

3. Caregiver Functions
- Assess client health status
- Derive nursing diagnosis
- Plan nursing intervention
- Implement plan of care
- Perform delegated medical treatments or provide primary care as needed

6. The community health nurse acts as a referral resource by directing clients to resources required to meet their needs. The referral process focuses on determining the need for a referral, identifying appropriate referral resources, making the referral, and following up on the referral.
7. The community health nurse acts as a role model by demonstrating healthy behaviors to clients and student or novice nurses. Health-related behaviors are influenced as the nurse responds to crises, in the treatment of clients and the types of client-focused activities selected, and in the professional display of competency.
8. The community health nurse acts as a case manager. This has been a proven cost-effective mechanism that enhances health outcomes through the coordination, selection, and use of health care services that meet the clients' needs. Case management maximizes the utilization of resources, minimizes the expenses of care, identifies high-risk/high-cost service needs clients, makes appropriate service choices, and ultimately controls costs.

3a Caregiver Functions (continued)
- Introduce other supportive services as needed
- Teach and supervise others
- Teach clients self-care
- Coordinate health care services
- Serve as liaison between client and system
- Evaluate the outcome of nursing intervention and modify plan

4 Educator Role
- Assess client's need for education
- Develop health education plan
- Present health education
- Evaluate outcome of health education

5 Counseling Role: Choose Viable Solutions to Health Problems
- Assist client to identify and clarify problem
- Help identify alternative solutions to problem
- Assist client to develop criteria for acceptable solution
- Assist client to evaluate alternative solutions
- Evaluate problem-solving process
- Point out use of problem-solving process for future use

6 Referral Resource: Direct Client to Resources Required to Meet Their Needs
- Obtain information on community resources
- Determine need for and appropriateness of referral
- Make and follow up on the referral

7 Role Model
- Demonstrate behaviors
  - Influence health related behaviors
  - Response to crisis
  - Treatment of clients
  - Types of client-focused activities
  - Display competence

8 Case Manager
- Identify need for case management
- Assess and identify client health needs
- Design plan of care
- Oversee implementation of care by others
- Evaluate outcome of care

SUGGESTIONS FOR CLASSROOM ACTIVITIES

Divide students into groups based on client-oriented roles. Have groups role-play as the community health nurse, with a client who is a homeless female who presents at 32 weeks pregnant with no prenatal care. Based on their specific group role, ask students to develop a course of action to address this client's needs. Share strategies with class.

SUGGESTIONS FOR CLINICAL ACTIVITIES

Have students identify the specific client-oriented roles they engage in during their care of specific clients in their clinical setting.

LEARNING OBJECTIVE 10

Describe at least three delivery-oriented roles performed by community health nurses.

CONCEPTS FOR LECTURE

1. Delivery-oriented roles enhance the operation of the health care delivery system through the roles of care manager, whose function is to coordinate care by a process of organizing and integrating services; collaborator, who resolves client health problems using communication skills and joint decision making with the client and other professionals and liaison; and liaison, who coordinates, refers, and advocates in order to connect the client to other providers, and later interprets and reinforces those provider's recommendations.

POWERPOINT LECTURE SLIDES

NOTE: The number on each PPT Lecture Slide directly corresponds with the Concepts for Lecture.

1 Delivery-Oriented Roles
- Enhance operation of health care delivery system
  - Coordinator/care manager
  - Collaborator
  - Liaison

1a Coordinator/Care Manager
- Determine who is providing care to client
- Communicate with other providers regarding client situation and needs
- Arrange case conferences as needed
- Assist in development of care networks

1b Collaborator
- Communicate with other health team members
- Participate in joint decision making
- Participate in joint action to resolve client problems
- Participate in joint activities to evaluate the outcome of care

1c Liaison
- Serve as initial point of contact between client and agency
- Facilitate communication between client and agency personnel
- Interpret and reinforce provider recommendations
- Serve as client advocate as needed

SUGGESTIONS FOR CLASSROOM ACTIVITIES

Have students role-play as coordinator/care manager, collaborator, and liaison for a suspected Hepatitis A outbreak in a local elementary school.

SUGGESTIONS FOR CLINICAL ACTIVITIES

1. Assign students to three groups. Each group will observe a community health nurse in the work setting from the perspective of coordinator/care manager, collaborator, and liaison and report during post conference specific behaviors that exemplify these delivery-oriented roles.
2. Have students provide examples of their enactment of delivery-oriented roles during their own clinical practice experiences.

LEARNING OBJECTIVE 11

Describe at least four population-oriented roles performed by community health nurses.

CONCEPTS FOR LECTURE

1. Population-oriented roles promote, maintain, and restore the health of the population through case finding, leadership, change agent, policy developer, community organizer/mobilizer, coalition builder, social marketer, and researcher roles.
2. Acting as a case finder, the community health nurse develops an index of suspicion, identifies individual cases or occurrences of specific diseases, and provides for follow-up services.
3. In a leadership role, the community health nurse identifies the need for action and leadership, assesses the leadership needs of followers, and selects and executes an appropriate style of leadership for followers and for the situation at hand.
4. As a change agent, the nurse plans, controls, and enhances health processes by recognizing the need for change, making others aware of hat need, motivating others to change, and initiating and directing desired change.
5. The community health nurse functions as a community mobilizer by assisting community members to identify issues and goals and develop action plans, mobilizing assets necessary to implement strategies, and participating in strategy implementation.
6. A coalition builder creates temporary or permanent alliances by identifying members for the coalition, presenting mutual benefits, delineating coalition goals, assisting in the development of coalition operating guidelines, and participating in the selection and implementation of means to accomplish those goals.
7. The community health nurse acts as a policy advocate by working for and arguing on behalf of policy formation and policy changes that affect the health of population groups.
8. As a social marketer, the nurse assumes a consumer-focused role in the development of social marketing approaches to achieve changes designed to improve population health.
9. Finally, as a researcher, the community health nurse reviews relevant research, identifies researchable problems, designs and conducts research, collects data, and disseminates those research findings to provide an evidence base for interventions to improve population health.

POWERPOINT LECTURE SLIDES

NOTE: The number on each PPT Lecture Slide directly corresponds with the Concepts for Lecture.

1 Population-Oriented Roles
- Promote, maintain, and restore the health of population
  - Case finder
  - Leader
  - Change agent
  - Policy developer

1a Population-Oriented Roles (continued)
- Community organizer/mobilizer
- Coalition builder
- Social marketer
- Researcher

2 Case Finder Role
- Develop knowledge of signs and symptoms of health-related conditions and contributing factors
- Use diagnostic reasoning process to identify potential cases of disease or other health-related conditions
- Carry out investigation of specific cases of disease as needed
- Provide follow-up care to identified cases

3 Leadership Role
- Identify need for action
- Assess situation and followers to determine appropriate leadership style
- Motivate followers to take action
- Coordinate group member activities in planning and implementing action
- Assist followers to evaluate the effectiveness of action taken

4 Change Agent
- Plans, controls, and enhances health processes
  - Recognizes need for change
  - Makes others aware of need
  - Motivates others to change
  - Initiates and directs desired change

5 Community Mobilizer
- Assists community members to identify health issues of concern
- Participates in data collection relevant to issues of concern
- Mobilizes community members to take action
- Assists with coalition development to foster community action
- Assists community members to identify achievable goals

POWERPOINT LECTURE SLIDES *continued*

- Participates in the development of strategies to accomplish identified goals
- Participates in the implementation of community strategies to achieve goals

6 Coalition Builder Creating Temporary/Permanent Alliances
- Functions include
  - Identify potential coalition members based on common interest, assets available, etc.
  - Present potential coalition members with the benefits to be achieved through alliance
  - Participate in the delineation of coalition goals
  - Assist in the development of operating guidelines for the coalition
  - Participate in the selection and implementation of strategies to accomplish coalition goals

7 Policy Advocate
- Determine need for policy development
- Analyze factors influencing the policy situation
- Identify key decision makers
- Assist in policy formation
- Communicate the proposed policy
- Monitor the progress of policy development

8 Social Marketer
- Identify the need for societal behavior change
- Analyze motivation and perceived benefits and barriers to the desired change
- Identify target markets and their unique features
- Develop and test social marketing strategies appropriate to target markets
- Assist with implementation strategies
- Evaluate the effectiveness of social marketing strategies in achieving the desired change

9 Researcher
- Critically review relevant research
- Apply research findings to practice
- Identify researchable problems
- Design and conduct research
- Collect and analyze data
- Disseminate research findings

SUGGESTIONS FOR CLASSROOM ACTIVITIES

Divide students into three groups: client oriented, delivery oriented, and population oriented. Ask students to prepare interview questions for community health nurses and leaders emphasizing the roles discussed in class.

SUGGESTIONS FOR CLINICAL ACTIVITIES

With an emphasis on client-oriented, delivery-oriented, and population-oriented roles, have students interview, prepare, and present a summary of discussion results with community health nurses and leaders.

The Population Context

RESOURCE LIBRARY

 COMPANION WEBSITE

Audio Glossary
Exam Review Questions
Case Study: Seatbelt Safety
MediaLink Applications: The Ruth Freeman Population
  Nursing Award

Media Links
Challenge Your Knowledge
Advocacy Interviews

LEARNING OBJECTIVE 1

Distinguish among neighborhoods, communities, and aggregates as populations served by community health nurses.

CONCEPTS FOR LECTURE

1. Differentiate population from neighborhoods, communities, and aggregates as subsegments of a population. A unique feature of community health nursing is the type of client served. Community health nurses provide services not only to individuals and families, but also to neighborhoods, communities, and targeted groups or aggregates of specific populations.

2. Neighborhoods are small, homogeneous groups of people with self-defined natural or human-made constraint factors. Neighborhoods are often characterized by face-to-face interactions and identification with others living in the neighborhood.

3. Communities are defined as groups of people who share common interests, interact with each other, and function collectively within a defined social structure to address common concerns. They can be geopolitical communities or communities of identity.

4. Defining aspects of communities include a social system or institutions, identity, commitment, common norms and values, common history or interests, common symbols, social interaction, and intentional action to meet common needs.

5. Aggregates are defined as subpopulations within a larger population who possess common characteristics, often related to high risk for specific health problems.

POWERPOINT LECTURE SLIDES

NOTE: The number on each PPT Lecture Slide directly corresponds with the Concepts for Lecture.

1 Community Health Nursing Clients
  • Neighborhoods
  • Communities
  • Aggregates
  • Populations

2 Neighborhood Characteristics
  • Small
  • Homogeneous
  • Self-defined
  • Constrained by:
    ○ Natural factors (e.g., a river or canyon)
    ○ Man-made factors (e.g., roads)

3 Community Characteristics
  • Groups of people
  • Share common interest
  • Interact with one another
  • Function collectively within defined social structure
    ○ Address common concerns
  • Types
    ○ Geopolitical
    ○ Communities of identity

4 Defining Aspects
  • Social system or institutions
  • Identity
  • Commitment
  • Common norms and values

4a Defining Aspects (continued)
- Common history or interests
- Common symbols
- Social interactions
- Intentional action

5 Aggregate Characteristics
- Subpopulations
  ○ Share common characteristics
    – May include high-risk for specific health problems

SUGGESTIONS FOR CLASSROOM ACTIVITIES

1. Neighborhoods, communities, and aggregate populations can have many different characteristics, issues, concerns, and interests. Divide students into groups. Have students list healthy and unhealthy qualities or characteristics of neighborhood, community, or aggregate groups.
2. Ask students to bring in newspaper clippings throughout the week that depict healthy or unhealthy characteristics of communities. Provide opportunity to discuss these characteristics.

SUGGESTIONS FOR CLINICAL ACTIVITIES

Arrange for students to work with a community health nurse who provides care in the community to specific aggregate populations. Have students observe the neighborhood and in post conference, discuss those observations.

LEARNING OBJECTIVE 2

Define population health.

CONCEPTS FOR LECTURE

1. Population health evolved as a result of limitations in individual-oriented care for improving the health of population groups. Population health is defined as the greatest possible level of health in the overall population and the distribution of health to its members.
2. Descriptive approaches to population health focus on the health status of a population utilizing specific summary indicators of health. Analytic approaches focus on broad factors that influence health and are used to direct interventions to improving health status.
3. The definition of population health developed from three conceptual models of health: a biomedical model (health problems), a holistic model (multiple factors), and a dynamic model (interaction of resources and physical capacities).
4. Healthy communities are characterized by their ability to foster dialogue among residents to develop a shared vision for the community, promote community leadership, engage in action based on a shared vision, embrace diversity among residents, assess needs and assets, link residents to community resources, foster a sense of responsibility and cohesion among residents, have an ability to change and adapt to changing circumstances, and manage conflict effectively.

POWERPOINT LECTURE SLIDES

NOTE: The number on each PPT Lecture Slide directly corresponds with the Concepts for Lecture.

1 Population Health
- Arose from limitations in individual-oriented care for improving the health of population groups
- Defined as highest possible level of health in the population
- Distribution of health among members of the population

2 Two Approaches to Population Health
- Descriptive approach
  ○ Focuses on the health status of a population
  ○ Utilizes specific summary indicators of health
  ○ Distribution of health indicators in that population

2a Two Approaches to Population Health (continued)
- Analytic approach:
  ○ Broad factors influencing health
  ○ Identifies factors contributing to health indicators
  ○ Direct interventions to improve health status

3 Population Health Conceptual Models
- Biomedical model
  ○ Present-focused on heath problems
- Holistic model
  ○ Multiple factors influence positive and negative states of health

- Dynamic model
  - Health is a process that improves quality of life
    - Health results from interaction with available resources

☐ 4 Characteristics of Healthy Communities
- Ability to foster dialogue among residents
- Promote community leadership
- Engage in action based on a shared vision
- Embrace diversity among residents

☐ 4a Characteristics of Healthy Communities (continued)
- Assess both needs and assets
- Link residents to community resources
- Foster a sense of responsibility and cohesion
- Change and adapt to changing circumstances
- Manage conflict effectively

SUGGESTIONS FOR CLASSROOM ACTIVITIES

1. Invite community leaders, health board members, and Chamber of Commerce or health providers to a roundtable discussion of healthy community concepts.
2. Divide students into two groups (descriptive and analytic). Using their selected approach, have students research a neighborhood or community using Internet resources, such as police reports, satellite photos of area, and state and local health reports, and present their research of as many community characteristics as possible to the class.

SUGGESTIONS FOR CLINICAL ACTIVITIES

Arrange for students to drive through selected communities or neighborhoods in teams of 3 or 4. Using their senses of vision and smell, and their cognitive skills of assessing resources, potential health risks, location to health resources, and other resources (bike paths, freeways, bridges, sites where homeless populations may cluster, parks and recreational areas, industrial areas, etc.) have students write down observations of those communities and report back to class.

LEARNING OBJECTIVE 3

Describe changes in approaches to population health.

CONCEPTS FOR LECTURE

1. Historically, the focus of population health was on the control of epidemics and communicable diseases through sanitation efforts. During the mid-1900s, the focus moved to disease prevention, which focused on personal behavior changes. Presently, population health emphasizes concepts of social justice and the creation of environments that foster health.

POWERPOINT LECTURE SLIDES

NOTE: The number on each PPT Lecture Slide directly corresponds with the Concepts for Lecture.

☐ 1 Population Health Trends
- Historical
  - Control of epidemics and communicable diseases:
    - Sanitation
    - Quarantine
- Mid-1900s
  - Disease prevention
    - Immunization
    - Personal behavior changes

☐ 1a Population Health Trends (continued)
- Present
  - Population health
    - Social justice
    - Healthy environments
    - Access to resources needed for health

SUGGESTIONS FOR CLASSROOM ACTIVITIES

1. Have students explore factors that led to changes in conceptualizations of population health and report their findings to the class.
2. Show the video, *The Most Dangerous Woman in America: Typhoid Mary.* Have the students discuss the video from the perspective of controlling disease, disease prevention, and social justice.
3. Arrange for an epidemiologist to discuss population health trends in the local area over the past 50 years.

SUGGESTIONS FOR CLINICAL ACTIVITIES

Have students identify population health issues they are encountering in the clinical setting and discuss how they might have been addressed using each of the three approaches discussed in the text.

LEARNING OBJECTIVE 4

Describe the three levels at which population health care occurs.

CONCEPTS FOR LECTURE

1. The three levels of population health care are primary prevention, secondary prevention, and tertiary prevention.
2. Primary prevention may be defined as measures designed to promote general optimum health and/or prevent illness. It includes actions taken prior to the occurrence of health problems with the general purpose of avoiding the occurrences altogether. The focus is on increasing resistance to illness, decreasing or eliminating the causes of health problems, or fostering a healthy environment.
3. Secondary prevention is defined as the early identification and treatment of existing health problems and takes place after the health problem has occurred. Activities include screening, early diagnosis and treatment, and development of programs to diagnose and treat at the community level.
4. Tertiary prevention aims to return the client to the highest level of function and to prevent health problem recurrences and further deterioration in health. Maintenance health programs and specific legislation that promotes a higher quality of life are examples.

POWERPOINT LECTURE SLIDES

NOTE: The number on each PPT Lecture Slide directly corresponds with the Concepts for Lecture.

1 Three Levels of Population Health Care
- Primary prevention
- Secondary prevention
- Tertiary prevention

2 Primary Prevention
- Promote general optimal health and prevent illness
- Actions occur prior to illness or disease
- Increase resistance to illness
- Decrease or eliminate the causes of health problems
- Foster a healthy environment

3 Secondary Prevention
- Early identification and treatment of existing health problems
- Actions take place after problem has occurred
- Screening, early diagnosis, and treatment
- Develop programs to diagnose and treat at community level

4 Tertiary Prevention
- Return client to highest level of function
- Prevent recurring health problems
- Prevent further deterioration of health:
  ○ Maintenance health programs

SUGGESTIONS FOR CLASSROOM ACTIVITIES

Assign students to teams to research one chronic disease (e.g., diabetes, hypertension, obesity) and one acute health problem (e.g., sexually transmitted disease, infectious disease). Addressing activities at the primary, secondary, and tertiary levels of prevention, have them present to the class the resources at local, state, and national levels that are available to community clients, neighborhoods, or aggregate groups.

SUGGESTIONS FOR CLINICAL ACTIVITIES

Have students interview community health nurses to assess programs and interventions that exist in various communities and report to the class the levels of prevention that are addressed by the programs or interventions during post conference.

LEARNING OBJECTIVE 5

Describe trends in national health objectives for 1990, 2000, and 2010.

CONCEPTS FOR LECTURE

1. The goal of the national health objectives as created in 1980 by the U.S. Department of Health and Human Services was to reduce mortality. These objectives set the goals and desired outcomes for population health in the United States and targeted 15 priority intervention areas in three strategic action categories: preventive health, health protection, and health promotion.

2. Developed in 1990, a second set of objectives focused on increasing the span of healthy life, reducing health disparities, and achieving uniform access to preventive health services.

3. Recent 2010 national objectives were systematically developed with input from many coalitions, agencies, and organizations, with two primary goals of increasing quality and length of healthy life and eliminating health disparities. Four elements were identified: goals, objectives, determinants of health, and health status. Two overarching goals are to increase quality of life and length of healthy life and to eliminate health disparities. The objectives specify the amount of progress expected in improving the health status of the population over the next 10 years. The determinants of health address various environments (individual, community physical and social) and the policies and interventions used to promote health, prevent disease, and ensure access to quality health care. Health status is the expected outcomes and measurements of success for each of the 467 objectives as well as reflected in the 10 leading health indicators.

4. The 2010 objectives cover 28 focus areas and 467 objectives. Each focus area identifies a lead agency responsible for monitoring progress, a concise goal statement, an overview of the context and background, data on progress, objectives related to the area, and a standard data table to monitor the progress.

5. Determinants of health are defined as the combined effects of individual and community physical and social environments and the policies and interventions used to promote health, prevent disease, and ensure access to quality health care.

6. Health status is described as the expected outcome and measure of success of the approach and includes the extent to which the objective is met.

POWERPOINT LECTURE SLIDES

NOTE: The number on each PPT Lecture Slide directly corresponds with the Concepts for Lecture.

1 National Health Objectives
- 1980 goals and desired outcomes
  - Reduce mortality

1a National Health Objectives (continued)
- 15 priority intervention areas
  - Three strategic action categories
    - Preventive health
    - Health protection
    - Health promotion
- Number of objectives

2 National Health Objectives for 2000
- Goals
  - Increase the span of healthy life
  - Reduce health disparities
  - Achieve uniform access to preventive health services
- Number of focus areas
- Number of objectives

3 National Health Objectives for 2010
- Input from coalitions, agencies, and organizations
- Two primary goals:
  - Increase quality and length of healthy life
  - Eliminate health disparities

3a Four Elements
- Goals
- Objectives
- Determinants of health
- Health status

4 2010 Objectives
- Cover 28 focus areas and 467 objectives
- Each focus area
  - Identifies a lead agency to monitor progress
  - Includes a concise goal statement
  - Provides an overview of the context and background
  - Provides data on progress
  - Delineates objectives related to the area
  - Provides a standard data table to monitor progress

5 Determinants of Health
- Individual and community physical and social environments
- Policies and interventions used to:
  - Promote health
  - Prevent disease
  - Ensure access to quality health care

Health Status
- Expected outcome
- Measure of success of approach
- Includes the extent to which objective is met

SUGGESTIONS FOR CLASSROOM ACTIVITIES

Provide students with a copy of the Healthy People 2010 National Health Objectives. Assign each student one focus area to review and summarize for class. Ask them to evaluate their focus area and the objectives based on several criteria: barriers to implementation, benefits to society and to the individual, stakeholders, and risks of not meeting the objectives.

SUGGESTIONS FOR CLINICAL ACTIVITIES

Have students interview community health nurses at a clinical site regarding programs or interventions that address their selected focus area. Ask students to report results of interviews during post conference.

The Historical Context

RESOURCE LIBRARY

COMPANION WEBSITE

Audio Glossary
Exam Review Questions
Case Study: Applying Lessons Learned from the Past
  to the Present
MediaLink Applications: Public Health Nursing
  History (Video)

Media Links
Challenge Your Knowledge
Advocacy Interviews

LEARNING OBJECTIVE 1

Describe the contributions of historical figures that influenced the development of community health nursing.

CONCEPTS FOR LECTURE

1. During the colonial period, early nursing care was a function of the women in a family. In Canada, public health was performed by Christian religious agencies with Jeanne Mance co-founding the Hotel Dieu in Montreal.

2. The Industrial Revolution, with overcrowding, migration from farms to city, and changes in technology spurred events resulting in poor nutrition, increased disease, and hazardous living and working conditions. These conditions did not go unnoticed by forward-thinking individuals who addressed and introduced concepts of sanitation engineering, early epidemiologic investigations by John Snow with the Cholera epidemic in London, and immunization development targeting smallpox and diphtheria.

3. District nursing and community health nursing evolved from the concern for the health of larger urban populations with Florence Nightingale endorsing health promotion and home care for the sick, and Elizabeth Fry founding the Institute of Nursing in London to provide care to the sick poor in their homes and in prisons.

4. The 1800s saw the creation of missionary nurses to provide nursing care and religious instruction for the sick poor, and visiting nurses associations to provide health teaching and illness care. Best known for their efforts to educate and deliver care to the sick, Lillian Wald and Mary Brewster established the Henry Street Settlement, recognized as the first American community health agency, with the purpose of delivering

POWERPOINT LECTURE SLIDES

NOTE: *The number on each PPT Lecture Slide directly corresponds with the Concepts for Lecture.*

1 Early Nursing Care
  • U.S. colonial period
    ○ Care part of family function
      – Home remedies
  • Canadian public health
    ○ Jeanne Mance

2 Industrial Revolution
  • Social ills contributed to:
    ○ Introduction of sanitation engineering
    ○ Epidemiologic investigations
      – Cholera
    ○ Immunizations
      – Diphtheria
      – Smallpox

3 District Nursing
  • Florence Nightingale
    ○ Community health nursing
  • Elizabeth Frye

4 Settlement Houses: Lillian Wald and Mary Brewster
  • Delivered health care to poor immigrant populations by living and working among them

CONCEPTS FOR LECTURE *continued*

care to poor immigrants. Wald and Brewster utilized germ theory as the foundation for nursing interventions, provided access to nursing services that was determined by the client and not the physician, cared for the sick in their homes, offered health education as a secondary focus of service, and sought to focus care to the whole community, not just individuals.

5. Other community health nurses active in the social change movement included Margaret Sanger, who argued for contraceptive services for women; Clara Barton, who provided nursing care to wounded soldiers in during the American Civil War, was active in locating missing Civil War soldiers, and established the American Red Cross; and Dorothea Dix, another community health nurse pioneer who not only provided care for wounded Civil War soldiers, but fought to improve conditions for inmates in U.S. prisons.

POWERPOINT LECTURE SLIDES *continued*

- First American community health agency
  - Established Henry Street Settlement in New York City
  - Utilized germ theory as foundation for interventions

 Settlement Houses: Lillian Wald and Mary Brewster (continued)
- First American community health agency
  - Access to nursing services determined by the client, not the physician
  - Cared for sick in their homes
  - Health education as a secondary focus
  - Focus of care to whole community

 Community Health Nurses: Social Change
- Margaret Sanger
  - Contraceptive services for women
- Clara Barton
  - Nursing care to wounded in American Civil War
  - Active in locating missing Civil War soldiers
  - Establishment of American Red Cross

 Community Health Nurses: Social Change (continued)
- Dorothea Dix
  - Active in improving conditions for inmates in U.S. prisons

---

SUGGESTIONS FOR CLASSROOM ACTIVITIES

Have students select and research one of the historical figures or time periods and provide a brief presentation to the class on how that person or period of time influenced the development of community health nursing.

SUGGESTIONS FOR CLINICAL ACTIVITIES

Arrange for students to spend time with a community health nurse during an investigation of a communicable disease and report observations to the class during post conference.

LEARNING OBJECTIVE 2

Discuss the contributions of community health nurses to social and health care reform.

CONCEPTS FOR LECTURE

1. Community health nurses, recognized by Lillian Wald as public health nurses, began to focus their services to the whole community. Poverty, social injustices, poor nutrition, and lack of health care services prompted nurses to become involved in social advocacy to promote social changes.

2. The Metropolitan Life Insurance Company was one of the first companies to offer nursing services to their policyholders with the intent to reduce mortality and limit death benefits paid by the company. This experiment proved extremely successful and continued for over 40 years.

3. A need to provide services and improve social conditions specific to mothers and children motivated community health nurses like Lillian Wald to bring

POWERPOINT LECTURE SLIDES

NOTE: The number on each PPT Lecture Slide directly corresponds with the Concepts for Lecture.

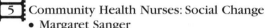 Community Health Nurses and Social Reforms
- Focus of services to the whole community
  - Addressing
    - Poverty
    - Social injustices
    - Poor nutrition
    - Lack of health care services

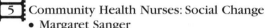 Metropolitan Life Insurance Company
- Successful social experiment
  - Provided nursing services to policyholder
    - Goal to reduce mortality

awareness to the national leaders. This attention resulted in the first White House Conference on Children in 1909 with the establishment of the U.S. Children's Bureau tasked to address the issue of child labor.

4. Rural nursing contributed to health care reform through the efforts of Mary Breckenridge and the Frontier Nursing Service, which provided midwifery services, assessed outcomes, and tracked case data. Rural health nursing also advocated care to Native American Indians and African Americans.

3 White House Conference on Children (1909)
- Lillian Wald and other social activists
  - Sought to improve social conditions that affected health
  - Resulted in U.S. Children's Bureau in 1912
    - Child Labor

4 Rural Nursing: Contributions to Health Care Reform
- Mary Breckenridge
  - Frontier Nursing Service
    - Provided midwifery services
    - Assessed outcomes
    - Tracked case data

4a Rural Nursing: Contributions to Health Care Reform (continued)
- Rural health focus
  - Native American Indians
  - African Americans

SUGGESTIONS FOR CLASSROOM ACTIVITIES

Divide students into groups to research and present in poster format the efforts, significant contributions, and other notable accomplishments of the early nursing leaders in social and health care reform.

SUGGESTIONS FOR CLINICAL ACTIVITIES

Have students compare and contrast social and health issues of today as seen in their clinical experiences with those of early community health nurses. What is similar? What has changed?

LEARNING OBJECTIVE 3

List significant historical events in the development of community health nursing in the United States.

CONCEPTS FOR LECTURE

1. The formation of early professional organizations such as the American Public Health Association in 1872 and the National Organization of Public Health Nurses in 1912 provided a format to advance the public health profession through standards and policies to promote population health.

2. Community health nursing as a distinct practice developed as a result of numerous events such as employment of public health nurses by government agencies in Alabama in 1907, the addition of a postgraduate course at Columbia University in 1910, and the establishment of the National Organization for Public Health Nursing in 1912.

3. Congress enacted legislation, such as the Sheppard-Tower Act of 1921, to help state and local agencies provide general health, maternity, prenatal, and child health services. As a result, community health nurses were hired. The National Institutes of Health was formed to address the need for federal support for health care research.

4. The Great Depression (1930s) created opportunities for the federal government to employ health and

POWERPOINT LECTURE SLIDES

NOTE: The number on each PPT Lecture Slide directly corresponds with the Concepts for Lecture.

1 Role of Early Professional Organizations
- American Public Health Association
- National Organization of Public Health Nurses
  - Advancing public health through standards and policies
  - Promoting population health

2 Community Health Nursing as a Profession
- Employment of public health nurses by government agencies in Alabama in 1907
- Postgraduate course at Columbia University in 1910
- Establishment of the National Organization for Public Health Nursing in 1912

3 Sheppard-Tower Act of 1921
- State and local agencies
  - General health, maternity, prenatal, child health services

social welfare programs to hire nurses under the Federal Emergency Relief Act (1933), the Civil Works administration (1933–34) and the Works Progress Administration (1935).
5. Functions of public health nurses and objectives related to the profession and critical to the advancement of the profession and education of community health nurses were developed in 1931, with numerous revisions as the profession developed.
6. Recognition of the contributions of community health nurses led the United State Public Health Service to employ their first public health nurse in 1934 with the establishment of a Division of Nursing in 1944.

4 Great Depression (1930s)
- Federal programs
  - Federal Emergency Relief Act
  - Civil Works Administration
  - Works Progress Administration

5 Functions of Public Health Nurses and Professional Objectives
- Critical to the advancement of the profession and education of community health nurses

6 United State Public Health Service
- Employed their first public health nurse
- Division of nursing established 10 years later

SUGGESTIONS FOR CLASSROOM ACTIVITIES

Assign students to research and bring in pictures or articles of local historical community health events. What have been some of the milestones in the community? When did the community receive public water and sewer services?

SUGGESTIONS FOR CLINICAL ACTIVITIES

Invite a community health nurse and a visiting home nurse to a post clinical conference to address the professional milestones that they have noted in their career. What do they see as their role in the advancement of community health nursing? What suggestions do they have for students interested in this career field? What opportunities exist for community health nurses?

LEARNING OBJECTIVE 4

Describe evidence for a shift in public health policy toward a greater emphasis on health promotion.

CONCEPTS FOR LECTURE

1. The shift in public health policy toward an emphasis on health promotion and illness prevention is evident in the changes in the U.S. national health objectives each decade beginning in 1980. Additionally, one of the focus areas for Healthy People 2010 is the development of the public health infrastructure, which includes the organizational structure of official government health agencies, the public health workforce, and the information systems in public health practice.
2. Another indicator of the growing emphasis on health promotion is the creation of the Center for Nursing Research in 1988 within the National Institutes of Health.
3. Further evidence is the passage of the Public Health Improvement Act of 2000 which provides funds for the development of public health activities at state and local levels.

POWERPOINT LECTURE SLIDES

NOTE: The number on each PPT Lecture Slide directly corresponds with the Concepts for Lecture.

1 Emphasis Changing to Health Promotion
- Changes in the U.S. national health objectives
  - Focus area for Healthy People 2010
    - Development of the public health infrastructure
      - Organizational structure of official government health agencies
      - Public health workforce
      - Information systems in public health practice

2 National Institutes of Health
- Creation of the Center for Nursing Research in 1988
  - Now called the National Institute for Nursing Research

3 Public Health Improvement Act of 2000
- Provides funds for the development of public health activities at state and local levels

SUGGESTIONS FOR CLASSROOM ACTIVITIES

Select examples from the 1980, 1990, 2000, and 2010 U.S. national health objectives. Working in pairs or larger groups, have students discuss the changes evident in the specific objectives and explain to the class how the health promotion and illness prevention focus has evolved.

SUGGESTIONS FOR CLINICAL ACTIVITIES

Have students examine specific health care services available in the local community. To what extent do they include health promotion and illness prevention services? Has the emphasis changed over time?

LEARNING OBJECTIVE 5

Describe national and international events that are shaping current and future community health nursing practice.

CONCEPTS FOR LECTURE

1. Population health problems received attention in Canada in the Canadian, LaLonde Report, *New Perspectives for the Health of Canadians* in 1974. Biological, environmental and lifestyle risks were recognized as determinants of health and shifting the focus from treatment to health promotion.
2. International focus resulted in the Declaration of Alma Alta in 1978, calling for access to primary health care for all; the 1984 Toronto Conference, which established two key health promotion concepts of healthy public policy and healthy cities; the U.S. National Health Objectives, which established a Behavior Risk Factor Surveillance System to systematically collect data; the World Health Organization, which addressed global strategies for the eradication of smallpox; the Ottawa Charter for Health Promotion (1986) that established the first International Conference on health promotion, which focused on social, economic, and political reform and empowerment, and the Jakarta declaration on health promotion, which focused efforts at global health promotion.
3. Public health practice changes began in 1988 when the Institute of Medicine report identified three core functions of public health as assessment, policy formation, and assurance.
4. Inadequacies in the U.S. public health infrastructure were recognized as a result of AIDS, SARS, and terrorist attacks.
5. Two recent developments projected to affect community health nursing are the Nursing Interventions Classification System that categorizes nursing services and facilitates direct reimbursements, and the Nursing Outcomes Classification, which allows nurses to document the effectiveness of interventions.

POWERPOINT LECTURE SLIDES

NOTE: The number on each PPT Lecture Slide directly corresponds with the Concepts for Lecture.

1 Population Health Problems
- Canadian, LaLonde Report (1974)
- *New Perspectives for the Health of Canadians*
  - Determinants of health risks
    - Biological
    - Environmental
    - Lifestyle

2 International Focus
- Declaration of Alma Alta (1978)
  - Access to primary care for all
- Toronto Conference (1984)
  - Key health promotion concepts
    - Healthy public policy
    - Healthy cities

2a International Focus (continued)
- U.S. National Health Objectives
  - Behavior Risk Factor Surveillance System
    - Data collection
- WHO
  - Smallpox eradication

2b International Focus (continued)
- Ottawa Charter for Health Promotion (1986)
  - First International Conference on Health Promotion
    - Focus on social, economic and political reform and empowerment
- Jakarta Declaration on Health Promotion
  - Global health promotion

3 Public Health Practice Changes
- Institute of Medicine (1988)
  - Three core functions
    - Assessment
    - Policy formation
    - Assurance

POWERPOINT LECTURE SLIDES *continued*

4 U.S. Public Health Infrastructure Inadequacies
- AIDS
- SARS
- Terrorist attacks

5 Recent Developments
- Nursing Interventions Classification
  - Categorizing nursing services
  - Facilitating direct reimbursement
- Nursing Outcomes Classification
  - Allows nurses to document the effectiveness of intervention

---

SUGGESTIONS FOR CLASSROOM ACTIVITIES

Invite a community health representative to class to discuss the impact of AIDS, SARS, and potential terrorist attacks on the U.S. public health infrastructure.

SUGGESTIONS FOR CLINICAL ACTIVITIES

Assign students to attend public health forums, meetings or committees that discuss AIDS, homeland security, or other broad general areas of concern and provide a summary of the meeting's mission, focus, goals or objectives at post conference.

Theoretical Foundations for Community Health Nursing

RESOURCE LIBRARY

COMPANION WEBSITE

Audio Glossary
Exam Review Questions
Case Study: Theory Application
MediaLink Applications: The Population Focus

Media Links
Challenge Your Knowledge
Advocacy Interviews

IMAGE LIBRARY

Figure 4-1 Elements of the Epidemiologic Triad Model

Figure 4-2 The Web of Causation for Adolescent Tobacco Use, Indicating the Interplay Between Multiple Direct and Indirect Causative Factors

Figure 4-3 A Composite Determinants-of-Health Model

Figure 4-4 Elements of Client in the Neuman Systems Model

Figure 4-5 Elements of the Dimensions Model of Community Health Nursing

Figure 4-6 The Intervention Wheel

Figure 4-7 The Los Angeles County Public Health Nursing Practice Model

LEARNING OBJECTIVE 1

Identify the need for a theoretical foundation for community health nursing.

CONCEPTS FOR LECTURE

1. Theoretical or conceptual models offer a systematic approach to assessing the health status of a population, and planning, implementing, and evaluating the effectiveness of nursing care. A conceptual model can be defined as a set of relatively abstract and general concepts that address the phenomena of central interest to a discipline and that direct attention to relevant client situations and interventions.

2. There are two types of models used by community health nurses. Epidemiologic models provide a means of examining factors that influence health and illness in populations, and nursing models suggest interventions to protect, improve, or restore health.

POWERPOINT LECTURE SLIDES

NOTE: The number on each PPT Lecture Slide directly corresponds with the Concepts for Lecture.

1 Theoretical and Conceptual Models
- Conceptual mode:
  - Set of relatively abstract and general concepts
  - Addresses phenomena of interest to a discipline
  - Directs attention to relevant client situations, interventions

1a Theoretical and Conceptual Models (continued)
- Systematic approach to
  - Assessing health status of a population
  - Planning nursing interventions
  - Implementing interventions
  - Evaluating effectiveness of nursing care

2 Two Useful Types of Models:
- Epidemiologic models
  - Examine factors that influence health and illness
- Nursing models
  - Suggest interventions to protect, improve, or restore health

LEARNING OBJECTIVE 2

Describe basic principles of epidemiology.

CONCEPTS FOR LECTURE

1. Epidemiology is the study of the distribution of health and illness within a population, factors that determine the population's health status, and use of the knowledge generated to control the development of health problems.

2. The four historical eras of epidemiologic thought are the sanitary era, the communicable disease era, the chronic disease era of multiple layers of personal risk, and the current ecosocial or molecular era.

3. The key concepts underlying epidemiologic perspectives on health and illness are causality, risk, and rates of occurrence.

4. The main purpose of epidemiology is to identify causal links between contributing factors and resulting states of health and illness. Causality refers to one event being the result of another event with concepts of causation evolving from the will of God, to natural causes, to specific causes, and recently, to multifactorial causes.

5. Epidemiologists must estimate the likelihood that a particular condition will occur. Risk is the probability that a given individual will develop a specific condition. Populations at risk are groups of people who have the greatest potential for developing a particular health problem as a result of the presence or absence of specific factors. Populations at risk become target groups for interventions designed to prevent the problem of interest.

6. Rates of occurrence are statistical measures that indicate the extent of health problems in a group and allow comparisons between groups of different sizes. Rates are computed by dividing the number of instances of an event during a specified period by the population at risk and multiplying by 1,000 or 100,000.

7. Morbidity and mortality, two important epidemiologic rates of interest, are used to assess the health status of populations, develop interventions, and evaluate long-term outcomes. Morbidity is the ratio of the number

POWERPOINT LECTURE SLIDES

NOTE: The number on each PPT Lecture Slide directly corresponds with the Concepts for Lecture.

1 Epidemiology
- Study of distribution of health and illness within a population
- Factors that determine population's health
- Use knowledge generated to control development of health problems

2 Four Eras:
- Sanitary era
- Communicable disease era
- Chronic disease era
  - Multiple layers of personal risk
- Ecosocial/molecular era

3 Epidemiologic Perspectives:
- Causality
- Risk
- Rates of occurrence

4 Causality
- Link between contributing factors and states of health and illness
- One event is the result of another event
- Evolution of concepts of causation
  - Will of God
  - Natural causes
  - Specific causes
  - Multifactorial causes

5 Risk
- Estimated likelihood a particular condition will occur
- Probability that a given individual will develop a specific condition
- Populations at risk
  - Groups with greatest potential to develop a particular health problem

CONCEPTS FOR LECTURE *continued*

of cases of a disease or condition to the number of people in the population. Morbidity is often described in terms of incidence, the number of new cases of a particular condition identified during a specific time period, and prevalence, the total number of people affected by a particular condition at a specified point in time. Mortality is the ratio of the number of deaths of a particular category to the number of people in a given population.

8. Case fatality and survival rates are additional epidemiologic statistics of concern. A case fatality rate for a particular condition reflects the percentage of persons with the condition who die as a result of it. Survival rates are the proportion of people with a given condition remaining alive after a specified period (usually 5 years). Related to survival rates is survival time, which is the average length of time from diagnosis to death.

POWERPOINT LECTURE SLIDES *continued*

○ Result of presence or absence of specific factors
○ Become target groups for interventions

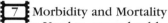 Rates of Occurrence
- Statistical measures
- Indicate extent of health problems in a group
- Allow comparison between groups of different sizes
- Computed by dividing the instances of an event by population at risk
- Multiplied by 1000 or 100,000

 Morbidity and Mortality
- Used to assess health status
- Develop interventions
- Evaluate long term outcomes
- Morbidity is ratio of number of cases to number in population

 Morbidity and Mortality (continued)
- Incidence and prevalence of a condition
  ○ Incidence
    - Number of new cases of a particular condition
    - Specified time period
  ○ Prevalence
    - Total number of people affected by a particular condition
    - Specified point in time
- Mortality is ratio of number of deaths of a particular category to number in population

8 Epidemiologic Statistics
- Case fatality rates
  ○ Percentage of persons with a condition who die of that condition
- Survival rates
  ○ Proportion of people with a condition remaining alive after a specified period
- Survival time
  ○ Average length of time from diagnosis to death

SUGGESTIONS FOR CLASSROOM ACTIVITIES

Prior to class, assign students a disease, health issue, or acute or chronic condition and ask them to research the incidence and prevalence rates, and the morbidity and mortality rates for those specific conditions or diseases. Have the students present findings to the class through discussion, poster presentation, or PowerPoint presentation format.

SUGGESTIONS FOR CLINICAL ACTIVITIES

Have students examine a common health problem encountered in their clinical setting and identify the local incidence and prevalence of the condition, mortality rates if relevant, risk factors involved, and population at risk.

LEARNING OBJECTIVE 3

Apply selected epidemiologic and nursing models to community health nursing practice with individuals, families, and populations.

CONCEPTS FOR LECTURE

1. Epidemiologic models direct community health nurses to strategies for interventions and for collection and interpretation of data and mechanisms for controlling health-related conditions. Three types of models dominate the field: the epidemiologic triad, the web of causation, and the determinants of health models.
2. The epidemiologic triad of disease collects data as it pertains to the host, agent, and environment as they contribute to the development of health problems.
3. The web of causation model emphasizes the interconnectedness of causal factors and explores multiple factors in terms of their interplay, both direct (proximal to condition) and indirect (distal to condition), as causes of an identified health problem.
4. Determinants of health models emphasize the various factors such as social, environmental, biological, psychological, behavioral/lifestyle, health care/health systems, and genetics that influence health and illness.
5. Nursing models, developed as the direct result of professional practice, utilize systematic, scientific inquiry to expand the profession's body of knowledge. Several models have application to the community health nursing practice, including: Neuman's health systems model; the dimensions model; the interventions wheel model; the Los Angeles County public health nursing practice model; and the community-as-partner model.
6. The types of models applied to the community health setting serve as a conceptual model for nurses to understand the interrelationships that exist among the specific concepts.
7. Neuman's health systems model involves a client system striving to prevent penetration or disruption of the system by a variety of stressors. The client is surrounded by three boundaries designed to protect the energy sources from environmental stressors. The core structure is composed of physiological, psychological, sociocultural, developmental, and spiritual variables. Neuman's model has numerous layers surrounding the core (client) that serve as lines of defense, lines of resistance, or stressors.
8. The Dimensions model of community health nursing consists of three elements: the dimensions of health, which guide the nurse's assessment of clients' health status, and the dimensions of health care and dimensions of nursing practice, which guide nursing interventions. The dimensions consist of six categories of factors that can be used to organize a community health assessment: the biophysical dimension, the psychological dimension, the physical environmental dimension, the sociocultural dimension, the behavioral dimension, and the health system dimension.

POWERPOINT LECTURE SLIDES

NOTE: The number on each PPT Lecture Slide directly corresponds with the Concepts for Lecture.

1 Epidemiologic Models
- Provide direction for community health nurses
  ○ Strategies for interventions
  ○ Collection and interpretation of data
  ○ Control health-related conditions

1a Three Types of Models:
- Epidemiologic triad
- Web of causation
- Determinants of health models

2 Epidemiologic Triad Model
- Agent
- Host
- Environment

2a See Figure 4-1

3 Web of Causation
- Emphasizes interconnectedness of causal components
- Multiple factors influence health
  ○ Direct causes
    – Proximal to health event
  ○ Indirect causes
    – Distal from health event

3a See Figure 4-2

4 Determinants of Health
- Various factors affect health and illness
  ○ Social
  ○ Environmental
  ○ Biological
  ○ Psychological
  ○ Behavioral/lifestyle

4a Determinants of Health (continued)
- Various factors affect health and illness
  ○ Health care/health systems
  ○ Genetics

4b See Figure 4-3

5 Community Health Nursing Models
- Developed as result of professional practice
- Utilize systematic, scientific inquiry

6 Types of Models Applied to Community Health Setting
- Serve as a conceptual model for nurses to understand the interrelationships that exist among the specific concepts

CONCEPTS FOR LECTURE *continued*

9. The Interventions Wheel model (previously known as the Public Health Nursing Interventions model) consists of 17 identified community health nursing interventions that cross over three levels of population-based practice: individual-focused, community-focused, and system-focused practice. Individual-level interventions are focused on change in individual health status, knowledge or skills. Community-level interventions address changes in community norms, awareness, attitudes, and behaviors in an entire community or in subgroups. Systems-level interventions focus on changes in the organizations and health care delivery structures that serve individuals and communities.

10. The Los Angeles County Public Health Nursing Practice model links public health nursing with principles of public health practice. Basic principles include: community health nursing is a multidisciplinary endeavor; clients must be active participants in the endeavor; community health nursing practice is population-based; community health nursing practice is based on the core functions and essential services of public health; and community health nurses engage in the interventions described in the intervention wheel model.

11 The Community-as-Partner model incorporates Neuman's health systems model and the nursing process. The client for nursing care is the community or population group. The inner core consists of the people comprising the community along with their belief, values, and history. The core is surrounded by eight community subsystems: physical environment, education, safety and transportation, politics and government, health and social services, communication, economics, and recreation. The community health nurse assesses the health status of the community core and factors within the eight subsystems as well as the strength of the normal and flexible lines of defense and the lines of resistance.

POWERPOINT LECTURE SLIDES *continued*

7 Neuman's Health System Model
- Client system striving to prevent penetration or disruption of the system by a variety of stressors

8 The Dimensions Model of Community Health Nursing
- See Figure 4-5

9 The Interventions Wheel Model
- Consists of 17 identified community health nursing interventions that cross over three levels of population-based practice
  - Individual-focused
  - Community-focused
  - System-focused practice

10 The Los Angeles County Public Health Nursing Practice Model
- Links public health nursing with principles of public health practice.
  - Community health nursing is a multidisciplinary endeavor; clients must be active participants in the endeavor.
  - Community health nursing practice is population-based.
  - Community health nursing practice is based on the core functions and essential services of public health.
  - Community health nurses engage in the interventions described in the intervention wheel model.

11 The Community-as-Partner Model
- Incorporates Neuman's health systems model and the nursing process

---

SUGGESTIONS FOR CLASSROOM ACTIVITIES

Assign students to work in groups. Give the groups one of the epidemiologic or community health nursing models and have them investigate and then explain a health condition or disease process in terms of the group theoretical model assigned.

SUGGESTIONS FOR CLINICAL ACTIVITIES

Assign students to attend a community support group. At post conference, have the students explain the health condition addressed by their assigned support group through the application of one of the theoretical models discussed in class.

The U.S. Health System Context

RESOURCE LIBRARY

COMPANION WEBSITE

Audio Glossary
Exam Review Questions
Case Study: Designing the Ideal Health Care System
MediaLink Applications: Educating about Obesity (video)

Media Links
Challenge Your Knowledge
Advocacy Interviews

IMAGE LIBRARY

Figure 5-1 Organizational Structure of the U.S. Health Care Delivery System

Figure 5-2 Typical Organizational Structure of a Local Health Department

Figure 5-3 Typical Organizational Structure of a State Health Department

Figure 5-4 Major Components of the National Institutes of Health

LEARNING OBJECTIVE 1

Describe the popular health care subsystem.

CONCEPTS FOR LECTURE

1. The popular health care subsystem is defined as the system in which care is provided by oneself, family members, or friends. Self-care and care by family and friends accounts for an estimated 70% to 90% of all illness care.

POWERPOINT LECTURE SLIDES

NOTE: The number on each PPT Lecture Slide directly corresponds with the Concepts for Lecture.

1. Popular Health Care Subsystem
   - Care provided by
     - Self
     - Family
     - Friends
   - Accounts for 70–90% of all illness care

SUGGESTIONS FOR CLASSROOM ACTIVITIES

Have students develop a list of self-care behaviors. Include symptoms, the common name/terminology for the ailment, and popular or common treatments. Using the blackboard, write information down in columns.

SUGGESTIONS FOR CLINICAL ACTIVITIES

Ask students to interview community health nurses about common popular health care practices noted from targeted populations in the community and report during clinical post conference.

LEARNING OBJECTIVE 2

Distinguish between the complementary and alternative subsystems of care.

CONCEPTS FOR LECTURE

1. The complementary and alternative health care subsystems are defined as care that is sought from other sources, providers, or practices that lie outside the scientific health care subsystem. Complementary health care practices are used in conjunction with scientific care to complement and enhance its effects. Alternative practices are used in place of scientific interventions.

POWERPOINT LECTURE SLIDES

NOTE: The number on each PPT Lecture Slide directly corresponds with the Concepts for Lecture.

1 Complementary and Alternative Health Care Subsystems
- Definition
  - Care sought from other sources/providers/practices
  - Considered outside scientific health care subsystem
- Complementary care
  - Used with scientific care
  - Complements/enhances effects of scientific care

1a Complementary and Alternative Health Care Subsystems (continued)
- Alternative practices
  - Used in place of scientific interventions

SUGGESTIONS FOR CLASSROOM ACTIVITIES

Have students make a list of practices that they consider are included in the complementary or alternative subsystems. Write responses on the blackboard under each column. Ask students to rate the effectiveness of each response on a scale of 1 to 5 with 5 representing "Extremely effective" and 1 representing "Not effective."

SUGGESTIONS FOR CLINICAL ACTIVITIES

Have students research in the professional journals or literature one complementary or alternative health care practice and prepare a brief report at post conference. Have students discuss the cultural implications of this practice, the potential benefits, and the potential harm. Ask them to describe the role of the community health nurse when presented with their alternative or complementary practice.

LEARNING OBJECTIVE 3

Identify six fundamental obligations of official public health agencies.

CONCEPTS FOR LECTURE

1. General goals for public health practice include improving population health, reducing health inequalities, and developing environments that support health.
2. These goals are met through noted fundamental obligations for official public health agencies, listed by the Institute of Medicine, which include adopting a population health approach with multiple determinants of health, strengthening governmental and public health infrastructure, building intersectoral partnerships, developing systems of accountability for quality assurance and availability of public health services, ensuring a foundation of evidence-based research, and enhancing and facilitating communication within the public health system.

POWERPOINT LECTURE SLIDES

NOTE: The number on each PPT Lecture Slide directly corresponds with the Concepts for Lecture.

1 General Goals for Public Health Practice
- Improving population health
- Reducing health inequalities
- Developing environments that support health

2 Fundamental Obligations of Public Health Agencies
- Adopt population health approach
- Multiple determinants of health
- Strengthen governmental and public health infrastructure
- Build intersectoral partnerships
- Develop systems of accountability

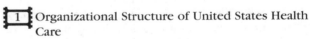

2a Fundamental Obligations of Public Health
Agencies (continued)
- Accountability for quality assurance
- Accountability for availability of public health services
- Ensure a foundation of evidence-based research
- Enhance/facilitate communication within the public health system

SUGGESTIONS FOR CLASSROOM ACTIVITIES

Assign each student one of the six fundamental obligations. Ask students to research their topic in the public health and community health journal articles and prepare a brief report to the class.

SUGGESTIONS FOR CLINICAL ACTIVITIES

Have students interview a community health nurse/manager/practitioner to discuss interventions or programs that are in place that meet the fundamental obligations. Report at next post conference.

LEARNING OBJECTIVE 4

Describe the organizational structure of the U.S. health care delivery system.

CONCEPTS FOR LECTURE

1. The three major organizational structure elements or subsystems in the U.S. health care system include the popular health care subsystem, the complementary or alternative health care subsystem, and the scientific health care subsystem, which consists of the personal health care sector and the public or population health care sector.

POWERPOINT LECTURE SLIDES

NOTE: The number on each PPT Lecture Slide directly corresponds with the Concepts for Lecture.

1 Organizational Structure of United States Health Care
- Three major subsystems
  - Popular health care subsystem
  - Complementary/alternative health care subsystem
  - Scientific health care system
    - Personal health care sector
    - Public/population health care sector

1a See Figure 5-1

SUGGESTIONS FOR CLASSROOM ACTIVITIES

Divide students into three subsystem groups. Each group is to use phone book and Internet sources to locate/list local and state examples of health care that represent their assigned subsystem.

SUGGESTIONS FOR CLINICAL ACTIVITIES

Arrange for students to have a clinical assignment at one of the three major health care delivery subsystems and present a summary of their assigned clinical experience at post conference.

LEARNING OBJECTIVE 5

Compare and contrast official and voluntary health agencies.

CONCEPTS FOR LECTURE

1. Official health agencies include local, state, and national governments, which share some aspects of the following characteristics: responsibility for the health of people in their jurisdictions, supported by tax revenues and public finding, accountable to the

POWERPOINT LECTURE SLIDES

NOTE: The number on each PPT Lecture Slide directly corresponds with the Concepts for Lecture.

 Official Public Health Agencies
- Governments

CONCEPTS FOR LECTURE *continued*

citizens of their jurisdiction, and often specific activities are mandated by law.

2. The key objectives of official public health agencies are to prevent epidemics and spread of disease, protect the public from environmental hazards, prevent injury, promote healthy behavior and good mental health, respond to disasters and assist with recovery from their effects, and ensure quality and accessibility of needed health care services.

3. The three core public health functions identified are assessment, policy development, and assurance. Assessment and surveillance includes regular and ongoing collection, analysis, and availability of information and statistics on health status, community health needs, and epidemiological health problems. Policy development involves advocacy and political action to develop local, state, and national policies conducive to population health. Assurance is described as the responsibility of the public health sector to ensure availability of and access to health care services essential to sustaining and improving the health of the population.

4. Voluntary health agencies are nonprofit organizations, funded primarily by donations and held accountable to their supporters that provide adjuncts to services provided by government agencies with a focus on a specific disease entity, an organ system, or a population group. These agencies have a primary emphasis of research, education, and policy development.

POWERPOINT LECTURE SLIDES *continued*

- Responsible for health of people in their jurisdictions
- Supported by tax revenues/public finding
- Accountable to citizens of their jurisdictions
- Mandate specific activities by law

2 Key Objectives of Official Public Health Agencies
- Prevent epidemics and spread of disease
- Protect public from environmental hazards
- Prevent injury
- Promote healthy behavior and good mental health
- Respond to disasters and assist with recovery
- Assure quality and accessibility of health care services

3 Core Public Health Functions
- Assessment and surveillance
  - Collection, analysis, and availability of information and statistics
    - Health status
    - Community health needs
    - Epidemiological health problems

3a Core Public Health Functions (continued)
- Policy development
  - Advocacy and political action
  - Policies conducive to population health
- Assurance
  - Availability of/access to essential health care services
  - Sustain and improve health of population

4 Voluntary Health Agencies
- Nonprofit organizations provide adjunct services to government agencies
- Focus
  - Specific disease entity
  - Organ system
  - Population group

4a Voluntary Health Agencies (continued)
- Funded by private donations
  - Accountable to supporters
- Activities determined by supported interests
- Primary emphasis
  - Research
  - Education
  - Policy development

SUGGESTIONS FOR CLASSROOM ACTIVITIES

Invite guest speakers that represent various official and voluntary health agencies to discuss services, funding sources, mission, and goals. Have students research prior to class each of the agencies and bring one or more questions for panel guests.

SUGGESTIONS FOR CLINICAL ACTIVITIES

Assign students to a local, state, or national health agency for a clinical assignment such as the American Lung Association, the American Red Cross, the March of Dimes, the Salvation Army, or other agencies. Discuss how each agency addresses one or more of the key objectives at post conference.

LEARNING OBJECTIVE 6

Describe at least five functions performed by voluntary health agencies.

CONCEPTS FOR LECTURE

1. Voluntary agencies perform eight basic functions within the scientific health care subsystem: pioneering, such as exploring poorly addressed areas of health concerns; demonstrating pilot projects; educating the public and health professionals; providing supplemental services, such as transportation to clinics, respite care, and special equipment; advocating for the public's health; promoting legislation related to health; assisting with health planning and organization; and assisting official agencies in developing community health programs.

POWERPOINT LECTURE SLIDES

NOTE: The number on each PPT Lecture Slide directly corresponds with the Concepts for Lecture.

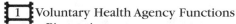 Voluntary Health Agency Functions
- Pioneering
- Explore poorly addressed areas of concern
- Demonstrate pilot projects
- Educate public and health professionals
- Supplemental services

[1a] Voluntary Health Agency Functions (continued)
- Advocacy for public's health
- Promote legislation
- Assist with health planning and organization
- Assist official agencies to develop community health programs

SUGGESTIONS FOR CLASSROOM ACTIVITIES

Have students research the Internet to locate Web pages for various voluntary health agencies or organizations such as the American Dairy Association, the March of Dimes, the American Diabetes Association, the American Red Cross, the American Heart Association, the American Cancer Association, or others. Ask them to locate examples of how these agencies meet the objectives of the core functions performed by voluntary health agencies. Have the students prepare a brief report to the class.

SUGGESTIONS FOR CLINICAL ACTIVITIES

Invite members of various local agencies to discuss their mission, goals and objectives, projects, and activities in a roundtable format. Ask students to research the background of these agencies and develop key questions on 3×5 cards to be addressed by guest speakers.

LEARNING OBJECTIVE 7

Identify ten essential public health services.

CONCEPTS FOR LECTURE

1. The Centers for Disease Control operationalized the public health core functions into ten essential services to include the following: monitoring health status to identify health problems; diagnosing and investigating health problems and hazards in the community; informing, educating, and empowering people regarding health issues; mobilizing community partnerships to identify and solve health problems; developing health policies and plans that support individual and community health efforts; enforcing laws and regulations that protect health and ensure safety; linking people to needed personal health care services and ensuring the provision of health care when unavailable; ensuring a competent health and personal health workforce; evaluating the effectiveness, accessibility, and quality of personal and population-based health services; and conducting research to develop new insights and innovative solutions to health problems.

POWERPOINT LECTURE SLIDES

NOTE: The number on each PPT Lecture Slide directly corresponds with the Concepts for Lecture.

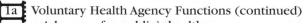 Essential Public Health Services
- Monitor health status to identify health problems
- Diagnose and investigate health problems and hazards in community
- Inform, educate, empower people
- Mobilize community partnerships to identify and solve health problems
- Develop health policies/plans that support individual/community health efforts

[1a] Essential Public Health Services (continued)
- Enforce laws/regulations that protect health and assure safety
- Link people to needed personal health care services

- Assure provision of health care when unavailable
- Assure competent public health and personal health workforce
- Evaluate effectiveness, accessibility, and quality of health services
- Conduct research on insights and innovative solutions

SUGGESTIONS FOR CLASSROOM ACTIVITIES

Assign students into groups to select and research a population health topic, such as tuberculosis, obesity, diabetes, or any infectious, chronic disease/health concern of interest and report briefly on one of the essential public health services.

SUGGESTIONS FOR CLINICAL ACTIVITIES

Have groups of students select one of the essential public health services. After interviewing staff at their community health clinical site, have students prepare a 5-minute report of how their agency addresses that essential service and present it at post conference.

LEARNING OBJECTIVE 8

Discuss the involvement of local, state, and national governments in health care in the United States.

CONCEPTS FOR LECTURE

1. There are three levels of health care delivery with specific responsibilities and official and voluntary agencies at each local, state, and national level.
2. A local government agency is defined as all entities that contribute to the delivery of public health services within a community. State agencies delegate responsibility to local health departments. Local health agencies receive authority from local health ordinances and funding from local taxes, states, federal subsidies, client fees, and private health insurance.
3. Responsibilities for local health departments vary from state to state, but generally include collection of vital statistics, communicable disease control, disease screening and surveillance, sanitation, school health, maternal–child health programs, and public health nursing services.
4. State government involvement includes state public health agencies and programs that contribute to public health services at the state level. State departments of health have the ultimate responsibility for the health of the public and possess essential power to make laws and regulations regarding health. Funding is derived from state tax revenues and federal government funds. State core functions include assessment of statewide health status and health care needs, development of statewide objectives related to health, assurance of adequate personnel and services to meet identified health care needs, guarantee of a minimum set of essential services to members of the population, and assistance to local jurisdictions.
5. National government agencies have no direct authority to regulate health. Indirect authority is derived from the power to regulate foreign and interstate

POWERPOINT LECTURE SLIDES

NOTE: The number on each PPT Lecture Slide directly corresponds with the Concepts for Lecture.

1 Levels of Health Care Delivery
- Specific responsibilities at each level
- Existence of both official and voluntary agencies
- Three levels
  ○ Local
  ○ State
  ○ National

2 Local Government
- All entities that deliver public health services within a community
- Local health department
- State delegates responsibility
- Receive authority from local health ordinances

2a Local Government (continued)
- Funding
  ○ Local taxes
  ○ State
  ○ Federal subsidies
  ○ Client fees
  ○ Private health insurance

3 Local Health Departments
- Responsibilities vary from state to state
  ○ Collection of vital statistics
  ○ Communicable disease control
  ○ Disease screening and surveillance
  ○ Sanitation

commerce and the power to levy taxes and spend to promote the general welfare. The United States Department of Health and Human Services is the official federal agency.

- ○ School health
- ○ Maternal-child health programs
- ○ Public health nursing services

3a See Figure 5-2

4 State Government
- • State agencies and programs that contribute to public health services
- • State department of health
- • Ultimate responsibility for health of public
- • Possesses essential power to make health laws and regulations
- • Funding
  - ○ State tax revenues
  - ○ Federal government funds

4a State Government (continued)
- • Core functions
  - ○ Assess statewide health status and health care needs
  - ○ Develop statewide objectives related to health
  - ○ Assure adequate personnel and services to meet identified needs
  - ○ Guarantee a minimum set of essential services to population
  - ○ Assist local jurisdiction

4b State Government (continued)
- • See Figure 5-3

5 National Government
- • No direct authority to regulate health
- • Indirect authority
  - ○ Power to regulate foreign and interstate commerce
  - ○ Power to levy taxes and spend to promote general welfare
- • Official agency
  - ○ United States Department of Health and Human Services

5a National Government (continued)
- • See Figure 5-4

Suggestions for Classroom Activities

Assign students to three groups to investigate one community health event or concern at each of the governmental levels. Each group is to report on specific responsibilities, funding sources, budget, programs, and interventions that address the health event or concern. Provide opportunity to compare and contrast how each governmental agency provides public health services.

Suggestions for Clinical Activities

Provide students an opportunity for a clinical assignment in local, regional, and state health departments. Have students interview a community health nurse or other health personnel about responsibilities, programs, and interventions. Discuss at post conference their observations, research, and interview results.

LEARNING OBJECTIVE 9

Identify outcomes of care at the primary, secondary, and tertiary levels of prevention.

CONCEPTS FOR LECTURE

1. Outcomes of care, such as access to care, are evaluated in terms of primary (availability of immunization services), secondary (access to prompt emergency services), and tertiary (access to rehabilitative services) levels of prevention.

POWERPOINT LECTURE SLIDES

NOTE: The number on each PPT Lecture Slide directly corresponds with the Concepts for Lecture.

 Outcomes of Care
- Levels of prevention
  - Primary
    - Availability of immunization services
  - Secondary
    - Access to prompt emergency services
  - Tertiary
    - Access to rehabilitative services

SUGGESTIONS FOR CLASSROOM ACTIVITIES

Divide students into six groups. Each group will be assigned one of the key objectives for a public health agency. Ask students to develop and present examples that apply to each of the levels of prevention for their objective.

SUGGESTIONS FOR CLINICAL ACTIVITIES

Have students investigate the services offered at their clinical site and categorize those services according to the levels of prevention for outcomes of care. Present at post conference.

LEARNING OBJECTIVE 10

Describe potential approaches to health system reform, including the possibility of a national health care system.

CONCEPTS FOR LECTURE

1. The Institute of Medicine offers six specific aims for improving a redesign of a health care system and ten rules to guide that redesign process.

POWERPOINT LECTURE SLIDES

NOTE: The number on each PPT Lecture Slide directly corresponds with the Concepts for Lecture.

1 Health System Reform
- Specific aims for improving health care systems
- Rules to guide health care redesign

SUGGESTIONS FOR CLASSROOM ACTIVITIES

Have students present suggestions for their ideal health care system with specific aims as they apply to their clinical setting.

SUGGESTIONS FOR CLINICAL ACTIVITIES

Ask students to evaluate their clinical setting in terms of the IOM specific aims for improvement. Present examples at post conference.

The Global Context

RESOURCE LIBRARY

COMPANION WEBSITE

Audio Glossary
Exam Review Questions
Case Study: Bird Flu: A Global Health Issue
Appendix E: Information on Selected Communicable
  Diseases

MediaLink Applications: WHO Measures Against Malaria
Media Links
Challenge Your Knowledge
Advocacy Interviews

IMAGE LIBRARY

Table 6-3 National Rankings for Health System Goal
  Attainment

Table 6-5 Comparison of Selected National Health
  System Features

LEARNING OBJECTIVE 1

Discuss the advantages of U.S. involvement in global health initiatives.

CONCEPTS FOR LECTURE

1. Globalization is defined as a complex process of increasing economic, political, and social interdependence that takes place as capital, traded goods, persons, concepts, images, ideas, and values diffuse across states' boundaries.
2. Advantages of U.S. involvement, cited by the CDC, are identified as protection of U.S. public from communicable disease threats, humanitarian efforts, economic/diplomatic benefits, and enhancement of U.S. security.
3. CDC priorities for U.S. involvement in global health initiatives include: response to disease outbreaks, global disease surveillance, global health research, dissemination of public health approaches to health problems, global disease control initiatives, and public health training and capacity building.

POWERPOINT LECTURE SLIDES

NOTE: The number on each PPT Lecture Slide directly corresponds with the Concepts for Lecture.

[1] Globalization
- Complex process of interdependence
  - Economic
  - Political
  - Social

[1a] Globalization (continued)
- Diffuses across states' boundaries
  - Capital
  - Traded goods
  - Persons
  - Concepts
  - Images
  - Ideas
  - Values

[2] Advantages of U.S. Involvement
- Protection of U.S. public from communicable disease threats
- Humanitarian efforts
- Economic/diplomatic benefits
- Enhancement of U.S. security

[3] Priorities for U.S. Involvement
- Response to disease outbreaks
- Global disease surveillance

- Global health research
- Dissemination of public health approaches to health problems
- Global disease control initiatives
- Public health training and capacity building

SUGGESTIONS FOR CLASSROOM ACTIVITIES	SUGGESTIONS FOR CLINICAL ACTIVITIES
Present case studies to the class, each involving examples that demonstrate the interdependence of health issues and globalization. Ask students to evaluate the potential impact of various assigned health conditions and their effect on neighboring countries or nations.	Have students identify and discuss ways in which global health issues affect the health of the local population.

LEARNING OBJECTIVE 2

Identify at least five policy dilemmas faced by national health care systems.

CONCEPTS FOR LECTURE

1. In general, national health care systems must address the following policy dilemmas: balancing the need for regional or national coordination with the requirement to meet local health needs; dealing with the problems of maldistribution of resources; providing services without impeding the voluntary health sector's work; balancing professional practice autonomy with accountability for population health outcomes; integrating primary care with hospital and specialty services; reconciling individual practice patterns with national standards; balancing individual and population foci with limited resources; assuring access to care in the face of cost constraints; balancing curative technology with allocations for prevention and promotion; maintaining a qualified health care workforce; ensuring community participation in policy making; and reaching hard-to-serve populations.

POWERPOINT LECTURE SLIDES

NOTE: The number on each PPT Lecture Slide directly corresponds with the Concepts for Lecture.

1 National Health Care System Policy Dilemmas
- Balancing regional/national needs with local health needs
- Dealing with maldistribution of resources
- Providing services without impeding voluntary work
- Balancing professional practice autonomy with outcomes accountability
- Integrating primary care with hospital and specialty services
- Reconciling individual practice patterns with national standards

1a National Health Care System Policy Dilemmas (continued)
- Balancing individual and population foci with limited resources
- Assuring access to care in the face of cost constraints
- Balancing curative technology with allocations for prevention and promotion
- Maintaining a qualified health care workforce
- Ensuring community participation in policy development

SUGGESTIONS FOR CLASSROOM ACTIVITIES	SUGGESTIONS FOR CLINICAL ACTIVITIES
Divide students into groups. Each group is to research one of the policy dilemmas faced by national health care systems and provide examples from the literature, both past and present, that exemplify approaches to dealing with their policy dilemma.	In a community health clinical setting, assign students to observe for examples that demonstrate the existence of specific policy dilemmas. Encourage students to interview community health nurses for suggestions and present at post conference.

LEARNING OBJECTIVE 3

Compare selected features of national health care systems.

CONCEPTS FOR LECTURE

1. In comparing health care systems, it has been noted that nations throughout the world organize their unique systems to address the following key features that include: locus of decision making (centralized versus decentralized), expenditures, funding mechanisms, consumer choice and professional autonomy, coverage and access, health outcomes, and consumer satisfaction.

POWERPOINT LECTURE SLIDES

NOTE: The number on each PPT Lecture Slide directly corresponds with the Concepts for Lecture.

1 Key Health Care Systems Features
- Locus of decision making
  - Centralized versus decentralized
- Expenditures
  - Percent of gross national product
  - Per capita expenditures
  - Out-of-pocket expenses

1a Key Health Care Systems Features (continued)
- Funding mechanisms
  - Out of pocket
  - Private insurance
  - Federal and state tax dollars
  - Social insurance funds
  - Payroll taxes

1b Key Health Care System Features (continued)
- Consumer choice and professional autonomy
  - Consumer choice of providers
  - Access to specialty care
  - Limitations of providers in treatment choices
  - Provider constraints on revenue sources

1c Key Health Care System Features (continued)
- Coverage and access
  - Universal access
- Health outcomes (Refer to Table 6–3)
  - Life expectancy
  - Health-adjusted life expectancy
  - Disability-adjusted life expectancy
  - Child survival
  - Disease incidence and prevalence

1d Key Health Care System Features (continued)
- Consumer satisfaction (Refer to Table 6–5)
  - Satisfaction studies

SUGGESTIONS FOR CLASSROOM ACTIVITIES

Divide students into groups to research, investigate, and analyze various countries and their health care systems based on the key features described. Compare available statistics of each country with those of the United States. When students have presented their comparisons, have them describe the "ideal" health care system based on identified features.

SUGGESTIONS FOR CLINICAL ACTIVITIES

In a community health clinical setting, have each student examine how their clinical setting addresses key features of health systems and present at post conference with case studies or examples.

LEARNING OBJECTIVE 4

Describe two types of international health agencies.

CONCEPTS FOR LECTURE

1. International agencies can be grouped as multilateral agencies or bilateral agencies. Multilateral agencies are those that involve several countries in joint activities related to health, such as the World Health Organization and the Pan American Health Organization. Bilateral agencies involve only two countries in any single project, such as specific initiatives undertaken by the United States Agency for International Development and ACTION.

POWERPOINT LECTURE SLIDES

NOTE: The number on each PPT Lecture Slide directly corresponds with the Concepts for Lecture.

1 Types of International Health Agencies
- Multilateral agencies
  - Involve several countries in joint activities related to health
    - World Health Organization
    - Pan American Health Organization

1a Types of International Health Agenices (continued)
- Bilateral agencies
  - Involve only two countries in any single project
    - United States Agency for International Development (USAID)
    - ACTION

SUGGESTIONS FOR CLASSROOM ACTIVITIES

Divide class into two groups and provide time to search the Internet for examples of past and current health-related projects of international agencies. Students should describe the countries involved, the health issues, the focus or mission of the initiative, and the funding sources. Students should also identify whether the organizations or initiatives are multilateral or bilateral.

SUGGESTIONS FOR CLINICAL ACTIVITIES

Arrange for students to spend a day with volunteers from local agencies such as the American Red Cross or other agencies or organizations that may have either a multilateral or bilateral focus. Invite speakers from these agencies to present their agency's health-related focus during post conference.

LEARNING OBJECTIVE 5

Distinguish between international and global health.

CONCEPTS FOR LECTURE

1. International health involves health matters that affect two or more countries and is distinguished by the authority of the specific nation-states to address health issues that affect both.
2. Global health involves multinational efforts to address health problems that cross national borders and is also concerned with factors that affect the capacity of individual nation-states to deal with the determinants of health and illness.

POWERPOINT LECTURE SLIDES

NOTE: The number on each PPT Lecture Slide directly corresponds with the Concepts for Lecture.

1 International Health
- Health matters that affect two or more countries
- Distinguished by the authority of the specific nation-states
- Addresses health issues that affect both

2 Global Health
- Multinational efforts to address health problems that cross national borders
- Concerned with factors that affect the capacity of individual nation-states to deal with the determinants of health and illness

SUGGESTIONS FOR CLASSROOM ACTIVITIES

Assign students two groups. Place 3 × 5 cards with the name of a disease or health concern/issue on each card into a box. Have each student select a card and discuss amongst his or her group the process by which the health concern could become an international or a global health matter. Each group will present a summary of its discussions to the class.

SUGGESTIONS FOR CLINICAL ACTIVITIES

Invite speakers to class who have volunteered or worked for various international agencies to share experiences from those countries during post conference.

LEARNING OBJECTIVE 6

Discuss positive and negative health effects of globalization.

CONCEPTS FOR LECTURE

1. Four key processes have occurred as a result of globalization. The first process is the change in the distribution of income. With the promotion of economic growth in some population sectors comes increasing inequalities within and between population groups. The second process is the change in production processes, which benefits some populations with greater employment but means loss of work for others. The third process is the liberalization of trade. Trade liberalization leads to greater financial prosperity and health in some areas, only to result in global marketing and sale of harmful products to regions not previously affected. The fourth process is the reshaping of nation-states, which can result in the erosion of traditional boundaries leading to a cross-border flow that strengthens state identity or circumvents boundaries.

2. Additionally, there are three dimensions of globalization: spatial, temporal, and cognitive. Negative effects of spatial dimensions include the ease of spread of communicable diseases and ease of illicit trade in harmful drugs and weapons. A positive effect is the broad dissemination of health knowledge. Temporal dimension includes the speeding up and slowing down of time. Negative effects include the rapid spread of disease, but positive effects include the rapid dissemination of surveillance and treatment information. The cognitive dimension reflects the changes and exchanges of ideas, beliefs, values, and cultural practices that affect our perceptions of the world. The cognitive dimension also includes the development of geocultures, the adoption of international health-related standards, and the dissemination of practices detrimental to health.

POWERPOINT LECTURE SLIDES

NOTE: The number on each PPT Lecture Slide directly corresponds with the Concepts for Lecture.

1 Globalization and Its Effects on Health
- Four key processes
  - Distribution of income
    - Economic growth in some sectors and inequalities within and between population groups

1a Globalization and Its Effects on Health (continued)
- Four key processes
  - Change in production processes
    - Greater employment opportunities for some population groups with concomitant loss of employment for others
- Liberalization of trade
  - Greater financial prosperity and health in some areas
  - Global marketing and sales of harmful products to regions not previously available

1b Globalization and Its Effects on Health (continued)
- Four key processes
  - Reshaping of nation-states
    - Erosion of traditional boundaries
- Cross-border flows
  - Strengthen state identity (international trade)
  - Circumvent boundaries (global warming and information technology)

2 Dimensions of Globalization
- Spatial
  - Spread of communicable diseases
  - Illicit trade in harmful drugs and weapons
  - Dissemination of health knowledge
- Temporal
  - Rapid spread of disease
  - Rapid dissemination of surveillance and treatment

2a Dimensions of Globalization (continued)
- Cognitive
  - Changes and exchanges of ideas, beliefs, values, and cultural practices
  - Development of geocultures
  - Adoption of international health-related standards
  - Dissemination of practices detrimental to health

SUGGESTIONS FOR CLASSROOM ACTIVITIES

Discuss examples of income disparities in developing nations, production processes (outsourcing to other countries), trade liberalization (HIV medication availability in African countries), and changes in nation-states (e.g., Yugoslavia) and the global health impact on the United States and other countries.

SUGGESTIONS FOR CLINICAL ACTIVITIES

Have students interview a community health nurse, epidemiologist, or infection control nurse with a focus on one communicable disease (Avian influenza, smallpox, tuberculosis) and address the potential for spread given spatial, temporal, and cognitive factors. Present a summary of their interview at post conference.

LEARNING OBJECTIVE 7

Identify elements of a global health policy agenda.

CONCEPTS FOR LECTURE

1. Global health policy is defined as the ways in which globalization may be affecting health policy and, alternatively, what health policies are needed to respond to the challenges raised by globalization processes. An adjunct to this definition is global governance, which sees the world as a single place and involves movement toward structures of international governance that manage a system of nation-states.

2. Elements of a global health policy agenda include: improving national health infrastructures; developing complementary health infrastructures at global and regional levels that address transborder determinants of health; fostering global cooperation; supporting participation in health policy development for disadvantaged populations, including health interests in other policy-making sectors; and using communication technology to support effective health policy making.

3. Indirect challenges to a global health policy agenda are that it is voluntary, with no mechanism for sanctioning countries that fail to comply, and that there are vested and conflicting interests from large companies and industries.

4. Direct challenges to a global health policy agenda include the following: improving societal conditions affecting health, improving child and adolescent health, providing better family planning services, reducing substance abuse incidence, preventing the spread of communicable diseases, managing physical and mental illness, linking health systems and social processes, and designing valid and economically feasible measures of health status.

POWERPOINT LECTURE SLIDES

NOTE: The number on each PPT Lecture Slide directly corresponds with the Concepts for Lecture.

1 Global Health Policy
- The ways in which globalization may be affecting health policy and, alternatively, what health policies are needed to respond to the challenges raised by globalization processes
- Global governance
  - World is a single place
  - Involves moving toward international governance of nation-states

2 Elements of a Global Health Policy Agenda Include:
- Improving national health infrastructures
- Developing complementary health infrastructures at global and regional levels that address transborder determinants of health
- Fostering global cooperation
- Supporting participation in health policy development for disadvantaged populations
- Including health interests in other policy-making sectors
- Using communication technology to support effective health policy making

3 Indirect Challenges
- No mechanism for sanctioning countries that fail to comply
- Vested and conflicting interests from large companies and industries

4 Direct Challenges
- Improving societal conditions
- Improving child and adolescent health
- Providing better family planning
- Reducing substance abuse

4a Direct Challenges (continued)
- Preventing spread of communicable diseases
- Managing physical and mental illness
- Linking health systems and social processes
- Designing valid measures of health status

SUGGESTIONS FOR CLASSROOM ACTIVITIES

Divide students into groups to research and design a flowchart that reflects the interrelatedness of the global health policy agenda and its challenges. Suggest the use of pictures, collages, and other visuals to emphasize key points. Direct students to provide examples of countries that would benefit most and countries that might benefit least from such a policy agenda.

SUGGESTIONS FOR CLINICAL ACTIVITIES

Invite speakers from nursing or other health profession who have conducted research that addresses one of the agenda items in other countries to discuss the results of their research.

LEARNING OBJECTIVE 8

Describe community health nursing involvement with respect to international terrorism.

CONCEPTS FOR LECTURE

1. Terrorism is defined as the unlawful use of force or violence against persons or property to intimidate or coerce a government, the civilian population, or any segment in furtherance of political or social objectives. Domestic terrorism is perpetrated by individuals or groups within a given country without foreign direction or involvement. International terrorism is directed by foreign groups and may transcend national boundaries, affecting people in several countries or perpetrated by residents of one country against another. Agroterrorism is the deliberate introduction of a disease agent, either against livestock or into the food chain, for purposes of undermining stability and/or generating fear.
2. The role of community health nurses may be to respond to terrorist attacks, to educate the public regarding preventive measures or actions to be taken in case of exposure, to prevent panic, and to identify symptoms of unusual illness in a population.

POWERPOINT LECTURE SLIDES

NOTE: The number on each PPT Lecture Slide directly corresponds with the Concepts for Lecture.

1 Terrorism
- Unlawful use of force or violence against persons or property to intimidate or coerce a government, civilian population, or any segment in furtherance of political or social objectives

1a Domestic Terrorism
- Perpetrated by individuals or groups within a given country without foreign direction or involvement

1b International Terrorism
- Directed by foreign groups
- Transcends national boundaries
- Affects people in several countries
- Can be perpetrated by residents of one country against another

1c Agroterrorism
- Deliberate introduction of a disease agent
  - Livestock
  - Food chain
  - Undermines stability and/or generates fear

2 Role of Community Health Nurse
- Respond to terrorist attacks
- Educate public on preventive measures or actions in case of exposure
- Prevent panic
- Identify symptoms of unusual illness

Suggestions for Classroom Activities

1. Arrange for a guest speaker from a community health committee to present local or state disaster preparedness plans. Provide students with historical data about the smallpox post event plans and other national efforts to prepare communities for identification of terrorist actions involving infectious diseases. Have students identify potential issues in the event of a terrorist attack in their community.

2. Assign students a biological or chemical agent that has potential for use as a terrorist weapon. Have students present information on their agent, such as mechanism of action or transmission, morbidity and mortality impact, treatment or vaccinations available, and potential areas for public education. Discuss the role of the community health nurse with respect to the agent.

Suggestions for Clinical Activities

Arrange for students to attend a local community health planning committee and report to the class the goals and objectives, community educational efforts, mechanisms for early detection of an outbreak, and responses of local, state, and national governments.

The Policy Context

RESOURCE LIBRARY

COMPANION WEBSITE

Audio Glossary
Exam Review Questions
Case Study: Political Action: New State Bill to Increase
  RN-to-Patient Ratios
MediaLink Applications: Preparing Effective Testimony

Media Links
Challenge Your Knowledge
Update *Healthy People 2010*
Advocacy Interviews

IMAGE LIBRARY

Figure 7-1 A Typical Legislative Process

Table 7-2 Community Health Nursing Roles and
Activities in Policy Development

LEARNING OBJECTIVE 1

Analyze potential community health nursing roles in policy development.

CONCEPTS FOR LECTURE

1. Policy is defined as a set of principles determining the direction for activity and allocation of resources toward achieving an identified prioritized group or organizational goal.
2. Public policy is defined as policy made on behalf of the public, developed or initiated by government, and interpreted and implemented by public and private bodies. Public policy includes laws or statues, regulations, executive orders, and court rulings.
3. Policy development is the process by which society makes decisions, selects goals and the best means for reaching them, handles conflicting views about what should be done, and allocates resources to address needs. Politics becomes the mechanism by which policy development is influenced by those with a vested interest in its outcomes.
4. Early nursing leaders became involved in policy development with political activism for social conditions, support for women's suffrage issues, and concern for the health of population groups. Stages of nursing involvement include the following: marginal participation in political activity with voting, collective policy development to improve the profession, coalition participation addressing societal issues, and more recently, leadership in mobilizing others to deal with health issues.

POWERPOINT LECTURE SLIDES

NOTE: The number on each PPT Lecture Slide directly corresponds with the Concepts for Lecture.

1 Policy
- Set of principles
- Determines direction for activity and allocation of resources
- Identifies prioritized group or organizational goals

2 Public Policy
- Policy made on behalf of the public
- Developed/initiated by government
- Interpreted/implemented by public and private bodies
  - Laws/statutes
  - Regulations
  - Executive orders
  - Court rulings

3 Policy Development Process
- Policy development
  - Process by which society makes decisions
  - Selects goals and best means for reaching them
  - Handles conflicting views
  - Allocates resources

CONCEPTS FOR LECTURE *continued*

5. The four spheres in which nurses influence policy development include the workplace, the governmental policy arena, within professional organizations, and the community sphere.

6. Community health nurses have four roles in their efforts to influence policy development: citizen, activist, politician, and researcher.

POWERPOINT LECTURE SLIDES *continued*

- Politics:
  - Policy development by those with a vested interest in its outcomes

4 Nursing Profession and Policy Development
- Early leaders
  - Activism for social conditions
  - Support for women's suffrage issues
  - Concern for health of population groups

4a Stages of Nursing Involvement
- Marginal participation in political activity
- Collective policy development
- Coalition participation
- Leadership in mobilizing others

5 Spheres of Nursing Influence
- Workplace
- Governmental policy arena
- Professional organizations
- Community

6 Community Health Nursing Roles (Refer to Table 7-2)
- Citizen
- Activist
- Politician
- Researcher

SUGGESTIONS FOR CLASSROOM ACTIVITIES

Referring to the case study at the end of the chapter, divide students into four groups (citizen, activist, politician, and researcher). As nurses, ask students to brainstorm ideas that would reflect each role as it pertains to the case study. Ask students to role-play and present ideas at an "emergency" community meeting.

SUGGESTIONS FOR CLINICAL ACTIVITIES

Provide students with an opportunity to attend community meetings, community health committee meetings, and meetings from various nonprofit health organizations. Ask students to identify opportunities for nurse involvement and share them at post conference.

LEARNING OBJECTIVE 2

Discuss three avenues for public policy development.

CONCEPTS FOR LECTURE

1. Health policies have many different categories, purposes, sources, and focuses. The five main categories include the following: substantive policies, which dictate action to be taken; procedural policies, which determine how the action will occur; distributive policies, which allocate goods and services; regulatory policies, which restrict or constrain behaviors; and redistributive policies, which take goods and services away from some members and give them to others.

2. Avenues for health policy development include four major forms: legislation and health programs created by legislation, rules and regulations for implementing legislation, administrative decisions, and judicial decisions. Legislation is usually created in the form of

POWERPOINT LECTURE SLIDES

NOTE: The number on each PPT Lecture Slide directly corresponds with the Concepts for Lecture.

1 Types of Health Policies
- Substantive policies
  - Dictate actions to be taken
- Procedural policies
  - Determine how those actions will occur
- Distributive policies
  - Allocate goods and services

1a Types of Health Policies (continued)
- Regulatory policies
  - Restrict or constrain behaviors

CONCEPTS FOR LECTURE *continued*

laws or statues utilizing the legislative branch of government at all three levels (federal, state, and local) to create legislative proposals for bills. Regulations, which are rules or orders that have the force of law to deal with procedures for implementing the legislation, are implemented by regulatory agencies. Administrative decisions such as executive orders are made by individuals or agencies and affect the implementation of health care policies or programs. Judicial decisions arise from the court system in response to the interpretation of laws.

POWERPOINT LECTURE SLIDES *continued*

- Redistributive policies
  - Take goods and services away from some and give to others

2 Avenues for Health Policy Development
- Legislation
  - Creates laws or statutes
- Rules and regulations
  - Orders that have the force of law
  - Deal with procedures to implement legislation

2a See Figure 7-1

2b Administrative Decisions
- Made by individual or agencies under executive orders

2c Judicial Decisions
- Interpret laws in the court system

SUGGESTIONS FOR CLASSROOM ACTIVITIES

Invite a local or state lawmaker or judge to discuss recent and upcoming health policy legislation. Have students use the Internet to research bills or legislation that is before the state legislature to discuss with the guest speaker. Have students prepare a pros and cons response to one legislative proposal for discussion with guest speaker.

SUGGESTIONS FOR CLINICAL ACTIVITIES

1. Arrange for students to attend local community or city planning committees, public forums, or school board meetings. Provide an opportunity at post conference for students to share observations about the political process, the decision-making process, community awareness and involvement, and the role of the community health nurse.
2. Have students identify policy issues in the institutions/agencies in which they are getting their clinical experience. Discuss the policy making process at the institutional level and the community health nurse involvement in that process.
3. Have students examine newspapers for articles dealing with local, state, or national health policy issues and present the pros and cons of the issue. Examine the position of nursing and involvement of nursing organizations with respect to these issues. Identify the implications of the issues for clients seen in the clinical practice setting.

LEARNING OBJECTIVE 3

Describe at least four aspects of the policy development process.

CONCEPTS FOR LECTURE

1. Nurses' involvement in the policy development process depends on their ability to assess the policy situation, plan and implement health care policy, and evaluate the effects of health policy development.
2. Aspects of the policy development process as influenced by community health nurses include use of a policy development model, setting a policy agenda, planning and implementing health care policy, and evaluating policy development. The first step in policy development is to understand available models. The rational or rational-comprehensive model includes defining a problem, identifying a goal, determining

POWERPOINT LECTURE SLIDES

NOTE: The number on each PPT Lecture Slide directly corresponds with the Concepts for Lecture.

1 Nursing Involvement
- Assess policy situation
- Plan and implement health policy
- Evaluate effects of health policy development

2 Models of Policy Development
- Rational or Rational-Comprehensive model
- "Garbage Can" model
- Kingdon's Policy Stream model
- Stage-Sequential model

and prioritizing social values, specifying criteria for problem resolution, examining alternative solutions, and implementing, monitoring, and evaluating alternative solutions. The "garbage can" model identifies problems, solutions, participants, and opportunities for choices. Kingdon's policy stream model addresses the problem stream, the policy stream, and the political stream. Finally, the stage-sequential model includes agenda setting, formulation of goals and programs, program implementation, and evaluation.

3. The second aspect of policy development is setting the agenda, which is the first stage in actual policy development. A policy agenda is the list of issues that become the focus for action by policy makers. The third aspect is planning health care policy, which provides opportunities for community health nurse involvement and includes the following activities: developing and evaluating alternative policy solutions, delineating policy, and planning strategies for policy adoption, including the use of traditional political strategies such as voting, campaigning, and holding office. The fourth aspect is evaluating the effectiveness of policy development.

3 Policy Development
- Agenda setting
  - Issue identification
  - Issue analysis
  - Consciousness raising regarding the issue

3a Plan Health Care Policy
- Develop/evaluate alternative policy solutions
- Delineate policy
- Plan for strategies for policy adoption

3b Strategies for Creating Support
- Stay informed and communicate with policy makers
- Network
- Build coalitions
- Create media support
- Organize community
- Lobby and advocacy
- Present testimony

3c Traditional Political Strategies
- Vote
- Campaign
- Hold office

SUGGESTIONS FOR CLASSROOM ACTIVITIES

Invite members of the local or state nursing organization to present current health policy issues with which the organization is involved. Discuss with guest speaker(s) in advance what issues are before the legislation. Have students investigate the health policy concern, identify the target population, and determine the political, economic, and social environment for the health policy legislation.

SUGGESTIONS FOR CLINICAL ACTIVITIES

Arrange for students to attend a local or state chapter of various nursing or health associations. Have students call the chairperson or secretary in advance to obtain a copy of the meeting's agenda. Provide an opportunity for students to relate their experiences in post conference. Ask students to assess the policy situation, develop a hypothetical plan to implement the health policy, and determine a hypothetical mechanism for evaluating the effects of the health policy.

LEARNING OBJECTIVE 4

Apply criteria for health policy evaluation.

CONCEPTS FOR LECTURE

1. Community health nurses have an opportunity to be involved in the health policy evaluation process by evaluating the extent to which all stakeholders have been involved in the policy development and in assessing the adequacy of strategic management of the policy development process.

2. Several criteria exist for evaluating health policies. They include: the adequacy of the policy for meeting the health needs of the public, safeguards for the rights of individuals, equitable allocation of resources, capacity for implementation, and finally, the effects of the policy on the target population.

POWERPOINT LECTURE SLIDES

NOTE: The number on each PPT Lecture Slide directly corresponds with the Concepts for Lecture.

1 Health Policy Evaluation
- Evaluate involvement of stakeholders' policy development
- Assess strategic management of policy development process

2 Criteria for Evaluating Health Policy
- Adequacy in meeting health needs of public
- Safeguards for the rights of individuals
- Equitable allocation of resources
- Capacity for implementation
- Effects of the policy on target population

SUGGESTIONS FOR CLASSROOM ACTIVITIES

Have students develop a health policy recommendation for the case study at the end of the chapter. Once the recommendation is developed, divide students into four groups to use the evaluation criteria to assess their newly developed health policy. Have students present evaluations to the class.

SUGGESTIONS FOR CLINICAL ACTIVITIES

Arrange for students to spend time with a local or state representative, community health nurse manager, or other persons who have a stake in health policy development. Have students develop questions about laws, policies, or regulations that affect a specific target population such as homeless populations, underinsured or uninsured populations, migrant populations, or other populations specific to the community. Discuss their experiences at post conference.

The Economic Context

RESOURCE LIBRARY

COMPANION WEBSITE

Audio Glossary
Exam Review Questions
Case Study: Helping Seniors with Medicare Plan D
MediaLink Applications: Universal Health Care in
  Massachusetts

Media Links
Challenge Your Knowledge
Update *Healthy People 2010*
Advocacy Interviews

IMAGE LIBRARY

Figure 8-1 Distribution of National Health Care
Expenditures, United States, 2003
Figure 8-2 Sources of Health Care Funding, United
States, 2003

Figure 8-3 Health Care Funding Through
Employment-Based Managed Care Plan Enrollment

Table 8-2 Differentiating Features of Medicare and
Medicaid

LEARNING OBJECTIVE 1

Analyze interrelationships among economic conditions, health care services, and health status.

CONCEPTS FOR LECTURE

1. Economics can be defined as the study of the ways in which societies make choices in how they address problems of scarcity. Economic principles that affect health and health care services include the following: resources are always more limited than what is needed, resources have alternative uses, and different people have different ideas about those uses.
2. Economic factors influence availability of and access to health care services, which, in turn, affects the health status of individuals/families and the overall population.
3. Societal productivity and stability are affected by a nation's overall health. Populations affected by chronic illness, poverty, and general ill health cost society in lost productivity and decreased revenues.

POWERPOINT LECTURE SLIDES

NOTE: The number on each PPT Lecture Slide directly corresponds with the Concepts for Lecture.

1. Health and Economic Factors
   - Economics
     ○ Study of how societies address problems of scarcity
   - Economic principles affecting health and health care services
     ○ Limited resources
     ○ Alternative uses for resources
     ○ Competing views on appropriate resource utilization

2. Economic Factors
   - Influence availability of health services
   - Influence access to available health services
   - Influence health status

3. Societal Productivity and Stability
   - Affected by nation's overall health
   - Chronic illness, poverty, and ill health result in:
     ○ Lost productivity
     ○ Decreased revenues

SUGGESTIONS FOR CLASSROOM ACTIVITIES

Divide students into groups to research information about state and local poverty statistics, chronic illness, and Medicaid utilization.

SUGGESTIONS FOR CLINICAL ACTIVITIES

Have students identify the health effects of economic factors for the clients they are seeing in the clinical setting.

LEARNING OBJECTIVE 2

Discuss factors contributing to escalating health care costs.

CONCEPTS FOR LECTURE

1. Factors that affect the escalating costs of health care include an aging population, greater use of technology, costly specialty care, costs of care for the uninsured, and the labor-intensive nature of health care delivery.

2. An aging population contributes to greater demand for and use of services, especially those services related to chronic health conditions. Chronic health conditions are associated with higher costs. The older population has increased in size from 8.1% in 1950 to a projection of 21.8% by 2030 and 25% of the total population by 2050.

3. Partially in response to fears of malpractice, U.S. physician are utilizing more expensive technology.

4. Nearly two thirds of U.S. physicians are specialists who tend to use more expensive technology to diagnose and treat health conditions. Additionally, greater use of technology is creating a demand for a better prepared health care workforce, which also comes with additional expenses.

5. The costs for uncompensated care and increasing prescription drug process also contribute to the rising costs of health care. Uncompensated care has lead to cost shifting, which is the passing on of the cost of uncompensated care to those who do pay for care, either through out-of-pocket or health insurance payments. In addition to higher prescription drug costs, decreased reimbursement from health insurance or employers affects older population groups as well as the underinsured population groups. There are large segments of the population who do not have assistance in paying for prescription medications.

6. Health care is considered a labor-intensive segment of the economy. Care is required for 24 hours a day and seven days a week in some settings. By 2010, the health care workforce will account for 13% of all wage and salary jobs.

POWERPOINT LECTURE SLIDES

NOTE: The number on each PPT Lecture Slide directly corresponds with the Concepts for Lecture.

1 Escalating Health Care Costs
- Aging population
- Greater use of technology
- Costly specialty care
- Costs of care for uninsured
- Labor-intensive nature of health care delivery

2 Aging Population
- Greater demand for and use of services
  - Increase in chronic diseases
    - High cost for disease management
- Size of population steadily increasing

3 Greater Use of Technology
- Response to fears of malpractice
- Demand for better prepared health care workforce

4 Costly Subspecialty Care
- Nearly 2/3 of U.S. physicians are specialists
  - Increased use of technology

5 Costs of Care For Uninsured
- Uncompensated care accounts for large percentage of all patient operating costs
  - Leads to cost shifting
- Increasing costs of prescription drugs
  - Affect large segments of population

6 Labor-intensive Nature of Health Care Delivery
- Amount of time required to provide care: 24/7
- By 2010, healthcare workforce will account for 13% of all jobs

SUGGESTIONS FOR CLASSROOM ACTIVITIES

Divide students into specific target population groups: women and infants, aging, homeless, migrant workers, disabled populations, and adolescents. Have students prepare a poster presentation to the class that depicts the effects of poverty on the nation's health respective to their population.

SUGGESTIONS FOR CLINICAL ACTIVITIES

Arrange for students to attend clinical settings that provide services to underserved or uninsured populations. Have students prepare a report about the agency or clinical setting that describes funding sources, changes in funding sources, mission, goals, and services provided.

LEARNING OBJECTIVE 3

Discuss the effects of economic factors on the provision of public health services.

CONCEPTS FOR LECTURE

1. Financing of pubic health services has been reduced to 3.2% of the total U.S. health care expenditures (2003) of $1.3 trillion. Public health agencies rely on government funding for personal services, care for uninsured populations, and safety net services.
2. Changes that have an affect on public health services include the following: emphasis on bioterrorism with funding to state and local public health agencies, decreased attention to and funding for routine public health programs, public health tailoring services based on funding availability rather than population needs, and private-sector care incorporating traditional public health functions.

POWERPOINT LECTURE SLIDES

NOTE: The number on each PPT Lecture Slide directly corresponds with the Concepts for Lecture.

1 Public Health Services and Economic Factors:
- Financing public health services
- U.S. health care expenditures (2003)
  ○ $1.6 trillion
- Public health expenditures
  ○ $53.8 billion (3.2%)

1a Public Health Agencies Provide
- Personal care services
- Traditional public health services
- Care for uninsured populations
- Safety net services

2 Changes that Affect Public Health Services
- Emphasis on bioterrorism
- Decreased attention to, and funding for, routine public health
- Pubic health tailoring based on funding availability
- Private sector care incorporates public health functions

SUGGESTIONS FOR CLASSROOM ACTIVITIES

Assign students to research and present economic and health conditions in various local communities, surrounding communities, or state regions. Provide students with access to public documents that discuss the economic base for the community, public health services, and local demographics.

SUGGESTIONS FOR CLINICAL ACTIVITIES

Have students explore state and local expenditures for public health versus personal health care costs.

LEARNING OBJECTIVE 4

Distinguish among selected approaches to financing health care services.

CONCEPTS FOR LECTURE

1. Four approaches to financing health care services are categorized based on the source of risk bearing for health care costs and include personal payment, government programs, commercial insurance, and self-funded insurance.
2. Personal payment, paying a provider directly out of pocket, is used by wealthy, by uninsured, or for services not covered by insurance; comprises 14% of health care funds; and includes insurance premiums, deductibles, and copayments.
3. In government-funded programs, the risk for the costs of care is borne by the government and accounts for approximately 44% of expenditures. The federal

POWERPOINT LECTURE SLIDES

NOTE: The number on each PPT Lecture Slide directly corresponds with the Concepts for Lecture.

1 Financing Health Care Services
- Four approaches based on source of risk
  ○ Personal payment
  ○ Government programs
  ○ Commercial insurance
  ○ Self-funded insurance

2 Personal Payment
- Paying a provider directly out of pocket
- Used by wealthy and uninsured

government funds approximately 33% and states fund 10.5%. The two major federal programs include Medicare and Medicaid. Medicare is designed to provide care for the elderly and disabled, and Medicaid, jointly financed by state and federal funds, provides health care to the poor.

4. Commercial or private insurance provides coverage of the costs of health care by an insurance company based on payment of premiums designed to cover costs. There are three general types: individual health insurance, wraparound or supplemental plans, and group health plans. Wraparound policies cover services not covered under other forms. Individual insurance is purchased directly by an individual, is expensive, and tends to have limited coverage. The group health plans are the largest and most popular service, are purchased by employers, and use employee pretax deductions.

5. Self-funded insurance, an approach used by employers to minimize the costs of commercial insurance benefits, involves a large employer collecting premiums from employees and paying for the cost of care. This option may use a self-insured program in which the employer hires a third party to administer the program and process the claims.

- Comprises 14% of health care funds
  - Insurance premiums
  - Deductibles
  - Co-payments

3 Government Programs (Refer to Table 8-2)
- Risk for cost of care borne by government
- Accounts for 44% of expenditures
  - Federal government: 33%
  - State government: 10.5%

3a Government Programs (continued)
- Two major programs
  - Medicare
    - Care for elderly and disabled
  - Medicaid
    - Care for poor

4 Commercial Insurance
- Payment of premiums covers health care costs
- Three types
  - Individual health insurance
    - Purchased directly by an individual
  - Wraparound/supplemental plans
    - Covers services not covered under other forms

4a Commercial Insurance (continued)
- Group health insurance plans
  - Purchased by employer

5 Self-funded Insurance
- Used by employers to minimize costs
- Employer collects premiums from employees to pay costs
- May use a self-insured program
  - Third party administers program and processes claims

SUGGESTIONS FOR CLASSROOM ACTIVITIES

Invite guest speakers from insurance companies, Medicare and Medicaid agencies, large hospitals, and small businesses to discuss health care reimbursement and policies that affect reimbursement.

SUGGESTIONS FOR CLINICAL ACTIVITIES

Arrange for students to visit various clinics that offer health services on sliding scale, no cost for services, and mixed payment services. Ask students to discuss at post conference which population groups use these services, gaps in health care services, and how services are advertised.

LEARNING OBJECTIVE 5

Analyze the effects of selected health care reimbursement mechanisms.

CONCEPTS FOR LECTURE

1. Approaches to reimbursing providers for health care services include out-of-pocket payments and third-party payments. Out-of-pocket payments, monies that health care recipients pay out of their own pockets for the services that they received, include direct payment for services and cost sharing with deductibles

POWERPOINT LECTURE SLIDES

NOTE: The number on each PPT Lecture Slide directly corresponds with the Concepts for Lecture.

1 Health Care Reimbursement
- Out-of-pocket payments
  - Health care recipient pays out of own pocket

CONCEPTS FOR LECTURE *continued*

and copayments. Third-party reimbursement mechanisms, designed to protect a person from financial devastation in the event of serious illness and to supplement client payment, may be either retrospective reimbursement or prospective reimbursement.

2. Retrospective reimbursement is payment for services rendered based on the cost of those services determined after the fact. Several types of retrospective reimbursements include fee-for-service, discounted fee-for-service payment, and per diem payments.

3. Prospective reimbursement is payment at a predetermined, fixed rate for a specific health care program or set of services and include diagnosis-related groups (DRGs), the Resource-Based Relative Value Scale (RBRVS), and capitation. DRGs are categories of client diagnoses for which typical costs of care have been calculated. Providers are paid a set fee based on client diagnosis. With RBRVS, the typical costs of a given health service are calculated based on the prevailing cost for that service in a particular locale for Medicare clients. Capitation is a prospective payment system that pays health plans or providers a fixed amount per enrollee per month to provide a defined set of health services based on enrollee needs.

POWERPOINT LECTURE SLIDES *continued*

  – Direct payment for services
  – Cost sharing with deductibles and co-payments
- Third-party payments
  ○ Protect from financial devastation
  ○ Supplements client payment
    – Retrospective reimbursement
    – Prospective reimbursement

2 Retrospective Reimbursement
- Payment for services determined after the fact
  ○ Fee-for-service
  ○ Discounted fee-for-service
  ○ Per diem payments

3 Prospective Reimbursement
- Payment at a predetermined, fixed rate
- Diagnosis-related groups (DRGs)
  ○ Categories of diagnoses with costs calculated
  ○ Providers paid a set fee

3a Prospective Reimbursement (continued)
- Resource-based relative value (RBRVs)
  ○ Similar to DRGs for Medicare clients
- Capitation
  ○ Pays health plans or providers fixed amount per enrollee

SUGGESTIONS FOR CLASSROOM ACTIVITIES

1. Invite guest speakers from local hospitals, clinics, and community health to discuss the impact of DGRs and the RBRVS on health care reimbursements and availability of services provided in the community.

2. Discuss with students the implications of the recent reduction in Medicare reimbursement rates for physician services. What was the impetus for the cuts? How might they affect access to care, quality of care, or other health-related outcomes?

SUGGESTIONS FOR CLINICAL ACTIVITIES

Arrange for guest speakers from hospital utilization review staff, local providers, and other agencies to discuss how DRGs and the RBRVS drive health care services, quality of services, and payments for services.

The Cultural Context

RESOURCE LIBRARY

COMPANION WEBSITE

Audio Glossary
Appendix B: Cultural Influences on Health and
  Health-related Behaviors
Exam Review Questions
Case Study: Care of the African American Muslim
  Patient

MediaLink Application: Racism and Powerlessness
  (video)
Media Links
Challenge Your Knowledge
Update *Healthy People 2010*
Advocacy Interviews

IMAGE LIBRARY

Table 9-1 Characteristics of Culture

Table 9-5 Elements of Selected Models of Cultural
Competence

LEARNING OBJECTIVE 1

Differentiate among culture, race, nationality, and ethnicity.

CONCEPTS FOR LECTURE

1. Understanding the influence of culture enables nurses to provide effective care, assists providers in modifying elements that impede effective health care, and helps in modifying health care systems to better meet client needs.

2. Culture is defined as the ways of thinking and acting developed by a group of people that permit them to interact effectively with their environment and to address concerns common to the human condition. Culture is generally unique to a group and is relatively stable and enduring.

3. Race is an artificial categorization of people based on genetic inheritance and physical characteristics such as skin color, blood type, hair color and texture, and eye color. Recent thoughts are that racial categorization does not adequately address the diversity of the U.S. population with suggestions that ethnicity replace race as categorizing health-related data.

4. Nationality refers to one's country of birth or a country adopted for permanent residence.

5. Ethnicity is defined as the aggregate of cultural practices, social influences, religious pursuits, and racial characteristics shaping the identity of a relatively homogenous community.

POWERPOINT LECTURE SLIDES

NOTE: The number on each PPT Lecture Slide directly corresponds with the Concepts for Lecture.

1 Understanding Culture
- Enhance effective care
- Modify elements that impede effective health care
- Modify health care systems to better meet client needs

2 Culture (Refer to Table 9-1)
- Ways of thinking and acting developed by a group of people
- Permits them to interact effectively with environment
- Permits them to address concerns common to the human condition
- Generally unique, stable, and enduring

3 Race
- Artificial categorization
- Based on genetic inheritance and physical characteristics
- Does not adequately address the diversity of the U.S. population

4 Nationality
- One's country of birth or a country adopted for permanent residence

5 Ethnicity
- Aggregate of cultural practices, social influences, religious pursuits, and racial characteristics
- Shape the distinctive identity of a relatively homogenous community

---

SUGGESTIONS FOR CLASSROOM ACTIVITIES

Write out four columns on the blackboard: culture, race, nationality, and ethnicity.

Using demographic data for the local community or region, ask students to describe the culture, race, ethnicity, and nationality of the surrounding population. Leave information on the board for students to refer to later in class.

SUGGESTIONS FOR CLINICAL ACTIVITIES

1. During the clinical assignment, have students identify one ethnic group receiving community health services. Ask students to bring in one research health article about that ethnic group and present a summary of the article at post conference that identifies cultural attitudes or behaviors that affect health.
2. Have students identify major ethnic groups in the community. Discuss with them the implications of ethnicity for their nursing interventions and how interventions might be modified based on client ethnicity.

LEARNING OBJECTIVE 2

Discuss direct and indirect influences of culture on health and health care.

CONCEPTS FOR LECTURE

1. The effect of culture on health and health care can be both positive and negative. Direct effects pertain to dietary practices, practices intended to promote health and prevent illness, or practices to restore health when ill. Indirect effects result from definitions of health and illness, acceptability of health care programs and providers, and cultural influences on compliance with suggested health or illness regimens.

POWERPOINT LECTURE SLIDES

NOTE: The number on each PPT Lecture Slide directly corresponds with the Concepts for Lecture.

1 Influences of Culture on Health
- Direct effects
  - Dietary practices
  - Practices intended to promote health and prevent illness
  - Practices to restore health when ill

1a Influences of Culture on Health (continued)
- Indirect effects
  - Definitions of health and illness
  - Acceptability of health care programs and providers
  - Cultural influences on compliance with health or illness regimens

---

SUGGESTIONS FOR CLASSROOM ACTIVITIES

Using the previous activity, divide students into groups to research cultural health articles that provide examples of the influences of culture on health. Have the students present results with pictures on poster board.

SUGGESTIONS FOR CLINICAL ACTIVITIES

1. Invite health provider guest speakers from various cultures, nationalities, or ethnicities to post conference to discuss their experiences of culture on health and health care in the community.
2. Assist students to identify the effects of culture on their own health and that of clients seen in the clinical setting.

LEARNING OBJECTIVE 3

Describe cultural competence.

CONCEPTS FOR LECTURE

1. Cultural competence is a dynamic, fluid, and continuous process whereby an individual, system, or health care agency finds meaningful and useful care delivery strategies based on knowledge of the cultural heritage, beliefs, attitudes, and behaviors of those to whom they render care.

2. Several models exist such as the ASKED, BE SAFE, and the Culturally Competent Community Care models. The ASKED model includes the following elements: A: cultural awareness based on examination of one's own prejudices and biases; S: cultural skill in collecting relevant cultural data; K: cultural knowledge of differences and similarities among cultural groups; E: cultural encounters in face-to-face cross-cultural encounters; and D: cultural desire and personal motivation to practice in a culturally competent manner.

3. The BE SAFE model includes: B: Barriers to the use of biomedical care such as prejudice, SES, stigma; E: Ethics: consideration of differences in ethical conceptualizations in the culture; S: Sensitivity: lack of provider bias, stigma, cultural imposition; A: Assessment of physical, emotional, spiritual, social, mental, and occupational factors affecting health; F: Facts about the cultural beliefs, values, and practices; E: Encounters: knowledge of behavioral dos and don'ts, communication.

4. The Culturally Competent Community Care model includes the following elements: interpersonal caring, cultural sensitivity, cultural knowledge, and cultural skill.

5. Characteristics of individual cultural competence include awareness of one's own culturally determined perspectives without letting them influence one's interactions with others, knowledge and understanding of another culture, acceptance of and respect for other cultures, and conscious process of adaptation of care to the cultural context.

6. Characteristics of cultural competence at the health system level include recognition of the complexities involved in language interpretation, awareness of the need to consider linguistic variation within cultural groups, facilitation of learning between providers and communities, involvement of communities in defining and addressing their health care needs, and promotion of interagency collaboration.

POWERPOINT LECTURE SLIDES

NOTE: The number on each PPT Lecture Slide directly corresponds with the Concepts for Lecture.

1 Cultural Competence (Refer to Table 9-5)
- A dynamic, fluid, continuous process
- Find meaningful and useful care delivery strategies
- Based on knowledge of cultural heritage, beliefs, attitudes, and behaviors

2 Models of Cultural Competence
- ASKED
  - A: Cultural awareness
  - S: Cultural skill in collecting relevant cultural data
  - K: Cultural knowledge of differences and similarities
  - E: Cultural encounters
  - D: Cultural desire and motivation to practice in a culturally competent manner

3 BE SAFE Model
- B: Barriers to the use of biomedical care such as prejudice, SES, stigma
- E: Ethics: consideration of differences in ethical conceptualizations in the culture
- S: Sensitivity: lack of provider bias, stigma, cultural imposition
- A: Assessment of physical, emotional, spiritual, social, mental, and occupational factors affecting health
- F: Facts about cultural beliefs, values, and practices
- E: Encounters: knowledge of behavioral dos and don'ts, communication.

4 Culturally Competent Community Care
- Interpersonal caring
- Cultural sensitivity
- Cultural knowledge
- Cultural skill.

5 Individual Cultural Competence
- Awareness of cultural perspectives
- Individual perspective does not influence interactions with others
- Knowledge and understanding of another culture
- Acceptance of and respect for other cultures
- Conscious process of adaptation of care to the cultural context

6 Health System Cultural Competence
- Recognize complexities involved in language interpretation
- Aware of need to consider linguistic variation within cultural groups

- Facilitate learning between providers and communities
- Involve communities in defining and addressing health care needs
- Foster interagency collaboration

SUGGESTIONS FOR CLASSROOM ACTIVITIES	**SUGGESTIONS FOR CLINICAL ACTIVITIES**
1. Divide students into three culturally competent models groups. Have students examine the model and present examples of how the community can benefit from a culturally competent health care system. 2. Have students provide examples of community health nurse behaviors that either do or do not exemplify cultural competence. How might the culturally incompetent behaviors be modified to be more culturally competent?	Assign students to observe and describe at post conference which cultures, nationalities, and ethnicities are served by their clinical agency. Using the characteristics of a culturally competent health care program, have the students interview the agency manager about program goals, mission, or objectives that meet these characteristics. Have the students *actually observe* the extent to which the characteristics are displayed by the organization.

LEARNING OBJECTIVE 4

Identify barriers to cultural competence.

CONCEPTS FOR LECTURE

1. A number of barriers in the form of challenges to cultural competence exist, such as clinical differences among cultural groups, communication among cultural groups, recognition of when it is appropriate to incorporate elements of culture in the plan of care, developing trust among members of different cultures, addressing stereotypes held by providers, a view of cultures as "them" not "me," confusing race, ethnicity, and culture, misdiagnosing ethnic medical concerns due to poor communication, and cultural mismatches between provider and client.

POWERPOINT LECTURE SLIDES

NOTE: The number on each PPT Lecture Slide directly corresponds with the Concepts for Lecture.

☐ 1 ☐ Barriers to Cultural Competence
- Recognizing clinical differences among cultural groups
- Communication among cultural groups
- Incorporating elements of culture in the plan of care
- Developing trust among members of different cultures

☐ 1a ☐ Addressing Stereotypes Held By Providers
- Viewing cultures as "them," not "me"
- Confusing race, ethnicity, and culture
- Misdiagnosing ethnic medical concerns
- Cultural mismatches

SUGGESTIONS FOR CLASSROOM ACTIVITIES	**SUGGESTIONS FOR CLINICAL ACTIVITIES**
Divide students into groups to discuss and discover examples of barriers to cultural competence and nursing actions that could diminish or remove those barriers. Share examples with the class.	Have students critically observe their community clinical setting and write down three or more examples of barriers that may be present. Share observations at post conference.

LEARNING OBJECTIVE 5

Conduct a cultural assessment of an individual, family, group, or health system.

CONCEPTS FOR LECTURE

1. A cultural assessment is guided by four basic principles: viewing the culture in the context in which it was developed, examining the underlying premise of culturally determined behavior, examining the meaning of behavior in the cultural context, and recognizing intracultural variation.

2. Conducting a cultural assessment requires obtaining cultural information in order to understand the process of cultural competence using the following steps: using personal insight and research to gain knowledge about a culture, interviewing colleagues who are members of the culture of interest, or living within the culture.

3. General guidelines useful for assessing another culture directly include looking and listening before asking questions, exploring how the group feels about being studied, discovering any special protocols, fostering human relations by putting the individual first before the need to obtain information, looking for similarities rather than differences, locating group leaders or elders, and being aware of acceptable or offensive questions.

4. Cultural assessment considerations include factors in the biophysical, psychological, physical environmental, sociocultural, behavioral, and health system dimensions.

5. Biophysical considerations include those related to attitudes about maturation and aging, genetic inheritance and physical differences, and physiologic function such as prevalent health problems, attitudes to body parts and functions, perceptions of health and illness and disease causation, and culture-bound syndromes.

6. Psychological considerations include the importance of group versus individual goals, attitudes toward change, and attitudes toward mental health and mental illness.

7. Physical environmental considerations include mastery over environment, beliefs about harmonious relationships with the external physical environment, and perceptions of space and time.

8. Sociocultural considerations include relationships with the supernatural, interpersonal roles and relationships, relationships with health care providers, socioeconomic status, sexuality and reproduction, coming of age, marriage, immigration, and death.

9. Biophysical considerations include dietary practices, consumption patterns, and health-related behaviors.

10. Health system considerations include factors related to health systems that affect the health of population groups such as design of health systems, health care providers, and health care practices.

POWERPOINT LECTURE SLIDES

NOTE: The number on each PPT Lecture Slide directly corresponds with the Concepts for Lecture.

1 Cultural Assessment
- Guided by four basic principles
  - View culture in the context in which it was developed
  - Examine underlying premise of culturally determined behavior
  - Examine meaning of behavior in the cultural context
  - Recognize intracultural variation

2 Conducting a Cultural Assessment
- Use personal insight and research to gain knowledge
- Interview colleagues who are members of the culture
- Live within the culture

3 Guidelines for Cultural Assessment
- Look and listen before asking questions
- Explore how the group feels about being studied
- Discover any special protocols
- Foster human relations

3a Guidelines for Cultural Assessment (continued)
- Put individual needs before the need to obtain information
- Look for similarities rather than differences
- Locate group leaders
- Be aware of acceptable or offensive questions

4 Cultural Assessment Considerations
- Biophysical
- Psychological
- Physical environmental
- Sociocultural
- Behavioral
- Health system dimensions

5 Biophysical Assessment
- Attitudes about maturation and aging
- Age composition of cultural group
- Genetic inheritance and physical differences
- Physiologic function:
  - Prevalent health problems
  - Attitudes to body parts and functions
  - Perceptions of health, illness, and disease causation
  - Culture-bound syndromes

6 Psychological Considerations
- Importance of group versus individual goals
- Attitudes toward change
- Attitudes toward mental health and mental illness

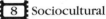 7 Physical Environmental
- Mastery over environment
- Beliefs about harmonious relationships with external environment
- Perceptions of space and time:
  - Personal space
  - Future-oriented versus past- or present-oriented

8 Sociocultural
- Relationships with supernatural
- Interpersonal roles and relationships
- Relationships with health care providers
- Socioeconomic status

8a Sociocultural (continued)
- Sexuality and reproduction
- Coming of age
- Marriage
- Immigration
- Death

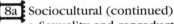 9 Behavioral/biophysical Considerations
- Dietary practices
- Consumption patterns
- Health-related behaviors

10 Health System Dimensions
- Health of population groups
- Design of health systems
- Health care providers
- Health care practices

SUGGESTIONS FOR CLASSROOM ACTIVITIES

Have students bring to class one or more articles that exemplify cultural nursing research. Using the focused assessment in the Appendix, ask students to answer as many questions as possible using their cultural article as their information base. Share responses with the class.

SUGGESTIONS FOR CLINICAL ACTIVITIES

Have students conduct a cultural assessment of an ethnic or other cultural group (gay, lesbian clients) encountered in the clinical setting and share the results at post conference.

LEARNING OBJECTIVE 6

Design, implement, and evaluate culturally competent care and health care delivery systems.

CONCEPTS FOR LECTURE

1. Providing culturally competent care requires that providers understand the need for culturally competent care and care systems, which arises from the increasing diversity of populations, the increasing provision of care in the home where cultural factors are influential, and the increasing disparities in health status among many ethnic cultural minorities.
2. Benefits of culturally competent care include promoting more appropriate and accurate diagnoses of health problems, improving compliance with treatment

POWERPOINT LECTURE SLIDES

NOTE: The number on each PPT Lecture Slide directly corresponds with the Concepts for Lecture.

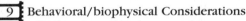 1 Rationale for Culturally Competent Care
- Increase in diverse populations
- Increase in home care where cultural factors are influential
- Increase in health disparities among ethnic cultural minorities

CONCEPTS FOR LECTURE *continued*

recommendations, reducing delays in care-seeking and use of services, enhancing client/provider communication, and enhancing compatibility of biomedical and traditional health care systems.

3. Leininger's transcultural nursing theory identifies three modes of providing culturally competent care, which include preservation, accommodation, and repatterning. Preservation is the attempt to maintain cultural resources that promote health or assist in recovery of health. Accommodation places emphasis on adjusting or adapting the actions of either client or provider to facilitate interaction designed to positively influence health. Repatterning involves changing attitudes and behaviors of providers or members of a culture of interest.

POWERPOINT LECTURE SLIDES *continued*

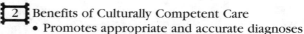 Benefits of Culturally Competent Care
- Promotes appropriate and accurate diagnoses
- Improves compliance with treatment recommendations
- Reduces delays in care-seeking and use of services
- Enhances client/provider communications
- Enhances compatibility of biomedical and traditional health care

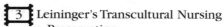 Leininger's Transcultural Nursing
- Preservation
  ○ Maintain cultural resources that promote health or assist in recovery
- Accommodation
  ○ Adjust or adapt client or provider actions
  ○ Facilitate interactions to positively influence health
- Repatterning
  ○ Change attitudes or behaviors of providers or clients

SUGGESTIONS FOR CLASSROOM ACTIVITIES

Divide students into three groups. Assign each group one of Leininger's transcultural nursing modes. Have each group research nursing articles that provide examples in the medical or nursing literature for their mode. Have groups prepare a presentation to the class.

SUGGESTIONS FOR CLINICAL ACTIVITIES

Assign students to work in groups to design, implement, and evaluate culturally competent care for their clinical setting community. One group will design, another group will develop implementation recommendations, and a third group will develop an evaluation tool.

The Environmental Context

RESOURCE LIBRARY

COMPANION WEBSITE

Audio Glossary

Exam Review Questions

Case Study: Advocacy in Environmental Health

MediaLink Application: Lead Poisoning Prevention (video)

Media Links

Challenge Your Knowledge

Update *Healthy People 2010*

Advocacy Interviews

IMAGE LIBRARY

Figure 10-1 Selected Environmental Components That Affect Health

Figure 10-2 Human Health Effects of Environmental Conditions

Table 10-2 Secondary Preventive Measures for Selected Environmental Hazards for Individuals, Families, and Populations

LEARNING OBJECTIVE 1

Analyze the interrelationships among environmental factors and human health.

CONCEPTS FOR LECTURE

1. Concern about the effects of the environment on health began as early as 2,500 years ago with Hippocrates. Nursing's and community health nurses' concern about the interactions of the physical and social environment continued with Florence Nightingale and Lillian Wald.

2. Environmental health, defined by the World Health Organization, is aspects of human health and disease determined by factors in the environment. It includes pathologic effects of chemicals, radiation, and some biological agents, as well as the effects that the physical, psychological, social, and aesthetic environment have on health and well-being.

3. Environmental forces on human health include climate change; microorganisms that cause communicable diseases; animals that contribute to the spread; plants that contribute to accidental poisoning and allergic reactions; industry, vehicles, and buildings that contribute to air, water, and noise pollution; and climate and terrain that contribute to natural disasters.

POWERPOINT LECTURE SLIDES

NOTE: The number on each PPT Lecture Slide directly corresponds with the Concepts for Lecture.

1 Effect of Environment on Health
- Concerns documented 2,500 years ago by Hippocrates
- Historical nursing involvement
  - Physical and social environment
    - Florence Nightingale
    - Lillian Wald

2 Environmental Health
- Definition (per WHO)
  - Human health and disease determined by factors in environment
  - Pathologic environmental effects
    - Chemicals
    - Radiation
    - Physical, psychological, social
    - Aesthetic

3 Environment and Health
- Climate change
- Microorganisms→Communicable diseases
- Animals→Spread diseases
- Plants→Accidental poisoning/allergic reactions

- Industry/vehicles/buildings→Air/water/noise pollution
- Climate/terrain→Natural disasters

SUGGESTIONS FOR CLASSROOM ACTIVITIES

Facilitate discussion on the effects and interrelationships between environmental factors and human health. Why should there be concern for the environment? What are examples of short- and long-term effects of the environment on health?

SUGGESTIONS FOR CLINICAL ACTIVITIES

Assign students to various environmental programs, settings, and clinical sites with health department and businesses. Have them determine objectives, mission, function, or purpose of programs and select one environmental factor that has the potential to affect health and report on it during post conference.

LEARNING OBJECTIVE 2

Discuss elements of the natural, built, and social environments that affect population health.

CONCEPTS FOR LECTURE

1. The natural environment consists of features that exist in a natural state, unmodified by humans. Examples include: weather, climate, terrain, natural flora and fauna, biological agents, and natural resources. All three elements interact with one another and are interdependent and interrelated. Elements of the natural environment interact with human development, human behavioral factors, and elements of the social environment to contribute to health problems. Elements of the built environment that pertain to food production affect the natural environment.

2. The built environment includes buildings, spaces, and products that are created or modified by people. Direct effects result from exposure to hazardous conditions arising from the built environment such as lead poisoning. Indirect effects occur as a result of the effects of the built environment on the natural environment or on human health-related behaviors.

3. Key elements of the built environment include urban sprawl with low density development outpacing population growth; land use mix, which is defined as the degree to which the environment has a mix of commercial, residential, and other noncommercial uses; and ecological footprints, which are areas of biologically productive space required per person in order to maintain current lifestyle.

4. Key elements of the social environment include social capital, which involves resources embedded in social networks that help individuals achieve goals that would otherwise be less attainable, and neighborhood quality, which includes socioeconomic status, deterioration, social organization or disorganization, safety, and noise. Social capital incorporates three elements: form, norms, and resources.

POWERPOINT LECTURE SLIDES

NOTE: The number on each PPT Lecture Slide directly corresponds with the Concepts for Lecture.

1 Natural Environment
- Features of the environment that exist in a natural state
- Unmodified by humans; examples:
  - Weather/climate
  - Terrain
  - Natural flora/fauna
  - Biological agents
  - Natural resources

2 Built Environment
- Buildings, spaces, and products created or modified by people
- Direct effects
  - Exposure to hazardous conditions
    - Lead poisoning

2a Built Environment (continued)
- Indirect effects
  - Effects of built environment on:
    - Natural environment
    - Human-related behaviors

3 Key Elements of Built Environment
- Urban sprawl
  - Low density development that outpaces population growth
- Land use mix
  - Environmental mix of commercial, residential, and other noncommercial uses
- Ecological footprints
  - Area of biologically productive space required per person

4 Key Elements of Social Environment
- Social capital
  - Resources embedded in social networks

    ○ Help individuals achieve otherwise unattainable goals
    ○ Form
    ○ Norms
    ○ Resources
- Neighborhood quality

SUGGESTIONS FOR CLASSROOM ACTIVITIES

Assign a neighborhood region to groups of students to research the natural, built, and social environment for that region.

SUGGESTIONS FOR CLINICAL ACTIVITIES

Have students prepare a written care plan for a neighborhood to identify potential areas for community health nursing interventions using the assessment done for classroom assignment.

LEARNING OBJECTIVE 3

Analyze the role of the community health nurse with respect to environmental health issues at the individual/family and population levels.

CONCEPTS FOR LECTURE

1. The community health nurse's role is assumed under one of the core public health functions to protect the environment. Five general nursing competencies related to environmental health include: knowledge of mechanisms for environmental exposure, prevention and control strategies and need for evidence-based approaches to dealing with environmental issues, the ability to make appropriate referrals for health care services, advocacy to support environmental justice and knowledge, and use of legislative and regulatory processes to address environmental conditions that jeopardize health.
2. Community health nursing activities at the individual/family level include preventing or minimizing public exposure to hazardous substances.
3. The National Institute of Nursing Research developed the following initiatives that emphasized nursing's role in environmental health research to include reducing environmental hazards for vulnerable populations, targeting specific settings for environmental research, and identifying infrastructure needs to support environmental health research.
4. Assessing environmental health in population groups involves assessing factors that contribute to environmental health problems and their effects on human health, assessing population factors that increase the risk or severity of health effects of environmental conditions, assessing individual and population groups for evidence of environmentally caused disease, assessing potential for exposure to hazardous environmental conditions created by local occupations and industries, and assessing health system factors that contribute to or exacerbate environmental health problems.

POWERPOINT LECTURE SLIDES

NOTE: The number on each PPT Lecture Slide directly corresponds with the Concepts for Lecture.

1 Core Public Health Functions
- Protecting the environment
- Nursing competencies for environmental health
    ○ Knowledge of mechanisms for environmental exposures
    ○ Prevention and control strategies
    ○ Referrals for health care services
    ○ Advocacy to support environmental justice
    ○ Use legislative process to address environmental concerns

2 Role of Community Health Nurse
- Individual and family level
    ○ Prevent or minimize exposure to hazardous substances

3 National Institute of Nursing Research Initiatives
- Nursing roles
    ○ Reduce environmental hazards for vulnerable populations
    ○ Target specific settings for environmental research
    ○ Identify infrastructure needs for environmental health research

4 Assess Environmental Health
- Factors that contribute to environmental problems
- Population factors that increase risk or severity of environmental health effects

- Evidence of environmentally-caused disease
- Potential for exposure to hazards
- Health system factors

SUGGESTIONS FOR CLASSROOM ACTIVITIES

1. Discuss students' feelings about nursing competencies for environmental health. What educational content would the nurse require? How can the nurse facilitate the community in protecting the environment with competing interests of individuals, families, and businesses or industries?

SUGGESTIONS FOR CLINICAL ACTIVITIES

1. Assign students into neighborhood groups. Have students prepare and present a written environmental health assessment of a community.
2. Using the National Institute of Nursing Research initiatives, assign students to groups to research one of the nursing roles, interview local community health resources, and present a written report on a community environmental health interest.

LEARNING OBJECTIVE 4

Identify factors in the natural, built, and social environments that influence the health of an individual/family or a selected population group.

CONCEPTS FOR LECTURE

1. The natural environment offers numerous opportunities to affect human health through climate effects such as hypothermia, poor weather, and accidents; global climate changes; greenhouse gases; increased ozone levels; rises in global temperatures; poor water quality; water contamination; and hazardous air quality.
2. Factors in the built environment that affect the health of individuals, families, and population groups include ingestion or inhalation of toxic chemicals used in buildings, air pollution created by businesses, and urban sprawl, which impacts resource use.
3. Factors in the social environment that influence human health include norms, attitudes, resources, and relationships.

POWERPOINT LECTURE SLIDES

NOTE: The number on each PPT Lecture Slide directly corresponds with the Concepts for Lecture.

1. Effects of Natural Environment
   - Climate
   - Water quality and contamination
   - Hazardous air quality
2. Factors in Built Environment
   - Ingestion or inhalation of toxic chemicals
   - Air pollution
   - Urban sprawl
3. Factors in Social Environment
   - Norms
   - Attitudes
   - Resources
   - Relationships

SUGGESTIONS FOR CLASSROOM ACTIVITIES

Divide students into three environmental groups. Have the students investigate and compare factors in each group that affect individuals/families and population groups for selected regions of the community. Have students prepare a poster presentation of results of their investigation for class.

SUGGESTIONS FOR CLINICAL ACTIVITIES

1. Invite a guest speaker to post conference from the county or regional health department to discuss local environmental concerns, assessment strategies, interventions, and community involvement.
2. Have students attend meetings of local environmental groups. What are the issues discussed? What are their implications for health?

LEARNING OBJECTIVE 5

Analyze the role of community health nurses in primary prevention measures for environmental issues that affect population health.

CONCEPTS FOR LECTURE

1. Primary prevention for the natural environment includes protection and preservation of natural resources through advocating for energy conservation and development of new energy sources. Examples include: initiating recycling campaigns and educating the public on safe vector control measures.
2. Primary prevention within the built environment includes developing well-designed communities that minimize urban sprawl, limit resource use, promote mixed land use, develop social capital, and foster healthy behaviors.
3. Primary prevention within the social environment includes nurses advocating for prevention legislation, funding for programs and public education to foster identification of risk groups, and interventions to reduce exposure risks.

POWERPOINT LECTURE SLIDES

NOTE: The number on each PPT Lecture Slide directly corresponds with the Concepts for Lecture.

1 Primary Prevention and Natural Environment
- Advocate for energy conservation
- Advocate for development of new energy sources
  ○ Initiate recycling campaigns
  ○ Educate public on safe vector control measures

2 Primary Prevention and Built Environments
- Develop well-designed communities
  ○ Minimize urban sprawl
  ○ Limit resource use
  ○ Promote mixed land use
  ○ Develop social capital
  ○ Foster health behaviors

2a Primary Prenvention and Built Environments (continued)
- Nurse's role
  ○ Educate on inexpensive water treatment measures

3 Primary Prevention and Social Environments
- Advocate role of community health nurses
  ○ Prevention legislation
  ○ Funding for programs
  ○ Public education
  ○ Identification of risk groups
  ○ Intervention to reduce exposure risks

SUGGESTIONS FOR CLASSROOM ACTIVITIES

Divide students into three environmental groups: natural, built, and social. Have students investigate community resources and prepare a community care plan that includes primary prevention measures for their specific environment. Have them discuss the community health nurse's role and present to class.

SUGGESTIONS FOR CLINICAL ACTIVITIES

Invite a local community health medical officer or epidemiologist to discuss primary environmental prevention measures for the local area.

LEARNING OBJECTIVE 6

Identify secondary and tertiary prevention measures for individuals or populations affected by environmental health problems and the role of the community health nurse in their implementation.

CONCEPTS FOR LECTURE

1. Secondary prevention with individuals and families includes identifying and resolving existing health problems caused by environmental conditions. Examples include: screening clients for potential contamination, referring for testing when contamination is suspected, referring for assistance with eliminating environmental hazards, referring for assistance in removing contaminants from homes, and monitoring responses to therapy and potential for continued exposure.

2. The community health nurse's role at the secondary prevention level for population groups is to promote targeted screening programs to identify prevalence of risk factors and encourage policy makers to adopt targeted screening practices.

3. At the tertiary individual or family prevention level, community health nurses work with individuals or families to prevent recurrence or complications of environmentally caused health problems by assisting families with housing and providing parents with referrals for assistance in coping.

4. Tertiary prevention at the population level includes political activity to mandate standards that prevent the recurrence of environmental contamination, to pass bond issues to renovate water treatment plants and prevent recontamination, or to advocate for passage of funds to remove contaminants from older homes.

POWERPOINT LECTURE SLIDES

NOTE: The number on each PPT Lecture Slide directly corresponds with the Concepts for Lecture.

1 Secondary Prevention With Individuals/Families
- Identify and resolve existing health problems from environmental conditions
  - Screen clients for potential contamination
  - Referrals for testing when contamination is suspected
  - Referrals for assistance with eliminating environmental hazards
  - Referrals for assistance in removing contaminants from home
  - Monitor responses to therapy and potential for continued exposure

2 Secondary Prevention at Population Level (Refer to Table 10-2)
- Community health nurse's role
  - Promote screening programs to identify risk factor prevalence
  - Encourage policy makers to adopt targeted screening practices

3 Tertiary Prevention With Individual/Families
- Prevent recurrence or complications of environmentally-caused health problems
  - Assist families with housing
  - Provide parents with referrals for assistance in coping

4 Tertiary Prevention at Population Level
- Political activity to prevent recurrence of environmental contamination
- Pass bond issues to renovate water treatment plants
- Prevent recontamination
- Advocate for passage of funds to remove contaminants from older homes

SUGGESTIONS FOR CLASSROOM ACTIVITIES

Divide students into four groups. Have each group select one environmental health concern or problem for the local area and develop secondary and tertiary prevention measures and recommendations. Present results at the next class.

SUGGESTIONS FOR CLINICAL ACTIVITIES

Arrange for students to research state legislative members' involvement in environmental issues to include any public presentations and voting on legislative issues or funding that affects the natural, built, or social environment. Have students prepare a short report on their legislative representative and develop a written community health nurse response to one environmental health concern.

Health Promotion

RESOURCE LIBRARY

COMPANION WEBSITE

Audio Glossary
Exam Review Questions
Case Study: Health Promotion through Education
MediaLink Application: Celebrity Health Promotion
(video)

Media Links
Challenge Your Knowledge
Update *Healthy People 2010*
Advocacy Interviews

IMAGE LIBRARY

Table 11-2 Phases of the Social Marketing Process

Table 11-6 Elements of a Community Health Education Program for Disaster Preparedness

LEARNING OBJECTIVE 1

Define health promotion.

CONCEPTS FOR LECTURE

1. Health promotion fostering the ability of populations to make informed health decisions is an aspect of the "new" public health era. Prior eras included health protection through religious, political, and cultural sanctions, and miasma control through sanitation, and contagion control was based on germ theory, preventive medicine, and primary health care.
2. Health promotion is defined as a process of enabling people to increase control over, and to improve, their health. It involves public policy formation, development of environments that support health, and promotion of community action.
3. Key elements of health promotion include: regulation of health via legislation, sanitation, immunizations, focus on risk modification, recognition of effects of social conditions on health, and preparation for informed decision making.

POWERPOINT LECTURE SLIDES

NOTE: The number on each PPT Lecture Slide directly corresponds with the Concepts for Lecture.

1 Evolution of Health Promotion
- Religious, political, and cultural sanctions
- Miasma control
- Contagion control
- Preventive medicine
- Primary health care movement

2 Health Promotion
- Enables people to increase control over, and improve, their health
- Policy formation
- Development of environments that support health
- Promotion of community action

3 Key Elements of Health Promotion
- Regulation of health via legislation
- Sanitation
- Immunization
- Focus on risk modification
- Recognition of effects of social conditions on health
- Preparation for informed decision making

SUGGESTIONS FOR CLASSROOM ACTIVITIES	SUGGESTIONS FOR CLINICAL ACTIVITIES
Have students develop their own definition of health promotion. Ask them to provide examples of health promotion from their clinical settings.	Have students work with a mentor at their clinical setting to select a health promotion topic or action for a target population. At post conference, have students discuss their topic and their proposed strategy for action.

LEARNING OBJECTIVE 2

Distinguish health promotion from health education.

CONCEPTS FOR LECTURE

1. Health education is one of the three health promotion strategies. Health education provides clients with the information and skills on which to base informed decisions regarding health-related behaviors. Health education uses education and motivation to affect behavioral changes by directly influencing values, beliefs, and attitudes.

2. Health promotion is a broad process that targets individuals, communities, and specific populations. Health education is one means by which health promotion is accomplished.

POWERPOINT LECTURE SLIDES

NOTE: The number on each PPT Lecture Slide directly corresponds with the Concepts for Lecture.

1 Health Education
- A health promotion strategy
- Provides clients with information and skills
  - Informed decisions regarding health-related behaviors

1a Health Education (continued)
- Uses education and motivation to change behaviors by influencing:
  - Values
  - Beliefs
  - Attitudes

2 Relationship Between Health Education and Health Promotion
- Health education is one means to accomplish health promotion

SUGGESTIONS FOR CLASSROOM ACTIVITIES	SUGGESTIONS FOR CLINICAL ACTIVITIES
Have students make a list of health education topics to reduce asthma or any other chronic health condition and targeted individuals or populations. Next, have students take their list of health education topics and discuss what specific health promotion process would be accomplished using their health education topics.	Arrange for students to identify opportunities for health education in their clinical settings. Have them write down when they observed or participated in health education, what the topic was, and the intended audience. During post conference, ask students to share experiences and then differentiate between educating about health and health promotion.

LEARNING OBJECTIVE 3

Describe selected models for health promotion practice.

CONCEPTS FOR LECTURE

1. Several models have been developed to explain why people do or do not engage in health-promoting activities. When community health nurses understand the motivations and factors involved in decision making, they can select appropriate strategies for promoting health in a population. The following models have been used extensively in the literature: the

POWERPOINT LECTURE SLIDES

NOTE: The number on each PPT Lecture Slide directly corresponds with the Concepts for Lecture.

1 Models for Health Promotion
- Precaution Adoption Process model
- The Theory of Reasoned Action/Planned Behavior

Precaution Adoption Process model, the Theory of Reasoned Action/Theory of Planned Behavior, the Health Belief model, Pender's Health Promotion model, and the PRECEDE-PROCEED model.

2. The Precaution Adoption Process model is a stage model that describes the stages that occur in the decision to adopt or not adopt a health-related behavior. The following stages describe the steps involved for this model: Stage 1, the person is unaware of the health-related issue; Stage 2, the person is aware, but is unengaged; Stage 3: the person is deciding whether to act or not act; Stage 4, the person has decided not to act; Stage 5, the person has decided to act, but has not taken any action; Stage 6, the person acts to engage in the behavior; and finally, Stage 7, the behavior becomes a routine part of their lifestyle.

3. The Theory of Reasoned Action and its related Theory of Planned Behavior, developed by Ajzen and Fishbein, contains two premises: attitudes to a health-related behavior reflect a person's attitudes to the expected consequences of the behavior, and attitudes are the product of subjective norms influenced by others. The intention to act is premised on one's own attitudes to a behavior, one's perceptions of the attitudes of others, and the value placed on others' judgments.

4. The Health Belief model, developed by Becker, Rosenstock, and others, has been the most widely used model for research and program development in health promotion. Elements of the model include individual perceptions of susceptibility and seriousness, modifying factors (demographic, sociopsychologic, and structural variables), perceptions of benefits and barriers to action, and cues to action.

5. The Health Promotion model was developed as a nursing model by Nola Pender. This model directs nursing intervention for health promotion. The conceptual components of the model state that behavior is influenced by individual characteristics and behavior-specific cognitions and affect (emotions) that result in a commitment to action. Commitment to action results in actual behavior but may be modified by competing demands and preferences.

6. The PRECEDE-PROCEED model has been extensively used in health education practice and consists of two components. The PRECEDE component reflects diagnostic activities that take place prior to planning health promotion activities and includes the following: predisposing, reinforcing, and enabling constructs in the education diagnosis and evaluation. The PROCEED component focuses on the development of health promotion interventions that will enhance the potential for healthy behavior and includes the following components: policy, regulatory, organizational constructs, and educational and environmental development.

- The Health Belief model
- Pender's Health Promotion model
- The PRECEDE-PROCEED model

2 Precaution Adoption Process Model
- Stages of health-related behavior decisions
  - Stage 1: Unaware of health-related issue
  - Stage 2: Aware but unengaged
  - Stage 3: Decision to act or not act
  - Stage 4: Decision to not act

2a Precaution Adoption Process Model (continued)
- Stage 5: Decision to act, but no action taken
- Stage 6: Act to engage
- Stage 7: Behavior becomes part of lifestyle routine

3 Theory of Reasoned Action/Planned Behavior
- Attitudes reflect attitudes to expected consequences
- Attitudes are a product of subjective norms influenced by others
  - Intention to act
  - Attitudes of person
  - Perceptions of others' attitudes
  - Value placed on others' judgments

4 Health Belief Model
- Individual perceptions of susceptibility and seriousness
- Modifying factors/variables
  - Demographic
  - Sociopsychological
  - Structural
- Perceptions of benefits and barriers to action
- Cues to action

5 Pender's Health Promotion Model
- Behavior is influenced by individual characteristics
- Behavior-specific cognitions and emotions result in a commitment to action
- Commitment to action results in actual behavior
- Behavior may be modified by competing demands and preferences

6 PRECEDE-PROCEED Model
- PRECEDE
  - Predisposing
  - Reinforcing
  - Enabling
  - Education
  - Diagnosis
  - Evaluation

6a PROCEED
- Policy
- Regulatory
- Organizational
- Educational and Environmental Development

SUGGESTIONS FOR CLASSROOM ACTIVITIES

Divide students into groups and assign a health promotion model to each group. Each group will choose one of the health problems for an elderly population mentioned in the case study at the end of the chapter. Using the elderly as their target population, and with their selected health problem, have them develop a schematic design of their model and present to the class.

SUGGESTIONS FOR CLINICAL ACTIVITIES

Have students review a health education program offered by their clinical site, present a summary of program, and discuss an appropriate health promotion model for the population.

LEARNING OBJECTIVE 4

Identify three strategies for health promotion.

CONCEPTS FOR LECTURE

1. The three strategies for health promotion include empowerment, social marketing, and health education. Empowerment focuses on the environmental conditions that affect people's abilities to act in ways that promote health. Social marketing emphasizes enhancing people's motivation to act. Health education is any activity that seeks to inform individuals or groups about health-related issues.

POWERPOINT LECTURE SLIDES

NOTE: The number on each PPT Lecture Slide directly corresponds with the Concepts for Lecture.

1 Strategies for Health Promotion
- Empowerment
  - Environmental conditions affect health promotion actions
- Social Marketing
  - Enhance people's motivation to act
- Health education
  - Activities that seek to inform

SUGGESTIONS FOR CLASSROOM ACTIVITIES

Divide students into three strategy groups: empowerment, social marketing, and health education. Have each group describe how they can use their strategy to design a health promotion focus that targets adolescent smoking at a local high school.

SUGGESTIONS FOR CLINICAL ACTIVITIES

Have students identify health promotion strategies used in their clinical setting. Ask students to design a health promotion strategy specific to their clinical practice setting and present it to the class during post conference.

LEARNING OBJECTIVE 5

Describe the four Ps of social marketing.

CONCEPTS FOR LECTURE

1. Social marketing uses commercial marketing technologies to analyze, plan, execute, and evaluate programs with the main objective of influencing voluntary behavior and improving personal or societal welfare.
2. Characteristics of social marketing include the concept of exchange, the use of research to direct action, the development of a marketing mix, and a positioning strategy.
3. Social marketing has three phases: phase 1, the preproduction or prepromotion stage of a health promotion initiative; phase 2, the research development and market testing strategies; and phase 3, the use of research methods to study the application and effectiveness of the marketing interventions.

POWERPOINT LECTURE SLIDES

NOTE: The number on each PPT Lecture Slide directly corresponds with the Concepts for Lecture.

1 Social Marketing
- Apply commercial marketing technologies
- Designed to influence voluntary behavior of target audiences
- Improve audiences' or society's personal welfare

2 Characteristics of Social Marketing
- Exchange
- Research to action
- Development of marketing mix
- Position strategy

---

4. The four Ps of social marketing include product (the need, service, or desired behavior such as not smoking, or starting an exercise program); price (the cost of or barriers to adopting the desired behavior such as specific physiological responses to nicotine withdrawal, or time and expense of exercising at a fitness center); place (the location where the product or service takes place such as where the smoking cessation programs or fitness centers are located); and promotion (the communication strategies and messages used to motivate such as television ads depicting smoker's breath, discolored hands and teeth, or ads that show the benefits and results of exercising).

3 Phases of Social Marketing (Refer to Table 11-2)
- Preproduction/prepromotion
- Research development and market testing
- Research methods to study applications and effectiveness of marketing

4 Four Ps of Social Marketing
- Product
  ○ Need, service, desired behavior
    - Not smoking
    - Beginning an exercise program

4a Price
- Cost of, or barriers to, adopting behavior
  ○ Physiologic responses to smoking cessation
  ○ Time and expense of joining fitness center

4b Place
- Location where product or service takes place
  ○ Location of smoking cessation programs in community
  ○ Location of fitness centers in community

4c Promotion
- Communication strategies and messages
  ○ Smoking cessation messages that focus on negative consequences
  ○ Exercise promotion messages that address health benefits, weight loss, increased energy

SUGGESTIONS FOR CLASSROOM ACTIVITIES

Have students select a health promotion focus such as lung cancer reduction, cardiovascular disease, diabetes, or obesity in children. Have students develop a social marketing plan using the four Ps that is specific to their topic using poster board and magazine pictures.

SUGGESTIONS FOR CLINICAL ACTIVITIES

Have students examine a health promotion campaign to analyze the four Ps of social marketing as included (or not included) in the campaign. Have students present and discuss at post conference.

LEARNING OBJECTIVE 6

Analyze the significance of empowerment for health promotion.

CONCEPTS FOR LECTURE

1. Empowerment is the process of enabling communities to pursue or obtain knowledge and skills necessary to make informed decisions and permitting communities to make those decisions.
2. Key requisites include motivating community participation through analytic and communication skills, using peer and organizational norms to support health promotion practice, having community agency managers who are empowerment-oriented, and having agencies with internal policies that permit and encourage empowerment of community members.
3. Community empowerment is an active process requiring community health nurses and other health

POWERPOINT LECTURE SLIDES

NOTE: The number on each PPT Lecture Slide directly corresponds with the Concepts for Lecture.

1 Empowerment
- Process of enabling communities to acquire knowledge and skills
- Allow communities to make informed decisions

2 Key Requisites of Empowerment
- Motivate community participation
- Peer and organizational norms that support health promotion practice
- Community agency managers who are empowerment-oriented

CONCEPTS FOR LECTURE continued

practitioners to engage community members in their own health education and health promotion needs. This process may occur along a five-point continuum that begins with empowering individuals for their own personal action, moving to empowering individuals to form small mutual assistance groups, progressing to empowering groups to create community organizations, then empowering community organizations to form partnerships, and finally, empowering communities to take social and political action to improve environmental conditions that affect health.

4. Empowerment fosters health promotion as individuals and communities become active participants in the health promotion process when they act on information and create knowledge and solutions from their own experiences, make informed decisions, and recognize that structural and behavioral changes are necessary to promote health and well-being.

POWERPOINT LECTURE SLIDES continued

- Agency internal policies for empowerment of community members

3 Community Empowerment
- Active process engaging community members in their own health education and health promotion needs
- Empower individuals for their own personal action
- Empower individuals to form small mutual assistance groups
- Empower groups to create community organizations
- Empowering community organizations to form partnerships
- Empower communities to take social and political action to improve environmental conditions that affect health

4 Fostering Health Promotion through Empowerment
- Individuals and communities become active participants in the health promotion process when they:
  ○ Act on information and create knowledge and solutions from their own experiences
  ○ Make informed decisions
  ○ Recognize that structural and behavioral changes are necessary to promote health and well-being

SUGGESTIONS FOR CLASSROOM ACTIVITIES	SUGGESTIONS FOR CLINICAL ACTIVITIES
None	During clinical experiences, have students identify opportunities to empower specific target populations. Assist students to develop strategies that might be effective in empowering the groups. Discuss the strategies at post conference.

LEARNING OBJECTIVE 7

Describe the health education process.

CONCEPTS FOR LECTURE

1. Health education is defined as an activity that seeks to inform the individual on the nature and cause of health/illness and that individual's personal level of risk associated with their lifestyle-related behavior. The health education process occurs within various learning domains including the cognitive, affective, psychomotor, and perceptual, and social interaction skills domains, which address specific types of learning expected to result from a health education encounter.

2. The purpose of health education is to assist clients in making health-related decisions about self-care, the use of health resources, and societal health issues.

POWERPOINT LECTURE SLIDES

NOTE: The number on each PPT Lecture Slide directly corresponds with the Concepts for Lecture.

1 Health Education Process
- Inform the individual on the nature and cause of health/illness
- Inform the individual of risk associated with lifestyle-related behavior
- Learning domains
  ○ Cognitive
  ○ Affective
  ○ Psychomotor
  ○ Perceptual

CONCEPTS FOR LECTURE continued

3. The goals of health education include client participation in health decision making, increased potential to comply with health recommendations, development of self-care skills, improved client and family coping, increased participation in continuing care for specific conditions, and adoption of healthier lifestyle.

4. The health education process includes assessing educational needs, planning and implementing health education programs, prioritizing learning needs, and developing goals and objectives.

POWERPOINT LECTURE SLIDES continued

2 Purpose of Health Education
- Assist clients in making health-related decision about:
  - Self-care
  - Use of health resources
  - Societal health issues

3 Goals of Health Education
- Client participation in health decision making
- Increased potential to comply with health recommendations
- Development of self-care skills
- Improved client and family coping
- Increased participation in continuing care for specific conditions
- Adoption of healthier lifestyle

4 Health Education Process
- Assess health education needs
- Plan and implement health education programs
- Prioritize learning needs
- Develop goals and objectives

SUGGESTIONS FOR CLASSROOM ACTIVITIES

During post conference, invite a guest speaker from a community health agency that offers health education services to discuss development of the health education process.

SUGGESTIONS FOR CLINICAL ACTIVITIES

Have students develop a plan for a health education opportunity at their clinical setting by describing the goals of their health education program, their target audience, audience characteristics, and how their program would meet the expectations of the goals.

LEARNING OBJECTIVE 8

Design and implement a health education program for a selected population.

CONCEPTS FOR LECTURE

1. Before designing a health education program, the community health nurse needs to perform an assessment of the audience, their health education needs, and the learning environment. Identification and selection of a target audience begins with an assessment of their level of need, resources available, or probability of success. A needs assessment is a planned process that identifies the reported needs of an individual or group.

2. After assessment, the nurse identifies characteristics of the audience that influence the learning situation such as considerations of biophysical, psychological, physical environmental, sociocultural, behavioral, and health system factors.

3. The health education process contains a planning process that includes prioritizing learning needs, developing goals and objectives, and selecting teaching/learning strategies.

POWERPOINT LECTURE SLIDES

NOTE: The number on each PPT Lecture Slide directly corresponds with the Concepts for Lecture.

1 Design and Implementation
- Needs assessment
  - A planned process
  - Identify the reported needs of an individual or group
  - Identify and select target audience
  - Assess health education needs
  - Assess learning environment

2 Identify Audience Characteristics
- Biophysical
- Psychological
- Physical environmental
- Sociocultural
- Behavioral
- Health system factors

3 Planning and Implementation
- Elements of planning process
  - Prioritize learning needs
  - Goals and objectives
  - Content selection
  - Teaching/learning strategies

SUGGESTIONS FOR CLASSROOM ACTIVITIES

1. Divide students into groups. Have each group select a target audience and develop an assessment of the target audience with questions that they will need to address about the audience, their health education needs, and the learning environment.
2. With their initial assessment questions, have students research the audience characteristics, prepare a report, and present the results to class.

SUGGESTIONS FOR CLINICAL ACTIVITIES

1. Arrange for students to attend a health education program in the community, local hospital, or local health department. Have students interview the program developer or coordinator about the target audience, needs assessment, and program design. Provide an opportunity for students to discuss and relate their assessment findings as well as the elements of the planning process in post conference.
2. Have students perform an assessment of a target audience from their clinical setting and present at post conference.

LEARNING OBJECTIVE 9

Analyze the implications of language and health literacy for health promotion.

CONCEPTS FOR LECTURE

1. Language considerations are essential in any health education program. Many non-English speakers have a higher need for preventive care and health promotion services. Health literacy is defined as the ability of individuals to obtain, interpret, and understand basic health information and services and to use such information and services in ways that enhance health.
2. The five basic principles that drive health literacy in health education include the following: the content of health-related materials should be based on written objectives for the health education encounter; reader involvement with the materials is critical; materials should be easy to read and understand; health-related materials should look easy to read; and visual features of health-related materials should clarify content and motivate reader action.

POWERPOINT LECTURE SLIDES

NOTE: The number on each PPT Lecture Slide directly corresponds with the Concepts for Lecture.

 1 Language and Health Literacy
- Considerations
  - Many non-English speakers need health preventive services
- Health literacy
  - Ability to obtain, interpret, and understand basic health information and services
  - Ability to use such information and services to enhance health

2 Basic Principles
- Content based on written objectives
- Reader involvement is critical
- Easy to read and understand
- Materials look easy to read
- Visual features clarify and motivate reader

SUGGESTIONS FOR CLASSROOM ACTIVITIES

1. After selecting a health topic based on an identified need in their clinical setting or community, have students develop a brief health brochure incorporating the five basic principles of health literacy.
2. Have students present a draft version of their health brochure for classmates to critique with comments for improvement.

SUGGESTIONS FOR CLINICAL ACTIVITIES

Have students bring to post conference samples of health education/health promotion brochures, handouts, or other materials from their clinical settings. Have students critique and discuss the qualities of the brochures or handouts.

LEARNING OBJECTIVE 10

Identify criteria for evaluating health information on the Internet.

CONCEPTS FOR LECTURE

1. The two major issues with Internet health information are accuracy and information bias.
2. Evaluative elements for Internet sites include the owner of the site and their reputability, sources of financial support for the site, purpose of the site, the sources of information provided, evidence provided to support the information given, the existence of an editorial group, and the currency of the information provided.

POWERPOINT LECTURE SLIDES

NOTE: The number on each PPT Lecture Slide directly corresponds with the Concepts for Lecture.

1 Evaluating Internet Information
- Major issues
  - Internet accuracy
  - Information bias

2 Evaluative Elements
- Owner of site and reputability
- Sources of financial support
- Purpose of site
- Sources of information provided

2a Evaluative Elements (continued)
- Evidence provided
- Editorial oversight
- Currency of information

SUGGESTIONS FOR CLASSROOM ACTIVITIES

Have students select a health-related concern or topic. Locate at least 4 or 5 Internet information sources. Have students describe and evaluate the Internet sources based on the evaluative elements. Discuss the results at the next class.

SUGGESTIONS FOR CLINICAL ACTIVITIES

Have students ask clients in the clinical setting if they have obtained any health-related information on the Internet. Determine what sites were used and the credibility of the information obtained.

LEARNING OBJECTIVE 11

Discuss criteria for evaluating health promotion programs.

CONCEPTS FOR LECTURE

1. Evaluation is an essential process in all health care professional and scientific endeavors. Evaluation of health education programs may occur at three different levels. The diagnostic level assesses the accuracy of the needs assessment upon which the health promotion program was based. Formative or process evaluation examines the manner in which the program was carried out. Summative evaluation focuses on program outcome and/or impact.
2. Programs may be evaluated using additional elements or criteria based on the extent to which they achieve empowerment, participation, holism (focusing on multiple aspects of health), intersectoral collaboration, equity, use of multiple strategies, and sustainability.

POWERPOINT LECTURE SLIDES

NOTE: The number on each PPT Lecture Slide directly corresponds with the Concepts for Lecture.

1 Evaluation of Health Promotion Programs (Refer to Table 11-6)
- Diagnostic evaluation
  - Accuracy of needs assessment
- Formative evaluation
  - How the program is carried out
- Summative evaluation
  - Program outcome and/or impact

2 Additional Elements for Evaluation
- Evaluations based on achieving criteria related to
  - Empowerment

POWERPOINT LECTURE SLIDES *continued*
- Participation
- Intersectoral collaboration
- Use of multiple strategies
- Sustainability

SUGGESTIONS FOR CLASSROOM ACTIVITIES	**SUGGESTIONS FOR CLINICAL ACTIVITIES**
Ask students to select and apply one evaluation process to a health education/health promotion program in their community or clinical setting. Prepare a report and discuss it in class.	1. Have students bring to post conference examples of program evaluation tools used at their clinical or community setting. Ask students to present and discuss the tool during post conference. 2. Have students conduct process and outcome evaluation of health education provided in the clinical setting.

Case Management

RESOURCE LIBRARY

COMPANION WEBSITE

Audio Glossary
Exam Review Questions
Case Study: Health Promotion through Case
  Management
MediaLink Application: Penalizing Obesity and
  Smoking (video)

Media Links
Challenge Your Knowledge
Advocacy Interviews

IMAGE LIBRARY

Figure 12-1 Sample Resource File Entry

LEARNING OBJECTIVE 1

Identify client-centered and system-centered goals of case management.

CONCEPTS FOR LECTURE

1. Case management is defined as a patient care delivery system that focuses on meeting outcomes within identified time frames using appropriate resources.
2. Early case management efforts focused on eliminating unnecessary cases, ensuring proper case selection, discharging when services were no longer needed, and making early referrals.
3. Case management has evolved along two tracks: individual or family case management and population case management. Individual or family case management is described as a one-to-one relationship development endeavor with specific clients or their families. Population case management is described as the development of systems of care, across multiple agencies, for specific groups of people with similar needs.
4. Case management programs are designed around their goals. Client-centered goals include promotion of optimal health and independence and client satisfaction, enhanced quality of life, prevention of deterioration in health status, decreased need for acute care services, and empowerment and advocacy. System-centered goals focus on equitable resource allocation, decreased utilization, cost containment, decreased fragmentation of care, and cost efficiency with the best possible care provided in the most efficient manner.

POWERPOINT LECTURE SLIDES

NOTE: The number on each PPT Lecture Slide directly corresponds with the Concepts for Lecture.

1 Case Management
  • A patient care delivery system
  • Focused on time-specific outcomes using appropriate resources

2 Early Case Management Efforts Focused on:
  • Eliminating unnecessary cases
  • Proper case selection
  • Discharging when services were no longer needed
  • Early referrals

3 Two Levels of Case Management Since Early Efforts
  • Individual/family case management
    ○ One-to-one relationship development endeavor
  • Population care management
    ○ Development of systems of care
    ○ Across multiple agencies
    ○ For specific groups of people with similar needs

4 Case Management Goals: Client-centered Goals
  • Promotes optimal health/independence and client satisfaction with care
  • Enhanced quality of life

POWERPOINT LECTURE SLIDES *continued*

- Prevention of deterioration in health status
- Decreased need for acute care services
- Empowerment and advocacy
- Promotion of optimal health through resource acquisition

 4a System-Centered Goals
- Equitable resource allocation
- Decreased utilization
- Cost containment
- Decreased fragmentation of case
- Cost-efficiency

SUGGESTIONS FOR CLASSROOM ACTIVITIES

Divide students into two groups and have them use the case study at the end of the chapter to develop client-centered and system-centered case management goals for the elementary school children.

SUGGESTIONS FOR CLINICAL ACTIVITIES

Assign students to develop two client-centered and two system-centered case management goals for one population group serviced by their clinical site or agency. Provide the opportunity to share goals and discuss with class during post conference.

LEARNING OBJECTIVE 2

Discuss standards and principles of case management practice.

CONCEPTS FOR LECTURE

1. Standards for case management are similar to those for community health nurses and include identifying and assessing the case, identifying the problem, planning, monitoring implementation of the case management plan, evaluating the effects of intervention, and modifying the plan to achieve appropriate, cost-effective outcomes.

2. General principles of effective case management include, but are not limited to, the following: people are not "case managed," rather the services and resources that they receive are the object of case management; assertive outreach is needed to identify clients; case managers should provide services rather than outsourcing the services; natural community resources are the primary partners for case management; case managers should have primary responsibility for services provided to clients; caseloads should be small; there should be unlimited time for management services, if needed; and case managers should foster choice and self-determination.

POWERPOINT LECTURE SLIDES

NOTE: The number on each PPT Lecture Slide directly corresponds with the Concepts for Lecture.

1 Standards of Case Management Practice
- Case identification and assessment
- Problem identification
- Planning
- Monitor implementation of case management plan
- Evaluate the effects of intervention
- Modify the plan to achieve appropriate, cost-effective outcomes

2 Principles of Case Management
- People are not "case managed"
- Assertive outreach to identify clients
- Provide services directly
- Natural community resources

2a Provide primary responsibility for services
- Small caseload size
- Unlimited time
- Foster choice and self-determination

SUGGESTIONS FOR CLASSROOM ACTIVITIES

Again, referring to the case study at the end of the chapter, have students write five population-specific examples that represent each of the general principles of effective case management. Statements will provide specific behaviors of how the case manager addresses the principle for the elementary school children.

SUGGESTIONS FOR CLINICAL ACTIVITIES

Invite a case manager from a community agency to present case studies that exemplify the principles and standards of case managers.

LEARNING OBJECTIVE 3

Analyze legal and ethical issues related to case management.

CONCEPTS FOR LECTURE

1. Ethical concerns expressed by case managers include the following: equity-related concerns, beneficence-related concerns, nonmaleficence-related concerns, and concerns related to autonomy, consent, and living at risk.

2. Equity-related concerns focus on the fair allocation of resources based on demographic elements such as age, gender, and socioeconomic status.

3. Beneficence-related concerns address the issues related to providing care over an appropriate time frame or rationing care to extend services over a longer period of time.

4. Non-maleficence is related to providing clients with choices and the need to prevent harm to clients or others providing care to clients.

5. Autonomy, consent, and living at risk pertains to clients' rights to engage in risk-related behaviors and the right to refuse services.

6. Additional concerns include legal and ethical issues related to confidentiality, denial of services, breach of contract, negligence, failure to follow clinical pathways or to individualize care, and dealing with reportable events.

7. Abandonment occurs when the case manager terminates services to a client with continuing needs without notifying the client or arranging for services from another provider.

8. Negligence is the failure to act in a situation as a reasonably prudent nurse would if faced with the same situation. Four conditions must exist for negligence to occur: there must be a duty to provide care; there must be a breach of duty; an injury must result from the breach of duty; and the injury must result in some form of quantifiable damage to the client.

POWERPOINT LECTURE SLIDES

NOTE: The number on each PPT Lecture Slide directly corresponds with the Concepts for Lecture.

1 Legal and Ethical Concerns
- Equity-related concerns
- Beneficence-related concerns
- Nonmaleficence-related concerns
- Concerns related to autonomy, consent, and living at risk

2 Equity-related Concerns
- Focus on the fair allocation of resources based on demographic elements
  - Examples: age, gender, and socioeconomic status

3 Beneficence-related Concerns
- Providing care over an appropriate time frame
- Rationing care to extend services over a longer period of time

4 Nonmaleficence
- Providing clients with choices
- The need to prevent harm to clients or others providing care to clients

5 Autonomy, Consent, and Living at Risk
- Pertains to clients' rights to engage in risk-related behaviors
- The right to refuse services

6 Additional Concerns: Legal and Ethical Issues
- Confidentiality
- Denial of services
  - Wrongful denial of services
  - Abandonment

6a Additional Concerns (continued)
- Breach of contract
- Negligent referral
- Failure to follow clinical pathways or to individualize care
- Dealing with reportable events

7 Abandonment
- Service termination without notifying the client or arranging for services

8 Negligence
- Failure to act in reasonably prudent manner
- Four conditions
  - Must be a duty to provide care
  - Must be a breach of duty
  - Injury must result from breach of duty
  - Damage must be quantifiable

LEARNING OBJECTIVE 4

Identify criteria for selecting clients in need of case management.

CONCEPTS FOR LECTURE

1. Case finding is an integral part of the case management process and may occur through one of three mechanisms: provider referral, population-based screening, or screening during health events.
2. Case selection involves identifying individual clients, families, and certain population groups that are in need of and can benefit most from case management services.
3. Criteria for population group case selection begin with indicators such as those with high-cost diagnoses, high-volume resource utilization, and poor coordination of services.
4. Criteria or indicators for individuals or families include the following: personal indicators such as diminished functional status, history of substance abuse or mental illness, poor cognitive abilities, prior noncompliance with treatment plans, age over 65 years, experience of a major life change or significant change in self-image, potential for severe emotional response to illness, or unrealistic expectations of potential outcomes of care.
5. Health-related indicators include the presence of specific medical conditions or diagnoses, multiple diagnoses, history of prolonged recovery or increased potential for complications, recent or frequent hospital readmissions or emergency department use, intentional or unintentional drug overdose, and involvement of multiple health care providers, agencies, or funding sources.
6. Social indicators include living alone or with a person who is disabled, being uninsured, evidence of family violence, homelessness or an unhealthy home environment, lack of support systems or financial resources, single parenthood, or living in an area where services are lacking.

POWERPOINT LECTURE SLIDES

NOTE: The number on each PPT Lecture Slide directly corresponds with the Concepts for Lecture.

1 Case Finding Mechanisms
- Provider referral
- Population-based screening
- Screening during health events

2 Case Selection
- Identify clients in need of, and can benefit most from, case management services

3 Population Group Case Selection
- Criteria begin with indicators
  - High-cost diagnoses
  - High-volume resource utilization
  - Poor coordination of services

4 Individual/Family Case Selection: Personal Indicators
- Diminished functional status
- History of substance abuse or mental illness
- Poor cognitive abilities
- Prior noncompliance with treatment plans
- Age over 65 years
- Experience of a major life change or significant change in self-image

5 Health-related Indicators
- Presence of specific medical conditions or diagnoses
- Multiple diagnoses
- History of prolonged recovery or increased potential for complications
- Recent or frequent hospital readmissions or emergency department use
- Intentional or unintentional drug overdose
- Involvement of multiple health care providers, agencies, or funding sources

6 Social Indicators
- Living alone or living with a person who is disabled
- Being uninsured
- Evidence of family violence

POWERPOINT LECTURE SLIDES *continued*

- Homelessness
- Lack of support systems, financial resources or single parenthood
- Living in an area where services are lacking

SUGGESTIONS FOR CLASSROOM ACTIVITIES

Divide students into three groups. Each group will develop criteria for selecting clients using the provider referral mechanism, the population-based screening, or the screen during health events mechanism. Referring to the case study at the end of the chapter, have students develop a hypothetical scenario and chart for selecting children in need of case management. Present results to the class for discussion and comments.

SUGGESTIONS FOR CLINICAL ACTIVITIES

Have students identify specific clients seen in the clinical setting for whom formal case management services are indicated.

LEARNING OBJECTIVE 5

Assess the need for case management and factors influencing the case management situation.

CONCEPTS FOR LECTURE

1. Assessment of the need for case management should include the client's health status, biophysical considerations such as age and functional ability in the individual, or increased incidence of chronic health conditions and comorbidity in specific populations.
2. Psychological factors include mental health status, coping abilities, and anxiety.
3. Physical environmental considerations include living conditions, neighborhood social capital, and environmental pollution.
4. Sociocultural factors address the client's educational level, economic status, occupation, transportation, and cultural beliefs or behaviors.
5. Behavioral factors include substance abuse, lack of physical activity, or poor diet.
6. Health system factors focus on assessing the types of services that the client may need, as well as the influences related to type and level of insurance coverage.

POWERPOINT LECTURE SLIDES

NOTE: The number on each PPT Lecture Slide directly corresponds with the Concepts for Lecture.

1. Factors Influencing Case Management
   - Client's health status
   - Biophysical considerations
     - Age
     - Functional ability
     - Physiologic health status
     - Populations with comorbid conditions

2. Psychological Considerations
   - Mental health status
   - Coping abilities
   - Anxiety

3. Physical Environmental Considerations
   - Living conditions
   - Neighborhood social capital
   - Environmental pollution

4. Sociocultural Factors
   - Client's education level
   - Support systems
   - Economic status
   - Occupation
   - Transportation
   - Cultural beliefs/behaviors

5. Behavioral Considerations
   - Substance abuse
   - Lack of physical activity
   - Poor diet

6. Health System Factors
   - Types of services client may need
   - Influences related to type and level of insurance coverage

LEARNING OBJECTIVE 6

Discuss aspects of developing a case management plan.

CONCEPTS FOR LECTURE

1. A case management plan is a timeline of patient care activities that includes expected outcomes of care and that also incorporates the plan of care of each discipline involved in the care of a particular patient or population group.
2. A case management plan is interdisciplinary, outcomes-based, clinically specific, and flexible, and incorporates a mechanism for provider documentation of their implementation.

POWERPOINT LECTURE SLIDES

NOTE: The number on each PPT Lecture Slide directly corresponds with the Concepts for Lecture.

1. Case Management Plan
   - A timeline of patient care activities and expected outcomes
   - Addresses the plan of care of each discipline involved in care

2. Elements of a Case Management Plan
   - Interdisciplinary
   - Outcomes-based
   - Clinically-specific
   - Flexible
   - Includes avenues for provider documentation of implementation

LEARNING OBJECTIVE 7

Identify advantages and disadvantages of clinical pathways.

CONCEPTS FOR LECTURE

1. A clinical pathway is defined as a tool for achieving coordinated care and desired health outcomes within an anticipated time frame, by using the appropriate resources available. It is a blueprint that guides the clinician in the provision of care.
2. Advantages of clinical pathways include the fact that they are often used as standards of care in malpractice or negligence suits. Legal challenges may be averted through careful documentation and periodic updates of the clinical pathway plan.
3. Disadvantages include the fact that deviations from clinical pathways may result in findings of negligence. Legal challenges can be avoided, though, through

POWERPOINT LECTURE SLIDES

NOTE: The number on each PPT Lecture Slide directly corresponds with the Concepts for Lecture.

1. Clinical Pathways
   - A tool for achieving coordinated care and desired health outcomes
     - Within an anticipated timeframe
     - Uses appropriate available resources
   - A blueprint that guides the clinician in the provision of care

2. Advantages of Clinical Pathways
   - Frequently used as standards for patient care

CONCEPTS FOR LECTURE *continued*

careful documentation of the implementation of clinical pathways. Case managers can be held legally liable for negligent referrals, though this can be avoided with follow-up on the outcomes of referrals that were made.

POWERPOINT LECTURE SLIDES *continued*

- Careful documentation can avoid legal challenges
- Periodic updates of plan may avoid legal action

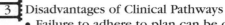 Disadvantages of Clinical Pathways
- Failure to adhere to plan can be considered negligence
- Case managers can be held legally liable for negligent referrals
- Deviations (variances) from plan may result in legal challenges

SUGGESTIONS FOR CLASSROOM ACTIVITIES

1. Divide students into groups and assign them to develop a clinical pathway for children with asthma, children with diabetes, and children with fetal alcohol spectrum disorder, all attending the same elementary school. Have them describe the advantages and disadvantages of their clinical pathway and present to the class.
2. Have students search for examples of existing clinical pathways for care of specific conditions. How are the pathways similar? How do they differ? What is the extent of the evidence base for specific pathways?

SUGGESTIONS FOR CLINICAL ACTIVITIES

Have students prepare a clinical pathway for a target population serviced at their clinical site. Have them list the resources that they used to develop their pathway and present to the class during post conference. What motivation and barriers would influence implementation of the pathway in the clinical setting?

LEARNING OBJECTIVE 8

Describe at least three considerations in delegation.

CONCEPTS FOR LECTURE

1. Delegation is defined as transferring to a competent individual the authority to perform selected tasks in a selected situation. Considerations that guide the delegation process include the stability of the client, the competence of the person to whom the task is being delegated, the level of decision making and problem solving required, and the need to supervise delegated tasks.

POWERPOINT LECTURE SLIDES

NOTE: The number on each PPT Lecture Slide directly corresponds with the Concepts for Lecture.

1 Delegation
- Transferring authority to a competent individual
- Considerations
  ○ Stability of the client
  ○ Competence of the person to whom the task is being delegated
  ○ The level of decision making and problem solving required
  ○ The need to supervise delegated tasks

SUGGESTIONS FOR CLASSROOM ACTIVITIES

Assuming that there is only one school nurse servicing a number of schools in the case study town, have students list the types of tasks that can be delegated, to whom the tasks would be delegated, and potential concerns for delegation.

SUGGESTIONS FOR CLINICAL ACTIVITIES

1. Invite a community health nurse and case manager to discuss the types of delegations that occur in their clinical setting, the legal grounds for delegation, and the control measures in place for monitoring the delegated tasks.
2. Have students identify instances of delegation in the clinical setting. Are tasks appropriately delegated? Why or why not?

LEARNING OBJECTIVE 9

Describe the benchmarking process and its use in case management.

CONCEPTS FOR LECTURE

1. Benchmarking is a process of comparing processes and outcomes among competing organizations to identify performance levels that a particular agency wants to exceed.

2. The benchmarking process follows nine basic steps: identify the area of practice involved; identify a patient-focused outcome; identify factors and processes that affect the outcome; identify benchmarks for the best practice for each factor; construct a scoring continuum for practice; score current practice with comments on why scores were assigned; compare results with the identified best practice; share results with others involved; and develop a plan of action for improving practice.

3. Examples of the benchmarking process include systems outcomes, such as client care outcomes, client satisfaction, length of stay, and costs of care.

POWERPOINT LECTURE SLIDES

NOTE: The number on each PPT Lecture Slide directly corresponds with the Concepts for Lecture.

1 Benchmarking
- A process of comparing processes and outcomes among competing organizations
- Identify performance levels to exceed

2 Benchmarking Process
- Identify the area of practice involved
- Identify a patient-focused outcome
- Identify factors and processes that affect the outcome
- Identify benchmarks for the best practice for each factor

2a Benchmarking Process (continued)
- Construct a scoring continuum for practice
- Score current practice with comments on why scores were assigned
- Compare results with the identified best practice
- Share the results with others involved
- Develop a plan of action for improving practice

3 Examples of the Benchmarking Process
- Systems outcomes
  ○ Client care outcomes
  ○ Client satisfaction
  ○ Length of stay
  ○ Costs of care

SUGGESTIONS FOR CLASSROOM ACTIVITIES

Have students search the journals for articles that discuss benchmarking and systems outcomes evaluations in the case management field. Have them prepare a brief summary of the article for class.

SUGGESTIONS FOR CLINICAL ACTIVITIES

1. Invite a case manager to provide examples of systems outcomes for the agency that they represent and the results of their evaluation methods during post conference. Has the agency developed benchmarks for outcomes of care? If so, what are they? How were they developed? To what extent are they achieved?

2. Have students develop potential benchmarks for evaluating the outcomes of care in the clinical setting.

Community Empowerment

RESOURCE LIBRARY

🌐 COMPANION WEBSITE

Audio Glossary
Exam Review Questions
Case Study: Planned Change
MediaLink Application: Grassroots Organizing (video)

Media Links
Challenge Your Knowledge
Advocacy Interviews

📖 IMAGE LIBRARY

Figure 13-1 The Relationship of Community Empowerment to Other Similar Concepts

Table 13-1 Elements of Selected Community Empowerment Models and Examples of Community Health Nursing (CHN) Involvement

LEARNING OBJECTIVE 1

Discuss the relationship of community empowerment to other similar concepts.

CONCEPTS FOR LECTURE

1. Community empowerment is described as the process of enhancing the capacity of communities to control their own lives, effect change, mobilize and use resources, and obtain services to address health problems and collectively counter health risk behaviors and conditions that produce and support them.
2. Community empowerment is closely linked to community development, community organization, community mobilization, community building, community capacity, and competence. Community development refers to the rejuvenation of communities through housing and business development. Empowerment occurs when communities take action and participate in decision making for disadvantaged groups.
3. Community organization is a process involving community groups that are helped to identify common problems or goals, mobilize resources, and develop and implement strategies for reaching the goals that they have collectively set. This process is more problem-specific than community empowerment where communities address more than one problem.
4. Community mobilization involves working with individuals and groups to provide population-based community-driven assessments, interventions, and evaluations. Again, this is problem-specific.
5. Community building is often a continuous, self-renewing effort by residents and professionals to engage

POWERPOINT LECTURE SLIDES

NOTE: The number on each PPT Lecture Slide directly corresponds with the Concepts for Lecture.

1 Community Empowerment
- Process of enhancing capacity of communities to:
  - Control their own lives
  - Effect change
  - Mobilize and use resources
  - Obtain services to address health problems
  - Collectively counter health risk behaviors/conditions

1a See Figure 13-1

2 Community Development
- Rejuvenation of communities
- Housing and business development
- Empowerment occurs when communities take action and participate in health related decision making for disadvantaged groups

3 Community Organization
- Aiding group to identify common problems/goals
- Mobilize resources
- Develop and implement strategies for reaching goals

in collective action aimed at problem solving and enrichment that creates new or strengthened social networks, new capacities for group action and support, and new standards for the life of the community. Community building efforts may lead to increases in community social capital, but may not focus specifically on health problems. This process is specific to collective problem-solving actions and may result in community empowerment as members begin to take control of their lives, learn to effect change, and address health problems.

6. Community capacity building involves three levels: developing the capacities of the health infrastructure to deliver needed services, maintaining and sustaining programs after initial funding is gone, and addressing a variety of health-related issues. Community empowerment results in increased community competence and capacity building.

- This process is more problem-specific compared to community empowerment where communities address more than one problem

4 Community Mobilization
- Population-based assessments, interventions, and evaluations
- Problem-specific
- May result in empowerment if actions and efforts are multifocal and health related

5 Community Building
- Continuous, self-renewing efforts
- Collective action aimed at problem solving and enrichment
- Creates new or strengthened social networks
- Creates new capacities for group action and support
- Creates new standards for the life of community
- Community building efforts may lead to increases in community social capital
- May not focus specifically on health problems

6 Community Capacity/Competence
- Develop capacities of health infrastructure
- Maintain and sustain programs after initial funding
- Address variety of health-related issues
- Community empowerment results in increased community competence and capacity building

---

SUGGESTIONS FOR CLASSROOM ACTIVITIES

Ask students to create a collage that depicts their interpretation of community empowerment. Have the students demonstrate relationships between the other community activities discussed in this objective.

SUGGESTIONS FOR CLINICAL ACTIVITIES

Have students identify opportunities at their community clinical site for community empowerment. Ask them to identify a problem, concern, or potential community goal. Have students use each of the community concepts (community, development, capacity building, mobilization and organization) to show how they anticipate the process of community empowerment will take place and present at post conference.

LEARNING OBJECTIVE 2

Identify levels of community empowerment.

CONCEPTS FOR LECTURE

1. Empowerment can occur at a variety of levels, including individual or community empowerment, horizontal or vertical empowerment, and continuum empowerment.
2. Individual empowerment involves improving individual skill and self-esteem and community empowerment results in increased civic participation.
3. Horizontal empowerment is a community's ability to problem solve by mobilizing its own resources, and vertical empowerment is described as efforts to change power structures outside the community.

POWERPOINT LECTURE SLIDES

NOTE: The number on each PPT Lecture Slide directly corresponds with the Concepts for Lecture.

1 Levels of Empowerment
- Individual and community empowerment
- Horizontal and vertical empowerment
- Continuum empowerment

2 Individual Empowerment
- Individual community member
- Focuses on improving individual skill and self-esteem

CONCEPTS FOR LECTURE *continued*

4. Continuum empowerment includes several levels: personal empowerment, support group development, community organization development, and coalition development. It is a gradual process of increasing individual and population group support to address community concerns.

POWERPOINT LECTURE SLIDES *continued*

2a Community Empowerment
- Community at large
- Addresses increased civic participation

3 Horizontal Empowerment
- Problem solving using community's own resources

3a Vertical Empowerment
- Change power structures outside the community

4 Continuum Empowerment
- Personal empowerment
- Development of small mutual support groups
- Development of community organizations
- Development of coalitions of community organizations and linking to outside resources

SUGGESTIONS FOR CLASSROOM ACTIVITIES

Divide students into groups to develop strategies that would promote empowerment at each of the continuum levels in the situation described in the case study at the end of the chapter.

SUGGESTIONS FOR CLINICAL ACTIVITIES

Assign students to develop an empowerment strategy for a population group served by their clinical agency or site. Have them choose one of the levels of empowerment and develop a detailed outline of the role of the community health nurse.

LEARNING OBJECTIVE 3

Apply selected models for community empowerment.

CONCEPTS FOR LECTURE

1. Rothman's framework addresses three levels of practice. Locality development involves development of a sense of community and a group identity. Social planning focuses on the resolution of specific problems identified in the community. Social action addresses activities that increase the problem-solving ability of the community.

2. The Community Action Model describes five steps for community organization. In Step 1 community health nurses help in identifying key community members for training, and assist community members to identify the issue and a focus for the issue through data collection and assessment. Step 2 addresses community diagnosis of root causes and assessment of the extent of the effect on the community. Community health nurses may assist community members to develop data categories and collection methods. Step 3 analyzes diagnostic results. Community health nurses may assist community members to analyze the data and identify key contributing factors as a target for action. In Step 4, the nurse assists community members to select, plan, and implement actions directed at the issue or problem, and identify desired outcomes. Finally, in Step 5, the CHN assists community members to develop mechanisms to monitor ongoing activities and results.

POWERPOINT LECTURE SLIDES

NOTE: The number on each PPT Lecture Slide directly corresponds with the Concepts for Lecture.

1 Rothman's Framework (Refer to Table 13-1)
- Locality development
- Social planning
- Social action

2 Community Action Model
- Step 1: Train key members and identify issues or concern
- Step 2: Conduct community diagnosis and assess extent of the effect on community
- Step 3: Analyze diagnostic results
- Step 4: Select, plan, and implement actions specific to the issue and identify desired outcomes
- Step 5: Enforce or maintain action or activity

3 Nursing Model of Community Organization for Change
- Assessment/reassessment
- Planning/design
- Implementation
- Evaluation/dissemination

3. The Nursing Model of Community Organization for Change has four main components with the community health nurse active in each step: assessing and reassessing of felt needs and assets; planning for and establishing goals and designing interventions; implementing the actions designed to achieve the identified goals; and evaluating, identifying successful and unsuccessful elements with dissemination of that information to the community.

4. The Community Organization Model focuses on community analysis and implementation. During the analysis phase, the community is defined, a community profile is developed, community capacity is assessed, barriers to action and readiness for change is assessed. During the implementation phase, interventions and a timeline are developed, community participation is solicited, media coverage is planned, financial and other support is sought, and evaluation plans are developed.

5. Another model for community empowerment is the Planned Approach to Community Health (PATCH) model. The five key elements of this model and the subsequent roles of the community health nurse include: 1) the community health nurse CHN mobilizes the community by helping to identify appropriate participants within the community; 2) the CHN assists the community members to collect and organize data related to the issue; 3) the CHN aids the community members in choosing health priorities; 4) the CHN assists the community members to develop a comprehensive intervention plan with multisectorial collaboration; and 5) the CHN assists the community members to evaluate the effectiveness of the interventions by developing criteria to measure success and data collection methods, as well as in analyzing evaluative data with the desired outcomes in mind.

6. The natural helper model focuses on the use of natural helpers who are individuals that others turn to, seek out, or rely on for advice, emotional support, and tangible aid. Examples include family, friends, neighbors, role-related helpers, and volunteers.

4 Community Organization Model
- Community analysis
- Design initiation
- Implementation
- Maintenance/consolidation
- Dissemination/reassessment
- Role of community health nurse

5 Planned Approach to Community Health (PATCH)
- Mobilize the community
  - Identify appropriate community members to participate
- Collect and organize data related to the issue
  - Assist community members to design and conduct community needs/asset assessment
- Choose health priorities
  - Assist community members to prioritize issues and select one for action

5a Planned Approach to Community Health (PATCH) (continued)
- Develop comprehensive intervention plan with multisectoral collaboration
  - Assist community members to determine desired outcome of action
  - Identify and evaluate possible alternative approaches to action
  - Develop specific strategies for selected alternative approach
- Evaluate the effectiveness of interventions
  - Assist community members in the development of criteria to measure success and data collection methods and in analyzing evaluative data

6 Natural Helper Model
- Use of natural helpers within the community to promote community empowerment
  - Those whom other turn to naturally for advice, emotional support, and tangible aid
  - Examples: family, friends, neighbors, role-related helpers, volunteers

---

SUGGESTIONS FOR CLASSROOM ACTIVITIES

Assign students to research a journal article that depicts one of the community empowerment models. Have students discuss and critique the utility of the model in promoting community empowerment in the situation described in the article.

SUGGESTIONS FOR CLINICAL ACTIVITIES

Have students define a health-related concern for a specific population group that they observed in their clinical experiences. Have them use the model that they selected from the literature to explain how that model might assist the community health nurse in developing strategies for empowerment.

LEARNING OBJECTIVE 4

Describe the process of community empowerment.

CONCEPTS FOR LECTURE

1. The key elements of the community empowerment process include assessment, planning, strategies for implementation, and evaluation.

2. Elements of the empowerment process include organizing for empowerment activity, planning and implementing empowerment strategies, and evaluating the outcomes of empowerment activities.

3. Organizing for empowerment begins with an assessment of the current situation. Community assessment may adopt a needs-based or an asset-based approach or a combination of both. The actual assessment of a community can be seen in terms of the dimensions of health or other types of community indicators (e.g. quality of life indicators, provocative indicators, community processes and their effects on health, and formal and informal leadership within the community).

4. Community assessment provides the basis for issue selection, the first step in planning strategies for community empowerment. Issue selection is the process of carefully identifying specific targets of change with the goal of unifying and building community strength. Four considerations surround the selection of an issue: identifying the constituents or interested parties, identifying their goals specific to the issue, identifying potential targets for action, and addressing the question of how leverage can be gained with respect to the issue. Team building focuses on actions and activities necessary to encourage member participation and commitment to the issue and the ability to work effectively together. Coalition development consists of four components: resource acquisition (e.g., recruiting coalition members and resources); development of a maintenance subsystem (e.g., the organizational control structure and strategies to maintain member commitment); production (e.g., action strategies to facilitate community empowerment and maintenance of the coalition's internal structure); and goal attainment (e.g., developing a track record of successes in community empowerment).

5. Implementation strategies include media advocacy and the use of community workers. Media advocacy is defined as strategic use of mass media to advance a social or public policy agenda and serves two functions: drawing public attention to an issue or to possible power inequities and focusing attention on factors contributing to issues of concern. Natural helpers, community volunteers, and community health workers can provide an opportunity to participate in conducting assessments or analysis of the evaluative findings.

POWERPOINT LECTURE SLIDES

NOTE: The number on each PPT Lecture Slide directly corresponds with the Concepts for Lecture.

1 Process of Community Empowerment
- Assessment
- Planning
- Strategies for implementation
- Evaluation

2 Empowerment Process
- Empowerment activity
- Planning empowerment strategies
- Implementation of strategies
- Evaluating the outcomes of empowerment activities

3 Community Assessment
- Selection of approaches
  - Community needs-based solutions
  - Assets-based approach
  - Dimensions of health and community indicators
    - Quality of life indicators
    - Provocative indicators

4 Community Assessment Planning Process
- Issue selection
  - Identify specific targets of change
    - Team building
      - Encourage member participation and commitment

4a Coalition Development
- Resource acquisition
- Development of maintenance subsystem
- Production
- Goal attainment

5 Implementation Strategies
- Media advocacy
  - Use of mass media to advance a social or public policy agenda
  - Functions
    - Drawing public attention to an issue/power inequities
    - Focus attention on factors contributing to issues of concern

5a Community Workers
- Natural helpers
- Community volunteers
- Community health workers

6 Evaluation
- Participatory evaluation
  - A partnership approach to evaluation
  - Engages those with interest in all aspects

6. Evaluation should be an integral part of the community empowerment process. Participatory evaluation is the involvement of community members in all steps of the empowerment evaluation process. Participatory evaluation is defined as a partnership approach to evaluation that engages those who have a stake in the project, program, or initiative in all aspects of evaluation design and implementation. The steps of evaluation include taking stock of community status, resources, capacities, challenges, and programs; setting goals for evaluation; developing evaluation strategies; and documenting the evaluation process and findings.

 Steps of Evaluation
- Take stock of community status, resources, capacities, challenges, and programs
- Set goals for evaluation
- Develop evaluation strategies
- Document evaluation process/findings

SUGGESTIONS FOR CLASSROOM ACTIVITIES

Divide students into groups. Assign each group one of the process steps for community empowerment. Have each group plan strategies that encompass a community empowerment process for a health related concern from their clinical experience.

SUGGESTIONS FOR CLINICAL ACTIVITIES

Arrange for students to attend and observe a community organizing group that is active in their locale. Have students focus on aspects of coalition building and report findings to class.

LEARNING OBJECTIVE 5

Apply criteria to evaluate community empowerment.

CONCEPTS FOR LECTURE

1. The basic principles of participatory evaluation include community participation and ownership, collaboration among all stakeholders, findings that promote change, and transformation of power relationships with community members in control of the evaluation.

POWERPOINT LECTURE SLIDES

NOTE: The number on each PPT Lecture Slide directly corresponds with the Concepts for Lecture.

1 **Participatory Evaluation Criteria**
- Basic principles
  - Community participation/ownership
  - Collaboration among stakeholders
  - Promote change on multiple levels
  - Transform power relationships

LEARNING OBJECTIVE 6

Analyze the role of community health nurses in community empowerment.

CONCEPTS FOR LECTURE

1. The role of the community health nurse in community empowerment is multipurpose and multilayered and includes the following activities: becoming active proponent of and participant in community empowerment, playing an advisory and facilitative leadership role, using their influence in discovery by making community members aware of the need for empowerment and decision roles to determine potential alternative strategies and evaluating them, and selecting strategies most likely to contribute to achievement of community-identified goals.

POWERPOINT LECTURE SLIDES

NOTE: The number on each PPT Lecture Slide directly corresponds with the Concepts for Lecture.

 Role of Community Health Nurse
- Active proponents of and participants in community empowerment
- Advisory role
- Facilitative role
- Discovery role
- Decision role

SUGGESTIONS FOR CLASSROOM ACTIVITIES

Have students refer to the case study at the end of the chapter and write examples of empowerment roles that the community health nurse can demonstrate for pregnant women in this community.

SUGGESTIONS FOR CLINICAL ACTIVITIES

1. Have students write a journal entry about the potential empowerment role of a community health nurse in their clinical setting, site, or agency. Have them select a health care topic and a target population and discuss the roles that can be utilized.

2. Have the students identify the extent to which nurses in the clinical setting engage in community empowerment activities. What factors promote or constrain such activities by community health nurses?

Care of Families

RESOURCE LIBRARY

COMPANION WEBSITE

Audio Glossary
Appendix F: Family Health Assessment and
   Intervention Guide
Exam Review Questions
Case Study: Family Health

MediaLink Application: Foster Parenting (video)
Media Links
Challenge Your Knowledge
Advocacy Interviews

IMAGE LIBRARY

Figure 14-1 Hierarchical Systems
Figure 14-2 Sample Family Genogram
Figure 14-3 Sample Family Ecomap
Figure 14-4 Family Communication Patterns

Table 14-2 Duvall's and Carter and McGoldrick's
   Stages of Family Development with Associated
   Developmental Tasks

LEARNING OBJECTIVE 1

Describe at least five family types and their characteristic features.

CONCEPTS FOR LECTURE

1. Family is defined as a social system consisting of two
   or more people who define themselves as a family
   and who share bonds of emotional closeness.
2. The nuclear conjugal family consists of husband, wife,
   and children. Children may be biological or adopted.
   Nuclear dyads are married couples without children
   under 18 years of age living in the home. Dual-earner
   families consist of two working parents with or without children.
3. Extended families include family members other than
   spouses and children and may include stepkin.
   Traditionally, extended families either shared household expenses and tasks or lived in close proximity
   and provided mutual support. Many extended families
   live in multigenerational households.
4. Single-parent families are among the most common
   family units served by community health nurses.
   A single-parent family, consisting of an adult woman
   or man and children, results from divorce, nonmarital
   pregnancies, absence or death of a spouse, or adoption by a single person.
5. Stepfamilies are composed of two adults, at least one
   of whom has remarried following divorce or death of

POWERPOINT LECTURE SLIDES

*NOTE: The number on each PPT Lecture Slide directly
corresponds with the Concepts for Lecture.*

1 Family
   • Social system of two or more people
   • Define themselves as a family
   • Share bonds of emotional closeness

2 Nuclear
   • Nuclear conjugal: husband, wife, and
     children
   • Nuclear dyads: married couple without children
     under 18 living in home
   • Children may be biological or adopted
   • Dual-earner: two working parents with or
     without children

3 Extended
   • Include family members other than spouses or
     children
   • May include stepkin
   • Share expenses and tasks
   • Live in close proximity and provide mutual
     support

a spouse and at least one of whom has children from a prior relationship. Stepfamilies can include children from either adult's previous relationship, as well as offspring from the new marriage.

6. Cohabiting families consist of a man and a woman living together without being married and may include teens to retired elderly persons. Each age group may have their own reason for cohabitation such as a desire for a trial marriage or increased safety and financial necessity. Cohabiting families may or may not include children.

7. Gay or lesbian families are a form of cohabitation in which a couple of the same sex live together and share a sexual relationship. In the United States, approximately 10% of unmarried partner households include partners of the same sex. There may or may not be children present in gay/lesbian families.

8. A grandparent-headed family is one in which the older person or grandparent is the head of the household. Approximately 7% of all U.S. families are headed by grandparents. Factors that contribute to this type of family are drug abuse, child abuse, AIDS, and nonmarital births.

9. Foster families consist of at least one adult and one or more foster children placed by the court system and also may contain the adult's own biological children or adopted children. Over 500,000 children may be in foster care in the United States. Foster children exhibit higher incidences of mental disorders such as depression, developmental disorders, and attention deficit hyperactivity disorders.

4 Single-parent
- Most common family served by community health nurse
- Consists of adult woman or man and children
- Many causes

5 Stepfamilies
- Two adults, at least one of whom has remarried
- Can include children from previous marriage
- Can include children from the new marriage

6 Cohabitating
- Man and woman living together without marriage
- Include anyone from teens to retired elderly
- Different reasons for cohabitation

7 Gay or Lesbian
- Form of cohabitation
- Same-sex couple who share a sexual relationship
- Comprise approximately 10% of unmarried couple households in U.S.

8 Grandparent-headed
- Older person or grandparent is head of household
- Comprise approximately 7% of U.S. families
- Many factors contribute to grandparent-headed families

9 Foster
- At least one adult and one or more foster children
- Children placed by the court system
- May contain the adult's own biological or adopted children
- Higher incidence of mental disorders in foster children

SUGGESTIONS FOR CLASSROOM ACTIVITIES

Have the class discuss the types of families that are represented by the students in the class.

SUGGESTIONS FOR CLINICAL ACTIVITIES

Assign students to identify and document the types of families that are served in their community health nursing clinical setting.

LEARNING OBJECTIVE 2

Describe elements of at least one theoretical model applied to families.

CONCEPTS FOR LECTURE

1. Family systems approaches evolved from a general systems theory that described biological and social systems. A system is defined as a complex of elements in interaction with each other in which the interaction is ordered rather than random. Systems theory features a number of components, such as a concept of hierarchial systems in which a given system is part of a suprasystem and is comprised of a variety of

POWERPOINT LECTURE SLIDES

NOTE: The number on each PPT Lecture Slide directly corresponds with the Concepts for Lecture.

1 Systems Approaches
- System is a complex of elements in interaction with each other
- Interaction is ordered, not random

subsystems. A family is a system within the suprasystem of a community or society. The family is, in turn, composed of individual member subsystems and their interrelationships. Boundaries define what part of the system is and what is not. System goals include a steady state and system growth. Systems have three processes designed to accomplish these goals. The first are those processes needed to regulate exchange with the environment and include: input (e.g., family system receives information about a member), throughput (e.g., process by which the family acts on the information), and output (e.g., what happens when the family acts or does not act on the information) processes. The second category of process includes those processes designed to limit expenditures of system energy and thus prevent overload. The third category are those internal processes which include subsystem change (a family accommodates a new member or loses a member) and adaptive (e.g., entropy, negentropy, and feedback) processes.

2. Developmental models maintain that human and social units develop in a logical fashion with predictable stages or milestones. Family development is defined as the unique path taken by any given family in its movement through the stages of growth. The family life cycle is a series of stages through which all families pass, which necessitates changes within the family and its interactions. When working with families, community health nurses focus on identifying the family's stage of development, assessing the degree to which the family has achieved the related developmental tasks, and developing strategies to assist families in task accomplishment.

3. Carter and McGoldrick's stages of family development include six stages: single young adult, new couple, family with young children, family with adolescents, launching children and moving on, and family in later life.

4. Structural functional approaches to family nursing are based on the principle that all families possess structure designed to allow them to perform specific functions essential to the health of the family. There are two basic concepts in this model which include: structure, which is the pattern of organization of the interdependent parts of a whole with the structural elements being family members and family interaction patterns related to roles, values, communication patterns, and power structure; and function, which is a group of related actions that lead to the accomplishment of specific goals. The five family functions include the affective, socialization, reproductive, economic, and provision of needs functions. Genograms and ecomaps are often used to diagram family structures and relationships within and outside the family.

1a System Components
- Hierarchal structure
- Suprasystem structure and subsystems
- Boundaries
- Mutual goals
  - Maintenance of a steady state
  - System growth

1b System Processes
- Those processes needed to regulate exchanges with the environment
  - Input, throughput, and output processes
- Processes involved in system operation
  - Designed to limit expenditures of system energy
- Internal processes
  - Subsystem and adaptive change processes

2 Developmental Approaches (Refer to Table 14-2)
- Humans and social units develop in a logical fashion
- Predictable stages or milestones
- Family development is a unique path through stages of growth

2a Nursing Focus
- Identify/assess family stage
- Assess degree that family has achieved developmental task
- Assess family engagement in action that promotes accomplishment of developmental tasks

3 Carter and McGoldrick's Stage of Family Development
- Stage I: Single young adult
- Stage II: New couple
- Stage III: Family with young children
- Stage IV: Family with adolescents
- Stage V: Launching children and moving on
- Stage VI: Family in later life

4 Structural Functional Approaches
- Family structure allows specific functions essential to health of family

4a Structural Elements Are Family Members and Interaction Patterns
- Roles
- Values
- Communication patterns
- Power structure
- Function

4b Family Functions
- Group of related actions to accomplish specific goals
  - Affective
  - Socialization
  - Reproductive

○ Economic
○ Provision of needs

 4c Genograms and Ecomaps
- Used to diagram family structures and relationships

SUGGESTIONS FOR CLASSROOM ACTIVITIES

Have students diagram their own family structures with a genogram including at least three generations and an ecomap.

SUGGESTIONS FOR CLINICAL ACTIVITIES

Have students use each theoretical model to develop a care plan for a family from their clinical setting. Compare and contrast the differences in the plan of care using the three models. Which model permits the most holistic approach to care of the family?

LEARNING OBJECTIVE 3

Identify family assessment considerations in the biophysical, psychological, physical environmental, sociocultural, behavioral, and health system dimensions.

CONCEPTS FOR LECTURE

1. The epidemiology of family health takes into consideration a number of biophysical factors such as the family's overall health status and how it affects family functions and relationships between family members. Family demographics are important in the identifying of problems and planning family care. Age, gender composition, race, and the presence of elderly family members may provide insight into family resource needs, family health problems, and family safety needs. The developmental status of individual family members provides insight into parental roles and needs.

2. Psychological considerations include communication patterns, relationships and dynamics, coping and emotional strengths, child-rearing practices, family goals, the presence of mental illness, and the existence of family crises.

3. Communication patterns are an important indicator of functioning in the psychological dimension. Communication patterns may also influence family relationships and dynamics and parental effectiveness.

4. Family relationships are bonds between family members that create identifiable patterns. They can be categorized as close, cohesive, and supportive, or distant, nonsupportive, or conflictual. Family dynamics includes the power structure within a family, which may be influenced by cultural beliefs and practices. Cultural beliefs and practices may also influence child-rearing attitudes and discipline practices. Family coping and emotional strengths are influenced by coping strategies that help a family to adapt to stress and defense mechanisms, which are tactics used for avoiding recognition of problems. Families may exhibit

POWERPOINT LECTURE SLIDES

NOTE: The number on each PPT Lecture Slide directly corresponds with the Concepts for Lecture.

1 Biophysical Considerations
- Family health status
- Family demographics
  ○ Age
  ○ Gender
  ○ Race
- Developmental status

2 Psychological Considerations
- Communication patterns
- Family relationships/dynamics
- Family coping/emotional strengths
- Child-rearing/discipline practices
- Family goals
- Presence of mental illness
- Family crisis

3 Communication Patterns
- Influence family relationships, dynamics, and parental effectiveness

4 Family Relationships
- Bonds between family members
  ○ Close, cohesive supportive
  ○ Distant, nonsupportive, conflictual
- Family dynamics
  ○ Cultural beliefs and practices
  ○ Coping and emotional strengths
  ○ Mental illness

certain strengths when faced with crises or stressors. These strengths are referred to as family resilience, which is described as the phenomenon of doing well in the face of adversity. Family goals evolve from family values and cultural backgrounds. Problems may arise when there is disagreement on family goals or when societal goals and expectations conflict with family goals. Mental illness affects both the individual and the family unit. Mental illness can trigger different types of crises and add to a family's stress level, financial needs, and inability to use effective coping mechanisms.

5. The physical environmental considerations that affect families come from both the internal environment of home and space and the external environment, which includes the neighborhood, existing industries, crime rates, and sanitation concerns.

6. A number of sociocultural considerations affect family health. Family roles of each family member must be understood. Knowledge of cultural and religious beliefs is essential to designing effective family interventions. A family's socioeconomic status can greatly affect the health of individual members as well as the overall family's health, access to health, and understanding of health practices. Employment or occupational factors can create stress-related illnesses, which also influence effective parenting and healthy relationships. External resources can include extended family, churches, or social organizations that can provide support, both emotional and financial, during crises or adversity. Refugee status affects the health and functional abilities of many families related to separation from other family members.

7. Behavioral considerations include family consumption patterns, which can be overconsumption, resulting in obesity and nutritional deficiencies. Consumption patterns also include use of alcohol and drugs and other substances (e.g., tobacco, caffeine). Cultural patterns also influence food choices and preparation. Rest and sleep patterns can be affected by a new infant or differing work schedules and can impact relationships, stress levels, and parenting practices. Safety practices are another element of the behavioral dimension in family health.

8. Health system considerations include a family's attitude toward health and its response to illness as well as its use of health care services. Families respond differently to illness, and certain family members may be the ones to determine who is ill. Families may be limited in their use of health care resources due to a lack of funds, language barriers, distance to facilities, and transportation limitations.

5 Physical Environmental Considerations
- Internal environment
  - Home
  - Space
- External environment
  - Neighborhood
  - Industry
  - Crime rate
  - Sanitation

6 Sociocultural Considerations
- Family roles
- Culture and religion
- Social and economic status
- Employment or occupational factors
- External resources
- Refugee status

7 Behavioral Considerations
- Family consumption patterns
- Cultural patterns
- Rest and sleep patterns

8 Health System Considerations
- Family attitudes toward health and response to illness
- Access to and use of health care services

SUGGESTIONS FOR CLASSROOM ACTIVITIES	**SUGGESTIONS FOR CLINICAL ACTIVITIES**
Allow students to explore ways that the community health nurse can conduct a family assessment.	Assign students to identify community resources and interventions for each of the family assessment considerations that they identified in their clinical setting family.

LEARNING OBJECTIVE 4

Differentiate between formal and informal family roles.

CONCEPTS FOR LECTURE

1. Roles are socially expected behavior patterns that are determined by a person's position or status within a family, such as the adult woman in a family may be a wife, mother, or cook.
2. Roles can be formal and informal. Formal roles are expected sets of behaviors associated with family positions, such as husband, wife, father, and child. Informal roles are those expected behaviors not associated with a particular position.
3. Family roles can be complementary or conflictual. Role conflict occurs when the demands of a single role are contradictory or when the demands attending several roles contradict or compete with each other. Role overload occurs when an individual is confronted with too many role expectations.

POWERPOINT LECTURE SLIDES

NOTE: The number on each PPT Lecture Slide directly corresponds with the Concepts for Lecture.

1 Family Roles
- Socially-expected behavior patterns
- Determined by a person's position or status within a family

2 Roles Are Formal or Informal
- Formal roles
  ○ Expected sets of behaviors associated with family positions
- Informal roles
  ○ Expected behaviors not associated with position

3 Complementary or Conflictual Roles
- Role conflict
  ○ Occurs when demands of role are contradictory or compete
- Role overload
  ○ Occurs with too many role expectations

SUGGESTIONS FOR CLASSROOM ACTIVITIES

Encourage active discussion and solicit volunteer information from students regarding their own roles in their lives and families, presence of role conflicts, and role overload situations.

SUGGESTIONS FOR CLINICAL ACTIVITIES

Have students describe a family situation from their clinical setting and identify roles (both formal and informal), role conflicts, and role overloads for that family.

LEARNING OBJECTIVE 5

Differentiate between situational and maturational crises.

CONCEPTS FOR LECTURE

1. Family exposure to stress may lead to the development of a crisis situation. A crisis occurs when a family faces a problem that is seemingly unsolvable.
2. Families may experience two types of crises: situational and maturational. Situational crisis can occur when the family experiences an event that is sudden, unexpected, and unpredictable. A maturational crisis can be viewed as a normal process or transition point where old patterns of communication and old roles must be exchanged for new patterns and roles. Examples of transition periods where maturational crises may occur are adolescence, marriage, parenthood, and first-time employment.

POWERPOINT LECTURE SLIDES

NOTE: The number on each PPT Lecture Slide directly corresponds with the Concepts for Lecture.

1 Family Crisis
- Occurs when family faces a seemingly insolvable problem

2 Types of Family Crises
- Situational
  ○ Family experiences an event that is sudden, unexpected, and unpredictable
- Maturational
  ○ Normal transition point
  ○ Exchange old patterns and roles for new

SUGGESTIONS FOR CLASSROOM ACTIVITIES	SUGGESTIONS FOR CLINICAL ACTIVITIES
Have students make a list of situational and maturational crises in their own lives and encourage students to share their experiences with the class.	Have students identify situational and maturational crises or potential or expected crises in a family from their clinical setting.

LEARNING OBJECTIVE 6

Discuss family-focused intervention at the primary, secondary, and tertiary levels of prevention.

CONCEPTS FOR LECTURE

1. Primary prevention interventions at the family level include health promotion and protection (such as educating family members about safety issues, safety in the home, nutrition, and the need for physical activity and rest) and illness prevention interventions (such as teaching effective hygiene and referring families for immunization services).

2. At the aggregate or population level, the community health nurse advocates for environmental protection, social justice, and availability of health promotion and illness prevention services, and provides education in coping skills.

3. Secondary prevention interventions at the family level include assisting families in obtaining needed care for existing health problems, helping families to deal with health problems, linking families with needed services, and initiating crisis intervention. At the population level, intervention strategies include alerting health policy makers about the need for family services and initiating plans for programs.

4. Tertiary interventions at the family level include assisting families in coping with long-term health problems, in dealing with the consequences of those health problems, and in dealing with the loss of a loved one. At the population level, the community health nurse advocates for the development of respite services for family caretakers and creates support groups for crisis-prone families.

POWERPOINT LECTURE SLIDES

NOTE: *The number on each PPT Lecture Slide directly corresponds with the Concepts for Lecture.*

1. Primary Prevention Family-focused Interventions
   - Family level
   - Health promotion and protection
     o Educate family members
       – Safety
       – Nutrition
       – Physical activity/rest
   - Illness prevention
     o Teaching effective hygiene
     o Referring for immunizations

2. Family-focused Interventions
   - Primary prevention–aggregate level
   - Advocate
     o Environmental protection
     o Social justice
     o Availability of health promotion and illness prevention services
   - Teach coping skills

3. Secondary Family-focused Interventions
   - Family level
     o Assist families in obtaining needed care
     o Help families deal with problems
     o Link families with services
     o Crisis intervention
   - Population level
     o Alert health policy makers to need for family services
     o Initiate plans for programs

4. Tertiary Family-focused Interventions
   - Family level
     o Assist families in coping with long-term health problems
     o Assist in dealing with consequences
     o Assist families with loss of loved one
   - Population/aggregate level
     o Advocate for development of respite services for family caretakers
     o Create support groups for crisis-prone families

SUGGESTIONS FOR CLASSROOM ACTIVITIES

Ask students to pair off. Assign a case scenerio and ask students to identify primary, secondary, and tertiary interventions for the family described.

SUGGESTIONS FOR CLINICAL ACTIVITIES

Have students select a family from their clinical setting, perform a family needs assessment, and develop primary, secondary, and tertiary intervention recommendations for that family.

15
CHAPTER

Care of Populations

RESOURCE LIBRARY

🌐 COMPANION WEBSITE

Audio Glossary
Appendix G: Community Health Assessment and
  Intervention Guide
Exam Review Questions
Case Study: Influencing the Health of a Community

MediaLink Application: Tobacco-Free Kids (video)
Media Links
Challenge Your Knowledge
Advocacy Interviews

📖 IMAGE LIBRARY

Figure 15-1 Partial Program Theory for a Smoking
  Cessation Program

LEARNING OBJECTIVE 1

Discuss the rationale for including members of the population in every phase of population health assessment
and health program planning.

CONCEPTS FOR LECTURE

1. Population health management is defined as "account-ability and management of the health of an entire community regardless of system membership or insurance status" (Greene & Kelsey, as quoted in Robertson, 2004, p. 495). It involves health promotion and illness prevention strategies.
2. Historically, identification of a population's health problems, and development and implementation of programs, was conducted by health professionals. More recently, health professionals have begun to involve members of the population of interest. It is important to include and involve members of the community in the population health assessment process for a number of reasons. Involvement in all phases of assessment, planning, implementation, and evaluation ensures that their interests are considered. It also facilitates development of an accurate and comprehensive appraisal of the health status of that population. Inclusion of the population members aids in offsetting organizational or agency agendas that may arise, and all participants are assured of a more comprehensive and balanced picture of the population's health.
3. Including population members may occur through the use of a rapid participatory appraisal process,

POWERPOINT LECTURE SLIDES

NOTE: The number on each PPT Lecture Slide directly corresponds with the Concepts for Lecture.

1 Population Health Management
- Accountability and management of health of entire community
- Regardless of system membership or insurance status
- Health promotion
- Illness prevention strategies

2 Population Health Assessment
- Benefits of including member of community
  - Ensures that their interests are considered
  - Accurate and comprehensive appraisal of health status
  - Aids in offsetting organizational or agency agendas that may arise
  - Assures a comprehensive/balanced picture of health

3 Rapid Participatory Appraisal
- Addresses community structure, composition, interest, and capacity
- Collects data regarding community needs and assets

CONCEPTS FOR LECTURE *continued*

which addresses information about community structure, composition, interest, and capacity; collects data regarding community needs and assets; identifies available services to meet those needs; and considers social policy as it affects capacity to meet population health needs.

4. A key concept to consider is that while a community is composed of individuals, families, organizations, and businesses that share a common language, values, history, or purpose, a target group is considered a subgroup within the community whose members exhibit particular health needs or who are at particular risk for the development of health problems. Community engagement is defined as the process of working collaboratively with and through groups of people affiliated by geographic proximity, special interest, or similar situations to address issues affecting the well-being of those people. Several community engagement principles have been developed and, if used, guide the process of population involvement and population health assessment.

POWERPOINT LECTURE SLIDES *continued*

- Identifies available services
- Considers social policy as it affects capacity to meet population health needs

4 Key Concepts
- Community
- Target group
- Community engagement

SUGGESTIONS FOR CLASSROOM ACTIVITIES

During class, have students discuss benefits and disadvantages of involving community members in a population health assessment.

SUGGESTIONS FOR CLINICAL ACTIVITIES

Arrange for students to attend a community forum. Have students note how many people attend, their interests in the meeting, their agendas (if any) and their contributions, and have students offer suggestions on how to involve more community members.

LEARNING OBJECTIVE 2

Describe factors in each of the six dimensions of health to be considered in assessing the health of a population.

CONCEPTS FOR LECTURE

1. The six dimensions of health frame the discussion of factors that affect the health of population groups. The biophysical considerations include age composition, which addresses annual birth rate and needs for specific services based on population age dynamics, and age-specific death rates, which provide information about health risks and risk behaviors. Genetic inheritance addresses the predisposition of the population to develop diseases with a genetic inheritance component such as diabetes, hypertension, and cancer. Racial or ethnic composition may alert health professionals to specific prevalent health problems such as sickle cell disease or diabetes. Disease incidence and prevalence and immunization levels are other biophysical considerations in community assessment.

2. Psychological considerations include those situations that increase or mediate exposure to stress and a population's ability to function effectively. Factors to consider are stressors affecting community members, suicide and homicide rates, relationships among groups

POWERPOINT LECTURE SLIDES

NOTE: The number on each PPT Lecture Slide directly corresponds with the Concepts for Lecture.

1 Factors Affecting Population Health: Biophysical Considerations
- Annual birth rate
- Age dynamics
- Age-specific death rates
- Genetics
- Race/ethnicity
- Disease incidence and prevalence

2 Psychological Considerations
- Community stressors
- Suicide and homicide rates
- Adequacy of law enforcement
- Communication patterns

3 Physical Environmental Considerations
- Geographical location
- Type and size of community

within the population, adequacy of law enforcement, and communication patterns within the community.

3. Physical environmental factors that affect a population's health include its geographical location, its type and size, topographical features, climate, type and adequacy of housing, water supply, and disaster potentials.

4. Sociocultural considerations include a community's government and leadership, language, income and education, employment levels and occupations, marital status and family composition, religion, transportation, and availability of goods and services. Understanding these elements provides insight into the success or failure of program implementation.

5. Behavioral considerations include consumption patterns, nutritional levels, use of harmful substances, and prevalent leisure activities.

6. Health system considerations that affect a population's health assessment include existing health services, the level of health system performance, the availability and adequacy of the health services, health care financing, and a community's definition of health and illness.

- Topographical features
- Climate

3a Physical Environmental Considerations (continued)
- Type and adequacy of housing
- Water supplies
- Disaster potentials

4 Sociocultural Considerations
- Community government and leadership
- Language
- Income and education
- Employment levels and occupations

4a Socioculutral Considerations (continued)
- Marital status/family composition
- Religion
- Transportation
- Availability of goods and services

5 Behavioral Considerations
- Consumption patterns
- Nutritional levels
- Use of harmful substances
- Prevalent leisure activities

6 Health System Considerations
- Existing health services
- Level of health system performance
- Availability and adequacy of services
- Health care financing
- Community's definition of health and illness

SUGGESTIONS FOR CLASSROOM ACTIVITIES

Have students review the community assessment plan for the region, county, or state where they are attending school.

SUGGESTIONS FOR CLINICAL ACTIVITIES

Have students conduct a community or target group assessment incorporating data related to each of the six dimensions of health.

LEARNING OBJECTIVE 3

Describe the components of a population nursing diagnosis.

CONCEPTS FOR LECTURE

1. A population health assessment is guided by several general principles, which include seeking multiple sources of information; addressing needs of specific subgroups; involving all potential stakeholders who are concerned with the outcomes of the evaluation; identifying population assets, needs, and problems; and using experts to conduct or direct the assessment.

2. Components of a population nursing diagnosis include: a potential adverse situation or risk; identification of a group or population subgroup at risk; group factors or characteristics that contribute to the risk; and indicators that support the conclusion that an increased risk is present.

POWERPOINT LECTURE SLIDES

NOTE: The number on each PPT Lecture Slide directly corresponds with the Concepts for Lecture.

1 Principles of Population Health Assessment
- Seek multiple sources of information
- Address needs of specific subgroups
- Involve all potential stakeholders
- Identify population assets, needs, and problems
- Use experts to conduct or direct assessment

2 Components of a Population Nursing Diagnosis
- A potential adverse situation or risk
- Identification of the group or population at risk

- Group factors or characteristics contributing to the risk
- Indicators that support the conclusion that an increased risk is present

---

SUGGESTIONS FOR CLASSROOM ACTIVITIES

Have students develop community nursing diagnoses from assessment information presented in class or in other case studies.

SUGGESTIONS FOR CLINICAL ACTIVITIES

Assign students to groups to conduct a community health assessment using the PROCESS steps. Have students search out references or resources needed to conduct their diagnosis of the community and share results with class.

LEARNING OBJECTIVE 4

Identify at least five tasks in planning health programs to meet the needs of populations.

CONCEPTS FOR LECTURE

1. Planning is defined as a collaborative and systematic process used to attain a goal. Collaboration means to involve community members and stakeholders. Systematic means that a process is intentionally used. Systematic planning utilizes three basic premises, which mandate that effective health systems respond to and are accountable to the needs of members of the population, limited resources must be used to the population's greatest advantage, and health is a societal value that should supersede other economic or social ends.

2. Program planning uses a five-step process that includes defining and prioritizing the issue to be addressed, creating the planning group, analyzing the issue, developing the program, and setting the stage for evaluation.

3. Defining and prioritizing the issue can be cumbersome and overwhelming. Using severity of the threat and degree of community's concern for the health problem as criteria may aid in prioritizing a population's health needs.

4. Five categories of participants should be included in creating a planning group: those in authority who must approve the program, people with expertise related to the issue, those who will implement the program, those who will benefit from the program, and those who might resist the program.

5. Analyzing the issue includes considering the contributing factors and potential alternative solutions as well as determining the level of prevention involved in its resolution; the costs, feasibility, acceptability, and availability of necessary resources; efficiency, equity, political advantages, and identifiability of the target group.

6. Program objectives are often the first step in the development of a program. Two types of program

POWERPOINT LECTURE SLIDES

NOTE: The number on each PPT Lecture Slide directly corresponds with the Concepts for Lecture.

1 Planning
- Collaborative, systematic process to attain a goal
- Collaboration through involving community and stakeholders
- Systematic process
  - Effective health systems respond to/are accountable to needs of population
  - Limited resources must be used to population's greatest advantage
  - Health supersedes other economic or social ends

2 Program Planning
- Utilizes five step process:
  - Define and prioritize issue to Be addressed
  - Create the planning group
  - Analyze the issue
  - Develop the program
  - Set the stage for evaluation

3 Define/Prioritize Issue to Be Addressed
- Severity of threat
- Degree of community's concern

4 Categories to Include When Creating a Planning Group
- Those in authority who approve program
- People with expertise related to issue
- Those who will implement program
- Those who will benefit from program
- Those who might resist program

5 Analyze Issue
- Contributing factors
- Alternative solutions

objectives must be considered: outcome objectives, which can include immediate, intermediate, and ultimate outcomes, and process objectives, which designate the level of expected performance of program staff in carrying out the program.

7. Evaluation involves four criteria, which include determining criteria to evaluate the program, determining types of data to be collected and the means used to collect the data, determining resources needed to carry out the evaluation, and determining who will evaluate the program.

- Determine level of prevention for problem resolution
- Determine costs, feasibility, and acceptability

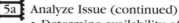 5a Analyze Issue (continued)
- Determine availability of necessary resources
- Determine efficiency
- Determine equity
- Identify political advantages

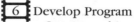 6 Develop Program
- Outcome objectives
  - Immediate, intermediate, and ultimate outcomes
- Process objectives
  - Designate level of expected staff performance

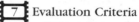 7 Evaluation Criteria
- Determine evaluation criteria
- Types of collection data
- Means of collecting data
- Resources needed to conduct evaluation
- Identify who will evaluate the program

SUGGESTIONS FOR CLASSROOM ACTIVITIES

Divide students into four groups. Each group is to identify a population health need or concern and develop a program for a community group outlining the steps involved in the process.

SUGGESTIONS FOR CLINICAL ACTIVITIES

Invite nurses who work with community programs to post conference to discuss the program's goals, objectives, and steps used to identify the need for the health program.

LEARNING OBJECTIVE 5

Analyze the elements of a program theory or logic model and its usefulness in health program planning.

CONCEPTS FOR LECTURE

1. A program theory or logic model is defined as an explanation of how elements of a program interact to produce the expected outcomes. It may also be a conceptual model of the interventions planned and how they work to achieve program outcomes. Generally, program theories are graphically displayed to demonstrate interrelationships among critical elements of the program and their relationship to expected outcomes.

POWERPOINT LECTURE SLIDES

NOTE: The number on each PPT Lecture Slide directly corresponds with the Concepts for Lecture.

1 Program Theory
- How elements of a program interact to produce outcomes
- Conceptual model of planned interventions and outcomes
- Graphically displayed interrelationships
  - Critical elements
  - Expected outcomes

1a Theory Types
- Theory of cause and effect
  - Links interventions with outcomes
- Theory of implementation
  - Describes strategies for program implementation

1b See Figure 15-1

LEARNING OBJECTIVE 6

Describe four levels of acceptance of a health care program.

CONCEPTS FOR LECTURE

1. Success of a health care program must have the acceptance and sanctioning of a number of groups. Acceptance of a planned program occurs at four levels, which include acceptance by community policy makers, acceptance by those who are tasked with implementing the program, acceptance and participation by members of the target group, and acceptance by potential resistors. Acceptance by policy makers may require the community health nurse to advocate for the plan or prepare community members to present the plan themselves. Acceptance by program implementers may only involve making the plan operational if they have been involved in all of the planning steps. Acceptance and participation of members of the target group may require marketing the program to that group. Acceptance by potential resistors is critical to the success or failure of a program. Early involvement in the planning process can positively influence this group of stakeholders.

POWERPOINT LECTURE SLIDES

NOTE: The number on each PPT Lecture Slide directly corresponds with the Concepts for Lecture.

1 Levels of Acceptance
- Community policy makers
- Program implementers
- Members of target group:
- Potential resistors:

1a Acceptance by Policy Makers
- May involve nurse as advocate

1b Acceptance by Program Implementers
- May only involve making plan operational

1c Acceptance by Members of Target Group
- May require marketing to that group

1d Acceptance by Potential Resistors
- Critical to success or failure of program
- Early involvement can positively influence this group

LEARNING OBJECTIVE 7

Describe three types of considerations in evaluating a health care program.

CONCEPTS FOR LECTURE

1. Programs are evaluated for a number of reasons including: to justify program continuation or expansion, to improve the quality of service, to determine future courses of action, to determine the impact of the program, to call attention to the program, to assess personnel performance, to assuage political expectation, and to make better programmatic decisions.

POWERPOINT LECTURE SLIDES

NOTE: The number on each PPT Lecture Slide directly corresponds with the Concepts for Lecture.

1 Program Evaluation
- Justify program continuation/expansion
- Improve quality of service

2. For program planners, there are several evaluation considerations in designing a health program. Planners must indentify the purpose and focus of the evaluation, such as how many people are served by the program. This, in turn, determines the type of data to be collected. Thirdly, planners must decide who will conduct the evaluation. Will the evaluators be the same individuals who designed the program, program beneficiaries, or outside experts? Fourth, the political context is essential in the timing for the implementation, and the amount and type of support received for the program. Ethical considerations include recognizing data that does not favorably support program implementation, and confidentiality considerations must be addressed early in the program design and evaluation process. Finally, program planners must consider the type of evaluation to be conducted. Prospective evaluation criteria are determined during the planning and development phase of the program, and retrospective evaluation is designed after the program is completed.

- Determine future courses of action
- Determine impact of program

 Program Evaluation (continued)
- Call attention to the program
- Assess personnel performance
- Assuage political expectations
- Make better programmatic decisions

 Considerations in Program Evaluation
- Purpose of the evaluation
- Who should conduct the evaluation
- Political considerations
- Ethical considerations
- Type of evaluation to be conducted
  ○ Prospective
  ○ Retrospective

SUGGESTIONS FOR CLASSROOM ACTIVITIES

Have students use the case study at the end of the chapter and develop an evaluation process for this community.

SUGGESTIONS FOR CLINICAL ACTIVITIES

Arrange for students to attend a health care program. Have students interview the program manager to determine types of evaluation methods designed for the program and results of those evaluation methods. Present interview results at post conference.

Meeting the Health Needs of Child and Adolescent Populations

RESOURCE LIBRARY

 COMPANION WEBSITE

Audio Glossary
Appendix C: Nursing Interventions for Common
  Health Problems in Children
Appendix H: Child and Adolescent Health Assessment
  and Intervention Guide
Exam Review Questions

Case Study: Promoting Children's Health and Safety
MediaLink Application: Adolescent Risk-Taking (video)
Media Links
Challenge Your Knowledge
Update *Healthy People 2010*
Advocacy Interviews

LEARNING OBJECTIVE 1

Identify factors affecting the health of children and adolescents.

CONCEPTS FOR LECTURE

1. Children and adolescents are an important demographic component of any society. In the United States, children under 18 years of age comprise 25% of the population. It is important to understand the health needs that are specific to this population.

2. Biophysical considerations for this population include understanding the effects of age and maturation, especially development and menarche. Development is a process of patterned, orderly, and lifelong change in structure, thought, or behavior that occurs as a result of physical or emotional maturation. Menarche is the first appearance of menstrual flow in adolescent girls. Abnormal conditions may occur as a result of early or delayed menarche. Children of different racial and ethnic groups are at higher risk of developing certain health conditions. Increased incidence and prevalence of specific health problems, accidents, congenital malformations, neoplasms, assault and homicide, and heart disease are all components of physiologic function as is the immunization level of the child and adolescent populations.

3. Psychological considerations include family dynamics, which can influence a child's self-image and self-esteem; parental expectations, which may lead to guilt and depression in children; discipline; parental coping or the presence of mental illness; mental

POWERPOINT LECTURE SLIDES

NOTE: The number on each PPT Lecture Slide directly corresponds with the Concepts for Lecture.

1 Child and Adolescent Populations
  • Comprise 25% of population
  • Health needs specific to population

2 Biophysical Considerations
  • Age and maturation
    ○ Development
    ○ Menarche
  • Genetic inheritance
    ○ Health problems specific to children

2a Child and Adolescent Populations (continued)
  • Physiologic function
    ○ Incidence/prevalence of specific physical
      health problems
    ○ Accidents
    ○ Congenital malformations
    ○ Neoplasms
    ○ Assault/homicide
    ○ Heart disease

3 Psychological Considerations
  • Family dynamics
  • Parental expectations

CONCEPTS FOR LECTURE continued

health problems in children, which affects approximately one in 10 U.S. children and adolescents; and physical, sexual, and psychological abuse, which can lead to drug and alcohol abuse, future prostitution, or increased sexual activity.

4. Physical environmental considerations include environmental health and safety issues related to age and physiology. Examples of increased risk include lead exposure, insecticide exposure, air pollution, safety hazards, accidents, and drownings.

5. Sociocultural considerations include factors affecting access to health care such as family income and employment, family educational level, parental work schedules, legislation, and the impact that media has in modeling healthy or unhealthy behaviors. Additional sociocultural considerations include childcare services and culturally defined roles and expectations of children and adolescents.

6. Behavioral considerations include nutrition and dietary practices, rest and exercise, exposure to hazardous substances resulting in conditions such as fetal alcohol syndrome and maternal smoking in pregnancy, tobacco and other drug use, sexual activity with outcomes such as unwanted pregnancy and sexually transmitted diseases, and violence by and against children and adolescents, and safety practices.

7. Health system considerations include attitudes toward health and health care; usual sources of health care, such as routine use of emergency departments as the primary source of care; and use patterns for health care services, which may be influenced by lack of insurance.

POWERPOINT LECTURE SLIDES continued

- Discipline
- Parental coping/mental health
- Mental health problems among children and adolescents
- Abuse

[4] Physical Environmental Considerations
- Susceptibility increased
- Lead exposure
- Insecticide exposure
- Air pollution
- Safety hazards
- Accidents/Drowning

[5] Sociocultural Considerations
- Factors affecting access to health care
  ○ Family income and employment
  ○ Family educational level
  ○ Parental work schedules
  ○ Legislation
  ○ Media impact on role models

[6] Behavioral Considerations
- Nutrition
- Rest and exercise
- Exposure to hazardous substances:
  ○ Fetal alcohol syndrome
- Sexual activity
- Violence

[7] Health System Considerations
- Attitudes toward health and health care
- Usual sources of health care
  ○ Routine use of emergency departments
- Use of health care services
  ○ Uninsured families

SUGGESTIONS FOR CLASSROOM ACTIVITIES

Have students research journal articles that discuss or address epidemiological factors for a child or adolescent health concern and provide a case summary of one those articles during class.

SUGGESTIONS FOR CLINICAL ACTIVITIES

Arrange for students to participate in well-child clinics, specialty clinics, or child find screening programs. Discuss at post conference the factors related to the health of the population represented in their clinical setting.

LEARNING OBJECTIVE 2

Describe at least five primary prevention measures appropriate to the care of children and adolescents and analyze the role of the community health nurse with respect to each.

CONCEPTS FOR LECTURE

1. Community health nurses have a number of interventions at the primary level that can support and promote the health of children and adolescents such as ensuring access to health care; reducing prematurity, low birth weight, and infant mortality; promoting growth and development; providing adequate nutrition; promoting safety; preventing communicable

POWERPOINT LECTURE SLIDES

NOTE: The number on each PPT Lecture Slide directly corresponds with the Concepts for Lecture.

[1] Primary Prevention Measures
- Ensure access to health care
- Reduce prematurity, low birth weight, and infant mortality

diseases; promoting optimal dental hygiene; and offering support for effective parenting resources. Other interventions may be employed to meet the primary prevention needs of children with special needs.

2. Ensuring access to health care is one of the most effective measures of promoting the health of children and adolescents. Several strategies are recommended such as ensuring that all children and adolescents have a regular source of primary health care, eliminating copayments and cost sharing for those services, establishing disincentives for seeking health care directly from specialists, including assessment of the adequacy of primary care services in quality assurance activities, supporting the education of primary providers, and developing information systems to monitor health activities among this population.

3. The community health nurse plays a vital role in reducing prematurity, low birth weight, and infant mortality by providing education about sexuality and contraception to the public and adolescents to prevent unintended pregnancies, advocating for effective and accessible contraceptive services, ensuring that health care services are available to pregnant teens and supporting teens in their role as parents, and providing prenatal nutritional education and making referrals for supplemental nutritional programs.

4. The community health nurse promotes growth and development by educating the public and families regarding developmental milestones that children and adolescents need to accomplish, alerting parents to the challenges posed by these milestones, advocating for community programs and environmental conditions that promote growth and development, and advocating for humanistic educational programs that promote emotional, cognitive, and physical development.

5. Community health nurses provide valuable nutritional support services through a number of activities: education of the public regarding the efficacy of breast-feeding and dietary needs and requirements for children and adolescents, promotion of policies that diminish access to "junk food" for children and adolescents, and advocating for nutritional supplemental programs and for adequate nutrition programs in schools and other institutional settings.

6. Community health nurses focus on safety when they promote the use of safety devices and equipment, educate families and children about the need for effective restraints, campaign for strict enforcement of restraint legislation for all vehicle occupants, educate the public about general safety behaviors and the use and storage of poisonous materials, advocate for effective labeling of hazardous substances, and become involved in suicide prevention activities with youth.

7. Community health nurses serve a vital role in preventing communicable diseases through immunization programs, campaigns, education of the general

- Promote growth and development
- Provide adequate nutrition

[1a] Primary Prevention Measures (continued)
- Promote safety
- Prevent communicable diseases
- Dental care
- Support for effective parenting

[2] Ensuring Access to Health Care
- Effective way to promote health
- Ensure regular source of primary health care
- Eliminate co-payments and cost sharing
- Establish disincentives for care directly from specialists

[2a] Ensuring Access to Health Care (continued)
- Assess adequacy of primary care services
- Support education of primary providers
- Develop information systems to monitor health activities

[3] Reducing Prematurity, Low Birth Weight, and Infant Mortality
- Provide education about sexuality and contraception to the public and adolescents to prevent unintended pregnancies
- Advocate for effective and accessible contraceptive services
- Ensure that health care services are available to pregnant teens
  ○ Support teens in their role as parents
- Provide prenatal nutritional education and make referrals for supplemental nutritional programs

[4] Promotion of Growth and Development: Role of Community Health Nurse
- Educate the public and families regarding developmental milestones that children and adolescents need to accomplish
- Alert parents to the challenges posed by these milestones
- Advocate for community programs and environmental conditions that promote growth and development
- Advocate for humanistic educational programs that promote emotional, cognitive, and physical development

[5] Providing Adequate Nutrition
- Educate the public regarding the efficacy of breastfeeding and dietary needs and requirements for children and adolescents
- Promote policies that diminish access to "junk food" for children and adolescents
- Advocate for nutritional supplemental programs and for adequate nutrition programs in schools and other institutional settings

CONCEPTS FOR LECTURE *continued*

public regarding practices to prevent specific communicable diseases such as HIV/AIDS, education about hygiene practices, and prevention of contamination of food and water supplies.

8. Dental hygiene is another focus area for community health nurses who educate parents about dental care in very young children, advocate for the need for preventive dental care, become involved in promoting fluoridation of community drinking water, educate parents about prevention of bottle-mouth syndrome, and provide referrals for financial assistance to families in need.

9. Community health nurses provide structural and functional support for effective parenting. Structural support is evidenced by establishing formal networks with families in need. Functional support is evidenced by education of families regarding the needs of children and adolescents (informational support), emotional support is demonstrated by interactions with parents who express the common frustrations of parenthood, instrumental support may be offered in referrals for respite services and childcare services for families in need, and appraisal support gives parents both positive and negative feedback on their performance as parents.

POWERPOINT LECTURE SLIDES *continued*

6 Promoting Safety: Role of Community Health Nurse
- Promote the use of safety devices and equipment
- Educate families and children about the need for effective restraints
- Campaign for strict enforcement of restraint legislation for all vehicle occupants
- Educate the public about general safety behaviors and the use and storage of poisonous materials
- Advocate for effective labeling of hazardous substances
- Become involved in suicide prevention activities with youth

7 Preventing Communicable Diseases: Role of Community Health Nurse
- Immunization programs and campaigns
- Educate the general public regarding practices to prevent specific communicable diseases such as HIV/AIDS
- Educate about hygiene practices
- Educate about the prevention of contamination of food and water supplies

8 Dental Care: Role of Community Health Nurse
- Educate parents about dental care in very young children
- Advocate for the need for preventive dental care
- Become involved in promoting fluoridation of community drinking water
- Educate parents about prevention of bottle-mouth syndrome
- Provide referrals for financial assistance to families in need

9 Effective Parenting Support: Role of Community Health Nurse
- Structural support for effective parenting
  - Establish formal networks with families in need
- Functional support
- Informational support: Educate families regarding the needs of children and adolescents

9a Effective Parenting Support: Role of Community Health Nurse (continued)
- Emotional support: Interact with parents who express the common frustrations of parenthood
- Instrumental support: Provide referrals for respite services and childcare services for families in need
- Appraisal support: Provide parents both positive and negative feedback on their performance as parents

LEARNING OBJECTIVE 3

Identify at least three approaches to providing secondary preventive care for children and adolescents and give examples of community health nursing interventions related to each.

CONCEPTS FOR LECTURE

1. Secondary prevention measures include screening for health problems soon after birth to improve outcomes and providing routine screening programs for children of all ages. Community health nurses may be involved in providing routine and specialized screening services or they may advocate for access to these services for child and adolescent populations.

2. The role of the community health nurse in the care of minor illnesses is evident when they educate the public about appropriate home treatment for minor illnesses and when professional care is required, educate parents about minor health problems in children and adolescents, educate on signs of illness in children, and assess the health status of specific children with recommendations for appropriate interventions or referrals for medical assistance.

3. Community health nurses perform secondary prevention services by providing care for children and adolescents with chronic conditions, which affect approximately 20 million U.S. children and increases family stressors. Specific interventions include: assisting families with medication management, behavioral modification, and advocating for environments that minimize the symptoms for children with ADHD, asthma or other conditions, as well as providing emotional support and recognizing the needs of those who care for children and adolescents with ADHD. Nurses may also provide referrals for services and counseling, provide education about the particular health condition, and promote healthy diets and physical activity.

4. Community health nurses provide secondary prevention services for the care of children and adolescents with terminal illnesses through their direct involvement in the provision of palliative care, the referral of clients for palliative care services, their work to assure the availability of palliative care services in the community and their accessibility to all those in need of them, and through their assistance with communication, emotional, and grief issues surrounding the dying child and their families.

POWERPOINT LECTURE SLIDES

NOTE: The number on each PPT Lecture Slide directly corresponds with the Concepts for Lecture.

1. Secondary Prevention Measures: Screen for Health Problems
   - Provide routine and specialized screening services
   - Advocate for access to these services for child and adolescent populations

2. Secondary Prevention Measures: Care of Minor Illnesses
   - Educate the public about appropriate home treatment for minor illnesses and when professional care is required
   - Educate parents about minor health problems in children and adolescents
   - Educate on signs of illness in children
   - Assess the health status of specific children
   - Make recommendations for appropriate interventions
   - Make referrals for medical assistance

3. Secondary Prevention Measures: Care of Children and Adolescents with Chronic Conditions
   - Assist with medication management
   - Advocate for environmental modification
   - Provide emotional support and recognize the needs of those caring for children and adolescents with chronic conditions
   - Provide referrals for services and counseling
   - Provide education about the particular health condition
   - Promote healthy diets and physical activity

4. Secondary Prevention Measures: Care of Children and Adolescents with Terminal Illnesses
   - Direct involvement in the provision of palliative care, the referral of clients for palliative care services, their work to assure the availability of palliative care services in the community and their accessibility to all those in need of them

POWERPOINT LECTURE SLIDES *continued*

- Assist with communication, emotional, and grief issues surrounding the dying child and their families

---

SUGGESTIONS FOR CLASSROOM ACTIVITIES

Assign students, as individuals or in groups, case studies of children or adolescents in need of or receiving secondary prevention interventions. Have students develop care plans with rationales for those interventions using evidence-based practice sources.

SUGGESTIONS FOR CLINICAL ACTIVITIES

Arrange for students to attend a genetics clinic, a cardiac clinic, an orthopedic clinic, or other clinics that provide services to children or adolescents with chronic or terminal illnesses. Assign students to develop a secondary prevention care plan using community resources and referrals that address family stressors and financial needs.

LEARNING OBJECTIVE 4

Describe three tertiary preventive considerations in the care of children and adolescents and analyze the role of the community health nurse with respect to each.

CONCEPTS FOR LECTURE

1. Tertiary prevention measures include preventing the recurrence of problems through education about bottle propping and otitis media, prevention of lead poisoning, and use of contraceptives; preventing further consequences through diabetic education and encouraging optimal self-care; and promoting adjustment for those children and adolescents with chronic illness or disability by preventing further loss of function and assisting families and children in the adaptation of lifestyles and behaviors in the presence of those chronic conditions.

POWERPOINT LECTURE SLIDES

NOTE: The number on each PPT Lecture Slide directly corresponds with the Concepts for Lecture.

1. Tertiary Prevention Measures
   - Prevent recurrence of problems
     - Educate about bottle propping and otitis media
     - Prevent lead poisoning
     - Promote use of contraceptives
   - Prevent further consequences
     - Diabetes education
   - Promote adjustment for those with chronic illness or disability
     - Prevent further loss of function

SUGGESTIONS FOR CLASSROOM ACTIVITIES

Divide students into groups. Assign each group a child or adolescent health-related concern or issue. Have groups develop a care plan using tertiary preventive measures and present a poster to the class for discussion.

SUGGESTIONS FOR CLINICAL ACTIVITIES

Arrange for students to work with a community health nurse to identify a child or adolescent health concern, and have students develop a teaching handout, a poster board, or any other project that addresses tertiary preventive measures for that target population.

Meeting the Health Needs of Women

RESOURCE LIBRARY

🌐 COMPANION WEBSITE

Audio Glossary
Appendix I: Adult Health Assessment and
  Intervention Guide
Case Study: Promoting Women's Health
Exam Review Questions

MediaLink Application: Discussing Menopause (video)
Media Links
Challenge Your Knowledge
Update *Healthy People 2010*
Advocacy Interviews

📖 IMAGE LIBRARY

Table 17-5 Routine Screening Recommendations for
Women

LEARNING OBJECTIVE 1

Identify at least two factors in each of the dimensions of health as they relate to the health of women.

CONCEPTS FOR LECTURE

1. Women's health is defined as health and illness issues that are unique to or more prevalent or serious in women. Women ages 20 to 64 comprise nearly 30% of the U.S. population. The national health objectives for 2010 include multiple objectives targeting the health needs of women. Even with recent attention to women's health needs, the American Association of Colleges of Nursing identified deficits in current knowledge of women's health care needs. Those areas include an understanding of the health consequences of trauma experienced by women; knowledge of gender-specific differences in development, manifestation, and treatment of specific conditions; lesbian and gay health issues; and health issues posed by women with disabilities.

2. Crucial to the understanding of women's health is our knowledge of the six dimensions of health. Biophysical considerations include genetically related or genetically linked conditions that affect women; maturation and aging issues such as premenopause, menopause, and postmenopause and conditions such as osteoporosis, heart disease, and cancer; physiologic

POWERPOINT LECTURE SLIDES

NOTE: The number on each PPT Lecture Slide directly corresponds with the Concepts for Lecture.

1 Women's Health
  • Definition
    ○ Health and illness issues unique to, more prevalent or serious in women

1a Women's Health (continued)
  • Demographics
  • Areas needing greater emphasis
    ○ Health consequences of trauma
    ○ Differences in development, manifestation, and treatment of specific conditions
    ○ Lesbian/gay health issues
    ○ Health issues specific to disabled women

2 Biophysical Considerations
  • Genetic inheritance
  • Maturation and aging
  • Physiologic functions
    ○ Physical illness and disability
      – Chronic illness

Concepts for Lecture *continued*

functions such as physical illness and disabilities resulting in chronic illness and its impact on women; reproductive issues such as contraception and infertility, and pregnancy; and immunization concerns for rubella, tetanus, and influenza.

3. Psychological considerations include the impact of stress on women's coping abilities, sexuality, and mental health and illness in women. Women's responses to life events may lead to increased stress, and distress related to interpersonal relationships, financial status, children, family health, and domestic violence. Depression is most common among women 18 to 44 years of age, but has been estimated to occur in 10% to 25% of all women.

4. Physical environmental considerations include repeated exposure to household chemicals, accidents and injuries in the home and workplace, and mineral deficiencies such as Vitamin D.

5. Sociocultural considerations include societal pressures regarding role and relationships, occupational and economic issues, and violence and abuse. Women's roles and responsibilities are culturally defined and may have an impact on women's health and well-being. Often, cultural groups place the needs of the family over the needs of the individuals, and women bear the consequences of limited access to health care. Women continue to earn less than three fourths of men's income even though 60% of adult females are employed in the United States. Women endure greater poverty issues related to delinquent child support, lower wages, and society's devaluing of traditional female jobs. An estimated 10% to 50% of women worldwide are assaulted by a male partner. Violence toward women is increased as a result of women's financial dependence on men, their partner's association with other women, and their partner's use of alcohol.

6. Behavioral considerations include dietary consumption patterns, such as fad diets, obesity, eating disorders, and nutrient deficiencies. Women's smoking patterns have failed to decline as rapidly as men's tobacco use. Smoking increases cancer incidence and cardiovascular disease, promotes urinary calcium excretion, and increases risks for osteoporosis. Women's substance abuse has seen increases in recent years. Physical activity and exercise can reduce the risk of hip fractures by 50%, yet over half of all U.S. women are sedentary. Sexual activity increases pregnancy and STD exposure risks.

7. Health system factors include a lack of attention to women's health needs except pertaining to reproductive issues, a lack of illness prevention and health promotion resources, disparities in health insurance coverage, a lack of support for the informal caregivers such as when women quit their jobs to care for sick children or elderly family members, and failure of health care providers to recognize signs of abuse.

PowerPoint Lecture Slides *continued*

2a Biophysical Considerations (continued)
- ○ Reproductive issues
  - – Contraception and infertility
  - – Pregnancy
- ○ Immunity

3 Psychological Considerations
- Stress and coping
- Sexuality
- Mental health and illness

4 Physical Environmental Considerations
- Exposure to household chemicals
- Accident and injury rates in home and workplace
- Vitamin D deficiencies

5 Sociocultural Considerations
- Roles and relationships
- Occupational and economic issues
- Violence and abuse

6 Behavioral Considerations
- Dietary consumption patterns
  - ○ Fad diets
  - ○ Obesity
  - ○ Eating disorders
  - ○ Nutrient deficiencies

6a Behavioral Considerations (continued)
- Tobacco, alcohol, and drug use
- Physical activity and exercise
- Sexual activity

7 Health System Considerations
- Lack of attention to women's health needs
  - ○ Focus primarily on reproductive issues
- Lack of illness prevention and health promotion resources
- Health insurance discrimination
- Lack of support for informal caregivers
- Failure of providers to recognize signs of abuse

LEARNING OBJECTIVE 2

Identify health problems common to women.

CONCEPTS FOR LECTURE

1. Health problems common to women include certain genetic predispositions to specific diseases such as thyroid disease, diabetes, asthma, dermatitis, and allergies.

2. Women also experience menarche with premenopausal, perimenopausal, menopausal, and postmenopausal physiologic health responses. For some cultures a women entering menarche is expected to submit to female genital mutilation. Approximately 3%–5% of women experience premenstrual dysphoric disorder (PMDD) during menstruation. For other women, perimenopause and menopause are accompanied by physical and psychological symptoms and discomforts.

3. There are physiologic function considerations that influence the health of women such as the incidence and prevalence of specific illnesses (e.g., heart disease, cancer, diabetes, stroke, Alzheimer's disease, rheumatoid arthritis, and osteoporosis) that place women as a population group at increased risk for multiple chronic physical illnesses and disability. Women also experience an increased incidence of disabilities and reported symptoms that affect self-care, self-image, and coping abilities.

4. While pregnancy-related mortality has decreased significantly in the United States, pregnancy-related deaths still occur each year. Maternal mortality worldwide can be a significant health issue in some countries. Perinatal transmission of HIV places women and their newborns at risk. While rates have decreased from 25% to 2% in the United States, other developing countries consider HIV infection endemic among women of childbearing age. Advanced maternal age at conception places women at risk for poor pregnancy outcomes. Pregnant women are also at risk for becoming victims of homicide with a homicide rate of 1.7 per 100,000 live births noted at one specific metropolitan hospital. Postpartum depression has been documented to affect not only women and their ability to care for and nurture their infant after delivery, but is correlated with delayed language development and behavior problems in their children.

5. Reproductive issues include contraception and infertility. Barriers to reproductive health include access to contraceptive methods and lack of education about contraception and pregnancy. Infertility may also have

POWERPOINT LECTURE SLIDES

NOTE: The number on each PPT Lecture Slide directly corresponds with the Concepts for Lecture.

1 Women's Health Problems
- Genetic predisposition to certain diseases
  - Thyroid diseases
  - Diabetes
  - Asthma
  - Dermatitis
  - Allergies

2 Menarche and Reproductive Concerns
- Cultural considerations
- Premenstrual dysphoric disorder (PMDD)
- Physiologic responses to menopause

3 Physiologic Functions Influencing Women's Health
- Incidence and prevalence of specific illnesses
  - Increased risk for multiple chronic diseases and disability
    - Examples: heart disease, cancer, stroke, Alzheimer's disease, diabetes, rheumatoid arthritis, osteoporosis
  - Increased incidence of disabilities and reported symptoms that affect self-care, self-image, and coping abilities

4 Pregnancy and Childbearing
- Pregnancy-related mortality
- Perinatal transmission of HIV
- Advanced maternal age at conception
- Pregnancy-related fatalities
  - Increased risk to become a victim of homicide
- Postpartum depression

5 Infertility and Contraception
- Access to and education about contraceptives
- Cultural implications of infertility
- Assistive reproductive technology and concomitant risks

6 Immunizations Levels
- Low immunization rates
  - Rubella
  - Tetanus
  - Influenza

strong cultural implications affecting a woman's social status, self-image, and stress level. For women with infertility concerns, assisted reproductive technology is associated with increased risk of complications of pregnancy.

6. While all adult immunization levels are cause for concern, immunizations of particular concern include rubella, tetanus, and influenza.

SUGGESTIONS FOR CLASSROOM ACTIVITIES

Divide students into groups. Assign each group to research a health problem frequently experienced by women and develop a poster board plan of care.

SUGGESTIONS FOR CLINICAL ACTIVITIES

1. Invite a women's health care practitioner to discuss health problems in women specific to the community. Have the guest speaker address referral resources and barriers to services.

2. Assign students to a women's health clinic or a clinic that serves specific target populations such as teenage girls. Have students perform an assessment by identifying at least two factors in each of the dimensions of health on a client from the clinical experience and present a case study to the class during post conference.

LEARNING OBJECTIVE 3

Describe at least three unique considerations in assessing the health needs of lesbian, bisexual, and transgender clients.

CONCEPTS FOR LECTURE

1. An estimated 1% of the U.S. female population is lesbian, and another 7% are believed to be bisexual. Women in these subpopulations may have health needs similar to their heterosexual counterparts, but they also have unique health needs that have been ignored by health providers and society. Biophysical considerations include varying risks for certain STDs and growing concern for reproductive health. Psychological considerations include feelings of isolation, coming out issues, and lack of societal understanding when relationship loss occurs. Sociocultural considerations include societal fears and misunderstandings such as homophobia and violence, discrimination, loss of social support, and legal issues. Behavioral considerations include varying use patterns of drugs, alcohol, and tobacco. Health system considerations include structural barriers, financial barriers, and personal and cultural barriers to health care access. Lesbian families may lack family insurance plans, which can limit use and access to health care. Health providers may not ask appropriate questions to identify health risks.

POWERPOINT LECTURE SLIDES

NOTE: The number on each PPT Lecture Slide directly corresponds with the Concepts for Lecture.

1 Health Needs of Lesbian Client
- Biophysical considerations
  - STD risks vary
  - Reproductive issues
- Psychological considerations
  - Feelings of isolation
  - Coming out issues
  - Lack of understanding about relationship loss issues

1a Health Needs of Lesbian Client (continued)
- Sociocultural considerations
  - Societal fears and misunderstandings
  - Discrimination
  - Loss of social support
  - Legal issues

1b Health Needs of Lesbian Client (continued)
- Behavioral considerations
  - Varying patterns of drug, alcohol, and tobacco use
- Health system considerations
  - Barriers to health care

SUGGESTIONS FOR CLASSROOM ACTIVITIES

Develop several short case studies that describe different types of health care issues pertaining to the lesbian client. Divide students into groups to discuss and develop a plan of care for their client.

SUGGESTIONS FOR CLINICAL ACTIVITIES

1. Arrange for students to spend time in a women's health clinic that offers services to lesbian, bisexual, or transgender clients. If services do not specifically address this subpopulation, then have students develop a plan of care for a lesbian client in the clinic.
2. Have students determine the extent to which services in the clinical setting are presented in a gender-neutral context. What changes might improve care for lesbian, bisexual, and transgender women in the setting?

LEARNING OBJECTIVE 4

Identify concerns in primary prevention for women and analyze the role of the community health nurse with respect to each.

CONCEPTS FOR LECTURE

1. Primary prevention for women is directed by four general wellness goals, which include maintaining balance, perspective, and priorities in life; developing and maintaining healthy relationships; developing and maintaining a healthy sense of self; and developing and maintaining a physically healthy body and preventing acute and chronic illness. Maintaining balance, perspective, and priorities in life means that women may need referrals to existing social service programs. Women, especially single mothers, may also need help in balancing multiple roles. Women caregivers may need assistance in learning to balance personal needs with those of family members or assistance with respite care. Developing and maintaining healthy relationships means that some women may need interventions in domestic violence prevention. Developing and maintaining a sense of self involves understanding specific developmental or maturational needs to maintain strong self-images, providing assistance for women in divorce or abuse situations, and providing anticipatory guidance in dealings with loss, guilt, or depression. Meeting the requirement of developing and maintaining a physically healthy body and preventing illness can involve prenatal care to underserved women, early case finding of pregnant women and referral for services, education about safety, immunizations, and benefits of abstinence from unhealthy behaviors.

POWERPOINT LECTURE SLIDES

NOTE: The number on each PPT Lecture Slide directly corresponds with the Concepts for Lecture.

1. Primary Prevention for Women
   - Maintaining balance, perspective, and priorities in life
   - Developing and maintaining healthy relationships
   - Developing and maintaining a healthy sense of self
   - Developing and maintaining a physically healthy body and preventing acute and chronic illness

---

SUGGESTIONS FOR CLASSROOM ACTIVITIES

Assign students to groups to prepare information on various primary prevention concerns in the community that are specific to women's health.

SUGGESTIONS FOR CLINICAL ACTIVITIES

Have students identify primary prevention services provided by their clinical agency or site that are specific to women's health and share them during post conference.

LEARNING OBJECTIVE 5

Describe areas of secondary prevention activity with women and design community health nursing interventions related to each.

CONCEPTS FOR LECTURE

1. Secondary prevention addresses screening, diagnosis, and treatment for existing health problems. Screening for existing health problems includes routine screening for breast and cervical cancer with PAP tests and mammograms, and education about the need for routine screening procedures in the female population.
2. The community health nurse can refer for medical assistance for diagnostic testing for infertility, fertility control, menopause, and physical abuse. Nurses can counsel, teach, and refer for all aspects of fertility control or pregnancy plans. Treatment for infertility requires a referral to a fertility specialist. Community health nurses provide case finding, referral, and support services.

POWERPOINT LECTURE SLIDES

NOTE: The number on each PPT Lecture Slide directly corresponds with the Concepts for Lecture.

1 Secondary Prevention for Women
- Refer to Table 17-5
- Existing health problems
- Screening
  - Breast and cervical cancer
  - Mammogram screening

1a Secondary Prevention for Women (continued)
- Diagnosis
  - Referral for medical or social assistance
    - Infertility/fertility control
    - Menopause
    - Physical abuse
- Treatment for existing problems

2 Role of Community Health Nurse
- Counsel, teach, and refer for all aspects of fertility control or pregnancy plans
- Referral to fertility specialist
- Provide case finding, referral, and support services

SUGGESTIONS FOR CLASSROOM ACTIVITIES

Have students work in groups to develop a plan of care for secondary prevention with a woman with a family history of breast cancer, a woman with health insurance with a new diagnosis of cervical cancer, a 40-year-old woman experiencing menopause, and a woman presenting to the clinic with signs of domestic abuse.

SUGGESTIONS FOR CLINICAL ACTIVITIES

Arrange for students to participate in a mobile mammogram service or women's health care clinic that offers fertility control services and cervical cancer screening services.

LEARNING OBJECTIVE 6

Describe two elements of secondary prevention of physical abuse of women and analyze the role of the community health nurse in addressing abuse.

CONCEPTS FOR LECTURE

1. Physical abuse of women has two dimensions. First, there are the physical and psychological effects of physical abuse, and second, there is the need to deal with the source of the problem. The first dimension requires recognition and education in the signs and symptoms of abuse.
2. The second dimension requires supportive counseling and reassurance to women of abuse when dealing with their own ambivalence and beliefs. Nurses can

POWERPOINT LECTURE SLIDES

NOTE: The number on each PPT Lecture Slide directly corresponds with the Concepts for Lecture.

1 Physical Abuse of Women: First Dimension
- Physical and psychological effects of abuse
  - Recognition of problem
  - Education in the signs and symptoms of abuse

assist women to explore alternative plans for solutions to the problem and help establish feelings of control and empowerment. Nurses also must be able to make appropriate referrals for medical care and counseling.

2 Physical Abuse of Women: Second dimension
- Dealing with source of problem
  - Supportive counseling
  - Reassurance
  - Establishing feelings of control and empowerment
  - Referrals for medical care and counseling

SUGGESTIONS FOR CLASSROOM ACTIVITIES

1. Have students bring in one article that pertains to domestic violence and physical abuse of women and present a summary of the article.
2. Divide students into groups to discuss common myths about women who experience abuse. Have them discuss how myths influence identification, treatment, and referrals for victims of abuse.

SUGGESTIONS FOR CLINICAL ACTIVITIES

1. Provide an opportunity for students to work in a shelter for women and children experiencing domestic violence. Have students identify and discuss secondary prevention elements provided at their clinical experience during post conference.
2. Invite a shelter staff person to present data on incidence and prevalence of domestic violence in the community, services provided, and safety concerns for women and staff.
3. Arrange for a police officer who deals with victims of violence to attend post conference to discuss how officers respond to domestic violence calls, current laws, and services available to women.

LEARNING OBJECTIVE 7

Describe at least two actions that the community health nurse can take to provide more sensitive and effective care to lesbian, bisexual, and transgender clients.

CONCEPTS FOR LECTURE

1. To provide more sensitive and effective care to lesbian, bisexual, and transgender clients, the community health nurse must gain an understanding of the similarities and differences between the subgroups and heterosexual population; identify support systems that are available; assist with referrals for legal support in the custody of children; gather data on lesbian, bisexual, and transgender perceptions and their use of health care services; and advocate for available screening services specific to this population.

POWERPOINT LECTURE SLIDES

NOTE: The number on each PPT Lecture Slide directly corresponds with the Concepts for Lecture.

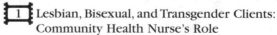 Lesbian, Bisexual, and Transgender Clients: Community Health Nurse's Role
- Gain understanding/insight into similarities and differences between subgroups and heterosexual population
- Identify support systems available
- Assist with availability of legal issues
- Gather data on their perceptions and use of health care services
- Advocate for available screening services
- Advocate for equitable treatment (e.g., inheritance laws, etc)

SUGGESTIONS FOR CLASSROOM ACTIVITIES

1. Have students bring in one research article that identifies community health nurse activities designed to gain understanding about this subgroup of women. Ask students to present a summary of their article.
2. Divide students into three groups. Each group is to compile a set of 10 questions that address a lesbian, bisexual, or transgender client's perception and use of health care services. Have each of the groups combine all 30 questions and discard questions that are redundant. Present final questions to class. Have students evaluate how these questions might be used during an initial health assessment.
3. Have students discuss their probable reaction and that of other family members if a sibling admitted to being lesbian or bisexual or experiencing gender dysphoria.

SUGGESTIONS FOR CLINICAL ACTIVITIES

If available, arrange for students to attend a support group for gay and lesbian couples. Have students identify common themes of concern, health issues, perceived or real barriers to health care, employment, family support or reactions, etc. During post conference, ask students to share their observations and responses, and to discuss the role of the community health nurse as an advocate for all population groups.

Meeting the Health Needs of Men

RESOURCE LIBRARY

 COMPANION WEBSITE

Audio Glossary
Appendix I: Adult Health Assessment and Intervention
 Guide
Exam Review Questions
Case Study: Promoting Men's Health

MediaLink Application: Prostate Cancer (video)
Media Links
Challenge Your Knowledge
Update *Healthy People 2010*
Advocacy Interviews

LEARNING OBJECTIVE 1

Describe major considerations in assessing the biophysical, psychological, physical environmental, sociocultural, behavioral, and health care system factors affecting men's health.

CONCEPTS FOR LECTURE

1. Adult males between the ages of 20 and 64 years comprise approximately 30% of the U.S. population. To understand men's health issues it is important to recognize differences in the incidence and prevalence of health conditions in men, differences in health-related habits and factors that create barriers to the use of health services, and differences in social roles, stress, and coping that contribute to specific health-related problems. Underscoring these factors is the lack of emphasis on holistic health for men and lack of recognition in the national health objectives for this approach to health care for men.

2. Biophysical considerations in understanding the health care needs of men include recognition that men have higher incidences of morbidity with the leading causes of death being heart disease, malignant neoplasms, unintentional injuries, cerebrovascular disease, chronic lower respiratory diseases, and diabetes mellitus. Additionally, men tend to have higher rates of sexually transmitted diseases. Testicular cancer is also the most common cancer in men 15 to 44 years of age and represents 2% of all cancers in men. Recent attention has been called to erectile dysfunction (ED), which occurs when a man cannot achieve or maintain an erection sufficient for satisfactory sexual activity. This condition affects approximately 35% of all men 40 to 70 years of age and rates increase with age.

POWERPOINT LECTURE SLIDES

NOTE: The number on each PPT Lecture Slide directly corresponds with the Concepts for Lecture.

1 Men's Health
- Men comprise approximately 30% of U.S. population
- Differences
  - Physiologic health differences
  - Differences in health-related habits/ health-seeking behaviors
  - Differences in social role, stress, and coping
- Lack of holistic approach to men's health

2 Biophysical Considerations
- Higher levels of morbidity
- Leading causes of death
  - Heart disease
  - Malignant neoplasms
  - Unintentional injuries

2a Biophysical Considerations (continued)
- Leading causes of death
  - Cerebrovascular disease
  - Chronic lower respiratory diseases
  - Diabetes mellitus

2b Biophysical Considerations (continued)
- Higher rates of STDs
- Testicular cancer
- Erectile dysfunction

3. Psychological considerations include socialization issues related to society's stereotype of male roles. This creates situations of social pressure to be strong and self-reliant. As a result, men may need to perceive themselves as healthy and invulnerable, which affects their willingness to seek or use health care services. Mental health problems arise from an inability to express healthy emotions, which can contribute to depression. Increased stress and diminished coping abilities contribute to higher incidences of suicide in men.

4. Health responses to pollution, overcrowding, and safety hazards are the same in men as for women, but men appear to have increased exposure to environmental hazards as a result of occupational and leisure activity choices.

5. Sociocultural considerations affecting men's health include family interactions such as parenting, lack of preparation for childcare experiences, and divorce, which may increase suicide risks resulting from diminished self-image and self-worth or homicidal behaviors if anger is directed outward. Economic and occupational issues affecting men's health include unemployment or joblessness and its association with lower educational levels. Violence in families, also known as intimate partner violence, affects men as victims of abuse, yet men are less likely to report physical or emotional abuse.

6. Behaviors affecting men's health include consumption patterns leading to higher obesity rates, substance use and abuse contributing to three times more alcohol-related motor vehicle accidents, physical risks related to competitive contact sports and leisure activities involving physical risk, socialization expectations resulting in reports of greater numbers of sexual partners than women, and other behavioral risk factors resulting in less use of seat belts and safety helmets. More recent behaviors include an increase in genital piercing and complications arising from this behavior.

7. In the health system dimension, men tend to define health as the ability to be employed and to be economically independent. This health perception affects men's readiness to utilize health care services. Other factors affecting men's use of health care systems include gender socialization, lack of trust in providers, language barriers, lack of health insurance, and perceived lack of need for health care. False perceptions of good health result in a delay in seeking assistance, delays in diagnosis and treatment, and potential for higher levels of poor outcomes.

3 Psychological Considerations
- Socialization
  - Male role social pressures
  - Perceptions of health/invulnerability

3a Psychological Considerations (continued)
- Mental health
  - Self-expression
  - Depression less likely to be diagnosed
- Stress and coping abilities
  - Suicide

4 Physical Environmental Considerations
- Effects of environment same as for women
  - Pollution
  - Overcrowding
  - Safety hazards
- Increased exposure to environmental hazards
  - Occupation/Leisure activity choices

5 Sociocultural Considerations
- Family interactions
- Economic/occupational issues
  - Unemployment/joblessness
- Issues related to violence/trauma
  - Intimate partner violence
  - Unintentional injuries

6 Behavioral Considerations
- Consumption patterns
  - Diet
  - Substance use/abuse

6a Behavioral Considerations (continued)
- Exercise and leisure
  - Competitive contact sports
  - Physical risk leisure activities
  - Sexual activity

6b Behavioral Considerations (continued)
- Other behavioral risk factors
  - Use of seat belts/safety devices
  - Increase in genital piercing

7 Health Care System Considerations
- Health perceptions
  - Ability to be employed
  - Economic independence

7a Factors Affecting Use of Health Care Services
- Gender socialization
- Lack of trust in providers
- Language barriers
- Lack of health insurance
- Perceived lack of need for health care

LEARNING OBJECTIVE 2

Describe factors that contribute to adverse health effects for gay, bisexual, and transgender men.

CONCEPTS FOR LECTURE

1. Definitions to clarify the use of the terms *gay, bisexual,* and *transgender* generally include three dimensions: one's sexual identity orientation, sexual behavior, and/or sexual attraction. Estimates are that 1 million to 3 million gay men are over 65 years of age. Due to their marginal status in society, this aging population may have more difficulty in obtaining assistance in old age and are reluctant to seek medical care.

2. Gay, bisexual, and transgender men tend to be at greater risk for a number of physical health problems, especially sexually transmitted diseases such as syphilis, lymphogranuloma venereum, and other conditions related to anal insertive sexual activity. This subpopulation of males has the usual immunization requirements with the additional requirements for hepatitis A and B. Barriers related to underutilization of health care services arise from discriminatory attitudes among health care providers and prior negative experiences with health professionals.

3. Psychological considerations to the understanding of gay, bisexual, and transgender health are gender dysphoria, which is defined as a sense of incongruity between one's physical gender and one's self-perceptions. This gender identity disorder increases men's risk for suicide, auto-castration, or substance abuse due to increased distress. This subgroup of men tends to be at risk for partner violence and depression, and they often have a history of child abuse. Suicide is higher in younger gay, bisexual, and transgender males, but overall suicide attempts are higher for this subpopulation.

4. Sociocultural considerations can have a profound impact on the health status and health-related behaviors of gay, bisexual, and transgender men. Sociological minority refers to any segment of the population subjected to negative acts and behaviors inflicted by the rest of society. Heterosexism is defined as an ideological system that denies, denigrates, and stigmatizes any nonheterosexual form of behavior. Both of these terms represent cultural conflicts that can have a negative impact on gay, bisexual, and transgender men. Compounding negative societal attitudes is the family reactions and responses to disclosure, which can result in isolation. Responses to disclosure vary according to the strength of traditional gender role conceptions,

POWERPOINT LECTURE SLIDES

NOTE: The number on each PPT Lecture Slide directly corresponds with the Concepts for Lecture.

1 Adverse Health Effects for Gay, Bisexual, and Transgender Men
- Definition
- Demographics
  - Estimates of 2.8% to 9% of U.S. men
  - 1 million to 3 million gay men over 65 years of age

2 Biophysical Considerations
- Physical health problems
  - STDs
  - Other conditions
- Immunization requirements
  - The usual requirements, plus hepatitis A and B

2a Barriers to Health Care Utilization
- Perceived or actual health professional discrimination
- Prior negative experiences

3 Psychological Considerations
- Gender dysphoria
  - Increased risks
    - Suicide
    - Auto-castration
    - Substance abuse

3a Psychological Considerations (continued)
- Partner violence
- Depression
- History of childhood abuse

4 Sociocultural Considerations
- Sociological minority
- Heterosexism
- Cultural conflicts
- Family Interactions
  - Response to disclosure

4a Societal Misperceptions
- Transmission to children

4b Occupational Risks of Self-disclosure
- Discrimination and rejection

perceptions of the probable attitudes of significant others in the family's social network, and parental age and educational level. Societal misperceptions that homosexuality can be transmitted to children has prompted significant research in the area, which has shown little impact of parental sexual orientation on children's gender identity. Occupational risks and concerns center on discrimination and rejection in the workplace.

5. Increased prevalence of drug abuse, increased risk of HIV, increased incidence of unprotected sexual activities with the potential for nondisclosure of HIV status to partner, sexual motivation, and sex trading behaviors are important to the community health nurse working with gay, bisexual, and transgender men. Sexual motivation includes pleasure-focused motivation, partner-focused motivation, and relationship-focused motivation with the latter more likely to have a steady partner. Sex trading is defined as engaging in sexual activity in return for money, drugs, shelter, or food and places men at risk for STDs.

6. The greatest impact on the use of health care systems by gay, bisexual, or transgender men is discrimination by health professionals, discrimination in health care settings, providers lacking knowledge about this subpopulation's health care needs, and the limited availability of transgender surgery.

5 Behavioral Considerations
- Prevalence of drug use
- Increased risk of HIV
- Unprotected sexual practices
  ○ Non-disclosure of HIV status
- Sexual motivation
- Sex trading

6 Health Care System Considerations
- Homophobia/heterosexism among health care workers
- Discrimination in health care settings
- Confidentiality issues
- Lack of providers knowledgeable about health care needs
- Transgender surgical availability

SUGGESTIONS FOR CLASSROOM ACTIVITIES

1. Provide students with an opportunity to discuss openly their beliefs about the health care needs of gay, bisexual, and transgender men.
2. Have students research one health care problem pertaining to gay, bisexual, or transgender men and discuss their findings in class.
3. Have students search the Internet for resources for gay, bisexual, and transgender men and discuss in class the credibility, usefulness, and potential agendas of those sources.

SUGGESTIONS FOR CLINICAL ACTIVITIES

1. Invite a guest speaker from a local support group or agency that serves gay, bisexual, and transgender men to post conference to discuss health issues pertaining to this population of men.
2. Examine the extent of support available (or lack of support) on campus for gay, bisexual, and transgender men.

LEARNING OBJECTIVE 3

Identify major considerations in primary prevention for men and analyze the role of the community health nurse with respect to each.

CONCEPTS FOR LECTURE

1. Primary prevention for men's health-related conditions focuses on common patterns of health behaviors. Nurses can develop strategies to change men's attitudes toward health and health-related behaviors by addressing reframing principles, which assist men in seeing the same situation from a different perspective, and emphasize alternative ways of coping with anxiety or fear.

POWERPOINT LECTURE SLIDES

NOTE: The number on each PPT Lecture Slide directly corresponds with the Concepts for Lecture.

1 Primary Prevention for Men
- Changing attitudes to health and health-related behaviors
  ○ Reframing

CONCEPTS FOR LECTURE *continued*

2. Nurses can promote the use of health-promoting behaviors by targeting injury prevention and safe sexual practices; promoting effective coping strategies for men with chronic illnesses; educating about chronic disease issues such as the importance of adequate nutrition, physical activity, weight control, and elimination of behaviors such as tobacco use; and advocating environmental modifications at the workplace to reduce work-related injuries and chronic diseases from exposure to hazardous substances.
3. Nurse can participate in immunization clinics and encourage other providers to provide immunization services for tetanus, hepatitis A and B, influenza, and pneumonia for high-risk male populations.

POWERPOINT LECTURE SLIDES *continued*

2 Increase Use Of Health-promoting Behaviors
- Injury prevention
- Safe sexual practices
- Educate for prevention/elimination of high-risk behaviors
- Environmental modifications
- Promote coping strategies

3 Immunizations

SUGGESTIONS FOR CLASSROOM ACTIVITIES

1. Have students develop a primary intervention care plan for a health-related concern for men.
2. Have students develop a health promotion or health education pamphlet that targets one health concern for men.

SUGGESTIONS FOR CLINICAL ACTIVITIES

Assign students to work in the occupational health branch of the local health department if available in the community. Ask students to note occupations at greater risk for morbidity and mortality and report their observations during post conference. Have students bring in health promotion or health-related materials targeted to men's health.

LEARNING OBJECTIVE 4

Describe secondary prevention considerations for men and related community health nursing roles.

CONCEPTS FOR LECTURE

1. Nursing goals at the secondary prevention level are to participate in health screening activities, providing or encouraging the male client's use of such health measures as blood pressure screening and cardiovascular risk-assessment programs. Other screening programs include rectal examinations, blood testing for prostate cancer, and chest x-rays for lung cancer.
2. Nurses can encourage other health care professionals to include secondary screening measures in their routine health services. Additional nursing interventions include teaching and motivating male clients to perform testicular self-exams, especially targeting young males. Community health nurses may advocate for routine health services, especially for low-income and uninsured men. Nurses may refer men with existing health problems for medical evaluation and treatment.
3. Treatment programs that identify high-stress clients during hospitalization, that track and reduce their stress levels after discharge, and that provide prompt assistance from community health nurses when episodes of increased stress occur can result in significant reduction of stress-related mortality.

POWERPOINT LECTURE SLIDES

NOTE: The number on each PPT Lecture Slide directly corresponds with the Concepts for Lecture.

1 Secondary Prevention for Men
- Effective screening
  - Rectal examinations
  - Blood testing for prostate cancer
  - Chest x-rays for lung cancer
  - Other screening procedures

2 Secondary Screening Measures
- Teach and motivate male clients to perform testicular self-exams

2a Advocate for Routine Health Services for Low-Income and Uninsured Men
- Referral for medical evaluation and treatment of health needs or disorders

3 Identification of High-stress Clients
- Treatment programs that track and reduce stress levels
- Can significantly reduce stress-related mortality

SUGGESTIONS FOR CLASSROOM ACTIVITIES

Provide students with case studies of men of varying ages with acute and chronic health-related conditions. Have students break out into groups to discuss secondary prevention strategies for intervention.

SUGGESTIONS FOR CLINICAL ACTIVITIES

Arrange for students to have a clinical experience with a community screening program such as health fairs for war veterans, health-department-organized health fairs, or community-organized, hospital-based health fairs. Have students perform blood pressures, blood testing, or other screening procedures.

LEARNING OBJECTIVE 5

Identify areas of emphasis in tertiary prevention for men and analyze the role of the community health nurse in each.

CONCEPTS FOR LECTURE

1. Nursing interventions at the tertiary level include assisting men in coping with continuing manifestations of illness and reducing the likelihood of future episodes of illness by encouraging men to join cancer, sexual dysfunction, or cardiac support groups.
2. Nurses may also advocate for development of and access to services for these health concerns. They may become instrumental in changing men's attitudes toward these problems and influence their willingness to seek help.

POWERPOINT LECTURE SLIDES

NOTE: The number on each PPT Lecture Slide directly corresponds with the Concepts for Lecture.

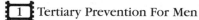 1 Tertiary Prevention For Men
- Assist men in coping with continuing manifestations of illness
  ○ Testicular cancer
  ○ Erectile/sexual dysfunction
  ○ Cardiovascular disorders
- Reduce likelihood of future episodes of illness
  ○ Encourage compliance with long-term treatment recommendations

2 Advocate for Access to Services
- Change men's attitudes toward health concerns
- Influence willingness to seek help

SUGGESTIONS FOR CLASSROOM ACTIVITIES

Divide students into three groups. Provide each group with a list of medications that are used for sexual dysfunction, cardiovascular disorders, and cancer treatment. Have students prepare 3 × 5 cards on these medications and develop a list of barriers to their access and use. Provide an opportunity for discussion about the role of the community health nurse in mitigating those barriers.

SUGGESTIONS FOR CLINICAL ACTIVITIES

Invite guest speakers from various support groups for men with chronic health conditions, representatives from a veteran's medical facility, and community health professionals to discuss service availability, barriers to access, and other issues or concerns for men's health.

19 CHAPTER

Meeting the Health Needs of Older Clients

RESOURCE LIBRARY

COMPANION WEBSITE

Audio Glossary
Appendix I: Adult Health Assessment and
  Intervention Guide
Exam Review Questions
Case Study: Caring for the Aged

MediaLink Application: Defying Ageism (video)
Media Links
Challenge Your Knowledge
Update *Healthy People 2010*
Advocacy Interviews

LEARNING OBJECTIVE 1

Describe three categories of theories of aging.

CONCEPTS FOR LECTURE

1. Aging is defined as maturation and senescence of biological systems. Senescence is defined as the progressive deterioration of body systems that can increase the risk of mortality as an individual gets older. While both may be associated with a gradual and progressive loss of function over time, they do not necessarily mean that there is an increase in disease.

2. The U.S. older population has been steadily increasing with 12.4% of the population over the age of 65, and projections to reach nearly 20% by 2030. The proportion of people over 65 years of age has increased as a result of two factors: increasing life expectancy and decreasing fertility. This phenomenon is mirrored worldwide as well.

3. With the world's older population increasing, societies must meet the demand for health care services. Of importance to understanding older client care is the fact that people over 65 years of age account for 45% of all hospital care and 38% of all hospital discharges. Costs for these services can create financial burdens on the individuals, families, and communities. The National Health Objectives for 2010 emphasize the need to reduce activity limitations that impair the quality of life for older persons.

4. Theories on aging originate from three distinct perspectives. Biological theories explain biophysical changes that occur in aging through programmed theories and error theories. Programmed aging theories

POWERPOINT LECTURE SLIDES

NOTE: The number on each PPT Lecture Slide directly corresponds with the Concepts for Lecture.

1 Aging
  • Maturation and senescence of biological systems

2 Aging Population
  • Over 12.4% of U.S. population is over 65
  • Projected increase to 20% by 2030
    ○ Increased life expectancy
    ○ Decreased fertility

3 Growing Demand for Services
  • Increased usage of hospital care services
  • Financial burdens
  • National Health Objectives
    ○ Emphasize reducing activity limitations that impair quality of life

4 Biological Theories of Aging
  • Biophysical changes
    ○ Programmed theories
      - Regulation by genetic codes
      - Address longevity, endocrine, and immune function
    ○ Error theories
      - Environmental assaults
      - Metabolic toxins accumulate and impair function

CONCEPTS FOR LECTURE *continued*

suggest that genetic codes regulate cell reproduction and death and that organ deterioration and eventual death are programmed into one's genetic makeup. Such theories address longevity, declining endocrine function, and declining immune function. Error theories hypothesize that cumulative environmental assaults stretch the body's ability to respond and cause accumulation of metabolic toxins that impair normal function.

5. Psychological theories of aging focus on psychological changes that occur with age. These theories suggest that effective aging requires development of effective coping strategies over time. Jung's theory of individualism, which proposes that an individual's mental focus changes from the external to the internal world, and Erikson's stage theory of development, which delineates eight stages of life, are two major psychological theories.

6. Sociological theories of aging focus on changes in roles and relationships that occur with advancing age. Disengagement theory proposes that individuals disengage from life as a means of making way for a younger generation in preparation for death. In activity and continuity theories, older persons maintain their interest in life, but their specific interests change.

POWERPOINT LECTURE SLIDES *continued*

5 Psychological Theories
- Effective aging results from development of effective coping strategies
- Jung's theory of individualism
- Erikson's stage theory of development

6 Sociological Theories
- Changes in roles and relationships
- Disengagement theory
- Activity and continuity theories

SUGGESTIONS FOR CLASSROOM ACTIVITIES

Using the case study at the end of the chapter, divide students into three groups. Assign each group to one of the aging theories and ask them to discuss how the theory applies to the case scenario.

SUGGESTIONS FOR CLINICAL ACTIVITIES

Assign each group to use a theory to develop a nursing care plan for the older client in the case study.

LEARNING OBJECTIVE 2

Describe biophysical, psychological, physical environmental, sociocultural, behavioral, and health system factors influencing the health of the elderly population.

CONCEPTS FOR LECTURE

1. Biophysical factors for the older client are those related to maturation and aging and physiologic function. One goal for community health nursing for older clients is to foster healthy aging and to promote active aging. Healthy and active aging is defined as the process of optimizing opportunities for health, participation, and security in order to enhance quality of life as people age.

2. Elderly populations must understand three essential requisites to healthy aging: accepting the limitations posed by bodily changes, modifying one's lifestyle as needed to accommodate these changes, and developing new personal standards of achievement and life goals consistent with the constraints imposed by the effects of aging.

POWERPOINT LECTURE SLIDES

NOTE: The number on each PPT Lecture Slide directly corresponds with the Concepts for Lecture.

1 Biophysical Considerations for Older Client
- Nursing goals
  - Foster healthy aging
  - Promote active aging

2 Essential Requirements to Healthy Aging
- Accept limitations posed by bodily changes
- Modify one's lifestyle
- Develop new personal standards

3. Community health nurses must be aware of mortality and morbidity rates for specific chronic health conditions such as heart disease, malignancies, arthritis, diabetes, and cerebrovascular disease. Chronic disease can lead to functional limitations and disability. Acute health conditions include accidental injuries such as falls and subsequent hip fractures. Vaccine-preventable diseases such as influenza and pneumonia constitute the fifth leading cause of death in people over 85 years of age.

4. Psychological considerations affecting the health of older clients that are important for the nurse to know include cognitive impairment such as Alzheimer's disease, stress and the effects of diminished resources for treatment, and depression, which is often undiagnosed due to co-morbidity with critical illness.

5. Physical environmental considerations affect the health of older populations by increasing safety hazards resulting from older housing, and exposure to heat and cold extremes. Older populations may experience quality of life issues resulting from living in older neighborhoods with increased crime rates, garbage, poor lighting, and inadequate transportation. There may also be direct effects from the physical environment such as the effects of ozone and pollution on health.

6. Sociocultural considerations that have an impact on older clients' health include changes in family roles and responsibilities, decreasing social support, economic and employment factors, and abuse and violence directed toward this population group. The incidence of elder abuse, both physical and financial, has coincided with the rise in this population, with rates increasing by 150%.

7. Nurses need to be aware of changing dynamics in families. With older people raising grandchildren there are indications of increased incidences of depression, insomnia, hypertension, diabetes, functional limitations, and poor self-reported health for these caregivers. Often older caregivers do not receive assistance for raising children, and nurses play a role in identifying community resources, financial assistance, and support networks. Economic factors such as income levels have a direct link to health. When older people have diminished economic resources, access to care and utilization of health services can be negatively impacted. Employment and retention of older people in the workforce has varying effects on this population as well as on society.

8. Behavioral factors include diet and consumption patterns, physical activity, sexuality, and medication use. Nutritional factors include proper dentition, diminished gastric secretions and motility, and diminished sense of taste and smell, all of which can lead to malnutrition, dehydration, and specific nutritional deficiencies. Dehydration is a leading diagnosis in emergency departments. Nutritional deficiencies can lead to osteoporosis. Exercise provides both physical and

3 Mortality and Morbidity Rates for Chronic Conditions
- Physiologic function
  - Acute and chronic conditions
  - Immunizations

4 Psychological Considerations
- Cognitive impairment
  - Dementia
    - Alzheimer's disease
- Stress
  - Fewer resources
- Depression
  - Undiagnosed

5 Physical Environmental Considerations
- Safety hazards
- Direct effects

6 Sociocultural Considerations
- Changes in family roles and responsibilities
- Social support
- Economic and employment factors
- Abuse and violence
  - Increased incidence of financial and physical abuse

7 Changing Dynamics in Families
- More older people are raising grandchildren
- Increased incidence of health problems for caregivers
- Impact of economic factors
  - Diminished access to care
  - Less utilization of health services
  - Employment and workforce retention of older population

7a Nurse's Role in Meeting the Health Needs of the Older Client
- Identify community resources
- Identify financial assistance resources
- Identify support networks

8 Behavioral Considerations
- Diet and consumption patterns
- Physical activity
- Sexuality
- Medication use

9 Health System Considerations
- Demand on health care services
- Health care access
- Costs of health care for uninsured
- Lack of appropriate medical services
- Societal response to high costs of medications
- Client-provider interaction

psychological benefits. Sexuality is important to older clients, with physical conditions and certain medications impacting healthy sexual functioning. Older clients are at risk for medication misuse and complications from multiple prescriptions for acute and chronic conditions and mixing of herbal medications with prescriptions. Other factors to consider are non-adherence in medications, cost of medications, and inappropriate medication use.

9. Health system factors include the increasing demand on health care services, access to health care, the cost of health care for uninsured older populations, lack of appropriate medical services, societal and governmental responses to high cost of medications, and the quality of provider knowledge about health care needs.

SUGGESTIONS FOR CLASSROOM ACTIVITIES

Divide students into six groups. Assign each group a health consideration category. Ask students to identify barriers to care and nursing actions.

SUGGESTIONS FOR CLINICAL ACTIVITIES

Have students work in various agencies in the community that provide health and mental health services to older people. Ask them to report on common health care needs for their target population.

LEARNING OBJECTIVE 3

Identify major considerations in primary prevention in the care of older adults and analyze community health nursing roles related to each.

CONCEPTS FOR LECTURE

1. The Centers for Disease Control has taken the lead in identifying roles for which health promotion should be directed for the older population. These roles include the following: provide high-quality information and resources to health care providers, support prevention activities by local providers and organizations, integrate public health prevention expertise with networks of services, identify and implement effective prevention efforts, and monitor changes in the health status of the older population.

2. Primary prevention of disability requires the interruption of three pathways: prevention or delay of fragility; prevention, recognition, and treatment of conditions that contribute to disability; and alteration of the environment to promote independence and prevent disability.

POWERPOINT LECTURE SLIDES

NOTE: The number on each PPT Lecture Slide directly corresponds with the Concepts for Lecture.

1 Strategies for Primary Prevention
- Provide high-quality information and resources to health care providers
- Support prevention activities by local providers and organizations
- Integrate public health prevention expertise with networks of services
- Identify and implement effective prevention efforts
- Monitor changes in health status of older population

2 Prevent Disability
- Prevent or delay fragility
- Prevent, recognize, and treat conditions that contribute to disability
- Alter environment to promote independence/prevent disability

LEARNING OBJECTIVE 4

Describe secondary preventive measures for at least four health problems common among older clients.

CONCEPTS FOR LECTURE

1. Secondary prevention strategies focus on screening and treatment of disease and self-management for conditions of chronic illness. Screening for older clients tends to be neglected, with reasons ranging from poor prognosis to lack of education of providers about the long-term benefits for screening and early treatment. Community health nurses can educate older clients about the need for routine screening and provider referral screening services. Nurses may also advocate for access to screening services.

2. Effective chronic disease control requires supportive care, self-management, maintenance of function, and prevention of further disability. Requisites for self-management include physical, environmental, mental, and socioeconomic factors that promote effective disease management. Older clients must also have the knowledge and skills needed to discontinue unhealthy behaviors and to learn and execute replacement behaviors and other related behaviors. Older clients must also have the desire to cope with their illness and take action.

3. Client activities for self-management include symptom response and monitoring, compliance with medical and lifestyle regimens such as managing medications, and development of the skills needed for self-management. Interventions to assist with effective medication management may include prompting devices, electronic dispensers, monitoring devices, and data management systems. Nurses may also provide information to clients about Web sites that provide comparisons of the effectiveness of specific medications.

4. For specific secondary interventions for common health problems, the nurse may recommend effective approaches, such as decreasing fluid intake after evening meals for urinary incontinence, noting dietary intake patterns, being prepared with supplies and extra clothing, and planning frequent stops when traveling. For other health problems such as substance abuse, depression, COPD, chronic pain, and mobility limitations, community health nurses can provide education, identify barriers to care and treatment, and advocate for access to care.

POWERPOINT LECTURE SLIDES

NOTE: The number on each PPT Lecture Slide directly corresponds with the Concepts for Lecture.

1. Secondary Prevention Strategies
   - Screening and treatment
     - Perceptions of poor prognosis
     - Need for education about long-term benefits

2. Chronic Disease Control
   - Supportive care
   - Self-management
   - Maintain function
   - Prevent further disability

2a. Chronic Disease Control (continued)
   - Self-management requisites
     - Promote effective disease management
     - Knowledge and skills needed to discontinue unhealthy behaviors
     - Desire to cope and take action

3. Client Activities for Self-Management
   - Symptom response/monitoring
   - Medical/lifestyle/medication compliance
     - Prompting and monitoring devices
     - Electronic dispensers
     - Data management systems
     - Provide Internet resources

4. Specific Secondary Interventions
   - Behavioral strategies
   - Dietary intake patterns
   - Psychological effects of preparation
   - Common health problems
   - Educate and identify barriers to care and treatment
   - Provide advocacy for access to care

SUGGESTIONS FOR CLASSROOM ACTIVITIES

Have students select one medical condition or health-related concern for older clients and research data about morbidity and mortality and factors that affect outcomes. Ask them to select one article from the nursing literature that addresses older population needs and intervention strategies for their health-related concern. Provide an opportunity for discussion of the role of community health nurse for screening and education.

SUGGESTIONS FOR CLINICAL ACTIVITIES

Arrange for students to work with a community health nurse who provides services for older clients. Assess available screening and treatment services for this population and identify four health concerns prevalent in the community. Discuss experiences and secondary prevention strategies during post conference.

LEARNING OBJECTIVE 5

Identify at least three foci for tertiary prevention with older clients and give examples of related community health nursing interventions.

CONCEPTS FOR LECTURE

1. Tertiary prevention strategies focus on the monitoring of health status by providing opportunities for education or advocating for provider interventions and self-management programs; providing palliative care that addresses pain and symptom relief in order to decrease suffering and improve quality of life; and advocating for and providing for effective end-of-life care to older clients and caring for caregivers.

POWERPOINT LECTURE SLIDES

NOTE: The number on each PPT Lecture Slide directly corresponds with the Concepts for Lecture.

1. Tertiary Prevention Strategies
   - Monitor health status
   - Palliative care
   - End-of-life care
     ○ Legislation
       – Advance directives
     ○ Respite care
   - Caring for caregivers

SUGGESTIONS FOR CLASSROOM ACTIVITIES

1. Have students research current state policies concerning advance directives and provide the opportunity for a discussion about the barriers and benefits of advance directives.
2. Assign students to three groups to address situations and examples of health-related concerns that would apply to each of the three tertiary strategies. Have students develop a plan of care for a client in each situation.

SUGGESTIONS FOR CLINICAL ACTIVITIES

1. Provide an opportunity for students to work with a nurse in a long-term-care facility or hospice.
2. Invite a hospice or respite care professional to post conference to discuss services available to older clients, legal issues, services to families, and the role of the community health nurse.

LEARNING OBJECTIVE 6

Identify considerations that may influence the community health nurse's approach to health education for older clients.

CONCEPTS FOR LECTURE

1. Two considerations that influence the community health nurse's approach to health education include the need to address specific auditory communication issues such as information that is too fast paced for comprehension, and sensory loss such as hearing or visual impairments requiring special devices, glasses,

POWERPOINT LECTURE SLIDES

NOTE: The number on each PPT Lecture Slide directly corresponds with the Concepts for Lecture.

1. Educational Considerations
   - Multisensorial presentations
   - Multiple repetitions

magnifying glasses, or large print for reading. Older clients may need information repeated, or provided in different mediums for retention; they may require lessons delivered at a slower pace with shorter times for each session.

- Reinforce verbal materials with written
- Memory aids
- Endurance or time considerations

SUGGESTIONS FOR CLASSROOM ACTIVITIES

Assign students to identify one health-related educational need for older clients and prepare a lesson plan that addresses barriers to learning.

SUGGESTIONS FOR CLINICAL ACTIVITIES

Have students work with a community nurse who provides services to the older client to identify an educational learning opportunity. Once the educational opportunity is identified, have students prepare materials about their health topic and provide an opportunity for students to present their materials to a group of older clients.

LEARNING OBJECTIVE 7

Analyze the influence of factors unique to older clients on evaluation of nursing care.

CONCEPTS FOR LECTURE

1. Evaluating the effectiveness of nursing care at the individual level focuses on assessing the client's health status and the effects of primary, secondary, and tertiary interventions in improving health status. Evaluation at the aggregate level should focus on criteria that measure the level of accomplishment of national health objectives.

POWERPOINT LECTURE SLIDES

NOTE: The number on each PPT Lecture Slide directly corresponds with the Concepts for Lecture.

 Evaluation of Nursing Care
- Individual level
  - Assess health status
  - Assess effects of interventions
- Aggregate level
  - Evaluate level of accomplishment of national health objectives

SUGGESTIONS FOR CLASSROOM ACTIVITIES

Have students work in groups to develop a detailed, comprehensive plan of care for the older client described in the case study in the text. Assign groups to research appropriate national health objectives that would be met if they were community nurses assigned to evaluate the impact of interventions to a larger group of clients with similar problems in the community. Provide students with an opportunity to present material for class discussion.

SUGGESTIONS FOR CLINICAL ACTIVITIES

Invite a community health nurse who works with older clients to discuss evaluation strategies used at the local health department in assessing primary, secondary, and tertiary interventions. Ask the guest to bring in publications used to deliver information to community members.

20

Meeting the Needs of Poor and Homeless Populations

RESOURCE LIBRARY

COMPANION WEBSITE

Audio Glossary
Appendix I: Adult Health Assessment and Intervention
  Guide
Exam Review Questions
Case Study: Promoting the Health of the Homeless
MediaLink Application: Lenny Kravitz on Poverty
  (video)

Media Links
Challenge Your Knowledge
Update *Healthy People 2010*
Advocacy Interviews

LEARNING OBJECTIVE 1

Analyze the effects of factors contributing to poverty and homelessness.

CONCEPTS FOR LECTURE

1. Poverty affects nearly 12.5% of the U.S. population. Poverty is defined as having insufficient money, goods, or means of support. Often poverty is defined in terms of the percent of one's income spent on essential goods and services, or income is compared to some median income for the local area.

2. An estimated 3.5 million people may be experiencing homelessness. These numbers are considered an underestimation. The Steven B. McKinney Homeless Assistance Act of 1987 defines homelessness as a situation in which an individual lacks a fixed, regular, and adequate nighttime residence and has a primary residence that is a supervised publicly or privately operated shelter designed to provide temporary accommodations, or is a temporary residence for individuals intended to be institutionalized, or is a public or private place not designed to be used as a regular sleeping environment.

3. Population factors affecting poverty and homelessness include ethnic minority, elderly, or veteran status. Ethnic minority groups may experience more poverty and homelessness in urban areas related to external socioeconomic factors such as unemployment. Elderly populations are becoming another segment of the U.S. population experiencing homelessness due to a

POWERPOINT LECTURE SLIDES

NOTE: The number on each PPT Lecture Slide directly corresponds with the Concepts for Lecture.

1 Poverty
- Affects 12.5% of U.S. population
- State of having insufficient money, goods, or means of support
- Percent of income
- Income is compared to local median incomes

2 Homelessness
- McKinney Homeless Assistance Act of 1987
- Lacking a fixed, regular, and adequate nighttime residence
  - Primary residence may be publicly supervised or privately operated
  - May utilize an institution that provides a temporary residence for individuals intended to be institutionalized
  - May use a public or private place not designed to be used as a regular sleeping accommodation
- Estimated 3.5 million people homeless, may be underestimated

CONCEPTS FOR LECTURE *continued*

loss of affordable housing for a population on a fixed income. Additionally, U.S. veteran populations account for approximately 23% of the total homeless population and 33% of homeless men with high rates of mental illness and addictive disorders as the root cause.

SUGGESTIONS FOR CLASSROOM ACTIVITIES

Assign students to groups to discuss feelings, perceptions, and myths about poverty and homelessness. Have them create a list of medical, social, economic, psychological, cultural, and legal factors that may contribute to poverty or homelessness.

POWERPOINT LECTURE SLIDES *continued*

 3 Contributing Factors
- Ethnic minorities
- Elderly
- Veterans

SUGGESTIONS FOR CLINICAL ACTIVITIES

Invite a guest speaker from the community who provides services for homeless population groups. Ask the guest to discuss what services are provided, how their services are funded, and what interventions are provided.

LEARNING OBJECTIVE 2

Identify biophysical, psychological, physical environmental, sociocultural, behavioral, and health system factors that influence the health of poor and homeless clients.

CONCEPTS FOR LECTURE

1. Biophysical factors that affect the health of the poor and homeless populations include health conditions that may contribute directly to economic stability or those health conditions that result from poverty and homelessness. Examples include hospitalization and fatigue that interrupts employment and chronic or infectious diseases that result from poverty or homelessness such as bronchitis, diabetes, STDs, heart disease, and hypertension.

2. Psychological factors influencing poverty and homelessness include family dynamics, such as limited support systems and coping abilities; mental illness, which affects approximately 20% to 25% of the homeless population; and deinstitutionalization of the mentally ill, which began in the 1950s and 1960s as an effort to move mentally ill persons back into their community environment.

3. Physical environmental considerations that affect the health of poor and homeless individuals include the effects of heat and cold exposure, overcrowding, poor sanitation, exposure to infectious diseases such as TB, unsafe physical environments, and rural areas lacking available shelters or access to assistance services.

4. Sociocultural factors that affect the health of poor or homeless populations include the lack of affordable housing, which can have a very direct effect on homelessness; social support through welfare programs and assistance have declined or have limitations on length and types of services; changes in the job market, often referred to as structural unemployment or deindustrialization, have shifted emphasis from heavy to light industry requiring different skills. Both unemployment and underemployment influence health outcomes for poor or homeless populations; school attendance is affected by poverty and homelessness, resulting in poor or inadequate attendance; and the effects of poverty and

POWERPOINT LECTURE SLIDES

NOTE: The number on each PPT Lecture Slide directly corresponds with the Concepts for Lecture.

1 Biophysical Factors
- Health conditions
  - Direct cause
  - Indirect result from poverty or homelessness

2 Psychological Factors
- Family dynamics
- Mental illness
- Deinstitutionalization

3 Physical Environmental Considerations
- Effects of exposure to natural elements
- Overcrowding
- Poor sanitation
- Exposure to infectious diseases
- Unsafe physical environments
- Rural areas lack services

4 Sociocultural Factors
- Lack of affordable housing
- Social support and welfare reform
- Employment
- School attendance
- Criminal justice
- Violence

5 Behavioral Factors
- Diet and nutrition
- Rest
- Substance abuse
- Sexual activity

homelessness have resulted in criminal behaviors to support basic needs, which results in overrepresentation in jails, higher incidences of criminalization, and susceptibility to violence or abuse.

5. Behavioral factors to consider are the effects of poor diet and nutrition and inadequate rest on the health of this population. Many homeless do not have access to kitchen facilities, and community food programs or kitchens provide limited services. Homeless children tend to exhibit anemia and growth failures. Without adequate sleep, poor or homeless children do not perform well in school, and adults are not prepared for work, if available. Substance abuse may cause individuals to spend limited monies for drugs and alcohol. Sexual activity can result in sex trading and injection drug use with additional risks of HIV and hepatitis B and C.

6. Health system factors may contribute to homelessness or limit access to care for poor or homeless persons. Catastrophic illness can result in depletion of financial resources, resulting in homelessness. Health systems often create financial barriers to health care such as when clinics are not targeting services to these populations, and the emergency departments become the routine provider of medical services for those unable to pay. Personal barriers to health care utilization include the need for survival over health needs, denial of illness, fear of loss of personal control, lack of money, and embarrassment over appearance and hygiene. Many communities lack preventive or comprehensive care services for this population.

6 Health System Considerations
- Catastrophic illness
- Barriers to care
- Lack of preventive services

SUGGESTIONS FOR CLASSROOM ACTIVITIES

Divide students into groups. Assign each group one factor to discuss, describe, and outline examples identified in the local community that pertain to the poor or homeless population. Ask each group to develop a poster board and present to the class.

SUGGESTIONS FOR CLINICAL ACTIVITIES

Provide an opportunity for students to work in a soup kitchen, a homeless shelter, a shelter for domestic violence, a community clinic that targets the homeless, or other available services in the community.

LEARNING OBJECTIVE 3

Describe approaches to primary prevention of homelessness and analyze related roles of community health nurses with respect to each.

CONCEPTS FOR LECTURE

1. Primary prevention may be directed at either preventing homelessness or preventing its health consequences at the individual or community level.

2. Of importance to nurses is to help prevent individuals and families from becoming homeless by helping them eliminate factors that contribute to homelessness such as unemployment and mental health issues and by addressing family communication and parenting skills for teens that run away.

3. At the community level, reducing the incidence of poverty and homelessness requires changes in societal

POWERPOINT LECTURE SLIDES

NOTE: The number on each PPT Lecture Slide directly corresponds with the Concepts for Lecture.

1 Primary Prevention
- Individual or community level
  o Prevent homelessness
  o Prevent health consequences

2 Role of Nurse (Individual Level)
- Prevent individuals and families from becoming homeless

CONCEPTS FOR LECTURE *continued*

structures and policies, as well as attitudes, such as creating employment opportunities, retraining opportunities, and social insurance programs. Advocacy and political action mean making policy makers aware of the needs of the homeless and participate in planning programs to prevent homelessness. Nurses can also promote adoption of sound housing policies to address unsafe housing, funding to ensure housing access, and local market conditions for available housing.

POWERPOINT LECTURE SLIDES *continued*

- Assist in eliminating contributing factors to homelessness
- Unemployment
- Mental health issues
- Address family communication/parenting skills

3 Role of Nurse (Community Level)
- Reduce incidence of poverty/homelessness
- Changes in societal structures, policies, attitudes
  - Employment opportunities
  - Retraining opportunities
  - Social insurance programs

3a Role of Nurse (Community Level) (continued)
- Advocacy and political action
  - Promote adoption of sound housing policies
  - Advocate funding to ensure housing

SUGGESTIONS FOR CLASSROOM ACTIVITIES

Divide students into small groups. Have students prepare a care plan for a homeless population of children, families, and veterans.

SUGGESTIONS FOR CLINICAL ACTIVITIES

Invite a social worker, a community health nurse, and a member of a volunteer agency that serves poor or homeless populations to have a roundtable discussion of the primary areas of concern for poor and homeless individuals.

LEARNING OBJECTIVE 4

Identify major areas of emphasis in primary prevention of health problems in poor and homeless clients.

CONCEPTS FOR LECTURE

1. Approaches to primary prevention include assessing the health of homeless individuals and groups of homeless persons and identifying factors that influence their health through data and information obtained from health professionals, church organizations, and social and governmental agencies that provide services for this population. Surveys can also be conducted on homeless populations by seeking out places where they congregate. Using the assessment, nursing diagnoses may be derived for individuals or groups of homeless individuals. Planning and implementation begins during the assessment phase, but becomes specific to population needs for both long-term and short-term solutions to problems.

POWERPOINT LECTURE SLIDES

NOTE: The number on each PPT Lecture Slide directly corresponds with the Concepts for Lecture.

1 Approaches to Primary Prevention
- Collect data
  - Health professionals, churches, social and governmental agencies
  - Conduct surveys of homeless populations
- Employ diagnostic reasoning
- Plan and implement health care
  - Short and long-term solutions

SUGGESTIONS FOR CLASSROOM ACTIVITIES

1. Show a video depicting the effects of poverty or homelessness on an individual or community. Direct the class to discuss cause and effect relationships in terms of factors that cause homelessness.
2. Assign students in small groups to research the efforts of state and local governments, health care agencies, and volunteer organizations to address poverty and homelessness in the local community.

SUGGESTIONS FOR CLINICAL ACTIVITIES

If one is available, schedule students to spend time with the local school homeless liaison to review school policies for homeless children and services available for families.

LEARNING OBJECTIVE 5

Identify areas in which secondary preventive interventions may be required in the care of poor and homeless individuals and analyze the role of the community health nurse in these interventions.

CONCEPTS FOR LECTURE

1. Secondary prevention strategies focus on the alleviation of existing homelessness and its health effects by assisting clients with shelter and basic necessities and assisting with governmental processes. Nurses may provide curative services such as food supplemental programs for pregnant women or treatment for skin conditions. They should also involve the runaway teen with long-term solutions to problems.

POWERPOINT LECTURE SLIDES

NOTE: The number on each PPT Lecture Slide directly corresponds with the Concepts for Lecture.

1. Secondary Prevention Strategies
   - Alleviate existing homelessness and its health effects
     ○ Shelter and basic necessities
       – Food supplemental programs
     ○ Assist with bureaucratic process
   - Provide curative services
   - Plan for long-term resolution for homeless runaways

SUGGESTIONS FOR CLASSROOM ACTIVITIES

Have students develop a care plan using secondary prevention approaches for a runaway teen; a homeless, pregnant women; and an unemployed farm worker with TB.

SUGGESTIONS FOR CLINICAL ACTIVITIES

Arrange for students to work with a nurse in a Women, Infant, and Children food supplemental clinic, a local food bank, or other agencies that provide shelter, food, and basic services for poor and homeless populations.

LEARNING OBJECTIVE 6

Identify strategies for tertiary prevention of poverty and homelessness at the aggregate level.

CONCEPTS FOR LECTURE

1. Tertiary prevention focuses on preventing recurrence of poverty and homelessness at all levels. Activities defined at the tertiary level include political activities to ensure the provision of services to relieve poverty and homelessness on a long-term basis, such as raising the minimum wage or designing programs to educate the homeless for employment. Other measures include preventing the criminalization of normal activities of life for homeless people, monitoring medication use in mentally ill clients, and encouraging clients to seek counseling or use rehabilitative services.

2. Tertiary prevention for individual homeless clients may entail referrals for employment assistance or for educational programs that allow homeless clients to eliminate the underlying factors associated with their homelessness. Community health nurses may assist clients to budget their income more effectively or develop ways to increase their buying power through cooperative buying. Nurses may assist families in obtaining respite care and other supportive services for family members with mental illness. Nurses also monitor medication use and encourage clients to receive counseling and other rehabilitative services.

POWERPOINT LECTURE SLIDES

NOTE: The number on each PPT Lecture Slide directly corresponds with the Concepts for Lecture.

1. Tertiary Prevention Strategies
   - Engage in political activities
   - Prevent criminalization of activities
   - Monitor medication use
   - Encourage counseling and rehabilitative services

2. Tertiary Prevention for Individual Homeless Clients
   - Referrals for employment assistance or for educational programs
   - Assist clients to budget their income more effectively or develop ways to increase their buying power through cooperative buying
   - Assist families in obtaining respite care and other supportive services for family members with mental illness
   - Monitor medication use
   - Encourage clients to receive counseling and other rehabilitative services

SUGGESTIONS FOR CLASSROOM ACTIVITIES

Ask students to research articles that address any of the recommendations made by the National Coalition for the Homeless and present a summary of one article to the class.

SUGGESTIONS FOR CLINICAL ACTIVITIES

Have students attend a community forum that addresses homelessness in the community. Invite local law enforcement to post conference to discuss strategies to reduce the criminalizing of homeless activities.

LEARNING OBJECTIVE 7

Describe considerations in implementing care for poor and homeless individuals.

CONCEPTS FOR LECTURE

1. Considerations in implementing care for poor and homeless individuals include focusing on prioritizing needs and identifying factors that affect the homeless in specific locales, specific population groups, and vulnerable populations.

POWERPOINT LECTURE SLIDES

NOTE: The number on each PPT Lecture Slide directly corresponds with the Concepts for Lecture.

[1] Implementation of Care
- Prioritize needs
- Identify factors that affect homeless
- Identify specific population groups or vulnerable populations

---

SUGGESTIONS FOR CLASSROOM ACTIVITIES

Have students work in groups and use their knowledge of the community to develop a priority needs list that addresses factors affecting the homeless in their community. Have students specify which populations are most at risk or in need of services and whether there are any vulnerable population groups.

SUGGESTIONS FOR CLINICAL ACTIVITIES

Using their clinical setting, have students identify barriers to implementing a care plan for homeless individuals or groups in their community. Provide the opportunity for discussion at post conference.

LEARNING OBJECTIVE 8

Identify the primary focus of evaluation for care of poor and homeless clients.

CONCEPTS FOR LECTURE

1. Evaluation occurs at the individual level by determining the effectiveness of interventions developed by both the nurse and the client. The nurse addresses the objectives with the client. Evaluation at the aggregate level determines whether programs in place are effective at preventing people from returning to poverty. A third level of evaluation can be accomplished by examining whether the national health objectives have been obtained using community, state, and national data for comparisons.

POWERPOINT LECTURE SLIDES

NOTE: The number on each PPT Lecture Slide directly corresponds with the Concepts for Lecture.

[1] Evaluation
- Individual level
  ○ Determine effectiveness of interventions by nurse and client
- Aggregate level
  ○ Determine effectiveness of poverty-prevention programs
- National health objectives
  ○ Determine results through comparative data

SUGGESTIONS FOR CLASSROOM ACTIVITIES

Have students research one national health objective that targets poor or homeless populations and identify specific opportunities for nurses in the community to develop evaluation techniques.

SUGGESTIONS FOR CLINICAL ACTIVITIES

Arrange for students to attend a local health department planning meeting that targets services for the poor or homeless. Provide guided discussion during post conference about possible evaluation strategies based on the meeting.

21

CHAPTER

Care of Clients in the Home Setting

RESOURCE LIBRARY

🌐 COMPANION WEBSITE

Audio Glossary
Exam Review Questions
Case Study: Home Health Nursing
MediaLink Application: Visiting Nurse Services,
  NYC (2 videos)

Media Links
Challenge Your Knowledge
Advocacy Interviews

📖 IMAGE LIBRARY

Figure 21-1 Maintaining Balance in Home Visiting

LEARNING OBJECTIVE 1

Describe the advantages of a home visit as a means of providing nursing care.

CONCEPTS FOR LECTURE

1. Historically, community health nurses have been providing home visits for decades. Recently, nurses have been providing services in many places and settings. A home visit is defined as a formal call by a nurse on a client at the client's residence to provide nursing care.
2. Home visiting offers distinct advantages over traditional services and includes six major aspects: convenience, access, information, relationship, cost, and outcomes.
3. Clients often prefer to be seen in their homes. A home visit is convenient in that clients do not incur transportation costs, nor do they have to wait for services that may occur in traditional health care settings.
4. Access has two parts and refers to clients who are immobile or lack transportation as well as the community health nurse, who has access to clients who may not necessarily present themselves for services in other settings. As a result, a home visit permits the nurse to identify clients in need of services.
5. The home visit permits the nurse to obtain information not readily available in other settings. Valuable information is obtained about family dynamics, physical environment, and psychological and sociocultural factors present that may have a bearing on the client's health status.

POWERPOINT LECTURE SLIDES

NOTE: The number on each PPT Lecture Slide directly corresponds with the Concepts for Lecture.

1 Home Visit
  - A nursing care visit in a client's residence
  - Historic background

2 Advantages of Home Visits
  - Convenience
  - Access
  - Information
  - Relationship
  - Cost
  - Outcomes

3 Convenience
  - Clients often prefer to be seen in their homes
  - Reduced transportation costs
  - No waiting for services

4 Access
  - Clients may be immobile or lack transportation
  - Community health nurse has access to clients who may not necessarily present themselves for services in other settings
  - A home visit permits the nurse to identify clients in need of services

6. In the home setting, the client exerts autonomy and control. This presents a unique situation for the nurse and the client and may aid the nurse in fostering a sense of empowerment for the client. The home visit also permits a sense of privacy and clients may offer more information, especially about sensitive issues. The home visit fosters a sense of continuity in the nurse-client relationship especially if there are repeated visits or a long-term purpose for the visits.
7. Home visits and home care are less expensive than hospital care or long-term facility placement.
8. Overall, home visitation programs have been documented to achieve a variety of health-related outcomes for many different populations.

5 Information
- The home visit permits the nurse to obtain information not readily available in other settings
- Valuable information is obtained about family dynamics, physical environment, psychological and sociocultural factors present that may have a bearing on the client's health status

6 Relationship
- In the home setting, the client exerts autonomy and control
- The nurse may foster a sense of empowerment
- Permits a sense of privacy
- Clients may offer more information, especially about sensitive issues
- The home visit fosters a sense of continuity in the nurse-client relationship, especially if there are repeated visits, or a long-term purpose for the visits.

7 Cost
- Home visits and home care are less expensive than hospital care or long-term facility placement

8 Outcomes
- Home visitation programs have been documented to achieve a variety of health-related outcomes for many different populations

SUGGESTIONS FOR CLASSROOM ACTIVITIES

Divide students into two groups. Provide a case study of a client needing services. Ask students to discuss differences in providing services in the hospital compared to a home setting.

SUGGESTIONS FOR CLINICAL ACTIVITIES

1. Invite a community health nurse or home health nurse to post conference to discuss the differences in providing care in the home, reasons for visits, and target populations or clients served by home visiting services.
2. Have students compare their own experiences of care for clients in home, hospital, and clinic settings. How are they similar? How do they differ? What advantages and disadvantages does each setting have?

LEARNING OBJECTIVE 2

Analyze challenges encountered by community health nurses making home visits.

CONCEPTS FOR LECTURE

1. Home visiting programs can bring about their own unique set of challenges that evolve from the diversity of the clients and the multiplicity of their problems.
2. Challenges come from the nurse's need to maintain a balance between often opposing agendas, including intimacy and professional distance, dependence and independence, risk and safety, cost containment and quality, health restoration and health promotion services, and task orientation and meeting the unique needs of the client.

POWERPOINT LECTURE SLIDES

NOTE: The number on each PPT Lecture Slide directly corresponds with the Concepts for Lecture.

1 Challenges of Home Visiting Programs
- Client diversity
  ○ Multiplicity of client problems

2 Need for Balance between Opposing Agendas
- Intimacy and professional distance
- Dependence and independence

POWERPOINT LECTURE SLIDES *continued*
- Risk and safety
- Cost containment and quality
- Health restoration and health promotion services
- Task orientation and meeting client needs

SUGGESTIONS FOR CLASSROOM ACTIVITIES	**SUGGESTIONS FOR CLINICAL ACTIVITIES**
Invite nurses who work in community-based programs to class to discuss their challenges in delivering care and successful strategies employed.	1. Arrange for students to make home visits to specific clients/families. 2. Have students identify challenges posed by home visits and strategies to address these challenges. During post conference, students will report their findings.

LEARNING OBJECTIVE 3

Identify the major purposes of home visiting programs.

CONCEPTS FOR LECTURE

1. Although various home visiting programs have their own goals, the major purposes of home visiting programs can be grouped into four categories: case finding and referral; health promotion and illness prevention; care of the sick; and care of the dying.
2. Case finding is designed to identify clients needing additional services and to provide referrals to appropriate sources of services. Typically, this involves only a single visit such as a lead abatement program in which nurses go house to house to identify homes with lead contamination.
3. Health promotion and illness prevention focuses on specific populations such as new mothers or families with children needing child developmental interventions.
4. Care of the sick frequently involves providing services to the elderly or populations with chronic conditions.
5. Care of the dying is a specialized service to people with terminal illnesses and includes palliative care, education and information for family members, caretaker respite services, physical therapy, counseling and spiritual care, and assistance with specialized equipment needs.

POWERPOINT LECTURE SLIDES

NOTE: The number on each PPT Lecture Slide directly corresponds with the Concepts for Lecture.

1 Purpose of Home Visiting Programs
- Four categories
  - Case finding and referral
  - Health promotion and illness prevention
  - Care of the sick
  - Care of the dying

2 Case Finding and Referral
- Identify clients needing additional services
- Provide referrals to appropriate sources of services
  - Example: Lead abatement program

3 Health Promotion and Illness Prevention
- Focuses on specific populations
  - Examples:
    - New mothers
    - Children needing child developmental interventions

4 Care of the Sick
- Providing direct services
- Examples:
  - Elderly
  - Populations with chronic conditions
  - Recent hospital discharges

5 Care of the Dying
- Specialized services to people with terminal illnesses
  - Palliative care
  - Education and information for family members
  - Caregiver respite services
  - Physical therapy
  - Counseling and spiritual care
  - Assistance with specialized equipment needs

SUGGESTIONS FOR CLASSROOM ACTIVITIES	SUGGESTIONS FOR CLINICAL ACTIVITIES
Provide students with a case study of a client in need of community health nursing services. Divide students into four groups, with each group developing a plan of care that addresses one of the major purposes: case finding, health promotion, care of sick, and care of dying. Provide the opportunity for discussion as to how the plan of care is different or similar in each group.	Have students identify the extent to which the home visits they make in the clinical setting address each category of purpose.

LEARNING OBJECTIVE 4

Describe major considerations in planning a home visit.

CONCEPTS FOR LECTURE

1. In planning a home visit, the community health nurse incorporates several steps or tasks to include: reviewing previous interventions, prioritizing client needs, developing goals and objectives, considering acceptance and timing, delineating nursing activities, obtaining necessary materials, and planning for evaluation.

2. The community health nurse reviews previous interventions and the efficacy of those interventions specific to the client's health needs in order to identify both successful and unsuccessful interventions.

3. The nurse prioritizes client health care needs based on either the potential threat to their health, the degree to which they concern the client, or the ability to resolve the health issue.

4. After prioritizing client specific interventions, the nurse develops goals and objectives related to each area of need. Goals and objectives may address primary, secondary, and tertiary levels of prevention. Goals are stated general expectations and objectives are specific or tangible outcomes desired. An example of a goal is for a parent to develop effective parenting skills. An example of an objective is that a client will display effective communication skills in relating to their children.

5. The nurse considers the client's readiness to accept interventions, the timing of the visit, and the introduction of the intervention. A component of acceptance is building trust and rapport with the client. In evaluating timing, the nurse must consider whether the client is open to the visit.

6. The community health nurse plans specific nursing activities for each nursing diagnosis based on practice guidelines, agency procedures, protocols or elements of clinical pathways. Nursing activities may focus on health promotion, the resolution of health-related problems, referrals, education, and technical procedures.

7. The nurse must obtain supplies and materials for the home visit such as educational materials, equipment, wound care supplies, or assessment equipment.

POWERPOINT LECTURE SLIDES

NOTE: The number on each PPT Lecture Slide directly corresponds with the Concepts for Lecture.

1 Planning a Home Visit
- Review previous interventions
- Prioritize client needs
- Develop goals and objectives
- Consider acceptance and timing
- Delineate nursing activities
- Obtain necessary materials
- Plan for evaluation

2 Review Previous Interventions
- Determine the efficacy of the interventions
- Identify successful and unsuccessful interventions

3 Prioritize Client Needs
- Potential threat to their health
- Degree to which the health threat concerns the client
- The ability to resolve the health issue

4 Develop Goals and Objectives
- Goals
  ○ Stated general expectations
    – Example: Develop effective parenting skills
- Objectives
  ○ Specific/tangible outcomes desired
    – Example: client will display effective communication skills in relating to their children

5 Consider Acceptance and Timing
- Client's readiness to accept intervention
  ○ Build rapport and trust
- Timing of the visit
  ○ Client must be open to the visit
- Introduction of the interventions

6 Delineate Nursing Activities
- Nursing diagnosis utilizes:
  ○ Practice guidelines
  ○ Agency procedures/protocols
  ○ Clinical pathways

CONCEPTS FOR LECTURE *continued*

8. Evaluation criteria are determined from the outcome objectives developed for the visit and may include long-term and short-term criteria. An example of short-term criteria is the client's receptiveness or response to nursing interventions. An example of long-term criteria is the actual accomplishment of the objective.

POWERPOINT LECTURE SLIDES *continued*

- Examples: health promotion, referral, education, technical procedures

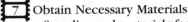 Obtain Necessary Materials
  - Supplies and materials for home visit
    ○ Educational materials
    ○ Health care equipment
    ○ Wound care supplies
    ○ Physical assessment equipment

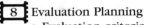 Evaluation Planning
  - Evaluation criteria obtained from outcome objectives
    ○ Long-term evaluation criteria
      – Client's receptiveness or response to nursing interventions
    ○ Short-term evaluation criteria
      – Actual accomplishment of objective

SUGGESTIONS FOR CLASSROOM ACTIVITIES

Provide students with different case studies. Discuss each of the elements in planning for the home visit. Provide examples for each of the major considerations.

SUGGESTIONS FOR CLINICAL ACTIVITIES

Have students describe how they have addressed each of the considerations in planning home visits in the clinical setting.

LEARNING OBJECTIVE 5

Identify tasks involved in implementing a home visit.

CONCEPTS FOR LECTURE

1. Tasks involved in implementing a home visit include the following: validating assessment and diagnosis, identifying additional needs, modifying the plan of care as needed, performing nursing interventions, and dealing with distractions.

POWERPOINT LECTURE SLIDES

NOTE: The number on each PPT Lecture Slide directly corresponds with the Concepts for Lecture.

1 Implementation of the Home Visit
  - Validate assessment and diagnosis
  - Identify additional needs
  - Modify the plan of care as needed
  - Perform nursing interventions
  - Deal with distractions

SUGGESTIONS FOR CLASSROOM ACTIVITIES

Have students role-play preparation for implementing a home visit. Provide various settings and family/client scenarios to provide a focus for the student home visit preparation.

SUGGESTIONS FOR CLINICAL ACTIVITIES

Have students describe a home visit from their clinical experiences and how they addressed each of the tasks involved in implementing their home visit.

Learning Objective 6

Analyze the effects of potential distractions during a home visit.

Concepts for Lecture

1. Nurses providing home services must contend with and anticipate potential distractions with service delivery. Distractions are categorized by three types: environmental, behavioral, and nurse-initiated.
2. Environmental distractions include background noise, crowded surroundings, and interruptions from other family members.
3. Behavioral distractions consist of behavior used by the client to distract the nurse from the purpose of the visit. Techniques employed by the nurse include exploring the reasons for distractions and working to establish trust.
4. Nurse-initiated distractions may result from fears, role preoccupation, and personal reaction to different lifestyles. Nurses may fear bodily harm, rejection by the client, or lack of control.

PowerPoint Lecture Slides

NOTE: The number on each PPT Lecture Slide directly corresponds with the Concepts for Lecture.

1 Distractions
- Environmental
- Behavioral
- Nurse-initiated

2 Environmental Distractions
- Background noise
- Crowded surroundings
- Interruptions

3 Behavioral
- Client behaviors
  - Explore reasons for behaviors
  - Work to establish trust

4 Nurse-initiated
- Fears
  - Bodily harm
  - Client rejection
  - Lack of control
- Role preoccupation
- Personal reactions to different lifestyles

Suggestions for Classroom Activities

Ask students to role-play situations in preparation for a home visit. Provide several scenarios that include distractions that may be encountered for students to practice communication skills.

Suggestions for Clinical Activities

Have students identify distractions encountered in home visits made in their clinical experiences, describe the strategies they used to address the distractions, and evaluate their effectiveness. Have classmates suggest other strategies that might have been employed to address the distractions.

Learning Objective 7

Discuss the need for both long-term and short-term evaluative criteria for the effectiveness of a home visit.

Concepts for Lecture

1. Long-term and short-term evaluative criteria are essential because the outcome of nursing interventions may not be immediately apparent. Without predetermined evaluative criteria, the community health nurse may not be able to determine if subsequent visits are required or if the appropriate level of prevention was implemented.

PowerPoint Lecture Slides

NOTE: The number on each PPT Lecture Slide directly corresponds with the Concepts for Lecture.

1 Evaluative Criteria
- Intervention outcomes not immediately apparent
- Need to determine if subsequent visits are needed
- Need to evaluate if appropriate level of prevention was implemented

LEARNING OBJECTIVE 8

Describe the relationship between home health nursing and community health nursing.

CONCEPTS FOR LECTURE

1. Home health nursing is considered a subspecialty of community health nursing because home health nurses work primarily with ill persons, yet continue to employ knowledge of environmental, social, and personal health factors.
2. Home health nursing is a specialized area of nursing practice with roots embedded in community health nursing. Characteristics of home health nursing include holism, care management, resource coordination, collaboration, and autonomous and interdependent practice. Interdependent practice means that nurses collaborate with other health care professionals, nonprofessionals, the client, and family members.
3. Home health care is defined as care provided to individuals and families in their place of residence for the purpose of promoting, maintaining, or restoring health or for maximizing the level of independence while minimizing the effects of disability and illness, including terminal illness. Services are generally provided through a home health agency with varying services offered from skilled nursing and therapy services to personal care and homemaking assistance.

POWERPOINT LECTURE SLIDES

NOTE: The number on each PPT Lecture Slide directly corresponds with the Concepts for Lecture.

1. Home Health Nursing
   - A subspecialty of community health nursing
2. Specialized Practice With Roots in Community Health Nursing
   - Holism
   - Care management
   - Resource coordination
   - Collaboration
   - Autonomous and interdependent practice
3. Home Health Care
   - Care provided in client's residence
   - Services provided
     - Skilled nursing and therapy
     - Personal care
     - Homemaking assistance

LEARNING OBJECTIVE 9

Discuss the need for collaboration in home health and hospice nursing.

CONCEPTS FOR LECTURE

1. Home care services are provided at the rate of approximately 16.4 per 10,000 people under the age of 65. For people over 65 years of age, the rate increases to 277 per 10,000 people. Types and percentages of services delivered include: 75% received skilled nursing; 44% received personal care services; 27% received physical therapy; 8% received occupational therapy; 4% received dietary and nutritional services; and 1.2% received respite care.
2. Home health care collaborates with other agencies, including hospice care, for durable medical equipment needs, for care to be holistic, and for referrals for additional services to meet client needs. Both services must be certified by the primary care provider.

POWERPOINT LECTURE SLIDES

NOTE: The number on each PPT Lecture Slide directly corresponds with the Concepts for Lecture.

1 Home Care Services
- 16.4 per 10,000 people under age 65
- 277 per 10,000 people over age 65

1a Home Care Services (continued)
- Services provided
  ○ 75% nursing
  ○ 27% physical therapy
  ○ 44% personal care
  ○ 8% occupational therapy
  ○ 4% dietary/nutritional services
  ○ 1.2% respite care

2 Collaboration
- Certified by primary care provider
- Essential for holistic care
- Used to obtain durable medical equipment
- Provide referral to additional services

SUGGESTIONS FOR CLASSROOM ACTIVITIES

Have students bring to class one article that depicts services from a home health care perspective and from a hospice care perspective. Ask students to provide a summary of the article and compare and contrast services, the nurse's approach to care, and other distinct features of the article.

SUGGESTIONS FOR CLINICAL ACTIVITIES

1. Invite a home health nurse and a hospice nurse to attend post conference to discuss similarities and differences in services and cases where collaboration was essential to the care of the client or family.
2. Arrange for clinical experience with a hospice care nurse and a home health nurse. Discuss differences in the nursing role in each setting from that in an official public health agency during post conference.

LEARNING OBJECTIVE 10

Discuss funding sources for home health and hospice care.

CONCEPTS FOR LECTURE

1. Since both home health care and hospice services must be certified by a primary care provider for reimbursement purposes, they fall under the domain of the primary care provider. Clients and families may contract independently for services, which means they can select which agency they want to deliver their services; but if services are not certified by a provider, the client or family must pay out of pocket. For some programs, clients may self-refer or the community health nurse may refer individual or families for services and in these situations, it is between the nurse and the client, not a third party, to determine if services will be delivered.

POWERPOINT LECTURE SLIDES

NOTE: The number on each PPT Lecture Slide directly corresponds with the Concepts for Lecture.

1 Reimbursement
- Contingent on provider certification of need
- Self-referral
  ○ Client pays out-of-pocket if not certified

2 Funding Sources
- Out-of-pocket
- Medicare
- Medicaid
- Private insurance

CONCEPTS FOR LECTURE *continued*

2. Medicare provides for about 52% of current home health client services and 80% of hospice client services. Medicaid pays for about 20% of home health care services and 7% of hospice services provided to clients. Another 17% of home health care services were reimbursed by private insurance. Both home health care and hospice services had expenditures that doubled in recent years and costs are expected to increase.

SUGGESTIONS FOR CLASSROOM ACTIVITIES

Divide students into small groups. Assign a case scenario for each group that describes the client, socioeconomic and demographic data about the client, family and community, the health condition, and the home environment. Ask students to discuss which services are needed in the home and possible funding sources.

SUGGESTIONS FOR CLINICAL ACTIVITIES

Ask students to research and identify funding sources primarily used by clients in their clinical agency. Ask students to investigate the typical cost of the services and the actual reimbursement provided. Discuss at post conference.

LEARNING OBJECTIVE 11

Apply evaluative criteria for home health and hospice care services.

CONCEPTS FOR LECTURE

1. Evaluation of home visiting services examines the care outcomes at both the individual and the aggregate level. One type of report is derived from the OASIS documentation system, which permits home care agencies to assess their care relative to that provided by other home care agencies. Two types of reports are generated by this system: the Outcome-Based Quality Monitoring system, which provides information on the types and frequency of adverse events experienced by clients, and the Outcome-Based Quality Improvement report, which assesses the outcomes of care across clients using specific health indicators. The final type of report generated by the OASIS system is the Case Mix report, which provides information on the types of clients served by the agency.

2. Another type of evaluation system is the Health Plan Employer Data and Information Set, which rates managed care organizations and provides purchasers with information needed to select a health care plan. Finally, home health agencies should evaluate the client's level of satisfaction with the care provided. Features to evaluate include indicators of good-quality and poor-quality care, ability to maintain independence and preserve dignity, decreasing emotional stress, provision of social support, facilitation of the learning of new skills, and assistance with navigating through complex health care systems.

POWERPOINT LECTURE SLIDES

NOTE: The number on each PPT Lecture Slide directly corresponds with the Concepts for Lecture.

1 Evaluation Criteria
- Types of reports
  - OASIS system
  - Outcome-Based Quality Monitoring report
  - Outcome-Based Quality Improvement report
  - Case Mix report

2 Additional Evaluation Criteria
- Health Plan Employer Data and Information Set
  - Rates managed care organizations
  - Provides purchasers with information needed to select a health care plan

2a Client Satisfaction Evaluation Criteria
- Indicators of good-quality and poor-quality care
- Ability to maintain independence and preserve dignity
- Decrease emotional stress
- Provide social support
- Facilitate learning new skills
- Assist with navigating through complex health care systems

SUGGESTIONS FOR CLASSROOM ACTIVITIES

Have students research articles on the topic of evaluating home health and hospice services. Ask students to identify measurement criteria used and the results of the evaluation.

SUGGESTIONS FOR CLINICAL ACTIVITIES

Assign students to investigate how services are evaluated and summarize any reports that are generated by their clinical agency. Provide an opportunity to discuss at post conference.

22 CHAPTER

Care of Clients in Official and Voluntary Health Agencies

RESOURCE LIBRARY

COMPANION WEBSITE

Audio Glossary

Appendix G: Community Health Assessment and
  Intervention Guide

Exam Review Questions

Case Study: A Nursing Experience in a Faith-Based
  Community

MediaLink Application: Nurse-Managed Services
  (video)

Media Links

Challenge Your Knowledge

Update *Healthy People 2010*

Advocacy Interviews

IMAGE LIBRARY

Table 22-1 Core Functions and Related Public
  Health Services

LEARNING OBJECTIVE 1

Discuss the legal and regulatory parameters of nursing in official health agencies.

CONCEPTS FOR LECTURE

1. Community health nurses working in official health agencies derive their roles and activities from federal or state legislative mandates or local ordinances with the ultimate purpose of protecting the health of the public. Under the auspice of official health agencies, community health nurses are charged with protecting the public. Examples of protective intervention include protection from communicable diseases by investigating reports of communicable diseases, assuring the public that those with infectious diseases are removed from public contact, and immunizing those at risk for exposure. Community health nurses also ensure that other health-related regulations are adhered to.

POWERPOINT LECTURE SLIDES

NOTE: The number on each PPT Lecture Slide directly corresponds with the Concepts for Lecture.

 Legal and Regulatory Parameters
  - Federal and state legislative mandates for protecting public health
  - Local ordinances
  - Other federal, state, or local health initiatives that address core public health functions

SUGGESTIONS FOR CLASSROOM ACTIVITIES

Assign students to small groups to research local, state, and federal health regulations that affect the role of community health nurses in protecting the health of the public. Have students select one regulation to discuss in class.

SUGGESTIONS FOR CLINICAL ACTIVITIES

1. Invite a community health nurse to discuss specific regulations and their impact on programs, services, and nursing activities.
2. Have students identify the services provided by the local health department and determine which of those services are mandated by law and which are based on local health status and needs.

LEARNING OBJECTIVE 2

Describe the core functions and essential services of local health departments.

CONCEPTS FOR LECTURE

1. The core functions of local health departments include assessment, policy development, and assurance.
2. Public health agencies are expected to regularly collect health-related information through on-going surveillance, and assemble, analyze, and make available information on the health of the community. This assessment function includes monitoring the community's health status, identifying community health needs, and diagnosing and investigating health problems and health hazards in the community.
3. Public health agencies serve as advocates and encourage the development of local, state, and national policies conducive to population health through political action and planning. This includes informing, educating, and empowering people regarding health issues, mobilizing community partnerships to identify and solve health problems, and developing policies and plans that support individual and community health efforts.
4. The public health sector serves its clients by assuring the availability of and access to health care services essential to sustaining and improving the health of the population.
5. The basic obligations of official health agencies are preventing epidemics and the spread of disease, protecting the public against environmental hazards, preventing injuries, promoting healthy behaviors and mental health, responding to disasters and aiding communities to recover from their effects, and ensuring the quality and accessibility of health services.
6. Ten essential services have been identified to address the obligations and core functions of public health: monitor health status to identify community health problems; diagnose and investigate health problems and health hazards in the community; inform, educate, and empower people about health issues; mobilize community partnerships to identify and solve health problems; develop policies and plans that support individual and community health efforts; enforce laws and regulations that protect health and ensure safety; link people to needed personal health services and ensure the provision of health care when otherwise unavailable; ensure a competent public health and personal health workforce; evaluate effectiveness, accessibility, and quality of personal and population-based health services; and research for new insights and innovative solutions to health problems.

POWERPOINT LECTURE SLIDES

NOTE: The number on each PPT Lecture Slide directly corresponds with the Concepts for Lecture.

1 Core Functions
- Assessment
- Policy development
- Assurance

2 Assessment Function
- Monitor health status
  - Regularly collect health-related information through on-going surveillance, and assemble, analyze, and make available information on the health of the community
- Diagnose and investigate health problems
  - Includes statistics on health status, community health needs, and epidemiological studies of health problems

3 Policy Development Function
- Encourage the development of local, state, and national policies conducive to population health through political action and planning

4 Assurance Function
- Assure the availability of and access to health care services essential to sustaining and improving the health of the population

5 Basic Obligations
- Prevent epidemics/spread of disease
- Protect the public against environmental hazards
- Prevent injuries
- Promote healthy behaviors and mental health
- Respond to disasters and help communities recover from their effects
- Ensure quality and accessibility of health services

6 Essential Services: Assessment (Refer to Table 22-1)
- Monitor health status
- Diagnose and investigate health problems

6a Essential Services: Policy Development
- Inform, educate, and empower people
- Mobilize community partnerships
- Develop policies and plans

6b Essential Services: Assurance
- Enforce laws and regulations
- Link people to needed personal health services
- Ensure a competent public health workforce
- Evaluate the effectiveness, accessibility, and quality of services
- Research new insights and innovative solutions

LEARNING OBJECTIVE 3

Discuss educational preparation for nursing in official health agencies.

CONCEPTS FOR LECTURE

1. In some jurisdictions, "*Public health nurse*" is a legal title that designates a registered nurse who meets specific educational requirements for state certification for aggregate-level practice. Educational preparation may differ slightly from one country to another, but the basic education includes a baccalaureate degree and PHN certification in some states. Certification is often based on demonstration of specific skills and competencies such as knowledge of physical, mental, and developmental assessment; surveillance and epidemiology; health promotion, health education, and disease prevention; multicultural health care; and research and statistics in a population-based practice with additional supervised clinical experiences varying in length of time.

2. Additional education may be needed in legal and financial issues, family violence, case management, and emergency preparedness and response.

POWERPOINT LECTURE SLIDES

NOTE: The number on each PPT Lecture Slide directly corresponds with the Concepts for Lecture.

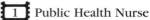 Public Health Nurse
- An RN who meets requirements for aggregate practice
- Educational preparation may require
  - Baccalaureate degree
  - Supervised clinical experience

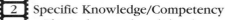 Specific Knowledge/Competency
- Physical, mental, and developmental assessment
- Surveillance and epidemiology
- Health promotion, disease prevention, health education
- Multicultural health care
- Research methodology and statistics
- Population-based practice

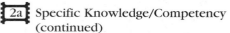 Specific Knowledge/Competency (continued)
- Legal and financial issues
- Family violence
- Case management
- Emergency preparedness and response

LEARNING OBJECTIVE 4

Analyze the core competencies of the public health workforce as they relate to nursing in official health agencies.

CONCEPTS FOR LECTURE

1. Core competencies for the public health workforce include: research and analytic skills to collect, analyze, and interpret community health data; communication skills related to presentation, advocacy, and leadership; policy development and program planning skills; skills derived from basic public health sciences; cultural skills; financial planning and management skills; and teaching skills.

POWERPOINT LECTURE SLIDES

NOTE: The number on each PPT Lecture Slide directly corresponds with the Concepts for Lecture.

 Core Competencies
- Research and analysis skills
- Communication skills related to presentation, advocacy, and leadership
- Policy development and program planning skills
- Skills derived from basic public health sciences
- Cultural skills
- Financial planning and financial management skills
- Teaching skills

SUGGESTIONS FOR CLASSROOM ACTIVITIES

Provide students with a community case study. Have students discuss how each of the core competencies can be applied to the case study and the role of the public health nurse.

SUGGESTIONS FOR CLINICAL ACTIVITIES

During clinical experience, ask students to describe behaviors they have exhibited in the clinical setting that reflect the core competencies of the public health nurse. Discuss at post conference.

LEARNING OBJECTIVE 5

Analyze community nursing diagnoses as they relate to nursing in official health agencies.

CONCEPTS FOR LECTURE

1. Community health nurses in official health departments have been found to address 65 nursing diagnoses contained in the NANDA diagnoses. These diagnoses most often address care of individuals and families. Six population-based community nursing outcomes included in NOC have been tested for their applicability to nursing in official public health agencies. These outcomes (which would result from care directed to community level nursing diagnoses) include: community competence, community health status, community health: immunity, community risk control: chronic disease, community risk control: communicable disease, and community risk control: lead exposure.

POWERPOINT LECTURE SLIDES

NOTE: The number on each PPT Lecture Slide directly corresponds with the Concepts for Lecture.

 Community Nursing Outcomes
- Community competence
- Community health status
- Community health: immunity
- Community risk control: chronic disease
- Community risk control: communicable disease
- Community risk control: lead exposure

SUGGESTIONS FOR CLASSROOM ACTIVITIES

Assign students to small groups. Provide a community case study or a journal article that describes a community and ask students to develop a nursing diagnosis or identify a potential nursing diagnosis and plan to address the health risk.

SUGGESTIONS FOR CLINICAL ACTIVITIES

Invite an official public health nurse manager or team leader to discuss how their agency addresses each of the nursing diagnoses within their agency.

LEARNING OBJECTIVE 6

Analyze the role of the community health nurse in carrying out the core functions and essential services in local health departments.

CONCEPTS FOR LECTURE

1. Community health nursing roles may be examined in relation to the essential services provided by public health agencies and directed by the three core functions of assessment, policy development, and assurance.

2. With assessment, community health nurses conduct community assessments, collect data to monitor the status of identified community health problems, identify assets and needs, identify factors that contribute to community health problems, and identify community health hazards and alert authorities.

3. To fulfill the policy development service of informing, educating, and empowering people about health issues, the community health nurse plans and implements health education programs, develops and disseminates health-related messages to the public, and assists with community organization and empowerment.

4. Under the policy development function of mobilizing community partnerships to identify and solve health problems, the community health nurse identifies key community members, assists those members to articulate needs and plans to address them, and identifies potential coalition members to address particular health issues.

5. Within the third element of policy development, the community health nurse participates in community health program planning based on identified needs, advocates for relevant and culturally sensitive health care programs, and advocates for involvement of community members in health program planning, implementation, and evaluation.

6. Guided by the assurance function of enforcing laws and regulations that protect health and ensure safety, the community health nurse identifies violations of health-related regulations and informs appropriate authorities, and educates the public regarding health-related regulations.

7. To fulfill the assurance function of linking people to health care services, the nurse makes referrals for health care services as needed, and often provides direct health care services.

8. Assurance entails assuring a competent public health and personal health workforce. The nurse assists in the education of community health nurses and other health care professionals.

9. Assurance also means to evaluate the effectiveness, accessibility, and quality of personal and population-based health services. The community health nurse carries out this function by participating in the planning and conduct of program evaluations to determine effectiveness, accessibility, and quality of services.

POWERPOINT LECTURE SLIDES

NOTE: The number on each PPT Lecture Slide directly corresponds with the Concepts for Lecture.

1 Public Health Nursing Roles
- Correlate to the three core functions
  - Assessment
  - Policy Development
  - Assurance

2 Assessment: Monitor and Diagnose
- Conduct community assessments
- Collect data
- Identify community assets and needs
- Identify factors that contribute to community health problems

3 Policy Development: Inform, Educate, and Empower
- Plan and implement health education programs
- Develop and disseminate health-related messages
- Assist with community organization and empowerment

4 Policy Development: Mobilize Community Partnerships
- Identify key community members
- Assist community members to articulate needs and plan to address them
- Identify potential coalition members

5 Policy Development: Develop Policies and Plans
- Participate in community health program planning
- Advocate for relevant and culturally sensitive health care programs
- Advocate for involvement of community members in health program planning, implementation, and evaluation

6 Assurance: Enforce Laws and Regulations
- Identify violations of health-related regulations and inform authorities
- Educate the public regarding health-related regulations

7 Assurance: Link People to Services
- Make referrals for health care services
- Provide direct health care services

8 Assurance: Assure Competent Public Health Workforce
- Assist in the education of community health nurses and other health care professionals

10. Assurance encompasses research for new insights and innovative solutions to health problems. The community health nurse identifies relevant research questions and participates in the design and conducts studies to answer those questions. The nurse also tests innovative practice models and delivery systems.

9 Assurance: Evaluate Effectiveness, Accessibility, and Quality of Health Services
- Participate in the planning and conduct of program evaluations to determine effectiveness, accessibility, and quality of services
- Use evaluative data to improve health care delivery

10 Assurance: Research
- Identify relevant research questions and participate in designing and conducting studies to answer them
- Test innovative practice models and delivery systems

SUGGESTIONS FOR CLASSROOM ACTIVITIES

Have students bring in an article from a public health or community health journal that addresses one of the core functions of public health and related community health nurse activities. Ask students to prepare a summary of the article and present it to class.

SUGGESTIONS FOR CLINICAL ACTIVITIES

Have students identify the activities of nurses in the local health department as they relate to each of the 10 essential functions.

LEARNING OBJECTIVE 7

Define faith community nursing.

CONCEPTS FOR LECTURE

1. A faith community is defined as an organization of families and individuals who share common values, beliefs, religious doctrine, and faith practices that influence their lives.
2. Some faith communities engage in health ministries, which is purposeful activity designed to help people in the congregation and surrounding community to achieve an optimal level of whole person health.
3. Whole person health is a holistic concept that conceives of health as an integration of physical, psychological, social, and spiritual well-being.

POWERPOINT LECTURE SLIDES

NOTE: The number on each PPT Lecture Slide directly corresponds with the Concepts for Lecture.

1 Faith Community
- Families and individuals with shared faith

2 Health Ministry
- Helps people in congregation and surrounding community
- Goal is to achieve optimal, whole person health

3 Whole Person Health
- Holistic concept
- Health is an integration of all aspects of well-being

SUGGESTIONS FOR CLASSROOM ACTIVITIES

1. Have students bring to class a faith-based nursing journal article to present to class.
2. Ask students to discuss the benefits of faith-based nursing care in small groups and present results of their discussion to class.

SUGGESTIONS FOR CLINICAL ACTIVITIES

1. Arrange for students to work with a faith-based agency that provides nursing services if available in the community.
2. Have students identify faith-based agencies in their community and describe the services offered.

LEARNING OBJECTIVE 8

Describe the philosophy of nursing in a faith-based community.

CONCEPTS FOR LECTURE

1. Faith community nursing is based on four philosophical premises: emphasis on the spiritual dimension as well as other dimensions of health; integration of science with theology, and combination of service with worship and nursing with pastoral care; the need for involvement of the faith community in health and healing; and the centrality of spiritual health to well-being, the coexistence of spiritual health with illness, and the possibility of healing in the absence of cure.

POWERPOINT LECTURE SLIDES

NOTE: The number on each PPT Lecture Slide directly corresponds with the Concepts for Lecture.

1 Philosophy of Faith-based Nursing
- Emphasize spiritual dimension as well as other dimensions
- Integrate science with theology
  - Combine service with worship
  - Combine nursing with pastoral care
- Facilitate involvement of faith community in health and healing

1a Philosophy of Faith-based Nursing (continued)
- Spiritual health is central to well-being
  - May coexist with illness
  - Healing may occur in absence of cure

SUGGESTIONS FOR CLASSROOM ACTIVITIES

Assign students to small groups to discuss the philosophical tenets of faith-based nursing. Ask students to compare faith-based and non-faith-based nursing services and discuss which population groups (if any) may be served by faith-based nursing.

SUGGESTIONS FOR CLINICAL ACTIVITIES

Arrange for students to participate in a faith-based nursing initiative. Have them describe how the agency exhibits the elements of the philosophy of faith-based care.

LEARNING OBJECTIVE 9

Describe the scope and standards of nursing in a faith-based community.

CONCEPTS FOR LECTURE

1. The standards of professional nursing practice in a faith-based community address the quality of care, performance appraisal, education for competent practice, collegiality, ethics, collaboration, research, and resource utilization.
2. The standards of care reflect the nursing process: assessment, diagnosis, outcome identification, planning, implementation, and evaluation.

POWERPOINT LECTURE SLIDES

NOTE: The number on each PPT Lecture Slide directly corresponds with the Concepts for Lecture.

1 Standards of Professional Nursing Practice
- Quality of care
- Performance appraisal
- Education for competent practice
- Collegiality

1a Standards of Professional Nursing Practice (continued)
- Ethics
- Collaboration
- Research
- Resource utilization

2 Standards of Care
- Reflect nursing process
  - Assessment
  - Diagnosis
  - Outcome identification
  - Planning
  - Implementation
  - Evaluation

Ask students to prepare a short response to the differences and similarities between the scope and standards of community health nursing and faith-based community nursing. Provide an opportunity for discussion in class.

SUGGESTIONS FOR CLINICAL ACTIVITIES

Have students interview a faith-based nurse about how they incorporate the scope and standards of nursing care.

LEARNING OBJECTIVE 10

Differentiate among models for nursing in a faith-based community.

CONCEPTS FOR LECTURE

1. Faith-based nursing may be provided using a variety of models. Models may be differentiated on the basis of financial arrangements or focus of services. Financial arrangement models include those in which faith-based nurses are paid employees or volunteers

2. Three focus-of-service models have been identified that categorize the approaches to faith-based nursing services: the mission-ministry model, where the focus is on a ministry of reconciliation, health, healing, wholeness, and discipleship; the marketplace model, where services are provided to members of a faith community by professional employees of a health care agency or organization who may or may not be members of a congregation; and the access models, which are political in nature and focus on advocacy for underserved populations where the nurse serves as a catalyst and social change agent to promote access to needed health care services.

POWERPOINT LECTURE SLIDES

NOTE: The number on each PPT Lecture Slide directly corresponds with the Concepts for Lecture.

1 Financial Arrangement Models
- Volunteer nurses
  - Resullts in long-term commitment
  - Nurse is a known and trusted member
- Paid employee

2 Service Focused Models for Faith-based Nursing
- Mission-ministry model
  - Reconciliation, health, healing, wholeness, discipleship focus
- Marketplace model
  - Health care agency provides services
  - Service providers may or may not be members of a congregation
- Access model
  - Political in nature
  - Focus on advocacy for underserved populations
  - Nurse is catalyst and social change agent

SUGGESTIONS FOR CLASSROOM ACTIVITIES

Assign students into three groups. Each group is to search the professional literature for one article that describes the use of a faith-based model for services and to present a summary to class. Encourage discussion on the differences of each of the models and the services provided. Ask students to identify populations served by each of the models.

SUGGESTIONS FOR CLINICAL ACTIVITIES

Invite guest speakers from each of the three categories of service models to discuss their focus, organizational structure, clients served, and role of health professionals.

LEARNING OBJECTIVE 11

Describe the roles and functions of community health nurses in a faith-based community.

CONCEPTS FOR LECTURE

1. The roles and functions of faith-based community nurses are dictated by the needs of the faith communities they serve. Five roles have been identified: health educator, personal health counselor, referral agent, coordinator of volunteers, and developer of support groups. Two additional roles are integrator of faith and health and health advocate.

POWERPOINT LECTURE SLIDES

NOTE: The number on each PPT Lecture Slide directly corresponds with the Concepts for Lecture.

1 Roles and Functions of Faith-based Community Nurses
- Health educator
- Personal health counselor

CONCEPTS FOR LECTURE *continued*

2. Additional responsibilities have been listed that focus on specific categories of services delivered by faith community nurses: basic physiologic care, behavioral care, safety, family care, health system-related care, and community care.

3. Roles for faith-based community nurses are similar to those of community health nurses, but have unique features such as the population served, the collaborative relationship with God and with individuals in the faith community, the emphasis on working with volunteers, the important role in end-of-life care, and grant writing emphasis.

POWERPOINT LECTURE SLIDES *continued*

- Referral agent
- Coordinator of volunteers
- Developer of support groups
- Integrator of faith and health
- Health advocate

 Additional Responsibilities
- Basic physiologic care
- Behavioral care
- Safety
- Family care
- Health system-related care
- Community care

 Unique Roles
- Population served
- Collaborative relationship with God
- Relationship with individuals in faith community
- Emphasis on working with volunteers
- Important role in end-of-life care
- Grant writing emphasis

SUGGESTIONS FOR CLASSROOM ACTIVITIES

Divide students into pairs. Assign each pair one role. Provide a case study of a community health nurse in a faith-based community and ask the students to develop specific actions, strategies, and plans that fulfill their specific role and address the needs of the case study community.

SUGGESTIONS FOR CLINICAL ACTIVITIES

Assign students to attend faith-based support groups in the community. Ask students to suggest a role or function for the community health nurse to promote or address the needs of their support group.

Care of Clients in the School Setting

RESOURCE LIBRARY

COMPANION WEBSITE

Audio Glossary
Appendix E: Information on Selected Communicable
   Diseases
Appendix G: Community Health Assessment and
   Intervention Guide
Exam Review Questions
Case Study: Safety at School

MediaLink Application: High School Stress (video)
Media Links
Challenge Your Knowledge
Update *Healthy People 2010*
Advocacy Interviews

IMAGE LIBRARY

Figure 23-1 Components of the School Health
   Program

LEARNING OBJECTIVE 1

Identify the overall goal of a school health program.

CONCEPTS FOR LECTURE

1. Over 45 million children attend schools in the United States. With students averaging 6 or more hours in those schools every day, it is significant that health factors can influence one's ability to learn and that education can affect one's ability to engage in healthful behaviors.
2. A school health program is defined as all the strategies, activities, and services offered by, in, or in association with schools that are designed to promote students' physical, emotional, and social development.
3. The overall goal of a school health program is to ensure children reach their full academic and health potential through health promotion, protection, and surveillance activities.

POWERPOINT LECTURE SLIDES

NOTE: The number on each PPT Lecture Slide directly corresponds with the Concepts for Lecture.

1. Impact of Schools on Health
   - 45 million children attend schools in the U.S.
   - Impact of health on learning

2. School Health Program
   - Strategies, activities, and services provided by schools
   - Promote students' physical, emotional, and social development

3. Goal of School Health Program:
   - Ensure children reach their full academic and health potential through:
     - Health promotion
     - Protection
     - Surveillance activities

SUGGESTIONS FOR CLASSROOM ACTIVITIES	SUGGESTIONS FOR CLINICAL ACTIVITIES
Divide the class into groups. Have students share their own views on the role of schools to provide health services, and the roles of the community, the state, and the federal government to support those services.	1. Have students investigate school policies and programs in local counties. Compare information about school health programs and services between jurisdictions. 2. Invite a school nurse to post conference to discuss how school health services are delivered in the local district.

LEARNING OBJECTIVE 2

Describe the components of a coordinated school health program.

CONCEPTS FOR LECTURE

1. Elements of a school health program include health services, health education, a healthy environment, physical education, nutrition services, counseling, and psychological services, staff health promotion, and parent and community involvement.

2. The activities that support the health services components of a school health program include assessment and screening, case finding, counseling, health promotion and illness prevention, case management, remedial or rehabilitative services, specific nursing procedures, and emergency care.

3. Health education is described as educating students for health awareness and healthful behaviors using both cognitive and affective learning.

4. The environmental component addresses the need for physical education, and nutritional services such as a school lunch program, counseling and psychological services, and the social environment of the school as well as the surrounding neighborhood and their effects on the health of school-age children.

5. Employee health provides assistance with health problems, reducing illness and absenteeism, enhancing interest in health issues, and role-modeling healthy behaviors.

6. The partnership component addresses the need to foster strong relationships among the school members, the family, and the community, and is directed at enhancing the health of the overall community.

POWERPOINT LECTURE SLIDES

NOTE: The number on each PPT Lecture Slide directly corresponds with the Concepts for Lecture.

1 Components of School Health Program
- Health services
- Health education
- Healthy environment
- Staff health promotion
- Parent and community involvement

1a Components of School Health Program
- See Figure 23-1

2 Health Services Activities
- Assessment and screening
- Case finding
- Counseling
- Health promotion and illness prevention
- Case management

2a Health Services Activities (continued)
- Remedial or rehabilitation services
- Specific nursing procedures
- Emergency care

3 Health Education
- Health awareness and healthful behaviors
- Uses both cognitive and affective learning

4 Environmental Component
- Physical education
- Counseling, psychological, and social services
- Nutritional services

5 Employee Health Component
- Reduce illness and absenteeism
- Role-model healthy behaviors

6 Partnership Component
- School
- Family
- Community

LEARNING OBJECTIVE 3

Describe considerations in assessing biophysical, psychological, physical environmental, sociocultural, behavioral, and health system factors influencing the health of the school population.

CONCEPTS FOR LECTURE

1. The six assessment considerations that are essential for the school nurse to have knowledge of are biophysical, psychological, physical environment, sociocultural, behavioral, and health system considerations.

2. Biophysical considerations include age and maturation, genetics, physiologic function such as obesity, asthma, and attention deficit hyperactivity disorders and immunization levels.

3. Psychological considerations include the relationships of students and staff, the relationship between the school and family, discipline practices of teachers, grading practices, and the presence of mental illness.

4. The physical environment includes the actual school building with its age and chemical and safety hazards, the distance the school is from the community, the potential for spread of disease in the facility, and the level of preparedness in the school setting for disaster events.

5. Sociocultural considerations include culture and ethnicity, economic resources, legislation, abuse and violence, and the potential for terrorism.

6. Behavioral considerations include school attendance factors, physical and recreational activities, diet and nutrition (including the adequacy of lunches brought from home and quality of school lunches), substance use and abuse, safety practices, and gambling habits of adolescents.

7. Health system considerations include assessments at the individual and community levels, such as the availability of health care services, the relationship between the school and the health care community, the organizational structure for delivering health services in the school setting, and the availability of mental health services in the school setting as well as the community.

POWERPOINT LECTURE SLIDES

NOTE: The number on each PPT Lecture Slide directly corresponds with the Concepts for Lecture.

1. Assessment of School Health Factors
   - Biophysical
   - Psychological
   - Physical environmental
   - Sociocultural
   - Behavioral
   - Health system

2. Biophysical Considerations
   - Age and maturation
   - Genetics
   - Physiologic function

3. Psychological Considerations
   - Student and staff relationships
   - School and family relationships
   - Teacher discipline practices
   - Mental illness presence

4. Physical Environment
   - School building age and hazards
   - Proximity of school to community
   - Potential for spread of disease
   - Disaster preparedness

5. Sociocultural Considerations
   - Culture and ethnicity
   - Economic resources
   - Legislation
   - Abuse and violence
   - Terrorism potential

6. Behavioral Considerations
   - School attendance
   - Physical and recreational activities
   - Diet and nutrition
   - Home and school lunch quality
   - Substance use and abuse
   - Safety practices
   - Gambling habits of adolescents

7 Health System Considerations
- Assessments at individual and community level
  ○ Availability of health and mental health services
  ○ Relationship between school and community
  ○ Structure for delivering health services

SUGGESTIONS FOR CLASSROOM ACTIVITIES

Divide students into three groups: elementary school, middle school, and high school. Have students develop an assessment tool or list of questions that incorporates each of the six areas of consideration that they would need to investigate in assessing the health status of their assigned population. Provide an opportunity for discussion.

SUGGESTIONS FOR CLINICAL ACTIVITIES

Assign students to work with a school nurse. During their clinical experience, ask students to assess the health of an individual student or the school population using the six assessment considerations.

LEARNING OBJECTIVE 4

Identify areas of emphasis in primary prevention in the school setting and analyze the role of the community health nurse in each.

CONCEPTS FOR LECTURE

1. Primary interventions include immunization services, safety, exclusion from school, health education, diet and nutrition, exercise, and illness prevention.

POWERPOINT LECTURE SLIDES

NOTE: The number on each PPT Lecture Slide directly corresponds with the Concepts for Lecture.

1 Primary Interventions
- Immunization
- Safety and injury/violence prevention
- Exclusion from school
- Health education
- Diet and nutrition
- Exercise and physical activity
- Illness prevention

SUGGESTIONS FOR CLASSROOM ACTIVITIES

Provide students with case studies based on a school setting with an outbreak of hepatitis A, rubella, or chickenpox. Have students identify primary prevention interventions that might have prevented the epidemic. Have students discuss interventions with the class.

SUGGESTIONS FOR CLINICAL ACTIVITIES

Assign students to work with a school nurse or community health nurse who provides immunizations to school age children. Have students review immunization records for the school nurse and identify adequacy of vaccination status of children.

LEARNING OBJECTIVE 5

Describe the facets of secondary prevention in the school setting and analyze related community health nursing roles.

CONCEPTS FOR LECTURE

1. Secondary interventions include screening for existing health conditions, referral, counseling, and treatment.
2. The goal of screening is to detect disease as well as children with special needs that require adjustment of the education program. Types of screening programs include dental screening, vision screening, hematocrit screening,

POWERPOINT LECTURE SLIDES

NOTE: The number on each PPT Lecture Slide directly corresponds with the Concepts for Lecture.

1 Secondary Interventions
- Screening
- Referral

height and weight measurements, and screening for scoliosis. School nurses recruit parents and volunteers to assist with screening and train them to participate effectively. School nurses also need to interpret the results of screening tests and inform parents of results.

3. Referral may occur as a result of the screening process when the data are interpreted by the nurse and discussed with parents. School nurses may also refer students or staff for care of other health problems identified in the course of a nursing assessment of an individual child or staff member.

4. Counseling involves assisting students, families, and staff to make informed health decisions.

5. Treatment can involve emergency care or medical management of minor illnesses, acute or chronic conditions, physical therapy, or care of special needs children.

- Counseling
- Treatment

[2] Screening
- Goal is to detect disease and special needs
- Types of screening services

[3] Referral
- Interpret data from screening and discuss with parents

[4] Counseling
- Assist in making informed health decisions

[5] Treatment
- Emergency care
- Medical management
- Special procedures

SUGGESTIONS FOR CLASSROOM ACTIVITIES

1. Assign students to perform vision, hearing, scoliosis, and height and weight checks on each other in the lab. Have students read about the procedures for performing vision and hearing screenings.

2. Assign students to read articles on hearing loss in school age children and types of vision problems that children may have.

SUGGESTIONS FOR CLINICAL ACTIVITIES

1. Invite a school nurse, a pediatrician, and a physical therapist to discuss scoliosis and techniques for performing this screening procedure on children.

2. Arrange for students to participate in a mass school health screening or to provide screening for children who were absent during the mass screening. Assign students to various screening stations.

LEARNING OBJECTIVE 6

Describe areas of emphasis in tertiary prevention in the school setting and analyze the role of the community health nurse with respect to each.

CONCEPTS FOR LECTURE

1. There are five aspects of tertiary prevention: preventing the recurrence of acute problems, preventing complications, fostering adjustment to chronic illness and handicapping conditions, dealing with learning disabilities, and sustaining school-based health services.

POWERPOINT LECTURE SLIDES

NOTE: The number on each PPT Lecture Slide directly corresponds with the Concepts for Lecture.

[1] Tertiary Prevention
- Prevent recurrence of acute problems
- Prevent complications
- Foster adjustment to chronic illness and handicapping conditions
- Address learning disabilities
- Sustain school-based health services

SUGGESTIONS FOR CLASSROOM ACTIVITIES

Ask students to investigate the types of acute and chronic conditions represented in their local school district. Assign students to various schools in the district to contact or interview school nurses. Provide an opportunity to share results of inquiry in class.

SUGGESTIONS FOR CLINICAL ACTIVITIES

Have students work with a school nurse in a school that serves medically fragile children or in a classroom with special needs children. Ask students to develop a nursing care plan for one child and family and present at post conference.

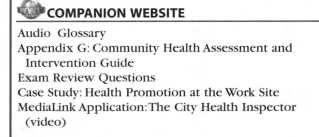

Care of Clients in the Work Setting

RESOURCE LIBRARY

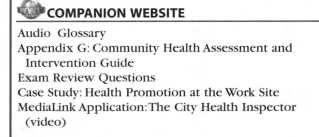

🌐 COMPANION WEBSITE

Audio Glossary
Appendix G: Community Health Assessment and
  Intervention Guide
Exam Review Questions
Case Study: Health Promotion at the Work Site
MediaLink Application: The City Health Inspector
  (video)

Media Links
Challenge Your Knowledge
Update *Healthy People 2010*
Advocacy Interviews

📖 IMAGE LIBRARY

Table 24-2 Primary Prevention Emphases and
  Interventions in Work Settings

LEARNING OBJECTIVE 1

Describe advantages of providing health care in work settings.

CONCEPTS FOR LECTURE

1. With nearly two thirds of the U.S. population over 16 years of age working, occupational or employee health has provided another focus for nurses to influence personal behaviors on and off the job.

2. Employer's interest in promoting and maintaining employee health has increased as a result of the effects of good health habits on productivity. With increasing costs of health insurance, employer support for health programs has been shown to be cost-effective.

3. Advantages of providing health care in work settings include the following: people spend a significant amount of their time at work; employees are a captive audience; individuals in the workforce may be at risk for a variety of health problems, and therefore motivated to maintain their health to ensure their continued ability to work; health promotion in work settings is efficient and cost-effective; health care services in the work setting may decrease both the visible costs of poor health (sickness, absenteeism, and employee turnover) and invisible costs related to low productivity, poor-quality work, poor customer services, accidents, and legal claims related to illness and injury.

4. The goal of occupational health services is to ensure that working adults reach and maintain their full

POWERPOINT LECTURE SLIDES

NOTE: The number on each PPT Lecture Slide directly corresponds with the Concepts for Lecture.

1 Clients in Work Settings
  • Two-thirds of U.S. population over 16 years of age work.

2 Employer Awareness of Benefits
  • Cost effectiveness
  • Impact on productivity

3 Advantages of Employee Health Programs
  • Amount of time at work
  • Captive audience
  • Risks for health problems
  • Motivation to maintain health
  • Health promotion efficient and cost-effective

3a Advantages of Employee Health Programs (continued)
  • Visible costs
    ○ Costs of poor health
      – Sickness
      – Absenteeism
      – Employee turnover

working potential through health promotion, protection, and surveillance activities.

3b Advantages of Employee Health Programs (continued)
- Invisible costs
  - Low productivity
  - Poor-quality work
  - Poor customer services
  - Accidents
  - Legal claims related to illness and injury

4 Goal of Occupational Health Services
- Ensure working adults reach and maintain full working potential
  - Health promotion
  - Protection
  - Surveillance activities

SUGGESTIONS FOR CLASSROOM ACTIVITIES

1. Ask students to contact local employers to inquire about availability of occupational health programs. Have students report their findings to the class.
2. Assign students to three groups. Have each group research local, state, and national occupational injury and illness rates.

SUGGESTIONS FOR CLINICAL ACTIVITIES

Assign students to work with an occupational health nurse in local hospitals, federal buildings, or other large businesses.

LEARNING OBJECTIVE 2

Identify types of health and safety hazards encountered in work settings.

CONCEPTS FOR LECTURE

1. The types of health and safety hazards encountered in work settings include occupational injuries such as musculoskeletal injuries, repetitive motion injuries, accidents, and chemical and noise exposure; agricultural injuries such as exposure to noise, heavy equipment accidents, and exposure to toxic chemicals; and occupational illnesses such as cancer, asthma, reproductive hazards, exposure to neurotoxins, noise, and skin ailments from chemicals.

POWERPOINT LECTURE SLIDES

NOTE: The number on each PPT Lecture Slide directly corresponds with the Concepts for Lecture.

1 Types of Health and Safety Hazards
- Occupational injuries
  - Musculoskeletal injuries
  - Accidents
  - Exposure to hazardous chemicals

1a Types of Health and Safety Hazards (continued)
- Agricultural injuries
  - Heavy equipment accidents
  - Exposure to hazardous chemicals
- Occupational illnesses

SUGGESTIONS FOR CLASSROOM ACTIVITIES

Provide students with a case study of an employee with a work-related illness or injury. Ask students to develop a nursing diagnosis and care plan.

SUGGESTIONS FOR CLINICAL ACTIVITIES

Have students explore several different types of businesses and industries and identify potential health and safety hazards that might be present in each type of industry. Be sure to include nursing in specific settings (e.g., hospital, nursing home, school) as some of the employment settings explored.

LEARNING OBJECTIVE 3

Identify biophysical, psychological, physical environmental, sociocultural, behavioral, and health system factors that influence health in work settings.

CONCEPTS FOR LECTURE

1. Biophysical considerations include the age of the employee with young adults having higher risks for injuries and older workers being at risk for occupational deaths due to age and preexisting conditions.

2. Workplaces that employee more females of childbearing age may need to provide prenatal care or contraceptive services and monitor the workplace for toxic or physical hazards.

3. Elements of physiologic function address the extent of injury and illness suffered by a population as well as their immunization levels. Occupational illnesses and work-related asthma may need to be monitored and assessed.

4. Psychological considerations relating to workplace health are stress in the workplace and mental health and illness.

5. Two models that explore the relationship between stress and health effects on the job are the job strain model, which states that job strain is the result of high job demands coupled with low ability to control demands and low levels of social support, and the effort-reward imbalance model, which states that job stress results from an imbalance between one's perceived work effort and the rewards received.

6. Another psychological consideration is mental health and illness in the work setting, especially depression, which can be a major risk factor for heart disease and other physical health conditions, as well as increasing health care costs to employer and employee.

7. Physical environmental factors affecting workers' health include physical hazards such as noise, lifting requirements, and equipment; chemical hazards such as toxins, lead, and heavy metals; electrical and magnetic field hazards; and exposure to metallic compounds, allergens, and molds.

8. Sociocultural considerations include those aspects of the social work environment that either positively or negatively affect the health status of workers, such as the quality of social interactions, attitudes toward work and health, and the presence or absence of racial tensions or other tensions.

9. Four major areas of sociocultural assessment include the effects of policy and legislation, the interactive effects of work and family life, workplace violence, and other sociocultural factors.

10. Behavioral factors that affect workplace health include the type of work performed, consumption patterns, patterns of rest and exercise, and use of safety devices.

11. Health system factors that the nurse must consider are the types of services used and the reasons for and appropriateness of their use, the availability of services, and the availability of health insurance.

POWERPOINT LECTURE SLIDES

NOTE: The number on each PPT Lecture Slide directly corresponds with the Concepts for Lecture.

1 Biophysical Considerations
- Age of employees determines health risks
  - Young adult risks
  - Older adult risks

2 Female Gender Composition
- Pregnancy
- Reproductive health

3 Physiologic Function
- Extent of injury and illness

4 Psychological Considerations
- Stress in workplace
- Mental health and illness

5 Stress in Workplace and Health Effects
- Job strain model
- Effort-reward imbalance

6 Mental Health and Illness in Workplace
- Depression
- Risk factor for health conditions
- Increase costs to employer and employee

7 Physical Environmental Considerations
- Physical hazards
  - Noise
  - Lifting
  - Equipment
- Chemical hazards
  - Toxins
- Electrical and magnetic field hazards
- Exposure to metallic compounds, allergens, molds

8 Sociocultural Considerations
- Positive or negative influences
  - Quality of social interactions
  - Attitudes toward work and health
  - Presence or absence of racial or other tensions

9 Major Areas of Sociocultural Assessment
- Policy and legislation
- Interactive effects of work and family life
- Workplace violence
- Other factors

10 Behavioral Considerations
- Lifestyle factors
  - Type of work performed
  - Consumption patterns
  - Patterns of rest and exercise
  - Use of safety devices

[11] Health System Considerations
- Types of services used
- Reasons for and appropriateness of use
- Availability of services
- Availability of health insurance

SUGGESTIONS FOR CLASSROOM ACTIVITIES

Assign students to six groups. With each of the epidemiological considerations, provide a case study for groups to identify factors in each dimension that are influencing the health status of the employee population in the case study.

SUGGESTIONS FOR CLINICAL ACTIVITIES

Have students identify factors in each dimension that are influencing the health status of the employee population at their clinical setting.

LEARNING OBJECTIVE 4

Analyze spheres of social influence and their effect on the health of employees.

CONCEPTS FOR LECTURE

1. The four spheres of social influence include the health-related behaviors of employees; the influence of coworkers on health; the influence of management's attitudes toward health and health-related policies and enforcement; and the influence of legal, social, and political actions on the health of employees.

POWERPOINT LECTURE SLIDES

NOTE: The number on each PPT Lecture Slide directly corresponds with the Concepts for Lecture.

[1] Four Spheres of Influence
- Individual health-related behaviors
- Coworkers' attitudes to and influence on health-related behaviors
- Management's attitudes and enforcement of health policies
- Legal, social, and political actions

SUGGESTIONS FOR CLASSROOM ACTIVITIES

Assign students to four spheres of influence groups. Provide a workplace case study and ask each group to identify influences and factors in each sphere that affect the health of employees.

SUGGESTIONS FOR CLINICAL ACTIVITIES

Have students assess and identify examples of the influences of each sphere on health-related behaviors of employees in their clinical setting, site, or agency. Discuss their observations at post conference.

LEARNING OBJECTIVE 5

Describe types of health care programs in work settings.

CONCEPTS FOR LECTURE

1. The types of health care programs in work settings are described as internal health care systems, which typically include toxic exposure programs, health promotion programs, comprehensive programs, and family care programs.
2. Toxic exposure programs are OSHA regulated and consist of two types: control programs or elimination programs.

POWERPOINT LECTURE SLIDES

NOTE: The number on each PPT Lecture Slide directly corresponds with the Concepts for Lecture.

[1] Types of Health Care Programs in Work Settings
- Internal health care systems
  - Toxic exposure programs
  - Health promotion programs

CONCEPTS FOR LECTURE *continued*

3. Control programs address engineering controls, work practice controls, and use of safety equipment or devices. The nurse may advocate on behalf of employees to make sure that employers comply with OSHA regulations.

4. The goal of health promotion programs is to limit hospitalizations and acute care expenses through education about improper body mechanics and other practices and development of company health policies.

5. The nurse has a variety of options and opportunities in employee health promotion programs, such as programs that are either illness oriented or wellness oriented.

6. Comprehensive programs incorporate a wellness approach through awareness of stress and stress management techniques, lifestyle changes such as exercise programs, and changes in environmental conditions to promote better health. Comprehensive programs address health problems encountered by employees beyond those strictly related to work. Nurses have an opportunity to offer stress or weight reduction classes or advocate for yoga and massage services to employees.

7. Family care responds to the premise that families and children are important to the productivity of the worker and may offer on-site child or elder care programs on-site, or counseling services.

8. The internal system of care interfaces with the external community health care system to address health care needs that cannot be met by the internal system.

POWERPOINT LECTURE SLIDES *continued*

- ○ Comprehensive programs
- ○ Family care

[2] Toxic Exposure Prevention Programs
- Control programs
- Elimination programs

[3] Control Programs
- Engineering controls
- Controlled work practices
- Safety equipment and devices
- Elimination programs
  - ○ Remove substances from workplace
  - ○ OSHA-regulated

[4] Health Promotion Programs
- Goal
  - ○ Limit hospitalizations and acute care expenses
- Types of services
  - ○ Education
    - – Proper body mechanics
    - – Company health policies

[5] Employee Health Promotion Programs
- Illness-oriented
- Wellness-oriented

[6] Comprehensive Programs
- Wellness approach
  - ○ Awareness
    - – Stress management programs
  - ○ Lifestyle changes
    - – Exercise programs

[6a] Comprehensive Programs (continued)
- Wellness approach
  - ○ Change environmental conditions to promote better health
    - – Yoga
    - – Massage services

[7] Family Care Programs
- On-site child care programs
- Counseling services
- On-site elder care services

[8] External System
- Internal system of care interfaces with the external community health care system
  - ○ Addresses health care needs that cannot be met by the internal system

---

SUGGESTIONS FOR CLASSROOM ACTIVITIES

Assign students to small groups. Ask groups to select local businesses, assess the health needs of employees at the business, and develop a health care program or service for that business.

SUGGESTIONS FOR CLINICAL ACTIVITIES

Arrange for students to participate in an employee health fair or screening program with an occupational health nurse or a community health nurse. Have students examine the types of health care programs that are available in their clinical setting and relate the goals and objectives of the employee health fair or screening program to potential benefits to both the employee and the employer.

LEARNING OBJECTIVE 6

Describe areas of emphasis in primary prevention in work settings and analyze the role of the community health nurse with respect to each.

CONCEPTS FOR LECTURE

1. Primary prevention includes health promotion, illness prevention, injury prevention, and violence prevention in the work setting.
2. Health promotion programs may focus on changing employee behavior or on creating conditions in the work environment that promote health. Specific initiatives may include employee education or the development of policies (and possibly facilities) that support health and a healthful environment. Providing prenatal care for pregnant employees is another example of health promotion in the work setting.
3. Illness prevention services may include immunization, risk factor modification, postexposure prophylaxis and stress reduction/management initiatives.
4. Injury prevention is often regulated by NIOSH workplace safety policies. Nurses may be responsible for monitoring hazardous conditions in the workplace or for planning and conducting environmental testing for hazardous levels of chemicals. Nurses may provide safety education for employees, make provisions for adequate safety equipment, develop policies and procedures that prevent injury, modify or eliminate injury risk factors in the work setting, and develop adequate management support for injury prevention policies and procedures.
5. Workplace violence prevention addresses the following elements: administrative support for violence prevention through policies and procedures for reporting violence or potential violence, assessment of company history and rates of violence, determination of violence patterns, and identification of workplace hazards that promote violence. The nurse is responsible for modification of worksite environments that promote violence, installing of security devices, development of processes and procedures for handling workplace violence or potential for violence, development of reporting procedures, development of disciplinary sanctions for violent behaviors in the work setting, and employee education on violence prevention, anger management, and recognition of potentially violent situations.

POWERPOINT LECTURE SLIDES

NOTE: The number on each PPT Lecture Slide directly corresponds with the Concepts for Lecture.

1. Primary Prevention in Work Setting (Refer to Table 24-2)
   - Health promotion
   - Illness prevention
   - Injury prevention
   - Violence prevention

2. Health Promotion
   - Exercise programs
   - Stress management
   - Programs to reduce negative effects of commuting
   - Reproductive health education and referral services

3. Illness Prevention
   - Immunization
   - Risk factor modification
   - Postexposure prophylaxis
   - Stress reduction/management education

4. Injury Prevention
   - Safety education
   - Make provisions for adequate safety equipment
   - Monitor effective use of safety equipment
   - Develop policies and procedures that prevent injury
   - Modify or eliminate injury risk factors in the work setting
   - Develop adequate management support for injury prevention policies and procedures

5. Violence Prevention
   - Modify worksite environments that promote violence
   - Encourage the installation of security devices
   - Develop processes and procedures for handling workplace violence or potential for violence
   - Develop reporting procedures
   - Develop disciplinary sanctions for violent behavior in the work setting
   - Employee education on violence prevention, anger management, and recognition of potentially violent situations

SUGGESTIONS FOR CLASSROOM ACTIVITIES

Have students examine primary prevention interventions in their clinical setting and identify if the interventions that emphasize health promotion, illness prevention, injury prevention, or violence prevention. Report findings at post conference.

SUGGESTIONS FOR CLINICAL ACTIVITIES

Have students identify workplace hazards at their clinical site or agency and report findings at post conference.

Describe major considerations in secondary prevention in work settings and analyze the contribution of community health nursing in each.

CONCEPTS FOR LECTURE

1. Secondary prevention strategies include screening and surveillance, treatment for existing conditions, and emergency care.

2. Screening and surveillance addresses the need for pre-employment screening, determination of work capacity, recommendations regarding work conditions or accommodations, periodic employee screening, periodic environmental screening programs, and reporting and interpreting screening findings and making referrals for care or environmental modification as needed.

3. Nurses may be involved in treatment for existing conditions by providing direct services for work-related illness or injury, providing immediate first aid, making referrals for medical assistance, developing health care delivery programs that address a high prevalence problem in the occupational setting, advocating for adequate employee health insurance coverage, and advocating for accessible internal or external health care services to meet employee health needs.

4. Emergency care provides on-site services for psychological and physical emergencies. Nurses may provide direct services to address coworkers' responses to homicide, suicide, and sexual assault, as well as referrals. Nurses respond to accidents and render aid for medical conditions such as worker heart attacks, strokes, seizure disorders, and insulin reactions. Nurses may also assist in the development of individual and disaster emergency response plans for the work setting, respond to individual physical or emotional emergencies, make referrals for continued treatment, respond to care needs in an occupational disaster, and evaluate the health effects of occupational disasters.

POWERPOINT LECTURE SLIDES

NOTE: The number on each PPT Lecture Slide directly corresponds with the Concepts for Lecture.

1 Secondary Prevention
- Screening and surveillance
- Treat existing conditions
- Emergency care

2 Screening and Surveillance
- Preemployment screening
- Determination of work capacity
- Recommendations regarding work conditions or accommodations
- Periodic employee screening
- Periodic environmental screening
- Reporting and interpreting screening findings and making referrals for care or environmental modification

3 Treat Existing Conditions
- Treat work-related illness or injury
- Provide immediate first aid
- Refer for outside medical assistance as needed
- Develop health care delivery programs to address high prevalence problems
- Advocate for adequate employee health insurance coverage
- Advocate for accessible internal or external health care services

4 Emergency Response
- Assist in developing individual and disaster emergency response plans in the work setting
- Respond to individual physical or emotional emergencies
- Refer for continued treatment
- Respond to care needs in an occupational disaster
- Evaluate the health effects of occupational disasters

SUGGESTIONS FOR CLASSROOM ACTIVITIES

Invite an employee health nurse, occupational health nurse, or community health nurse to present information on employer programs aimed at secondary prevention. Discuss gaps in services available in the local community.

SUGGESTIONS FOR CLINICAL ACTIVITIES

Have students identify secondary prevention services for their clinical experience. Ask students to discuss the role of the nurse in their clinical work setting.

LEARNING OBJECTIVE 8

Describe emphases in tertiary prevention in work settings and analyze the role of the community health nurse with respect to each.

CONCEPTS FOR LECTURE

1. Tertiary prevention in the work setting is directed toward preventing the spread of communicable diseases, preventing the recurrence of other acute conditions, preventing complications of chronic conditions, and assessing fitness to return to work.

2. The nurse is involved in the prevention of the spread of communicable diseases by providing employee immunization programs and providing education on infection control procedures.

3. Prevention of the recurrence of other acute conditions requires the nurse to educate employees to prevent recurrent health problems, and advocate for environmental modification to prevent recurrent problems.

4. Prevention of complications of chronic conditions means that the nurse must monitor treatment effects and disease status, educate employees for disease self-management, and ensure that modifications of the work environment are in place to accommodate limitations due to disability.

5. Finally, the nurse assesses an employee's fitness to return to work by following up on worker's compensation claims, assessing the recovery status of an employee, and ensuring that modifications of the work environment are in place to promote return to work for an injured employee.

POWERPOINT LECTURE SLIDES

NOTE: The number on each PPT Lecture Slide directly corresponds with the Concepts for Lecture.

1 Tertiary Prevention
- Prevent the spread of communicable diseases
- Prevent recurrence of acute health problems
- Prevent complication of chronic conditions
- Assess fitness to return to work

2 Preventing the Spread of Communicable Diseases
- Employee immunization programs
- Education on infection control procedures

3 Preventing the Recurrence of Acute Conditions
- Education of employees
- Advocacy for environmental modifications

4 Preventing Complications of Chronic Conditions
- Monitor treatment effects and disease status
- Educate employees for disease self-management
- Ensure modification of the work environment to accommodate limitations due to disability

5 Assessing Fitness to Return to Work
- Follow-up on worker's compensation claims
- Assess recovery status
- Ensure modification of work environment as needed to promote return to work

SUGGESTIONS FOR CLASSROOM ACTIVITIES

Have students examine the sick-leave policies at their clinical setting and evaluate the effectiveness of the sick-leave policy in terms of prevention of the spread of communicable diseases. Discuss results of findings in class.

SUGGESTIONS FOR CLINICAL ACTIVITIES

1. If available, arrange for students to participate in an employee immunization program such as for influenza, tetanus, or hepatitis A or B. What incentives are in place, if any, to encourage participation in an employee immunization program? What are the barriers to participation?

2. Ask students to develop recommendations for engineering measures for an identified safety hazard at their clinical site or agency, at the college, or any other workplace. Present the recommendations to the class.

25 CHAPTER

Care of Clients in Urban and Rural Settings

RESOURCE LIBRARY

 COMPANION WEBSITE

Audio Glossary
Appendix G: Community Health Assessment
  and Intervention Guide
Exam Review Questions
Case Study: Community Health Care in a Rural Area
MediaLink Application: Choosing a Career in Rural
  Health (video)

MediaLink Application: The Urban Health Initiative
  (video)
Media Links
Challenge Your Knowledge
Update *Healthy People 2010*
Advocacy Interviews

📖 **IMAGE LIBRARY**

Table 25-1 Approaches to Defining Urban and Rural

LEARNING OBJECTIVE 1

Describe various approaches to defining *rural* and *urban*.

CONCEPTS FOR LECTURE

1. Essential to understanding the importance that rural or urban settings have on population health is the number of people affected by their geographical and residential locations. Approximately 83% of the U.S. population lives in urban areas, and 30% live in cities with populations of 5 million or more.
2. Definitions for rural and urban have been used by various organizations or entities to capture specific features. One approach that has been used is that of the U.S. Census Bureau, which defines areas as rural, urban clusters, or urbanized.
3. Another approach is the U.S. Department of Agriculture's which defines urban regions in terms of three categories of metropolitan counties based on population size; rural regions are classified as non-metropolitan based on eight population size continuum classifications.
4. The Office of Management and Budget (OMB) system classifies areas based on population as metropolitan counties (large, medium, and small) and nonmetropolitan counties (micropolitan and non-micropolitan).
5. The Montana State University rurality index uses a person-based approach to defining rurality as an

POWERPOINT LECTURE SLIDES

NOTE: The number on each PPT Lecture Slide directly corresponds with the Concepts for Lecture.

1 Importance of Setting on Population Health
  • 83% of U.S. population live in urban areas
  • 30% live in cities of 5 million of more

2 Approaches to Defining Rural and Urban Settings (Refer to Table 25-1)
  • U.S. Census Bureau
    ○ Rural
    ○ Urban cluster
    ○ Urbanized

3 U.S. Department of Agriculture
  • Metropolitan counties
    ○ Four designations
  • Non-metropolitan counties
    ○ Eight designations

4 Office of Management and Budget (OMB)
  • Metropolitan
    ○ Large: 1 million or more

CONCEPTS FOR LECTURE *continued*

index for an individual resident based on the population density of the county and the distance to the nearest emergency services for both urban and rural classifications.

POWERPOINT LECTURE SLIDES *continued*

- ○ Medium: 250,000 to 1 million
- ○ Small: 50,000-250,000
- Non-metropolitan

 Montana State University Rurality Index
- Urban
  - ○ An index for an individual resident based on the population density of the county and the distance to the nearest emergency services
- Rural
  - ○ Same index

SUGGESTIONS FOR CLASSROOM ACTIVITIES

Have students find and discuss their community of residence classification using the U.S. Census Bureau, the OMB, and the U.S. Department of Agriculture approaches. What are some of the benefits and disadvantages of each of the classification systems?

LEARNING OBJECTIVE 2

Analyze barriers to effective health care in urban and rural areas.

CONCEPTS FOR LECTURE

1. Barriers to effective health care in urban and rural areas can be categorized into provider, scope of practice, types of health care services available, proximity to health care resources, beliefs and health beliefs, and economic or financial resources.

POWERPOINT LECTURE SLIDES

NOTE: The number on each PPT Lecture Slide directly corresponds with the Concepts for Lecture.

 Barriers to Effective Health Care
- Provider
- Scope of practice
- Types of services
- Proximity to services
- Health beliefs
- Economic and financial resources

SUGGESTIONS FOR CLASSROOM ACTIVITIES

Have students develop a list of examples for each of the barriers to health care for rural and urban areas, either from personal experiences or the literature. Provide an opportunity for students to discuss their examples.

SUGGESTIONS FOR CLINICAL ACTIVITIES

Assign students to a rural health department, clinic, or other appropriate setting, such as working with a community health nurse who provides services to rural clients. Have students make a journal entry about their observations of client needs, barriers to health care, and the role of the rural health nurse.

LEARNING OBJECTIVE 3

Identify differences in biophysical, psychological, physical environmental, sociocultural, behavioral, and health system factors as they affect health in urban and rural areas.

CONCEPTS FOR LECTURE

1. Factors influencing the health status of rural and urban populations include compositional and contextual factors. Compositional factors arise from the characteristics of the people who compose the population in a given area. Contextual factors are derived from the characteristics unique to the rural or urban setting.

2. A key term is *health disparity population*, which is defined as a population where there is a significant disparity in the overall rate of disease incidence, prevalence, morbidity, mortality, or survival rates in the population compared to the health status of the general population.

3. Biophysical factors include differences in age and aging distributions and the physical health status of individuals living in rural and urban settings. Rural populations tend to have more elderly people because people in rural areas are growing older, younger people are moving out of rural areas, and older people are returning to rural areas to retire. Age disparities are associated with different patterns of disease prevalence. Differences in physical health between rural and urban settings include differences in stress levels, higher rates of premature mortality in rural areas, higher rates of COPD and cancer in urban areas, higher rates of accident mortality in rural areas, and higher rates of dental problems, diabetes, and obesity in rural regions.

4. Psychological factors include higher rates of firearm-related suicide mortality in rural areas due to a rural cultural value on self-reliance, travel to and availability of mental health services, and social stigma of mental illness. The community health nurse's role for both areas includes advocating with providers to increase diagnosis and effective treatment of mental illness.

5. Physical environmental factors include differences between the built and natural environment. The built environment consists of buildings, spaces, and products created or modified significantly from their natural state by people. The natural environment involves natural features of the area, including plants and animal life, and terrain. Examples of urban built environments impacting health include noise exposure, overcrowding, and environmental pollutants. Examples of the natural environment that may affect health risks include specific plants and animals that are vectors of disease, sources of allergens, and weather conditions that can diminish access to health facilities or the ability to receive home care services. Community health nurses in urban areas can advocate for planned development that promotes physical activity, and in rural areas, the nurse can advocate for increased access to needed transportation services or safety of road systems.

POWERPOINT LECTURE SLIDES

NOTE: The number on each PPT Lecture Slide directly corresponds with the Concepts for Lecture.

1. Factors Influencing Health
   - Compositional
     - People characteristics
   - Contextual
     - Setting characteristics

2. Health Disparity Population
   - A population where there is a significant disparity in the overall rate of disease incidence, prevalence, morbidity, mortality, or survival rates in the population compared to the health status of the general population

3. Biophysical Factors
   - Age and aging
   - Physical health status

4. Psychological Factors
   - Variations in stress levels
   - Mental health services
   - Suicide
   - Role of nurse

5. Physical Environmental Factors
   - Built environments
     - Noise
     - Overcrowding
     - Sanitation
     - Pollutants/chemical exposures
   - Natural environment
     - Plants/animals
       - Disease
       - Allergens
     - Physical barriers to health services

6. Sociocultural Factors
   - Social values/conditions
     - Gender roles
     - Sustained relationships
   - Economic issues
     - Poverty

6a. Sociocultural Factors (continued)
   - Cultural factors
   - Occupational factors
   - Health knowledge and value differences
     - Self-reliance
       - Rejection of needed health care services

7. Behavioral Factors
   - Dietary consumption patterns
   - Use of tobacco/drugs/alcohol
   - Physical activity

6. Sociocultural considerations include differences in social values and conditions, economic issues, cultural factors, occupational factors, and health knowledge and values that are different for each area and that affect health. Rural cultures are described as high-context cultures in which they value sustained relationships, whereas urban cultures may be low-context cultures resulting from social isolation, greater mobility, and high turnover in friends and coworkers. Yet, rural elderly populations tend to experience more social isolation as a result of transportation and distance situations. Rural cultures may also have a sense of self-reliance that rejects or hesitates to utilize or delays treatment from health care services. Community health nurse roles include advocating for public assistance for low-income families, addressing legislation affecting migrant workers, and joining advocacy groups to address the inequities of workers' compensation legislation in their states.

7. Behavioral considerations include similar risk factors for diabetes and obesity but resulting from different causal factors. Rural populations consume more fat and calories, have limited access to nutritionists or weight control programs, use different meal patterns, and tend to use tobacco and alcohol at higher rates than urban populations. Urban populations may use tobacco and alcohol, but have higher use rates for drugs. Rural populations tend to have 50% less leisure-time physical activity, less physical education in school curriculums, or less access to exercise facilities. Rural populations are less likely to engage in the use of complementary or alternative medicines or to engage in health-promotive behaviors such as immunizations for influenza and pneumonia or routine pap tests.

8. Health system considerations include limited access, narrower scope of practice, limited resources, and higher costs for health care in rural regions, which can create health professional shortage areas and medically underserved areas or populations. A key solution to health care disparities is the use of organized indigenous caregiving strategies, which involves training local laypeople for specific provider extender roles.

- Sexual activity
- Health-related behaviors

 Health System Factors
- Accessibility/availability
- Cost of care
- Scope of practice issues
- Organized indigenous caregiving strategies

SUGGESTIONS FOR CLASSROOM ACTIVITIES

1. Ask students to research a nursing journal that features delivery of nursing care to rural populations. Have students present a summary of their article and discuss the factors that affect health in a rural area.

2. Assign students into two groups: urban and rural. Ask the groups to list physical, sociocultural, economic, and other advantages for their area. Have the groups define their term. Provide an opportunity for discussion.

SUGGESTIONS FOR CLINICAL ACTIVITIES

1. Assign students to either an urban or rural health clinic, then rotate students the following clinical period. Have students write a comparison journal entry and document observed differences based on the six health considerations.

2. If available, invite the program coordinator for any organized indigenous caregiving program that may exist in the region, or arrange for a teleconference with a provider or program coordinator to discuss key elements of a training program for laypeople.

LEARNING OBJECTIVE 4

Analyze differential effects of government policy on urban and rural community health.

CONCEPTS FOR LECTURE

1. The effects of governmental policies on urban and rural health include incentives that direct health care providers to specialize in care of specific populations, identification and labeling of medically underserved areas, funding for rural health care through such legislation as the Rural Health Services Act or the Migrant Health Program, and funding improvements for road services in rural areas.

POWERPOINT LECTURE SLIDES

NOTE: The number on each PPT Lecture Slide directly corresponds with the Concepts for Lecture.

1. Governmental Policy Effects
   - Incentives to providers
   - Identification of medically underserved areas
   - Funding for rural health care
   - Improvements in services

SUGGESTIONS FOR CLASSROOM ACTIVITIES

Have students write a sample letter to their local legislator that identifies a rural or urban population group at risk for health-related problems. The letter should address one specific request or recommendation for their targeted groups for the legislator to address, such as widening or paving a section of a highway to a medically underserved area so that ambulances can access the community more easily and safely.

SUGGESTIONS FOR CLINICAL ACTIVITIES

Have students prepare a written care plan that includes one governmental policy recommendation that would have either a direct or indirect effect on a high-risk rural or urban population group identified from their clinical experiences.

LEARNING OBJECTIVE 5

Discuss assessment of health needs in urban and rural settings.

CONCEPTS FOR LECTURE

1. Assessment of rural and urban health needs begins with collection and interpretation of data from numerous local, state, and national sources. Valuable information can also be obtained from census data and voluntary organizations that monitor the health of rural populations.

POWERPOINT LECTURE SLIDES

NOTE: The number on each PPT Lecture Slide directly corresponds with the Concepts for Lecture.

1. Population Health Assessment
   - Population composition
     - Local, state, and national agencies
     - Voluntary organizations
     - Census data
   - Morbidity and mortality

SUGGESTIONS FOR CLASSROOM ACTIVITIES

Present a case study on a rural client experiencing a health problem. Divide students into small groups to identify assessment data that they need to collect in order to provide services to their client.

SUGGESTIONS FOR CLINICAL ACTIVITIES

Have students conduct their own assessment of a rural area. Encourage students to use the Internet and Web sites, social service agencies, and the local library for data pertaining to their region.

LEARNING OBJECTIVE 6

Describe goals for intervention in urban and rural settings.

CONCEPTS FOR LECTURE

1. Goals designed for interventions may differ between rural and urban settings, but can be generally summed up as including the following measures: increase access to health care services and decrease barriers to their use, eliminate or modify environmental risk factors, modify social conditions that adversely affect health, increase clients' abilities to make informed health decisions, develop systems of care that are population appropriate, and develop equitable health care policies that address the diverse needs of urban and rural populations.

2. Key to the success of intervention goals is using the appropriate model of care for each setting that may direct the type of intervention or strategy developed. An example is the use of school-based clinics in urban areas and the use of parish or locally based nursing services for rural areas.

POWERPOINT LECTURE SLIDES

NOTE: The number on each PPT Lecture Slide directly corresponds with the Concepts for Lecture.

 Intervention Goals in Rural and Urban Settings
- Increase access to health care services and decrease barriers to their use
- Eliminate or modify environmental factors
- Modify social conditions
- Increase clients' abilities to make informed health decisions
- Develop systems of care that are population-appropriate
- Develop equitable health care policies for rural and urban populations

2 Success of Interventions
- Appropriate model of care

SUGGESTIONS FOR CLASSROOM ACTIVITIES

Refer students to the case study at the end of the chapter as an example of a population health need. Assign students to small groups to develop coalition building and empowering strategies to address each of the goals of care for a migrant population.

SUGGESTIONS FOR CLINICAL ACTIVITIES

Invite community health nurses who provide services to a rural population and to an urban population. Ask the guests to discuss formalized goals for interventions, if available, and policies, procedures, and protocols that guide their delivery of services to their respective population groups.

LEARNING OBJECTIVE 7

Analyze approaches to evaluating the effectiveness of health care in rural and urban settings.

CONCEPTS FOR LECTURE

1. Evaluating the effectiveness of health care can begin with examining the national health objectives and the priority areas delineated in the *Rural Healthy People 2010* objectives. Nurses must also be aware of the similarities and differences for rural and urban health evaluation strategies.

POWERPOINT LECTURE SLIDES

NOTE: The number on each PPT Lecture Slide directly corresponds with the Concepts for Lecture.

 Evaluating Effectiveness of Health Care
- National health objectives
- Acknowledge need for setting specific evaluation methods

SUGGESTIONS FOR CLASSROOM ACTIVITIES

Have students research the CDC Web site for the *Healthy People 2010* national health objectives. Ask students to select one objective and plan to evaluate the achievement of the objective in a specific urban or rural setting.

SUGGESTIONS FOR CLINICAL ACTIVITIES

Invite a community health nurse manager to present evaluation strategies used for both urban and rural populations. Ask the guest speaker to describe the evaluation process used and the role of community health nurses in the evaluation process.

Care of Clients in Correctional Settings

RESOURCE LIBRARY

 COMPANION WEBSITE

Audio Glossary

Appendix G: Community Health Assessment and
  Intervention Guide

Exam Review Questions

Case Study: Penitentiary Nursing

MediaLink Application: Puppetry in Prison (video)

MediaLink Application: Interview with Author of
  Acres of Skin (video)

Media Links

Challenge Your Knowledge

Update *Healthy People 2010*

Advocacy Interviews

LEARNING OBJECTIVE 1

Discuss the impetus for providing health care in correctional settings.

CONCEPTS FOR LECTURE

1. On any given day, between 2 and 10 million people are either housed in or passing through local, state, and federal correctional systems.
2. Inmates are particularly vulnerable to all types of health problems; they are highly vulnerable to exploitation as research subjects. Unlike any other population group, they have a constitutional right to health care. Primary prevention in correctional settings is cost effective.
3. Because of the environmental settings and behavioral factors, there is significant risk of transmission of communicable diseases within the correctional setting and to the outside community.
4. In addition, the correctional setting predisposes inmates to social isolation, boredom, stress, hostility, and depression.

POWERPOINT LECTURE SLIDES

NOTE: The number on each PPT Lecture Slide directly corresponds with the Concepts for Lecture.

1 Health Care in Correctional Settings
- Between 2 and 10 million people are in correctional system

2 Health Needs Due to
- Vulnerability to health problems
- Potential for exploitation
- Constitutional right to health care

3 Risk for Transmission of Communicable Diseases
- Within the correctional setting
- To the outside community

4 Predisposition for Other Health Concerns
- Social isolation
- Boredom
- Stress
- Hostility
- Depression

SUGGESTIONS FOR CLASSROOM ACTIVITIES

Assign students to explore one health concern in a correctional setting. Have students present a brief summary of findings and provide an opportunity for discussion.

SUGGESTIONS FOR CLINICAL ACTIVITIES

Invite a correctional nurse to post clinical to discuss health care in a correctional setting, services provided, common health concerns, and the role of the nurse.

LEARNING OBJECTIVE 2

Differentiate between basic and advanced nursing practice in correctional settings.

CONCEPTS FOR LECTURE

1. Basic nursing practice in a correctional setting focuses on care to individuals and families and includes disease prevention and health promotion, recognition and treatment of disease and injury, and counseling.
2. Advanced nursing in correctional settings involves basic nursing practice as well as policy formation and the development, implementation, and evaluation of care for groups of people. Advanced practice may include supervision of the practice of others, advanced clinical practice, management, and evaluation of the effects of correctional health care programs.

POWERPOINT LECTURE SLIDES

NOTE: The number on each PPT Lecture Slide directly corresponds with the Concepts for Lecture.

1 Basic Nursing in Correctional Settings
- Focus on care to individuals and families
- Disease prevention
- Health promotion
- Recognition and treatment of disease and injury
- Counseling

2 Advanced Nursing in Correctional Settings
- Focus on policy formulation and program development, implementation, and evaluation
- Supervision
- Management
- Clinical practice
- Program evaluation

SUGGESTIONS FOR CLASSROOM ACTIVITIES

Invite a nurse and nurse practitioner who work in a correctional setting, preferably from the local jail or prison if available. Ask guest speakers to discuss nursing roles in their settings.

SUGGESTIONS FOR CLINICAL ACTIVITIES

Arrange for students to work in a correctional facility with a nurse or nurse practitioner. Have students write a journal entry about their experience addressing the level(s) of practice observed.

LEARNING OBJECTIVE 3

Describe biophysical, psychological, physical environmental, sociocultural, behavioral, and health system factors that influence health in correctional settings.

CONCEPTS FOR LECTURE

1. Biophysical factors that affect health and the need for health care services in correctional facilities include the age composition of the inmate population and age-related health concerns, gender and ethnic composition, and existing acute and chronic physical health problems, pregnancy, and immunization levels. Inmates tend to be 35 to 39 years of age, but there are growing numbers of youth and elderly in U.S. correctional facilities. Each age group has associated health risks, such as juvenile inmates having higher prevalence of physical and mental health conditions and a history of substance abuse. Juveniles have different nutritional needs and treatment requirements. Community health nurses may need to advocate for the recommendations made by the American Academy of Pediatrics regarding incarcerated youth. Women constitute 10% of the state and federal incarcerated population and 12% of the local jail population. These numbers are increasing although the types of crimes may differ than for men. This presents

POWERPOINT LECTURE SLIDES

NOTE: The number on each PPT Lecture Slide directly corresponds with the Concepts for Lecture.

1 Biophysical Considerations
- Age and aging
- Gender and ethnic composition
- Existing health problems
- Pregnancy
- Immunization status

2 Psychological Considerations
- Preexisting conditions
  - Drug and alcohol abuse
  - Mental illness
- PTSD
  - Women and juveniles
- Suicide

3 Physical Environmental Considerations
- Confined spaces
- Poor ventilation

specific requirements to address their health care needs, such as gynecological services, nutritional requirements, and mental health services. Nurses need to recognize that men and women differ in their physical and emotional responses to incarceration. Ethnic minority groups tend to be disproportionately represented in correctional settings. Inmates enter correctional settings with existing conditions, or as a result of the environmental conditions and behavioral patterns, stressors can exacerbate health problems such as TB, hepatitis, HIV/AIDS, and MRSA, and a variety of chronic health problems.

2. Preexisting mental health conditions such as women and juveniles with PTSD and inmates with psychiatric conditions, drug or alcohol abuse, or learning disabilities contribute to the psychological factors that correctional nurses must address. Incarceration can exacerbate existing mental health illness or create additional stressors increasing risks for suicide attempts.

3. The physical environment for a correctional facility results in confined spaces, poor ventilation, lack of temperature control, and unsanitary conditions.

4. Sociocultural factors that may cause incarceration are homelessness and socioeconomic conditions. Being incarcerated in a setting with its own correctional culture may create opportunities for additional violence and abuse. Nurses need to balance health care needs in a traditionally nontherapeutic setting with diligence for safety and security. Family relationships are affected by incarceration especially for women with children. Separation from family and children may contribute to additional stress. Nurses need to advocate for parenting classes for incarcerated women.

5. Nurses need to assess several behavioral factors that affect health and the need for health care services in a correctional setting. Inmates tend to use more tobacco, alcohol, and drugs than the general public. With limited distractions, inmates may increase these behaviors within the correctional setting. Sexual behaviors prior to incarceration may influence behaviors in the correctional setting with the added concern for increased consensual and nonconsensual sexual activity as well as violence and risks for STD.

6. Health system considerations include the adequacy of the correctional health care system, the need for health promotion and illness prevention services, medical and dental services, mental health services, and emergency response capabilities. Correctional facilities may provide in-house services with staff employed by the facility or contract with other provider agencies for needed services. Minimal screening services provided at any correctional facility include screening for evidence of infectious disease, existing health problems, current medications, evidence of disability or limitations, and suicide risk.

- Lack of temperature control
- Unsanitary conditions

 Sociocultural Considerations
- Socioeconomic factors
- Homelessness
- Family relationships
- Correctional culture
- Violence and abuse
- Security issues

 Behavioral Considerations
- Diet
- Substance abuse
- Exercise/recreational opportunities
- Sexual activity
- Medication use and dispensing practices

 Health System Considerations
- Funding for and organization of services
- Health promotion/illness prevention services

Health System Considerations (continued)
- Medical/dental services
  - Minimal screening services
    - Evidence of infectious disease
    - Existing health problems
    - Current medications
    - Disabilities/limitations
    - Suicide risk

 Health System Considerations (continued)
- Mental health services
- Emergency response capabilities
- Provisions for continuity of care

SUGGESTIONS FOR CLASSROOM ACTIVITIES

Divide students into six health consideration groups to research and investigate examples or case studies that address their health risk factor or consideration in a correctional setting. Ask groups to present similarities and differences for inmates and clients in community settings. Have groups present a summary with evidence that supports their findings for discussion with the entire class.

SUGGESTIONS FOR CLINICAL ACTIVITIES

Assign students to work with a correctional nurse and assess the health status of a particular inmate or the correctional population addressing the six dimensions of health.

LEARNING OBJECTIVE 4

Identify major aspects of primary prevention in correctional settings and analyze the role of the community health nurse in each.

CONCEPTS FOR LECTURE

1. Primary prevention services in a correctional setting include health promotion services such as assessment of nutritional status, advocacy of exercise and rest, health education for self-care and risk factor modification, and prenatal care for pregnant inmates or contraception.
2. Illness prevention services include preventing communicable diseases, beginning with screening for TB and administering TB medications; assessing an inmate's risk for suicide; and advocating and providing for violence prevention activities.
3. Primary prevention may also include advocacy for the availability of health promotion and illness/injury prevention services.

POWERPOINT LECTURE SLIDES

NOTE: The number on each PPT Lecture Slide directly corresponds with the Concepts for Lecture.

1. Primary Prevention in Correctional Settings
   - Health promotion
     - Adequate nutrition
     - Rest and exercise
     - Health education
       - Self-care
       - Risk factor modification
     - Prenatal care and contraception

2. Illness Prevention
   - Communicable disease prevention
   - Suicide prevention
   - Violence prevention

3. Primary Prevention: Advocacy
   - Availability of health promotion services
   - Availability of illness/injury prevention services

SUGGESTIONS FOR CLASSROOM ACTIVITIES

Assign students to three groups. Give each group a case study that involves an incarcerated individual who is a teen, a pregnant woman, or an adult male with a history of drug abuse. Have groups develop primary prevention interventions for their individual. Provide an opportunity for presentation and discussion.

SUGGESTIONS FOR CLINICAL ACTIVITIES

Arrange for students to work with a nurse in a correctional clinic. If safety permits, have students participate in a health promotion activity.

LEARNING OBJECTIVE 5

Describe approaches to secondary prevention in correctional settings and analyze community health nursing roles with respect to each.

CONCEPTS FOR LECTURE

1. Secondary prevention activities include screening, diagnosis, and treatment.
2. Screening has three purposes: identify and address the health needs of inmates such as pregnancy or acute or chronic illness, promote early identification of key problems such as suicide risk factors, and identify and isolate potentially communicable inmates such as individuals with hepatitis, TB, STDs, or HIV/AIDS. Screening may also include identifying pre-existing mental illness, and specialized screening for conditions such as diabetes, or hypertension.
3. Diagnostic services include addressing existing health, mental health, and medical or dental needs.
4. Once screening and diagnostic services identify health needs of inmates, treatment begins with medications for existing conditions, infectious diseases such as TB or HIV, and medical treatment for chronic health conditions, mental illness, or substance abuse. Treatment also includes emergency care services and provisions for disaster care.

POWERPOINT LECTURE SLIDES

NOTE: The number on each PPT Lecture Slide directly corresponds with the Concepts for Lecture.

1 Secondary Prevention in Correctional Settings
- Screening
- Diagnostic services
- Treatment

2 Screening Foci
- Identify and address health needs of inmates
- Pregnancy screening
- Promote early identification of key problems
- Identify and isolate potentially communicable inmates
- Pre-existing mental illness
- Specialized screening

3 Diagnostic Services
- Medical conditions
- Mental illness

4 Treatment
- Medications
  - TB treatment
  - HIV therapies
- Medical treatments
  - Chronic health conditions
  - Substance abuse/Mental health

4a Treatment (continued)
- Emergency care
- Disaster care

SUGGESTIONS FOR CLASSROOM ACTIVITIES

Assign students to small groups to identify nursing interventions for inmates with a medical problem, a mental health/illness concern, or a substance abuse condition. Ask the groups to write out questions that they need to address to assess the inmate before providing secondary prevention services.

SUGGESTIONS FOR CLINICAL ACTIVITIES

Invite a medical or nursing provider who works at a correctional facility to discuss secondary prevention services, safety concerns, and prevalent health concerns in the facility.

LEARNING OBJECTIVE 6

Discuss considerations in tertiary prevention in correctional settings and analyze related community health nursing roles.

CONCEPTS FOR LECTURE

1. Tertiary prevention in correctional settings includes long-term care planning, reentry planning, and end-of-life care.
2. Nurses must plan for the care of elderly inmates and those with chronic conditions or disabilities, which

POWERPOINT LECTURE SLIDES

NOTE: The number on each PPT Lecture Slide directly corresponds with the Concepts for Lecture.

1 Tertiary Care in Correctional Settings
- Long-term care planning

may require transfer to facilities that can accommodate their health needs such as specialized hospice units or facilities with assisted living capabilities. Long-term care planning also includes providing for assistance by a personal care attendant, adult day care services, making provisions of home care in the general population, and monitoring treatment compliance.

3. Reentry is defined as the process of leaving prison and returning to society. Reentry planning takes into consideration risks to the community for spread of communicable disease and is based on individualized needs assessments for health care and social and financial resources. Reentry as tertiary prevention foci includes: development of systematic discharge protocols, development of an individual discharge plan and assistance with family reintegration as needed, provision for continuity of health care, arrangment for a supply of necessary medications on discharge, arrangement for health insurance coverage, and advocacy for prerelease planning, community infrastructure to support reentry, and civil rights of released inmates.

4. End-of-life care issues are similar to, but may be more complicated than, those outside prison. Nurses may need to assist with advanced directives, advocate adherence to advance directives, and consider referral for hospice services or compassionate release. Additionally, end-of-life care can mean addressing psychological issues and stressors associated with death sentences, and advocacy for medical parole and arrangements for follow-up care.

- Reentry
- End-of-life care

 Long-term Care Planning
- Assistance by a personal care attendant
- Inmates with chronic conditions
- Provision of home care in general population
- Monitoring treatment compliance
- Transfer to appropriate facility as needed
- Adult day care services

 Reentry Planning
- Development of systematic discharge protocols
- Development of individual discharge plan and assistance with family reintegration as needed
- Provision for continuity of health care
- Arrange for a supply of necessary medications on discharge
- Arrangement for health insurance coverage
- Advocacy for prerelease planning, community infrastructure to support reentry, and civil rights of released inmates

 End-of-life Care
- Advanced directives
- Palliative care
- Compassionate release
- Referral to hospice care
- Inmates under sentence of death
- Advocacy for medical parole and arrangement for follow-up care

---

SUGGESTIONS FOR CLASSROOM ACTIVITIES

Divide students into two groups to investigate ethical considerations in tertiary prevention. Have students list their personal beliefs and feelings and locate any articles or case studies published about the nurses' role for elderly or inmates under sentence of death.

SUGGESTIONS FOR CLINICAL ACTIVITIES

Invite a nurse manager or medical officer for the local prison system to discuss tertiary strategies that address reentry of inmates with chronic or communicable diseases, health needs of inmates under sentence of death, and policies and procedures regarding advanced directives.

Care of Clients in Disaster Settings

RESOURCE LIBRARY

🌐 COMPANION WEBSITE

Audio Glossary
Exam Review Questions
Case Study: Disaster Care
MediaLink Application: Student Nurses in the
  Aftermath of Katrina (video)

Media Links
Challenge Your Knowledge
Advocacy Interviews

📖 IMAGE LIBRARY

Figure 27-1 Areas of Disaster Impact
Figure 27-2 The Federal Process of Disaster
Declaration
Figure 27-3 Sample Community Risk Map

Figure 27-4 Sample Community Resource Map
Figure 27-5 Areas of Operation in Immediate Care

LEARNING OBJECTIVE 1

Describe ways in which disaster events may vary.

CONCEPTS FOR LECTURE

1. A disaster can be a natural or man-made situation that results in human suffering and creates human needs that victims cannot alleviate without assistance.
2. An emergency is a serious threatening event that falls within the coping abilities of the individual, family, or community.
3. Disasters vary based on such characteristics as frequency, predictability, preventability, imminence, duration, and extent of their effects.
4. Certain regions of the United States and the world experience disasters more frequently; as a result, people in those areas may be more knowledgeable of preparedness activities.
5. Some disasters are more predictable, such as rivers flooding or snow blizzards in northern regions. Other types of disasters may not be anticipated or predictable, such as chemical spills or explosions. Certain disasters are more easily preventable, such as rerouting waterways or building dams to prevent flooding disasters.
6. Disasters can also vary according to their imminence; with respect to their speed of occurrence. Advanced warning, when possible, can minimize the impact of the event.

POWERPOINT LECTURE SLIDES

NOTE: The number on each PPT Lecture Slide directly corresponds with the Concepts for Lecture.

1 Disaster
  - Man-made
  - Natural
  - Results in human suffering
  - Victims needing assistance

2 Emergency
  - Serious threatening event
  - Individual, family, or community able to cope with situation

3 Characteristics of a Disaster
  - Frequency
  - Predictability
  - Preventability
  - Imminence
  - Duration
  - Extent of effects

4 Disaster Frequency
  - Determines amount of knowledge and experience that a community may have to react and respond
  - Affects preparedness

7. Disasters can vary according to their overall impact and their destructive potential with some having limited geographical scope affecting only small numbers of people and other disasters affecting large areas and great numbers of people.

5 Disaster Predictability
- River flooding
- Snow blizzards
- Situations that are not predictable
  - Explosions
  - Chemical spills
- Situations that are preventable

6 Disaster Imminence
- Speed of occurrence
- Advanced warning can minimize the impact of the event

7 Disaster Impact
- Destructive potential
- Geographical scope

SUGGESTIONS FOR CLASSROOM ACTIVITIES

1. Have students list the various types of disasters likely to occur in their own locale and the potential health impact that disasters can have on a human population.
2. If appropriate, provide video or news clips of recent disasters and provide an opportunity to discuss the impact on human lives.

SUGGESTIONS FOR CLINICAL ACTIVITIES

1. Invite a Red Cross disaster volunteer to discuss services provided to individuals, families, and communities.
2. Have students observe the community and identify potential disaster hazards in the community.

LEARNING OBJECTIVE 2

Describe the elements of a disaster.

CONCEPTS FOR LECTURE

1. Disasters have four main elements: the temporal element, the spatial element, the role element, and the effects element.
2. The temporal element describes the stages of disaster response beginning with the non-disaster/inter-disaster stage. Activities that correspond with this stage include: identification of potential disaster risks and mapping their locations; conducting a vulnerability analysis of groups within the population that may be particularly vulnerable; developing a resource capability inventory and assessing stockpiling capabilities; and developing primary prevention strategies for preparedness and mitigation as well as public and professional education.
3. The pre-disaster stage is described as when a disaster event is imminent but has not yet occurred. Crucial to this stage are effective warning systems, pre-impact mobilization (actions aimed at averting the disaster) and evacuation activities.
4. At the impact stage, the disaster event has occurred. At this point, a damage inventory and injury assessment must be accomplished to determine the immediate needs of the community.
5. The emergency stage focuses on saving lives through search and rescue efforts, first aid, relief assistance,

POWERPOINT LECTURE SLIDES

NOTE: The number on each PPT Lecture Slide directly corresponds with the Concepts for Lecture.

1 Elements of a Disaster
- Temporal
- Spatial
- Role
- Effects

2 Temporal Element: Stages of Disaster Response
- Non-disaster/inter-disaster stage
  - Disaster risk identification and vulnerability analysis
  - Capability inventory and stockpiling
  - Prevention and mitigation
  - Response planning and plan dissemination
  - Public and professional education

3 Temporal Element: Pre-disaster Stage
- Warning
- Pre-impact mobilization
- Evacuation

4 Temporal Element: Impact Stage
- Damage inventory
- Injury assessment

restoring communication and transportation routes for needed supplies and communication of needs. An overall public health surveillance must be conducted to determine potential infectious disease exposures and mental health problems that may arise.

6. The recovery stage describes activities directed at returning equilibrium to a community through restoration of the community's functional capabilities, reconstruction of physical and social environments, reuniting families that became separated, reconstitution of some sense of normalcy, and mitigation activities aimed at preventing subsequent disasters.

7. The spatial element refers to the extent of the effects of a disaster on specific geographic regions, which includes the area of total impact (where the most severe effects of the disaster occurred), the area of partial impact where there is some evidence but less magnitude of effects from the disaster, and outside areas that may not be directly affected but may be a source of assistance in response to the disaster.

8. The role element describes the two basic roles for people: the victim and the helper. Disaster victims have six levels. Primary victims are those who experience maximum exposure to the disaster event. Secondary victims are affected indirectly as friends and family members of primary victims. Third-level victims include the first responders and health care professionals involved in rescue and recovery efforts. Fourth through sixth level victims are affected vicariously as a result of the disaster or the responses of the primary victims. Refugees and internally displaced persons are special categories of primary victims. The helper role includes rescue and recovery personnel as well as other community members who may be exposed to post-disaster stresses or injury.

9. The effects element distinguishes between primary or direct effects and those secondary or indirect effects resulting from a disaster event. Primary effects may be more obvious such as death, injury, and destruction of property. Secondary effects may not be as evident and include malnutrition and psychological distress that may arise.

5. Temporal Element: Emergency Stage
   - Search and rescue
   - First aid
   - Relief assistance
   - Restoration of communication and transportation
   - Public health surveillance

6. Temporal Element: Recovery Stage
   - Restoration of functional capabilities
   - Reconstruction of physical and social environments
   - Reunification of families
   - Reconstitution
   - Mitigation of future disaster events

7. Spatial Element
   - Area of total impact
   - Area of partial impact
   - Outside areas

8. Role Element
   - Victim
     ○ Primary victims
       – Refugees and internally displaced persons
     ○ Secondary victims
     ○ Third-level victims
     ○ Fourth-sixth level victims
   - Helper

9. Effects Element
   - Primary/direct effects
     ○ Death
     ○ Injury
     ○ Destruction of property
   - Secondary/indirect effects
     ○ Psychological problems

SUGGESTIONS FOR CLASSROOM ACTIVITIES

Have students discuss the role of the community health nurse with respect to each of the elements of a disaster. Using a case scenario, divide students into temporal stage groups to role-play as community health nurse teams responding to each temporal element stage. What would be their primary role? What would be their secondary role? What about their friends and family who may be in the disaster region?

SUGGESTIONS FOR CLINICAL ACTIVITIES

Have students examine a disaster preparedness plan for their clinical setting. Ask students to compare the disaster plan to the temporal stages and describe the plan to the class.

LEARNING OBJECTIVE 3

Describe two aspects of disaster-related assessment.

CONCEPTS FOR LECTURE

1. Disaster-related assessments begin with a pre-disaster risk and capacity assessment, followed by a post-disaster rapid assessment.
2. For a pre-disaster risk assessment, community health nurses may utilize community risk maps to identify potential disaster risks in a community from industry activities, civil unrest, or forecastable situations likely to cause a disaster.
3. Assessment of response capability examines the attitudes of community members toward disaster preparedness, the actual extent to which individuals or families are prepared, emergency routes, and community resources that can affect preparedness. Capacity assessment may employ creation of community resource maps of resources that can be brought to bear in response to a disaster situation.
4. Community health nurses may be key responders to assess the extent of health-related disaster effects such as deaths, injuries, and potential illnesses.

POWERPOINT LECTURE SLIDES

NOTE: The number on each PPT Lecture Slide directly corresponds with the Concepts for Lecture.

1. Disaster-related Assessment
   - Pre-disaster risk and capacity assessment
   - Post-disaster rapid assessment

2. Pre-disaster Risk and Capacity Assessment
   - Community risk and resource map

3. Assessment of Response Capability
   - Attitudes of community members
   - Extent of preparations
   - Emergency routes
   - Community resources

4. Role of Community Health Nurses
   - Key responders
     - Assess the extent of health-related disaster effects
       - Death
       - Injuries
       - Potential illnesses

SUGGESTIONS FOR CLASSROOM ACTIVITIES

Have students brainstorm the types of potential disasters that could occur in their community, resources available, strengths of the community that could be used in the event of a disaster, and available sources of information to report the aftermath of a disaster.

SUGGESTIONS FOR CLINICAL ACTIVITIES

1. Invite a community health nurse or member of a disaster preparedness team to discuss planning and assessment processes in the community, region, and state.
2. Have students create disaster risk and resource maps for their community.

LEARNING OBJECTIVE 4

Identify biophysical, psychological, physical environmental, sociocultural, behavioral, and health system considerations to be assessed in relation to a disaster.

CONCEPTS FOR LECTURE

1. Biophysical factors that affect the forecasting of potential disasters include awareness of groups of individuals more vulnerable in the event of disaster, such as the very young and the elderly in an influenza epidemic, people closest to a chemical plant in the event of an explosion, or people with chronic medical conditions or illnesses. Physiologic responses to disaster can result in death classified as direct deaths, indirect deaths, and disaster-related natural deaths.

POWERPOINT LECTURE SLIDES

NOTE: The number on each PPT Lecture Slide directly corresponds with the Concepts for Lecture.

1. Biophysical Considerations
   - Vulnerable populations
     ◦ Very young
     ◦ Elderly
     ◦ Groups with disabilities or illnesses

2. Four psychological factors that influence the effects of a disaster on health include the individual's perceived ability to remove him- or herself from direct impact of the event, a person's prior experience in evacuation, individual decision making about evacuation, and how disaster event information is disseminated that directly affects evacuation decisions. Factors that influence a community's response to a disaster include the occurrence of extreme and widespread property damage, realization of serious and ongoing economic impact, extent of death and traumatic injuries, and perception of human carelessness or intent as the cause of the disaster.

3. The community health nurse identifies the physical features in the environment that could contribute to the occurrence of a disaster, such as flooding, heavy rain, geographical features that contribute to isolation, or industries with explosive hazards. The nurse would also evaluate features that inhibit or impair a community's response to a disaster such as access to shelters, sanitation and facilities for adequate hygiene, and environmental conditions that imperil health during the disaster event.

4. The community health nurse identifies social factors that can influence the way people respond to a disaster or that might contribute to a disaster. Social features could be racial tension or some type of community violence, such as terrorism. Poverty, power imbalances, social or environmental injustice, and media coverage can either positively or negatively act as a precursor to terrorism. Many other features of a community, such as language barriers, social responses, social effects on specific groups, and cultural and occupational factors, can affect a community's susceptibility to a disaster or its ability to prepare or react effectively to a disaster.

5. Behavioral factors that apply to a community's response or susceptibility to a disaster include consumption patterns, leisure activities, and the extent of disaster preparedness among members of the community. Individuals may be malnourished, which can affect their survivability in the event of a disaster, or post-disaster; individuals may increase consumption of alcohol, tobacco, or drugs as a result of stressors created by the disaster. Leisure activities need to be considered as part of a community assessment if people are not prepared for strenuous activity during a disaster. It is also important to consider groups that may have the skills needed for search and rescue during and after a disaster.

6. The community health nurse is involved in assessing the adequacy and availability of existing health care services and facilities prior to a disaster, assisting with education of providers about unusual diseases, and assessing the damage to facilities after a disaster.

- Proximity to potential situations
- Types of deaths

2 Psychological Considerations
- Response to warning
  - Perceived evacuation capability
  - Prior experience with disasters
  - Concern about actual evacuation
  - Information dissemination

2a Psychological Considerations (continued)
- Response to actual disaster
  - Extent of property damage
  - Realization of economic impact
  - Extent of deaths and traumatic injuries
  - Perceptions of human carelessness or intent to cause event

3 Physical Environmental Considerations
- Features in physical environment
- Adequacy of community's response
- Conditions that imperil health during disaster

4 Sociocultural Considerations
- Presence of tensions in community
- Terrorism susceptibility
- Social responses
- Social effects

5 Behavioral Considerations
- Consumption patterns
  - Malnourished
  - Post-disaster consumption patterns
- Leisure activities
  - Inability to perform strenuous labor
  - Special skills of certain groups
- Extent of preparedness

6 Health System Considerations
- Adequacy of health system response
- Available facilities
- Damage to existing facilities
- State and local health department preparedness
  - Educating providers to recognize unusual disease pattern

SUGGESTIONS FOR CLASSROOM ACTIVITIES

1. Have students search the Internet for a disaster preparedness plan for any state, region, or health care system. In reviewing the plan, ask students to select one feature of the plan that corresponds to one of the six health considerations and present a summary to the class.
2. Assign students to small groups. Have each group use one of the six dimensions and develop a disaster assessment for the college that they attend. Have groups apply the same questions and assessment strategies to the community of student nurses, instructors, etc.

SUGGESTIONS FOR CLINICAL ACTIVITIES

1. Arrange for students to attend a disaster preparedness meeting or a mass casualty event sponsored by the local hospital or joint organizations.
2. Invite the local Red Cross representative to discuss disaster preparedness planning and available assessment tools during post conference.

LEARNING OBJECTIVE 5

Describe two aspects of primary prevention related to disasters.

CONCEPTS FOR LECTURE

1. Two aspects of primary prevention related to disasters include prevention of disasters and minimizing the effects of a disaster. Prevention strategies include identifying and eliminating factors that contribute to the effects of a disaster, such as building fortification or security against terrorism, reporting employee behaviors that could create occupational hazards, routing hazardous material transports away from densely populated regions, educating the public, and immunizing against diseases that could pose bioterrorist threats. Disaster minimization strategies can occur before, during, and after a disaster with public education and training at the individual, neighborhood, and advanced level and immunizations being the primary areas of focus.

POWERPOINT LECTURE SLIDES

NOTE: The number on each PPT Lecture Slide directly corresponds with the Concepts for Lecture.

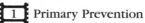 1 Primary Prevention
- Preventing disasters
  - Security
  - Reporting behaviors
  - Rerouting hazardous materials
  - Education
  - Immunizations

1a Primary Prevention (continued)
- Minimizing disaster effects
  - Individual training
  - Neighborhood training
  - Advanced level training

SUGGESTIONS FOR CLASSROOM ACTIVITIES

1. Assign students to small groups. Divide the county into regions for each group to identify potential geological, geographical, environmental, industrial, or human-made hazards. Ask groups to develop primary strategies for preventing potential disasters for their regions.
2. Ask students to develop a poster for education related to disaster preparedness for various population groups such as schools, community neighborhoods, or other areas.

SUGGESTIONS FOR CLINICAL ACTIVITIES

1. Arrange for students to work with a community health or volunteer agency involved in disaster prevention. Ask students to identify resources, goals, and areas of geographical responsibility.
2. Assign students to work with a school nurse to develop an educational tool for disaster preparedness that is age or developmentally specific.

LEARNING OBJECTIVE 6

Discuss the principles of community disaster preparedness.

CONCEPTS FOR LECTURE

1. Disaster preparedness is defined as the set of measures that ensure the organized mobilization of personnel, funds, equipment, and supplies within a safe environment for effective relief. There are two purposes for disaster preparedness: to limit morbidity and mortality and to ensure that resources are available for effective response in the event of a disaster.

2. Principles of disaster preparedness provide guidelines for effective planning. Disaster plans should be formulated based on flexibility, familiar procedures, and knowledge of human behavior. Their success is grounded in being locally focused, enlisting support from the community, and keeping responsibility based on position and not a particular individual. Other principles for a disaster plan include ensuring provisions for casualties, recognizing the need to care for the mental and physical health of the population, providing for resource acquisition and management, disseminating the plans to the public, and using disaster drills as a means of evaluating the effectiveness of the developed plan.

POWERPOINT LECTURE SLIDES

NOTE: The number on each PPT Lecture Slide directly corresponds with the Concepts for Lecture.

1 Disaster Preparedness
- Definition
- Purpose
  - ○ Limit morbidity and mortality
  - ○ Ensure availability of resources

2 Principles of Disaster Preparedness
- Flexible response plans
- Base plans on everyday methods and procedures
- Provide for extended authority
- Use existing knowledge of human response to disasters
- Use plans with local focus
- Enlist support and coordinate efforts of entire community

2a Principles of Disaster Preparedness (continued)
- Specify personnel roles by titles
- Ensure that plans are acceptable to all
- Include provisions for casualty distribution
- Provide for resource acquisition and management
- Include provisions for mental as well as physical health
- Disseminate plan to public
- Implement plans into disaster drills

SUGGESTIONS FOR CLASSROOM ACTIVITIES

Have students develop a table-top disaster drill. Give each student five 3×5 cards to write down ideas to consider in response to the disaster drill, such as resources needed and who should be involved in the planning. Use the principles of community disaster preparedness as guidelines.

SUGGESTIONS FOR CLINICAL ACTIVITIES

Invite a disaster drill coordinator to post conference to discuss the after-action report from the last community disaster drill. Ask students to write one question from the principles to address to the guest speaker about the development of the disaster drill process.

LEARNING OBJECTIVE 7

Identify the component elements of an effective disaster response plan.

CONCEPTS FOR LECTURE

1. An effective disaster response plan should have a systematic mechanism for notifying the person(s) who set the plan in motion. Once notified, the community needs a disaster warning system, which is usually issued by local radio or television or some type of alarm system. After a community is warned, there

POWERPOINT LECTURE SLIDES

NOTE: The number on each PPT Lecture Slide directly corresponds with the Concepts for Lecture.

1 Elements of an Effective Disaster Response Plan
- Notification
- Warning

CONCEPTS FOR LECTURE *continued*

should be a control mechanism in place that includes procedures, materials, and personnel needed to carry out the control measures specific to the disaster, Logistical coordination is used to procure, maintain, and transport needed materials. An evacuation plan is necessary that identifies who is needed, what is needed, and how they are notified. The plan must specify how search and rescue efforts are to be activated and by whom.

2. A disaster plan should include protocols for immediate care of the injured, usually through some triage system, and which individuals or what agencies will provide supportive care such as food, water, and shelter. Recovery and evaluation are considered a component of tertiary prevention, but must be addressed in any disaster plan.

POWERPOINT LECTURE SLIDES *continued*

- Control
- Coordination
- Evacuation
- Rescue

 Additional Elements
- Immediate care
- Supportive care
- Recovery
- Evaluation

SUGGESTIONS FOR CLASSROOM ACTIVITIES

Have students research articles from the nursing literature that describe the role of nurses in disasters. Ask students to summarize the article and identify the elements of a disaster response plan in their summary. Allow for discussion.

SUGGESTIONS FOR CLINICAL ACTIVITIES

Have students prepare a 5-page disaster response plan for their community or their educational institution that includes the elements of an effective plan and the role of the community health nurse in prevention strategies. Ask students to outline the plan on a poster board and present at post conference.

LEARNING OBJECTIVE 8

Analyze the role of community health nurses in primary, secondary, and tertiary prevention related to disaster situations.

CONCEPTS FOR LECTURE

1. In a primary prevention role, nurses focus on disaster prevention and minimization of disaster effects. Disaster prevention includes identification of contributing factors, political activism to eliminate or modify risk factors, advocacy regarding identification of potential terrorist targets, providing immunization services, and supervising shelter activities. Nurses involved in minimizing disaster effects focus on communicating community disaster response plans to the public, educating the public to support "community-as-resource" strategies, advocating for the availability and use of PPE by disaster responders, educating responders on the use of PPE, and initiating post-disaster immunization campaigns.

2. Secondary prevention activities include immediate care and supportive care. Immediate care includes triage and treatment of injuries. Supportive care focuses on shelter supervision, surveillance and screening activities, and treatment of disease and injury or referral for care.

3. Community health nurses' role in tertiary prevention include providing follow-up care for injuries, physical

POWERPOINT LECTURE SLIDES

NOTE: The number on each PPT Lecture Slide directly corresponds with the Concepts for Lecture.

 Primary Prevention Activities
- Disaster prevention
  - Identification of contributing factors
  - Political activism to eliminate or modify risk factors
  - Advocacy regarding identification of potential terrorist targets
  - Immunization
  - Public education for preparedness

 Primary Prevention (continued)
- Minimizing disaster effects
  - Assist in communicating community disaster response plans to the public
  - Educate the public to support "community-as-resource" strategies
  - Advocate for availability and use of PPE by disaster responders

Concepts for Lecture *continued*

and psychological; assisting with recovery via referrals for services and financial assistance; and preventing future disasters through advocacy and education.

PowerPoint Lecture Slides *continued*

- ○ Educate responders on use of PPE
- ○ Initiate post-disaster immunization campaigns

 Secondary Prevention Activities
- • Immediate care
  - ○ Triage
  - ○ Treatment of injuries
- • Supportive care
  - ○ Shelter supervision
  - ○ Surveillance and screening
  - ○ Treatment of disease and injury or referral for care

 Tertiary Prevention Activities
- • Follow-up care for injuries
- • Follow-up care for psychological problems
- • Recovery assistance
- • Prevention of future disasters and their consequences

Suggestions for Classroom Activities

Assign students to three groups: primary, secondary, and tertiary prevention teams. Provide the groups with case scenarios and ask the students to develop case-specific nursing diagnoses and intervention activities for their assigned level of prevention. Present for discussion.

Suggestions for Clinical Activities

Invite several community health nurses or providers to post conference to discuss the role of community health nurses in all three levels of prevention. Ask guest speakers to provide examples from recent disasters, if possible.

Communicable Diseases

28
CHAPTER

RESOURCE LIBRARY

COMPANION WEBSITE

Audio Glossary
Appendix E: Information on Selected Communicable
  Diseases
Exam Review Questions
Case Study: TB, a Communicable Disease
MediaLink Application: Old Bugs, New Threats (video)

Media Links
Challenge Your Knowledge
Update *Healthy People 2010*
Advocacy Interviews

IMAGE LIBRARY

Table 28-1 Modes of Disease Transmission and
  Typical Diseases

LEARNING OBJECTIVE 1

Analyze major trends in the incidence of communicable diseases.

CONCEPTS FOR LECTURE

1. Key terms important in understanding communicable diseases include endemic disease, which is a disease that demonstrates a consistent chain of transmission from person to person for 12 months or more in a particular geographical area; an epidemic, which involves the occurrence of a great number of cases of a disease, beyond what is normally expected; and disease outbreak, which is an increased number of cases in the population that does not approach epidemic proportions.

2. A number of major trends in the incidence of communicable disease have been noted. Of significance is the eradication of smallpox, the near-eradication of poliomyelitis, and the targeted eradication of rubella, measles, and dracunculiasis (Guinea worm disease). The emphasis on vaccine-preventable diseases has shown significant results, greatly reducing epidemic and endemic incidences of such diseases. Several other communicable diseases have seen an increase in their incidence and prevalence such as HIV/AIDS, chlamydia, and Rocky Mountain spotted fever. Other diseases have decreased in incidence and prevalence, such as syphilis and hepatitis. Diseases that have noted fluctuations are tuberculosis, influenza, and pneumococcal disease. A few diseases have emerged as a concern including avian influenza and West Nile

POWERPOINT LECTURE SLIDES

NOTE: The number on each PPT Lecture Slide directly corresponds with the Concepts for Lecture.

 Key Terms
- Endemic disease
  - Demonstrates a consistent chain of transmission from person to person for 12 months or more in a particular geographical area
- Epidemic
  - Occurrence of a great number of cases of a disease, beyond what is normally expected
- Outbreak
  - An increased number of cases in the population that does not approach epidemic proportions

 Major Trends
- Eradication
  - Smallpox
- Near eradication
  - Poliomyelitis
- Targeted eradication
  - Rubella
  - Dracunculiasis

 Major Trends: Vaccine Preventable Diseases
- Measles/Mumps/Rubella

Chapter 28/Learning Objective 1   **195**

CONCEPTS FOR LECTURE continued

virus, and finally, there are diseases that continue to emerge or reemerge such as methicillin-resistant *Staphylococcus aureus* (MRSA).

POWERPOINT LECTURE SLIDES continued

- Tetanus/Diptheria/Pertussis
- Hepatitis A and B
- Varicella
- Influenza
- Pneumococcal pneumonia

 Major Trends (continued)
- Increased incidence and prevalence
  - HIV/AIDS
  - Chlamydia
  - Rocky Mountain spotted fever
- Decreased incidence and prevalence
  - Syphilis
  - Hepatitis

 Major Trends (continued)
- Diseases with noted fluctuations
  - Tuberculosis
  - Influenza
  - Pneumococcal disease

 Major Trends (continued)
- Diseases of interest
  - Diseases of concern
    - Avian influenza
    - West Nile virus
  - New emerging/reemerging diseases
    - MRSA

SUGGESTIONS FOR CLASSROOM ACTIVITIES

Divide students into groups to research and present on the local, state, national, and global trends such as incidence, prevalence, and populations at risk for their communicable disease group.

SUGGESTIONS FOR CLINICAL ACTIVITIES

Have students interview a community health nurse, infection control nurse, or epidemiologist about a disease of interest for their agency. Provide an opportunity for discussion of the interview at post conference.

LEARNING OBJECTIVE 2

Identify the modes of transmission for communicable diseases.

CONCEPTS FOR LECTURE

1. The mode of transmission refers to the means by which the infectious agent or organism that causes a disease is transferred from an infected person or animal to an uninfected one.
2. Common modes of transmission include airborne transmission, fecal–oral transmission, direct contact, sexual transmission, transmission by direct inoculation, transmission by insect or animal bite, and transmission by other means.
3. Airborne transmission occurs when the infectious organism is present in the air and is inhaled by a susceptible host during respiration. Examples of airborne disease include exanthems, infections of the mouth and throat, and infections of the upper and lower respiratory system.

POWERPOINT LECTURE SLIDES

NOTE: The number on each PPT Lecture Slide directly corresponds with the Concepts for Lecture.

 Mode of Transmission
- Means by which the infectious agent or organism that causes a disease is transferred from an infected person or animal to an uninfected one

2 Common Modes of Transmission (Refer to Table 28-1)
- Airborne transmission
- Fecal–oral transmission
- Direct contact
- Sexual transmission

CONCEPTS FOR LECTURE continued

4. Fecal–oral transmission (gastrointestinal) occurs by direct or indirect inoculation of hands with human feces containing an infectious organism such as salmonella, shigella, and botulism.

5. Direct contact involves skin-to-skin contact or direct contact with mucous membrane discharges between an infected person and another person. Typical diseases include mononucleosis, impetigo, scabies, and lice.

6. Sexual transmission is a subtype of direct contact that is specific to a category of diseases transmitted by means of sexual intercourse, such as HIV/AIDS, gonorrhea, syphilis, genital herpes, and hepatitis B, C, and D.

7. Transmission by direct inoculation refers to when the infectious agent is introduced directly into the bloodstream of the new host such as by transplacentally from mother to fetus, contaminated needles, or transfusion, or splashing of contaminated body fluids to mucous membranes.

8. Infectious disease transmission can also occur from insect or animal bites such as mosquito transmission of malaria and West Nile virus, rabies from warm-blooded animals, ticks that transmit Lyme disease and Rocky Mountain spotted fever, and fleas that transmit plague.

9. Other modes of transmission include contact with spores present in the soil or with inanimate objects such as exposure to the bacillus that causes tetanus, which occurs through a dirty puncture wound. Hookworm is an intestinal parasite that can infect humans through direct contact with contaminated soil by walking barefoot or by ingesting contaminated soil.

POWERPOINT LECTURE SLIDES continued

2a Common Modes of Transmission (continued)
- Transmission by direct inoculation
- Transmission by insect or animal bite
- Transmission by other means

3 Airborne Transmission
- Infectious organism is present in the air and is inhaled by a susceptible host during respiration
  - Exanthems
  - Infections of mouth and throat
  - Infections of upper and lower respiratory system

4 Fecal–Oral Transmission
- Direct transmission
- Indirect transmission

4a Fecal-Oral Transmission (continued)
- Examples
  - Salmonella
  - Shigella
  - Botulism

5 Direct Contact
- Skin-to-skin contact
- Direct contact with mucous membrane discharges
- Examples
  - Mononucleosis
  - Impetigo
  - Scabies
  - Lice

6 Sexual Transmission
- Sexual contact (direct contact transmission)
- Examples
  - HIV/AIDS
  - Gonorrhea
  - Syphilis
  - Genital herpes
  - Hepatitis B, C, and D

7 Transmission by Direct Inoculation
- Infectious agent is introduced directly into the bloodstream of the new host
  - Transplacentally
  - Contaminated needles or blood products
  - Splashing of contaminated body fluids
- Examples
  - HIV/AIDS

8 Transmission by Insect/Animal Bite
- Mosquito - Malaria
- Warm-blooded animals - Rabies
- Ticks - Lyme disease and Rocky Mountain spotted fever
- Fleas - Plague

9 Transmission by Other Means
- Spores in soil
- Examples
  - Tetanus
  - Hookworm

LEARNING OBJECTIVE 3

Describe the influence of biophysical, psychological, physical environmental, sociocultural, behavioral, and health system factors on communicable diseases.

CONCEPTS FOR LECTURE

1. Considerations that influence the development and effects of any communicable disease include biophysical factors, which include age, gender, race/ethnicity, and physiologic health status including immunity. Each of these factors can influence one's chances of exposure to specific diseases.
2. Psychological considerations include the effects of stress, risk-taking behaviors, and depression.
3. The physical environment can impact the development of disease through poor sanitation, overcrowding, climates with extreme winds and dust, contaminated waters, and regions with infectious insects or animals.
4. Sociocultural considerations that contribute to communicable disease risk factors include poverty, poor nutrition, unemployment, homelessness, cultural beliefs, and gender socialization.
5. Behavioral considerations, which include diet, sexual activity, drug use, use of mosquito nets or swimming in contaminated water, can increase one's risk of disease.
6. A country's health care system can impact or influence the course of communicable diseases as well. Health care providers may fail or be unable to screen for diseases; they may fail to recognize or diagnose certain diseases; or they may have certain attitudes about diseases that can influence care.

POWERPOINT LECTURE SLIDES

NOTE: The number on each PPT Lecture Slide directly corresponds with the Concepts for Lecture.

1. Epidemiological Factors: Biophysical
   - Age
   - Gender
   - Race/ethnicity
   - Physiologic health status
     ○ Immunity

2. Epidemiological Factors: Psychological
   - Effects of stress
   - Risk-taking behaviors
   - Depression

3. Epidemiological Factors: Physical Environmental
   - Poor sanitation
   - Overcrowding
   - Climates with extreme winds and dust
   - Contaminated waters
   - Regions with infectious insects or animals

4. Epidemiological Factors: Sociocultural
   - Poverty
   - Poor nutrition
   - Unemployment
   - Homelessness
   - Cultural beliefs
   - Gender socialization

5. Epidemiological Factors: Behavioral
   - Diet
   - Sexual activity
   - Drug use
   - Use of mosquito nets
   - Swimming in contaminated water

6. Epidemiological Factors: Health Systems
   - Failure or inability to screen for diseases
   - Failure to recognize or diagnose certain diseases
   - Attitudes about diseases that can influence care

<table>
<tr>
<td>

SUGGESTIONS FOR CLASSROOM ACTIVITIES

Have students investigate a communicable disease and provide examples of how epidemiological factors influence the course of the disease, the prevalence of the disease, and the outcomes of the disease.

</td>
<td>

SUGGESTIONS FOR CLINICAL ACTIVITIES

Invite a guest speaker from the health department to present information on the epidemiological factors of a communicable disease of interest.

</td>
</tr>
</table>

LEARNING OBJECTIVE 4

Analyze the potential effects of epidemics due to bioterrorist activity.

CONCEPTS FOR LECTURE

1. Epidemics related to bioterrorist activities are important because of the potential for significant morbidity and mortality, the psychological and economic impacts on populations and communities, the impact on production and transportation of foods and essential goods, the burden placed on current health care systems, and the problem of inadequate facilities and supplies needed to address widespread communicable disease incidence.

POWERPOINT LECTURE SLIDES

NOTE: The number on each PPT Lecture Slide directly corresponds with the Concepts for Lecture.

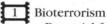 Bioterrorism
- Potential for significant morbidity/mortality
- Psychological and economic impacts on populations/communities
- Impact on production and transportation of foods/essential goods
- Burden health care systems
- Problem of inadequate facilities/supplies needed to address widespread communicable disease incidence

<table>
<tr>
<td>

SUGGESTIONS FOR CLASSROOM ACTIVITIES

Assign groups of students to research the different types of organisms that could be used to create an epidemic as a result of bioterrorist activity such as smallpox, anthrax, or botulism. Guide students to use the CDC Web site for organisms and their transmission routes, signs and symptoms, prevalence, and incidence, and primary prevention treatment. Have groups present their findings and discuss the differences in impact on the health care community and the population, and the role of the community health nurse.

</td>
<td>

SUGGESTIONS FOR CLINICAL ACTIVITIES

Arrange for students to attend a community planning meeting/community forum that addresses bioterrorism or pandemic preparedness.

</td>
</tr>
</table>

LEARNING OBJECTIVE 5

Analyze the role of community health nurses in controlling communicable diseases as it interfaces with those of other health professionals.

CONCEPTS FOR LECTURE

1. Community health nurses provide a number of roles in controlling communicable diseases in individual clients and in population groups. Using the nursing process, community health nurses assess factors contributing to communicable diseases, identify the presence and extent of communicable disease in individuals or populations, plan and implement control strategies for communicable diseases, evaluate the

POWERPOINT LECTURE SLIDES

NOTE: The number on each PPT Lecture Slide directly corresponds with the Concepts for Lecture.

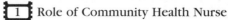 Role of Community Health Nurse
- Assess factors contributing to communicable diseases
- Identify presence and extent of communicable disease

effectiveness of communicable disease interventions, conduct epidemiological research to identify factors contributing to disease, and may also administer entire communicable disease programs.

2. Roles specific to interfacing with other health professionals include receiving postexposure client referrals for contact information, identification, and notification; making referrals to health care providers for postexposure prophylaxis; and collaborating with environmental specialists to address issues of food or water contamination.

- Plan/implement control strategies
- Evaluate effectiveness of disease interventions
- Conduct epidemiological research
- Administer communicable disease programs

 Interfacing with Health Professionals
- Receiving postexposure client referrals
  - Information
  - Identification
  - Notification
- Making referrals to health care providers for postexposure prophylaxis
- Collaborating with environmental specialists

SUGGESTIONS FOR CLASSROOM ACTIVITIES

Divide students into role-playing groups, with each group assigned a community health nurse role. Have students refer to the case study at the end of the chapter and write out questions that they might need to ask at the hospital and the dormitory, people that they need to interview, and health professionals that they need to contact. Have students present to the class how they would address the problem of rubella, and their actions and roles.

SUGGESTIONS FOR CLINICAL ACTIVITIES

Assign students to identify community resources and health care providers that would be involved when conducting a communicable disease intervention.

LEARNING OBJECTIVE 6

Provide examples of approaches to primary prevention of communicable diseases.

CONCEPTS FOR LECTURE

1. The purpose of primary prevention interventions is to prevent the occurrence of disease, guided by several prevention measures and specific community health nursing interventions.

2. Primary prevention strategies include immunization. Community health nurses educate clients and the public regarding the need for immunizations, refer clients for immunization services, provide direct immunization services, and advocate for access to immunization services for all segments of the population.

3. Contact notification is another focus of community health nursing interventions. Nurses educate providers regarding the legal requirements for reporting communicable diseases, interview clients with communicable diseases for names and locating information, inform contacts of their exposure, refer clients for testing and postexposure prophylaxis (PEP), educate clients about preventive measures, and advocate for and plan effective contact notification services.

4. Postexposure prophylaxis involves referring clients for PEP services, providing PEP under established protocols, monitoring and promoting compliance with PEP, monitoring for adverse effects and side effects of

POWERPOINT LECTURE SLIDES

NOTE: The number on each PPT Lecture Slide directly corresponds with the Concepts for Lecture.

1 Primary Prevention Strategies
- Prevent the occurrence of disease
- Specific prevention measures
- Community health nursing interventions

2 Immunization
- Educate clients and the public
- Refer clients for immunization services
- Provide immunization services
- Advocate for access to immunization services

3 Contact Notification
- Educate providers regarding the legal requirements for reporting communicable diseases
- Interview clients with communicable diseases
- Inform contacts of their exposure
- Refer clients for testing and PEP
- Educate clients regarding preventive measures
- Advocate for and plan effective contact notification services

PEP, and advocating for the availability of PEP for clients in need.

5. Other primary prevention measures include but are not limited to: promoting adequate nutrition, rest, and other facets of good health, educating clients and the public about effective wound care, educating clients and the public on safe sexual practices, preventing drug abuse or referring clients for drug abuse treatment, promoting use of universal precautions for bloodborne diseases, and advocating for adequate sanitation.

6. Primary prevention measures also address pandemic and bioterrorism preparedness. Community health nurses assist in identifying the potential for a pandemic or bioterrorist event, assist in identifying vulnerable populations and factors influencing their vulnerability, participate in planning community response to a pandemic or bioterrorist event, educate the public and other health providers regarding prevention of illness or self-care during a pandemic or bioterrorist event, and educate the public regarding the signs and symptoms of disease during a pandemic or bioterrorist event.

4 Postexposure Prophylaxis
- Refer clients for PEP services
- Provide PEP under established protocols
- Monitor and promote compliance
- Monitor for adverse effects
- Advocate for PEP for clients in need

5 Other Primary Prevention Measures
- Promote adequate nutrition, rest, and other facets of good health
- Educate clients and the public regarding effective wound care
- Educate clients and the public on safe sexual practices
- Prevent drug abuse or refer clients for drug abuse treatment
- Promote use of universal precautions
- Advocate for adequate sanitation

6 Pandemic and Bioterrorism Preparedness
- Assist in identifying the potential for a pandemic or bioterrorist event
- Assist in identifying vulnerable populations and factors influencing their vulnerability
- Participate in planning community response
- Educate the public and other health care providers regarding prevention of illness or self-care during a pandemic or bioterrorist event
- Educate the public regarding signs and symptoms of disease from these events

SUGGESTIONS FOR CLASSROOM ACTIVITIES

Divide students into groups and have them develop primary prevention strategies for the community, college, and students in the case study at the end of the chapter who may have been exposed to rubella. Have them assess which groups are at highest risk. Have students present their findings.

SUGGESTIONS FOR CLINICAL ACTIVITIES

Assign students to analyze primary prevention strategies employed at their clinical site or agency. Have students identify the strategies used for specific communicable diseases and the target populations. Have students present at post conference.

LEARNING OBJECTIVE 7

Describe major considerations in secondary prevention for communicable diseases.

CONCEPTS FOR LECTURE

1. Secondary prevention strategies include case finding and surveillance. Case finding involves being familiar with the signs and symptoms of communicable diseases for the region. Surveillance occurs at the population level and involves gathering and analyzing data that reflects trends in disease incidence and prevalence.

2. Screening, which can occur through either individual or selective screening or population or mass screening, is the presumptive identification of asymptomatic

POWERPOINT LECTURE SLIDES

NOTE: The number on each PPT Lecture Slide directly corresponds with the Concepts for Lecture.

1 Secondary Prevention Strategies
- Case finding
  ○ Signs and symptoms of diseases
- Surveillance
  ○ Gather and analyze data

2 Screening and Reporting
- Selective or mass screening

persons with disease. Screening can be based on interest in specific diseases and CDC recommendations. Reporting requirements are integral to the effective control of communicable diseases and may require forwarding information to state, federal, and international agencies. Case reports and outbreak reports are two categories of communicable disease reports. Reportable communicable diseases are classified into five categories, which dictate which agency is notified. Class 1 diseases such as cholera, plague, and yellow fever are reportable to the World Health Organization. Class 2 diseases are reportable to the CDC and to any other state or local agencies that have jurisdictional requirements. Class 3 diseases are required to be reported in selected endemic areas. Class 4 diseases are required to be reported in the instance of outbreaks only. Class 5 diseases are not ordinarily reportable because they are rare or are not directly transmissible from person to person.

3. Diagnosis involves diagnostic testing for the presence of specific antibodies in the blood of infected persons. Treatment for communicable diseases is accomplished through antibiotic or antiviral medications or provision of supportive care, and can often require timely identification of people in need of treatment, supervising or monitoring compliance, and motivating people who need medications.

- Diseases of interest
- CDC recommendations

 Diagnosis and Treatment
- Diagnostic testing
- Reporting requirements
  ○ Reportable disease categories

 Diagnosis and Treatment (continued)
- Treatment
  ○ Medications
  ○ Supportive care
  ○ Timely identification
  ○ Supervising/monitoring compliance

SUGGESTIONS FOR CLASSROOM ACTIVITIES

Invite a community health nurse or regional health department medical provider who works with the secondary prevention programs to discuss interventions, programs available, and reporting requirements.

SUGGESTIONS FOR CLINICAL ACTIVITIES

1. Arrange for students to participate in a case finding visit with a community health nurse or other personnel responsible for case finding of a reportable communicable disease.
2. Provide students with a clinical opportunity at a communicable disease treatment clinic such as a tuberculosis, STD, or AIDS clinic. Have students discuss their experiences at post conference.

LEARNING OBJECTIVE 8

Discuss tertiary prevention of communicable diseases.

CONCEPTS FOR LECTURE

1. Tertiary prevention strategies occur at the individual or population level. At the individual level, emphasis is placed on preventing complications and long-term sequelae, monitoring treatment compliance and its effects, monitoring for side effects, assisting clients in handling the side effects, providing assistance with coping with long-term consequences, and educating about ways to prevent complications.

2. Tertiary prevention at the population level is directed at preventing the spread of communicable diseases

POWERPOINT LECTURE SLIDES

NOTE: The number on each PPT Lecture Slide directly corresponds with the Concepts for Lecture.

 Tertiary Prevention Strategies: Individual Level
- Preventing complications and long-term sequelae
- Monitoring treatment compliance
- Monitoring for side effects
- Assisting clients in handling side effects

CONCEPTS FOR LECTURE *continued*

through isolation or quarantine measures; outbreak response, such as managing those with disease and interrupting disease transmission; or social distancing measures, such as closing schools and businesses or restricting access to certain areas.

POWERPOINT LECTURE SLIDES *continued*

- Providing assistance with coping with long-term consequences
- Educating about ways to prevent complications

 Tertiary Prevention Strategies: Population Level
- Preventing the spread of disease
  - Isolation or quarantine
  - Outbreak response
    - Management of those with disease
    - Interrupting disease transmission
  - Social distancing
    - Closing schools and businesses
    - Restricting access to certain locations

SUGGESTIONS FOR CLASSROOM ACTIVITIES

Referring to the case study at the end of the chapter, assume that 30 more cases of suspected rubella have been identified through the local hospital. Assign students to two groups. Each group will have 15 minutes to develop tertiary prevention strategies for a rubella outbreak and 10 minutes to present their strategies to the class.

SUGGESTIONS FOR CLINICAL ACTIVITIES

1. Invite a community health nurse or local health department official to discuss tertiary prevention strategies for specific diseases for the community. Ask the guest speaker to address: What resources, policies, funding, and programs are available? What examples can they provide of local or state case studies? What data are available to evaluate tertiary prevention outcomes?

2. Have students explore the availability of tertiary prevention services for communicable diseases in the local community.

Chronic Physical Health Problems

RESOURCE LIBRARY

 COMPANION WEBSITE

Audio Glossary
Appendix J: Factors in the Epidemiology of Selected
  Chronic Physical Health Problems
Exam Review Questions
Case Study: Health Promotion for the Chronically Ill
MediaLink Application: Living with Crohn's Disease
  (video)

Media Links
Challenge Your Knowledge
Update *Healthy People 2010*
Advocacy Interviews

IMAGE LIBRARY

Table 29–8 Goals for Secondary Prevention and
  Related Community Health Nursing Interventions in
  the Control of Chronic Physical Health Problems

LEARNING OBJECTIVE 1

Describe personal and population effects of chronic physical health problems.

CONCEPTS FOR LECTURE

1. Chronic disease affects roughly 90 million people in the United States and accounts for three fourths of the U.S. health care expenditures each year. Chronic disease is defined as a physical or emotional condition that requires ongoing medical care, limits what one can do, and is likely to last longer than one year. Chronic health conditions arise from a variety of sources and have personal and family effects, population effects, societal costs, and morbidity and mortality consequences.

2. Personal effects of chronic illness include pain, suffering, impairment, and disability. Other effects include required changes in lifestyle and social isolation. Disability, as a culturally defined concept, is seen as a multidimensional phenomenon resulting from the interaction between people and their physical and social environment and leading to inability to function in expected roles.

3. Family effects of chronic illness include changes in family roles and relationships, stress, and financial burden.

4. Population effects include the financial costs to society and the overall impact of morbidity and mortality on each society.

POWERPOINT LECTURE SLIDES

NOTE: The number on each PPT Lecture Slide directly corresponds with the Concepts for Lecture.

1 Chronic Disease
  • Definition
  • Types
    ○ Physical
    ○ Emotional

2 Personal Effects of Chronic Physical Health Problems
  • Pain and suffering
  • Impairment
  • Disability
  • Changes in lifestyle
  • Social isolation

3 Family Effects
  • Changes in family roles and relationships
  • Stress
  • Financial burden

4 Population Effects
  • Financial costs to society
  • Impact of morbidity and mortality

LEARNING OBJECTIVE 2

Identify biophysical, psychological, physical environmental, sociocultural, behavioral, and health system factors that influence the development of chronic physical health problems.

CONCEPTS FOR LECTURE

1. Biophysical considerations include the presence, impact of, or risk of developing a chronic condition as a result of maturation and aging, gender, race and ethnicity, and physiologic function such as obesity, hypertension, and predispositions to cancer. The very young and the elderly are often at higher risk for accidental injuries, accidental death, or epilepsy. Some chronic diseases are more prevalent in adults, such as arthritis, COPD, and certain cancers. Strokes tend to double for every decade after age 65.

2. Psychological considerations include the impact of stress, depression, anxiety, and the effect of chronic debilitating conditions on the individual and family.

3. The physical environmental contributes to chronic health problems through its effects of environmental pollutants, global climate, and seasonal variation changes on conditions such as asthma and allergies, blood pressure, and stroke. When certain populations or communities must travel considerable distances to reach health care services, the outcomes of chronic health conditions may be more severe. Environmental hazards may either cause or exacerbate chronic health conditions as a result of living in a low-income neighborhood.

4. Sociocultural factors contributing to the effects of chronic health conditions include social norms, role modeling, media messaging, cultural factors, social participation, and socioenvironmental factors. Certain social norms and role modeling may promote the use of tobacco and alcohol, and media messaging may work to reduce smoking in targeted groups. Culture plays a role in the extent of support for healthy or unhealthy behaviors and low social participation may be associated with increased risk of coronary heart disease. The social environmental factors such as low income, low educational levels, and unemployment may prevent access to health care services.

5. Behavioral factors include dietary consumption patterns that contribute to obesity, high cholesterol, or

POWERPOINT LECTURE SLIDES

NOTE: The number on each PPT Lecture Slide directly corresponds with the Concepts for Lecture.

1 Biophysical Considerations
- Maturation and aging
- Gender
- Race and ethnicity
- Genetic inheritance
- Physiologic function

2 Psychological Considerations
- Stress
- Depression/anxiety
- Effects of chronic debilitating conditions

3 Physical Environmental Considerations
- Environmental pollutants
- Global climate changes
- Seasonal variations
- Distance to treatment
- Environmental hazards

4 Sociocultural Considerations
- Social norms
- Role modeling
- Media messaging
- Cultural factors
- Social participation
- Socioenvironmental factors

5 Behavioral Considerations
- Consumption patterns
- Exercise
- Other behaviors
  - Self-assessment behaviors
  - Use of safety devices and precautions

6 Health System Considerations
- Lack of access to care
- Failure of providers to educate about risk behaviors

insufficient intake of Vitamin D, which may be associated with certain forms of cancer. Lack of exercise can influence the development and course of some chronic conditions such as diabetes. Other behaviors such as sunbathing may lead to skin cancer, or use patterns for safety devices such as seat belts and helmets may affect the severity of accident outcomes.

6. Health system factors contribute to the development or the prognosis of chronic health conditions. Lack of access to care, failure of health care professionals to educate their clients on the effects of lifestyle behaviors, the availability of screening services, and the availability and quality of treatment obtainable for persons with chronic conditions all have varying effects on morbidity and mortality outcomes.

- Availability of screening services
- Availability and quality of treatment

SUGGESTIONS FOR CLASSROOM ACTIVITIES

Assign students to small groups to research one or more epidemiological considerations for a selection of chronic health conditions provided to them. Have students present their findings to class.

SUGGESTIONS FOR CLINICAL ACTIVITIES

Arrange for students to work in a chronic disease section of the local health department. Ask students to identify programs that are available, services provided, and types of populations and conditions most served. Ask students to identify gaps in service for specific health concerns and provide an opportunity for discussion at post conference.

LEARNING OBJECTIVE 3

Describe strategies for primary prevention of chronic physical health problems and analyze the role of the community health nurse related to each.

CONCEPTS FOR LECTURE

1. Primary prevention strategies for chronic health conditions most used by nurses include health promotion and risk factor modification. Health promotion interventions include promoting healthy lifestyles, such as educating individuals and community members about basic nutrition and specific nutritional age requirements and about the benefits of exercise. Nurses may assist individuals to develop ways to incorporate physical activity into their daily routine. Nurses may also teach coping skills to high-risk individuals or groups. Political activity by community health nurses might also be required to establish and enforce policies and legislation that foster healthy behaviors, such as enforcing laws related to the sale of tobacco to minors or monitoring smoking in public facilities. Nurses also provide immunization services to children and high-risk groups.

2. Risk factor modification is another primary prevention focus and includes modifying factors such as smoking, obesity, hypertension, and safety and environmental hazards.

POWERPOINT LECTURE SLIDES

NOTE: The number on each PPT Lecture Slide directly corresponds with the Concepts for Lecture.

1 Primary Prevention: Health Promotion
- Promoting healthy lifestyles
- Political activity
- Immunization

2 Risk Factor Modification
- Smoking
- Obesity
- Hypertension
- Safety precautions and environmental modification

SUGGESTIONS FOR CLASSROOM ACTIVITIES

Have students research information on the incidence and prevalence of chronic conditions in the community to develop primary prevention nursing interventions such as health promotion or risk factor modification opportunities at their clinical setting. Suggest sources of information such as the local health department, online published reports by state health agencies, and local agencies that target chronic conditions by providing specific services to at-risk groups such as the local diabetes association. Provide an opportunity for students to discuss their research and suggested interventions in class.

SUGGESTIONS FOR CLINICAL ACTIVITIES

1. Arrange for students to work in an immunization clinic. Ask students to identify population groups where immunization services are lacking. Have students develop a nursing intervention to reach their target group.

2. Assign students to develop one health promotion and one risk modification nursing intervention for an individual or group served by their clinical agency or setting.

LEARNING OBJECTIVE 4

Identify the major aspects of secondary prevention of chronic physical health problems and analyze community health nursing roles with respect to each.

CONCEPTS FOR LECTURE

1. Secondary prevention activities focus on three areas: screening for the existence of chronic health problems, such as breast or cervical cancer, colorectal cancer, or prostate cancer; developing screening programs that may be lacking for targeted populations; or advocating for the availability and accessibility of screening programs for underserved groups in the community. Early diagnosis is another secondary prevention strategy, which involves case finding, case referral, and surveillance at both the individual and population level.

2. Prompt treatment can influence the severity and the overall outcomes of certain chronic conditions and requires promotion and monitoring treatment standards for chronic disease. Prompt treatment addresses the need to stabilize the client's condition, establish a treatment regimen, motivate for compliance, and eventually promote self-management.

POWERPOINT LECTURE SLIDES

NOTE: The number on each PPT Lecture Slide directly corresponds with the Concepts for Lecture.

 Secondary Prevention (Refer to Table 29–8)
- Screening
  - Existing chronic conditions
  - Programs for targeted populations
  - Programs for underserved groups
- Early diagnosis
  - Case finding
  - Case referral
  - Surveillance

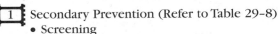 Secondary Prevention: Treatment
- Prompt treatment
  - Stabilizing client's condition
  - Establishing treatment regimen
  - Motivating compliance
  - Promoting self-management

SUGGESTIONS FOR CLASSROOM ACTIVITIES

Assign students to small groups to examine and discuss the impact of secondary intervention strategies for a chronic condition. Ask them to identify specific nursing actions and identify the national health objective that corresponds to their chronic condition.

SUGGESTIONS FOR CLINICAL ACTIVITIES

Arrange for students to participate in a screening program for a chronic health problem at the local health department. Have students discuss their experiences during post conference.

Analyze community health nursing roles in tertiary prevention of chronic physical health problems.

CONCEPTS FOR LECTURE

1. Tertiary prevention involves preventing further loss of function in affected and unaffected systems; restoring function; monitoring health status; assisting the client to adjust functionally and psychologically to the presence of a chronic condition with appropriate pain control and other measures; assisting clients with survivorship care; and providing end-of-life care as needed.

POWERPOINT LECTURE SLIDES

NOTE: The number on each PPT Lecture Slide directly corresponds with the Concepts for Lecture.

1 Tertiary Prevention
- Preventing loss of function in affected and unaffected systems
- Restoring function
- Monitoring health status

1a Tertiary Prevention (continued)
- Promoting adjustment
  - Functional adjustment
  - Psychological adjustment
  - Pain management
- Providing end-of-life care
- Assisting clients with survivorship care

SUGGESTIONS FOR CLASSROOM ACTIVITIES

Provide students with a case study to develop a nursing care plan that incorporates tertiary prevention strategies. Allow class time for discussion.

SUGGESTIONS FOR CLINICAL ACTIVITIES

Invite a breast cancer or other cancer survivor to post conference to discuss life experiences, support networks, impact on life and quality of life, and perceived needs in the community.

Community Mental Health Problems

RESOURCE LIBRARY

 COMPANION WEBSITE

Audio Glossary
Exam Review Questions
Case Study: Providing Nursing Care for the Mentally Ill
MediaLink Application: Beyond the Black Hole of
   Depression (video)

Media Links
Challenge Your Knowledge
Update *Healthy People 2010*
Advocacy Interviews

LEARNING OBJECTIVE 1

Analyze the personal, family, and societal impact of mental illness and mental health problems.

CONCEPTS FOR LECTURE

1. Key concepts for understanding community mental health problems include the following definitions: Mental health is the ability to successfully perform mental functions, to engage in productive activities and meaningful interpersonal relationships, and to adapt to change and cope with adversity. Mental illness includes a variety of diagnosable mental disorders that are characterized by changes in thinking, moods, or behavior associated with stress or impaired function. Serious mental illness is defined as an intensity that disables people, preventing them from functioning adequately on the basis of their culture and background. Mental health problems involve signs and symptoms of mental distress that are of insufficient duration or intensity to qualify as mental disorders diagnoses on the basis of accepted criteria. Finally, community mental health problems are those that occur with sufficient frequency in the community or population group to be of serious concern in the overall health status of the population.

2. The effects of mental health problems on the individual include suffering and disability with physical and social impairments, and premature death.

3. The effects of mental health problems on families are both economic and emotional. Individual family members with mental health problems may experience unemployment or underemployment, which affects income and access to and payment for mental health services. Families may also experience emotional stress due to disruption in normal life patterns, communication patterns, and guilt or fear of social stigma.

POWERPOINT LECTURE SLIDES

NOTE: The number on each PPT Lecture Slide directly corresponds with the Concepts for Lecture.

1 Key Concepts
- Mental health
- Mental illness
- Serious mental illness
- Mental health problem
- Community mental health problems

2 Effects on Individual
- Suffering
- Disability
- Physical/social impairments
- Premature death

3 Effects on Family
- Economic strain
- Emotional stress
- Changes in family roles
- Caregiver stress

4 Societal Effects
- Economic burdens
  - Costs for mental health care services and treatment
  - Lost worker productivity

Caregiver stress is an additional family effect of mental illness in a member.

4. The effects on society are the economic burdens for communities and countries as a result of costs for mental health care services and treatment and lost worker productivity.

SUGGESTIONS FOR CLASSROOM ACTIVITIES

1. Assign students to three groups to investigate the costs, both economic and emotional, of mental health problems at the community, state, and national level. Have groups identify national health objectives that address mental health concerns for the nation. Ask each group to identify the top five most common mental health diagnoses for their geographic region. Provide the opportunity for discussion of findings.

2. Have students share feelings and beliefs about mental health illness in class and what the perceived costs of mental illness might be for them and their families.

SUGGESTIONS FOR CLINICAL ACTIVITIES

Invite a local mental health provider to discuss mental health concerns in the community, available services, and the impact of mental illness on the individual, family, and community.

LEARNING OBJECTIVE 2

Analyze factors influencing the development of mental health problems.

CONCEPTS FOR LECTURE

1. Biophysical factors influencing mental health problems include genetics and gender, maturation and aging, race and ethnicity, and physiologic function. Family history of mental health disorders such as schizophrenia present a 10 times greater risk for individuals within that family, and women are 70% more likely to report serious psychological distress and have a lifetime prevalence of major depression, nearly twice that of men. Mental health problems are distributed differently among various age groups with 20% of children diagnosed with neuropsychiatric disorders and 4.2% of men between 45 and 54 years of age reporting serious psychological distress. Depression is reported across the age spectrum, but is more common in older people. Mental illness and mental health problems vary among racial and ethnic populations with American Indians and Alaska Natives reporting the highest incidence. Comorbidity with other chronic medical conditions, infections, malnutrition, and hormonal imbalances impacts the overall effects of physiologic functioning on mental health problems. Nurses need to be aware of the effects of pregnancy and postpartum on the incidence of depression.

POWERPOINT LECTURE SLIDES

NOTE: The number on each PPT Lecture Slide directly corresponds with the Concepts for Lecture.

1 Biophysical Considerations
- Genetics and gender
- Maturation and aging
- Race and ethnicity
- Physiologic function
  - Comorbidity
  - Depression and pregnancy

2 Psychological Considerations
- Personality traits and temperament
- Stressful life events
- Below average intelligence
- Existing health problems
- Lack of coping skills
- Suicide potential

3 Physical Environmental Considerations
- Environmental exposure
- SAD

CONCEPTS FOR LECTURE *continued*

2. The psychological factors affecting mental health include the effects of personality traits and temperament, stressful life events, below average intelligence, existing health problems, lack of effective coping skills, and suicidal ideations.

3. Physical environmental factors that increase one's risk of acquiring a mental health problem include exposure to environmental toxins such as lead and arsenic, and the direct effects of climate and geography on conditions such as seasonal affective disorder, which as a form of depression tends to occur in the fall and winter when exposure to natural light diminishes.

4. Sociocultural factors that influence risk for and treatment of mental health problems include societal disorganization brought about by disasters and wars; social and economic factors, such as poverty and homelessness; family relationships, such as communication difficulties with parents and the correlation with schizophrenia; social support, which can hinder or help with recognition, treatment, and compliance with therapeutic interventions; culture where mental health problems may not be recognized or are defined as normal or abnormal; and societal attitudes toward mental illness, which can lead to criminalization of behaviors and incarceration.

5. Behavioral factors that can impact the presence or severity of mental health problems include lack of physical activity, alcohol and drug use, and sexual activity, especially high-risk sexual activity displayed by individuals with particular types of diagnoses.

6. A number of health system issues affect the recognition, diagnosis, treatment, and preventive actions taken by a society. These issues include the lack of adequate mental health care services, lack of insurance coverage, lack of a unified mental health care system, and discrepancies in provider practice as evidenced by nonadherence to established clinical guidelines for treatment. Currently, the United States has four sectors that provide services for mental health care and present their own focus of care: the general medical or primary care sector, the specialty mental health care sector, the social services sector, and the volunteer support network sector.

POWERPOINT LECTURE SLIDES *continued*

4 Sociocultural Considerations
- Societal disorganization
- Social/economic factors
- Family relationships
- Social support
- Culture
- Societal attitudes

5 Behavioral Considerations
- Lack of physical activity
- Alcohol and drug use
- Sexual activity

6 Health System Considerations
- Lack of adequate mental health care services
- Lack of insurance coverage
- Lack of unified mental health care system
  - General medical/primary care sector
  - Specialty mental health care sector
  - Social services sector
  - Volunteer support network sector

6a Health System Considerations (continued)
- Discrepancies in provider practice
  - Nonadherence to established clinical guidelines

SUGGESTIONS FOR CLASSROOM ACTIVITIES

Assign students to small groups to research one or more category of health considerations as they influence the development or course of mental illness. Have students select several journal articles that address or represent their specific health consideration and summarize findings in class.

SUGGESTIONS FOR CLINICAL ACTIVITIES

Assign students to a mental health setting that offers outpatient or inpatient services. Have students select one client to develop an assessment of the six health considerations. Ask students to present a case summary that addresses a nursing diagnosis for each health dimension if relevant.

LEARNING OBJECTIVE 3

Identify symptoms characteristic of common mental health problems.

CONCEPTS FOR LECTURE

1. Depression affects nearly 21 million people in the United States. Bipolar disorder is characterized by shifts in mood, energy, and functional ability with people cycling through periods of depression alternating with periods of energy, excitability, and irritability. Schizophrenia can present with many signs and symptoms with three types of symptoms prominent: positive symptoms with unusual thoughts or perceptions that are not present in other people, negative symptoms with an absence of normal behaviors and emotional states, and cognitive symptoms that reflect deficits in attention, memory, and executive functions that permit planning and organizing thoughts and behaviors. Anxiety disorders include a group of illnesses that result in chronic and overwhelming fear and anxiety that tend to grow progressively worse with time. Up to 5% of the female population suffers from eating disorders, which include anorexia nervosa, bulimia nervosa, and binge eating disorders. Anorexia nervosa is characterized by a strong resistance to maintaining a minimal weight for one's height and body type, by intense fear of gaining weight, and by a distorted body image. Bulimia nervosa is characterized by uncontrollable eating followed by compensatory purging and other behaviors to prevent weight gain. Binge eating is excessive overeating without compensatory purging and other behaviors. Borderline personality disorder is characterized by rapidly changing moods and resulting difficulty with interpersonal relationships and an inability to function effectively in society. Autism spectrum disorders occur in young children, with Asperger syndrome being the mildest and Rhett syndrome being the most severe and rarest form. Clinical symptoms include lack of interactive behaviors, not responding to their name, failing to maintain eye contact, not playing with toys, not smiling, and not liking to be cuddled.

POWERPOINT LECTURE SLIDES

NOTE: The number on each PPT Lecture Slide directly corresponds with the Concepts for Lecture.

1. Common Mental Health Problems
   - Depression
   - Bipolar or manic-depressive disorder
   - Schizophrenia
   - Anxiety disorders
   - Eating disorders
   - Borderline personality disorders
   - Autism spectrum disorders

SUGGESTIONS FOR CLASSROOM ACTIVITIES

Assign students to select one mental health problem and present a description of that problem and its characteristic features.

SUGGESTIONS FOR CLINICAL ACTIVITIES

If appropriate, invite an individual with a mental health condition, or a family member to discuss the impact of mental health diagnosis on the family. Ask the speaker to describe personal experiences of the characteristics of his or her disorder. Have students compare the description to the textbook features of the disorder.

LEARNING OBJECTIVE 4

Analyze the role of the community health nurse in strategies to prevent mental health problems.

CONCEPTS FOR LECTURE

1. Community health nurses have a number of opportunities to affect mental health services and problems in the community. Nurses begin with assessing individual, family, and population risk factors, and include an assessment of the incidence and prevalence of specific mental health problems. Nurses may survey community members or community informants who are knowledgeable about the attitudes to mental health problems. Nurses can determine the availability of mental health services, both the actual services and the barriers to services. They also assess clients for evidence of mental health problems.

2. Direct prevention roles include promoting protective factors and risk factor reduction strategies that foster supportive environments and individual and family resilience. Nurses may develop programs that promote coping in school, work, or other settings; advocate for societal stress minimization by identifying existing sources of stress; and assist with development of mental health services.

POWERPOINT LECTURE SLIDES

NOTE: The number on each PPT Lecture Slide directly corresponds with the Concepts for Lecture.

1 Role of Community Health Nurse
- Assess risk factors
- Assess incidence and prevalence of specific mental health problems
- Survey community members about attitudes toward mental health problems
- Determine availability of mental health services
- Assess clients for evidence of mental health problems

2 Prevention Role
- Promote protective factors/risk factor reduction
- Promote coping abilities and resilience
- Advocate for societal stress minimization
- Assist with development of mental health services

SUGGESTIONS FOR CLASSROOM ACTIVITIES

Assign students to select a client from their clinical setting with a mental health diagnosis, assess the incidence and prevalence of the disorder, and investigate the availability of mental health services in the community with the client in mind.

SUGGESTIONS FOR CLINICAL ACTIVITIES

Have students develop a nursing intervention strategy for one client from their clinical setting. Provide an opportunity for discussion at post conference.

LEARNING OBJECTIVE 5

Discuss approaches to community treatment of mental health problems and analyze the community health nurse's role in each.

CONCEPTS FOR LECTURE

1. Community treatment of mental health problems is considered secondary prevention, which begins with screening or a mental health evaluation of a client's psychiatric history, use of current psychotropic drugs, presence of suicidal ideation or attempt, drug and alcohol abuse, and a history of sex offenses, victimization, or violence. A client's motivation for treatment, as part of the screening assessment, includes perceptions of the seriousness of the mental health problem, desire for and perceived importance of treatment, and past attempts at treatment and their effects.

2. A mental health evaluation may also include a history of special education placement, history of traumatic brain injury, incarceration, and evidence of mental retardation.

POWERPOINT LECTURE SLIDES

NOTE: The number on each PPT Lecture Slide directly corresponds with the Concepts for Lecture.

1 Secondary Prevention
- Mental health evaluation
  - Psychiatric history
  - Use of psychotropic drugs
  - Suicidal ideation/attempt
  - Drug/alcohol abuse
  - History of sex offenses/victimization/violence

1a Secondary Prevention (continued)
- Motivation for treatment
  - Perceptions of the seriousness of the mental health problem

3. The role of community health nurses is to be knowledgeable about and alert to signs and symptoms of mental illness, make appropriate and effective referrals, and assist clients in their decision-making process.

4. Approaches to treatment include pharmacotherapy, individual or group therapy, family intervention, and self-help groups.

5. Pharmacotherapy uses medications alone or in conjunction with other treatment approaches to mental illness. Medications include antipsychotics, antidepressants, stimulants, mood stabilizers, anxiolytics, and cholinesterase inhibitors.

6. The role of the nurse is to monitor and motivate medication compliance, monitor therapeutic effects, assist with side effects, and identify adverse effects.

7. Community health nurses need to be aware of ethnopsychopharmacology, which is the study of ethnic and cultural alterations in response to medication as a result of genetic differences in drug metabolism. Cultural practices related to medication adherence and the use of traditional therapies may affect response to and compliance with medications.

8. Psychotherapy involves an individual or group in therapy and is designed to develop an understanding of one's problems and ways of dealing with them. Family intervention is directed toward alleviation of inappropriate family dynamics that promote stress and result in mental distress. The nurse's role in both psychotherapy and family intervention is one of referral for services. Self-help groups are designed to promote mutual support, education, and personal growth for individuals with similar mental health problems. The community health nurse can be actively involved in initiating and supporting self-help groups in the community, and in promoting client and family empowerment in treatments for mental health problems.

- ○ Desire for and perceived importance of treatment
- ○ Past attempts at treatment and their effects

2 Additional Components
- Special education placement
- History of traumatic brain injury
- Incarceration
- Evidence of mental retardation

3 Role of Community Health Nurse
- Knowledge about/alert to signs/symptoms of mental illness
- Make appropriate/effective referrals
- Assist clients in their decision-making process

4 Approaches to Community Treatment
- Pharmacotherapy
- Individual/group psychotherapy
- Family intervention
- Self-help groups

5 Pharmacotherapy
- Neurotransmitters
  - ○ Antipsychotics
  - ○ Antidepressants
  - ○ Stimulants
  - ○ Mood stabilizers

6 Role of Community Health Nurse
- Monitor/motivate medication compliance
- Monitor therapeutic effects
- Assist with side effects
- Identify adverse reactions

7 Ethnopsychopharmacology
- Study of ethnic and cultural alterations in response to medication as a result of genetic differences in drug metabolism
- Cultural practices
  - ○ Medication adherence
  - ○ Traditional therapies
  - ○ Response to/compliance with medications

8 Community Health Nurse's Role in Treatment Modalities
- Psychotherapy/family intervention
  - ○ Referral
- Self-help groups
  - ○ Initiate/support self-help groups
  - ○ Empowerment

SUGGESTIONS FOR CLASSROOM ACTIVITIES

Divide students into four treatment groups with a corresponding case scenario. Ask groups to develop a care plan for their case study and delineate interventions and roles for the community health nurse. Have groups present for discussion.

SUGGESTIONS FOR CLINICAL ACTIVITIES

Invite a community health nurse, a mental health nurse, and a hospital psychiatric nurse to post conference to discuss treatment modalities in their clinical setting, available services in the community, and barriers to those services.

LEARNING OBJECTIVE 6

Describe areas of emphasis in maintenance therapy for mental health problems and analyze the role of the community health nurse in maintenance.

CONCEPTS FOR LECTURE

1. Tertiary prevention for mental health conditions is considered maintenance therapy. The goal of maintenance therapy is to maintain the client's level of function and to prevent recidivism or frequent rehospitalization.

2. The role of the community health nurse is to follow clients with chronic mental illness to provide support, encourage compliance, and monitor the effects of treatment. Nurses may assist clients with planning regular lifestyles, such as sleeping and waking patterns, and to minimize sources of stress in their lives.

POWERPOINT LECTURE SLIDES

NOTE: The number on each PPT Lecture Slide directly corresponds with the Concepts for Lecture.

1 Tertiary Prevention
- Maintenance
  - Maintain client's level of function
  - Prevent recidivism/frequent rehospitalization

2 Role of Community Health Nurse
- Follow clients with chronic mental illness to provide support
- Encourage compliance
- Monitor effects of treatment
- Assist clients with planning regular lifestyles
- Minimize sources of stress

SUGGESTIONS FOR CLASSROOM ACTIVITIES

Have students select a client with a mental health problem and develop a nursing care plan for tertiary prevention for that client.

SUGGESTIONS FOR CLINICAL ACTIVITIES

Assign students to work with a community health nurse, a mental health nurse, or a hospital-based psychiatric nurse. Have students research prevalent mental health conditions in the community or at their clinical setting and the availability of tertiary prevention services such as maintenance therapy. Present findings at post conference.

Substance Abuse

RESOURCE LIBRARY

 COMPANION WEBSITE

Audio Glossary

Exam Review Questions

Case Study: The Effects of Substance Abuse

MediaLink Application: Overcoming Addiction: Combined Therapies (video)

Media Links

Challenge Your Knowledge

Update *Healthy People 2010*

Advocacy Interviews

LEARNING OBJECTIVE 1

Identify signs and symptoms of psychoactive substance dependence.

CONCEPTS FOR LECTURE

1. Substance-related disorders are defined as disturbances of behavior, cognition, and/or mood caused by the taking and/or abuse of a drug, alcohol, or tobacco; the side effects of medication; or exposure to toxins. Psychoactive substances are drugs or chemicals that alter ordinary states of consciousness, including mood, cognition, and behavior. Drug use is the taking of a drug in the correct amount, frequency, and strength for its medicinal purpose. Drug abuse or misuse is the deliberate use of a drug for other than medicinal purposes in a manner that can adversely affect one's health or ability to function.

2. With more than 1 million people in the United States seeking treatment for substance abuse problems, the magnitude of the problem has been recognized by the more than 40 national health objectives for 2010. Unfortunately, the process of moving from abuse to dependence is not well understood.

3. Signs and symptoms of psychoactive substance dependence include: an increase in the amount of substance used, or extended over a longer period than intended; persistent desire for the substance or one or more unsuccessful attempts to control its use; an increase in the amount of time spent in obtaining, using, or recovering from the effects of the substance; frequent symptoms of intoxication or withdrawal interfacing with obligations; elimination or reduction of important occupational, social, or recreation activities as a result of substance use; continued use of the substance despite recurrent problems caused; increased tolerance to the substance; experience of

POWERPOINT LECTURE SLIDES

NOTE: The number on each PPT Lecture Slide directly corresponds with the Concepts for Lecture.

1 Substance-Related Disorders
- Definition
- Psychoactive substances
- Drug use
- Drug abuse

2 Prevalence
- 1 million people in the United States sought substance abuse treatment
- Magnitude recognized by *Healthy People 2010* objectives
- Process of abuse to dependence not well understood

3 Signs and Symptoms of Psychoactive Substance Dependence
- Increase amount of substance used, or extended over a longer period than intended
- Persistent desire for the substance or one or more unsuccessful attempts to control its use
- Increased time spent in obtaining, using, or recovering from the effects of the substance
- Frequent symptoms of intoxication or withdrawal interfacing with obligations

3a Signs and Symptoms of Psychoactive Substance Dependence (continued)
- Elimination or reduction of important occupational, social, or recreational activities as a result of substance use

CONCEPTS FOR LECTURE *continued*

characteristic withdrawal symptoms; and an increase in substance use to decrease withdrawal symptoms.

POWERPOINT LECTURE SLIDES *continued*
- Continued use of the substance despite recurrent problems caused
- Increased tolerance to the substance
- Experience of characteristic withdrawal symptoms
- An increase in substance use to decrease withdrawal symptoms

---

SUGGESTIONS FOR CLASSROOM ACTIVITIES

Arrange tables in the classroom so that groups are seated together. Provide various magazines at each table, along with supplies such as scissors, tape, glue, and poster paper. Ask groups to find pictures, words, or symbols that represent substance dependence or abuse. Put together a collage and share with the class.

SUGGESTIONS FOR CLINICAL ACTIVITIES

Invite a drug treatment facility professional, a community health nurse, and law enforcement to post conference to discuss the prevalence of substance abuse in the community and encourage a discussion of how nurses can identify signs and symptoms of substance abuse in the client.

LEARNING OBJECTIVE 2

Distinguish between psychoactive substance dependence and abuse.

CONCEPTS FOR LECTURE

1. Psychoactive substance dependence is a cluster of cognitive, behavioral, and physiologic symptoms that indicate impaired control over the use of a psychoactive substance and continued use despite adverse consequences.
2. Psychoactive substance abuse involves maladaptive patterns of substance use that do not meet the criteria for dependence, but include the continued use of a substance despite persistent or recurrent physical, psychological, or social problems related to its use, or recurrent use of the substance in physically dangerous situations.

POWERPOINT LECTURE SLIDES

NOTE: The number on each PPT Lecture Slide directly corresponds with the Concepts for Lecture.

1 Psychoactive Substance Dependence
- Impaired control over the use of a psychoactive substance and continued use despite adverse consequences
  - Symptoms involve
    - Diminished cognitive functioning
    - Behavioral symptoms
    - Physiologic symptoms

2 Psychoactive Substance Abuse
- Maladaptive patterns of substance use
- Does not meet criteria for dependence
  - Continued use despite problems related to its use
    - Physical
    - Psychological
    - Social
  - Recurrent use in physically dangerous situations

SUGGESTIONS FOR CLASSROOM ACTIVITIES

Encourage students to share ideas and feelings about the difference between substance dependence and substance abuse. Ask students to discuss ethical, medical, and legal implications of a nurse working with clients with substance dependence or abuse problems.

SUGGESTIONS FOR CLINICAL ACTIVITIES

Arrange for students to work with a community health nurse in a drug intervention program, with staff at a methadone clinic, or with other agencies and compare symptoms seen in clients with textbook descriptions of symptoms.

LEARNING OBJECTIVE 3

Identify substances that lead to dependence and abuse.

CONCEPTS FOR LECTURE

1. The top 10 substances associated with abuse or dependence include alcohol; sedatives, hypnotics, or anxiolytics; opioids; cocaine; amphetamines; hallucinogens; cannabis; inhalants; steroids; and nicotine. Alcohol is the most used and abused substance with over 50% of the U.S. population age 12 and older reporting use, nearly 23% reporting binge drinking, and almost 8% of the population meeting the criteria for dependence or abuse. Sedatives, hypnotics, and anxiolytics are CNS depressants used for a number of different reasons such as anxiety and inability to sleep. Nearly 7% to 8% of the male and female population report misuse of these prescription medications. Opioids are also CNS depressants derived from the opium poppy or created synthetically. Opioid use has been reported by almost 3.3% of the high school population. Cocaine is a stimulant causing euphoria and a sense of competence. It is derived from the leaves of the coca plant and its use and abuse puts it second behind alcohol. Amphetamines are CNS stimulants, chemically manufactured, and often obtained through prescription for weight loss and fatigue. Its derivative, methamphetamine, is highly addictive and highly dangerous to manufacture, and its use is increasing among middle school and high school students. Hallucinogens such as PCP can create either a stimulant or a depressant effect. Almost 15% of the U.S. population over 12 years of age has reported using hallucinogens. Cannabis may be inhaled or ingested, and its general use ranges from 6% of the U.S. population to almost 40% of high school students reporting using marijuana. Inhalants are abused by sniffing products to create a sense of euphoria, loss of inhibition, or excitement. Its use is common among adolescents, and its danger is one of suffocation, organ damage, and potential for explosion. Steroids are generally obtained through prescription for their immunosuppressant qualities for conditions such as arthritis or joint injury. Its abuse has been reported to be almost 4% of high school students for nonmedical purposes, and its physiologic dangers include enlargement of sexual organs, liver impairment, G.I. problems, and growth impairment. Nicotine is highly addictive, and tobacco use occurs in approximately 21% of the U.S. population.

POWERPOINT LECTURE SLIDES

NOTE: The number on each PPT Lecture Slide directly corresponds with the Concepts for Lecture.

1 Substances Commonly Involved in Abuse or Dependence
- Alcohol
- Sedatives, hypnotics, anxiolytics
- Opioids
- Cocaine
- Amphetamines
- Hallucinogens

1a Substances Commonly Involved in Abuse or Dependence (continued)
- Cannabis
- Inhalants
- Steroids
- Nicotine

SUGGESTIONS FOR CLASSROOM ACTIVITIES

Have students select one commonly abused substance and present a summary of the prevalence of the problem and local resources for individuals and families.

SUGGESTIONS FOR CLINICAL ACTIVITIES

Invite a community health nurse and a school counselor to discuss trends in substance use and abuse in the community.

LEARNING OBJECTIVE 4

Analyze personal, family, and societal effects of substance abuse.

CONCEPTS FOR LECTURE

1. Substance abuse affects all aspects of life, from the individual to the family to the community.
2. The effects on the individual include physical effects such as increased morbidity resulting from exposure to communicable diseases, unintentional injury, unintended pregnancy, and fetal alcohol syndrome. Individuals may also experience withdrawal syndrome caused by drugs. Individuals afflicted with substance abuse problems may undergo personality disturbances, anxiety, and depression.
3. The social impact of substance abuse is the effects on family relationships and employment, which can lead to impaired support networks and financial difficulties. Families experience conflict, anger, violence, and many other problems as a result of substance abuse. Family members may exhibit co-dependence, which is maladaptive behaviors arising out of a need to cope with the problem of abuse. Children suffer from the direct and indirect effects of substance abuse, such as physical and psychological abuse, irritability, disruptions in school, and direct exposure to unhealthy substances.
4. Societal effects include increased morbidity and mortality as a result of accidents, exposure to acute and chronic diseases, higher economic costs from treatment and prevention measures, increased law enforcement needs in a community, and increased crime arising out of a need to support the abuse patterns.

POWERPOINT LECTURE SLIDES

NOTE: The number on each PPT Lecture Slide directly corresponds with the Concepts for Lecture.

1. Effects of Substance Abuse
   - Individual
   - Family
   - Community

2. Individual Effects
   - Increased morbidity
     - Exposure to communicable diseases
     - Unintentional injury
     - Unintentional pregnancy
     - Withdrawal symptoms
     - Personality changes

3. Effects on Family
   - Disruption of family relationships
   - Conflicts
   - Impaired social networks
   - Financial difficulties
   - Co-dependence
   - Effects on children

4. Societal Effects
   - Increased morbidity and mortality
   - Exposure to acute and chronic diseases
   - Higher economic costs
     - Treatment
     - Prevention measures
   - Increased law enforcement
   - Increased crime

SUGGESTIONS FOR CLASSROOM ACTIVITIES

Assign students to select one research or nursing journal article that addresses the effects of substance abuse on the individual, the family, or the community. Have students present a summary of the article to the class.

SUGGESTIONS FOR CLINICAL ACTIVITIES

Have students analyze the effects of substance abuse on a client from their clinical setting, the client's family members, and the community.

LEARNING OBJECTIVE 5

Analyze biophysical, psychological, sociocultural, behavioral, and health systems factors that influence substance abuse.

CONCEPTS FOR LECTURE

1. Biophysical factors that contribute to the overall effects of substance abuse include genetic inheritance, maturation and aging, and the direct physiologic effects of the substances on the human body. Some evidence supports a genetic predisposition for substance abuse, especially with stronger evidence toward the

POWERPOINT LECTURE SLIDES

NOTE: The number on each PPT Lecture Slide directly corresponds with the Concepts for Lecture.

1. Biophysical Factors
   - Genetic inheritance

male gender. Certain ethnic groups are more likely to abstain from using alcohol, and other ethnic groups may have a higher incidence of use and abuse. Use or misuse of substances varies also by age, peer influence, and risk-taking behaviors. Perinatal exposure of the fetus to alcohol can have a lifelong negative affect, resulting in a need for medical and educational or learning interventions. Physiologic function can affect the use of substances and the use of substances can affect physiologic function. Individuals with chronic health conditions may misuse or abuse medications, alcohol, or other substances in order to cope with disabilities or pain. On the other hand, substance abuse may create chronic health problems such as serious infections, cancer, and HIV/Aids.

2. Psychological factors to consider are the personality traits that place an individual at risk for substance abuse, the underlying psychiatric disorders that predispose a person to misuse, and the personality changes or defense mechanisms that result from substance abuse. Substance abusers tend to display denial, projection, rationalization, conflict minimization, and avoidance as a result of coping with their abuse behaviors.

3. There are three spheres of influence that need to be considered in the sociocultural factors: Family influences include their perceptions of substance abuse harm, the individual's perception of disapproval from the family, and the families who experience multiple stressors posing increased risk of substance misuse and violence. Peer influences may contribute to substance abuse, such as smoking or alcohol consumption, especially with adolescents and preadolescents. Certain social factors may influence an individual or community's risk of substance abuse such as poverty, unemployment, and discrimination. Societal attitudes also influence drug use and abuse, especially attitudes that promote incarceration versus treatment strategies, or legislation that restricts public behaviors such as smoking restrictions.

4. Behavioral factors include recreational activities that contribute to the use of psychoactive substances, high-risk behaviors, and subsequent comorbidity associated with poly-drug use such as needle sharing.

5. Providers often pay little attention to educating clients and the public about the hazards of substance abuse. The U.S. health care system has inadequate treatment facilities and programs that are not specific for targeted groups, thus decreasing the likelihood of successful treatment.

- Maturation and aging
- Physiologic function

 Psychological Factors
- Personality traits
- Underlying psychiatric disorders
- Defense mechanisms
  - Denial
  - Projection
  - Rationalization
  - Conflict minimization
  - Avoidance

 Sociocultural Factors
- Family influence
  - Reductions in perceived harm
  - Family stressors
- Peer influence

 Sociocultural Factors (continued)
- Societal influence
  - Poverty
  - Unemployment
  - Discrimination
  - Attitudes

 Behavioral Factors
- Recreational activities
- Comorbidity of polydrug use
- High-risk behaviors

 Health System Factors
- Education about hazards of substance abuse
- Inadequate treatment
- Treatment programs not specific for targeted groups

SUGGESTIONS FOR CLASSROOM ACTIVITIES

Assign students to small groups. Provide case studies about individuals with substance abuse problems. Ask groups to list at least three or four health considerations for each of the dimensions. Provide an opportunity for discussion and sharing of ideas about the case studies.

SUGGESTIONS FOR CLINICAL ACTIVITIES

Ask students to select one client from their clinical setting with a substance abuse problem and assess the client situation from the perspective of each of the health dimensions.

Learning Objective 6

Discuss aspects of community health nursing assessment in relation to substance abuse.

CONCEPTS FOR LECTURE

1. The World Health Organization (WHO) has developed a community health substance abuse assessment called rapid assessment and response (RAR) that includes guidelines for increasing the timely response capabilities with health issues. The RAR is a pubic health assessment tool that addresses the characteristics of the health problem, population groups affected, settings and context, health and risk behaviors, and social consequences. The four steps for the RAR are to gather information about the nature and extent of the problem, its adverse health and social consequences, a population's protective factors, and community-based intervention proposals for the problem at hand.

2. A community health nurse assessment at the individual level includes identifying the persons or groups most at risk, assessing the risk factors for substance abuse, and assessing for signs and symptoms of substance abuse such as intoxication, withdrawal, and long-term effects.

POWERPOINT LECTURE SLIDES

NOTE: The number on each PPT Lecture Slide directly corresponds with the Concepts for Lecture.

1 Community Assessment
- WHO rapid assessment and response (RAR) guidelines
- Increases timely response capabilities in dealing with health issues
  - Nature/extent of problem
  - Adverse health/social consequences
  - Protective factors
  - Intervention proposals

2 Individual Assessment
- Identify persons/groups at risk
- Assess risk factors for substance abuse
- Assess for signs of substance abuse
  - Intoxication
  - Withdrawal
  - Long-term effects

SUGGESTIONS FOR CLASSROOM ACTIVITIES

Provide students with 3×5 cards. Ask each student to write down individuals and groups at risk in the immediate community. Have students identify protective factors for nonrisk groups or individuals. Collect the cards and write down the results on the board.

SUGGESTIONS FOR CLINICAL ACTIVITIES

Have students complete a community health nursing assessment of their clinical agency and its targeted population.

Learning Objective 7

Identify major approaches to primary prevention of substance abuse and analyze the role of the community health nurse with respect teach.

CONCEPTS FOR LECTURE

1. Primary prevention goals for substance abuse include preventing nonusers from initiating use of psychoactive substances, preventing progression from experimentation to chronic use, and preventing expansion to the use of other substances.

2. Primary prevention methods use education and risk factor modification as the basis for their focus on substance abuse reduction or minimization. Education begins with the public and is best if community health nurses target specific groups, such as developing school-based education campaigns. Addressing knowledge and attitudes about the use of psychoactive substances is part of the community health nurse's role. Risk factor modification can occur at all three levels: individual, family, or society. Nurses can evaluate an individual's stress level, or assist families

POWERPOINT LECTURE SLIDES

NOTE: The number on each PPT Lecture Slide directly corresponds with the Concepts for Lecture.

1 Primary Prevention Goals
- Prevent nonusers from initiating use
- Prevent progression from experimentation to chronic use
- Prevent expansion to use of other substances

2 Primary Prevention Methods
- Education
- Risk factor modification

3 Nurse's Role
- Individual level
  - Refer to social services
  - Refer for respite care

with stress to eliminate or modify the source of stressors, or assist with developing effective coping skills.

3. Nurses can refer clients and families experiencing financial stress to social services or to other needed services, such as respite care. By reducing sources of stress or modifying their reactions to stressors, individuals or families may reduce their risk for self-medication through psychoactive substances. At the societal level, nurses may become politically involved to advocate for control or limited access and availability of psychoactive substances.

- Societal level
  - Advocate for control of or limited access to psychoactive substances

---

SUGGESTIONS FOR CLASSROOM ACTIVITIES

Have students select a target population to address substance abuse prevention and education measures. Have students select one primary goal. Have students develop a nursing care plan for their target audience that outlines an educational strategy and a risk factor modification strategy.

SUGGESTIONS FOR CLINICAL ACTIVITIES

1. Arrange for students to work with a health educator, a community health nurse, or a school nurse. Ask students to identify an at-risk population, develop a primary prevention goal, select one method, and prepare a written care plan for substance abuse prevention.
2. Have students work with a school nurse to develop a health education lesson plan for an age-specific group of students.

LEARNING OBJECTIVE 8

Describe the components of the intervention process in secondary prevention of substance abuse.

CONCEPTS FOR LECTURE

1. Secondary prevention incorporates screening, intervention, and treatment for psychoactive substance use. Intervention is the act of confronting the substance abuser with the intent of making a referral for assistance in dealing with the abuse. The goal is to elicit an agreement from the individual to be evaluated for possible substance abuse problems.
2. The community health nurse aids in the intervention process by aiding families to view themselves as clients, reinforcing the idea that substance abuse is a family disorder, and providing families with basic information about substance abuse and the defense mechanisms used by both the abuser and significant others, which may result in a co-dependent or enabling relationship. Nurses educate families about the intervention process, their responsibilities for the process, and some of the feelings that they may experience during the intervention.
3. Nurses prepare families for the intervention process by assisting them to determine who should be involved, who may be able to influence the abuser's behavior in a positive way, and those who are able to engage in the intervention.
4. The intervention process continues with bringing the individual to an agreed upon site, and if the individual agrees to evaluation, the nurse encourages the family

POWERPOINT LECTURE SLIDES

NOTE: The number on each PPT Lecture Slide directly corresponds with the Concepts for Lecture.

1 Secondary Prevention
- Intervention
  - Confront the substance abuser with the intent of making a referral for assistance in dealing with the abuse
- Goal
  - Elicit an agreement from the individual to be evaluated for possible abuse problems
  - Facilitate intervention process
    - Assist family members in planning responses

2 Role of Community Health Nurse
- Aid families to view themselves as clients
- Reinforce the idea that substance abuse is a family disorder
- Provide families with basic information about substance abuse and defense mechanisms used by both the abuser and significant others, which may result in a co-dependent or enabling relationship

2a Role of Community Health Nurse (continued)
- Educate families about the intervention process
  - Family responsibilities for the process

CONCEPTS FOR LECTURE *continued*

to accompany the individual to the evaluation appointment. The nurse may meet with family members to discuss feelings about the process and its outcome. If the intervention is not successful, the nurse reassures the family members and aids them in planning a subsequent intervention.

POWERPOINT LECTURE SLIDES *continued*

○ Feelings that they may experience during the intervention

3. Intervention Process: Family Role
   - Assist family to determine who should be involved
   - Who may be able to influence the abuser's behavior in a positive way
   - Those who are able to engage in the intervention

4. Intervention Process
   - Client agrees to intervention
     ○ Bring the individual to an agreed upon site
     ○ Encourage family to accompany the individual to the evaluation appointment
     ○ Meet with family members to discuss feelings about the process and its outcome
   - Client does not agree to intervention
     ○ Reassure family members and aid them in planning a subsequent intervention

---

SUGGESTIONS FOR CLASSROOM ACTIVITIES

Have students research different treatment modalities and assess available treatment options in the community. Provide case scenarios for students to develop a nursing care plan based on available screening and treatment services in the community.

SUGGESTIONS FOR CLINICAL ACTIVITIES

Invite a treatment facility provider, social worker, substance abuse counselor, or community health nurse to post conference to discuss treatment options for substance abusers in the community.

LEARNING OBJECTIVE 9

Identify general principles in the treatment of substance abuse.

CONCEPTS FOR LECTURE

1. Treatment for substance abuse must be tailored to the specific drug or substance abuse, but there are general principles that guide the various treatment modalities. There should be multi-treatment modalities that are individually tailored, using both professionals and laypersons. The families should be involved, and there should also be a detoxification or sobriety component built in to the program.

2. Additionally, treatment should address the underlying psychopathology and anticipate the guilt that arises when an individual relapses. There should also be social and vocational rehabilitation services to aid the individual in returning to the community and finding employment. Treatment should be available for other unforeseen consequences, such as health conditions that arise from the use of the psychoactive substance.

POWERPOINT LECTURE SLIDES

NOTE: The number on each PPT Lecture Slide directly corresponds with the Concepts for Lecture.

1. General Principles in Treatment
   - Multi-treatment modalities
   - Individually tailored
   - Use of professional and laypersons
   - Involvement of family
   - Detoxification/sobriety

2. General Principles in Treatment (continued)
   - Treat underlying psychopathology
   - Address guilt with relapses
   - Social/vocational rehabilitation
   - Treatment for other consequences

LEARNING OBJECTIVE 10

Describe treatment modalities in substance abuse control and analyze the role of the community health nurse in their implementation.

CONCEPTS FOR LECTURE

1. The three treatment modalities include biological methods such as medications and physiologically based therapies; psychosocial methods such as individual, group, or family therapy, behavior modification, contracting, or aversion or relaxation therapies; and sociotherapies such as therapeutic communities, residential programs, self-help therapies, and mutual-help groups. Medications such as Valium or Librium may be used to treat the physical symptoms of withdrawal. Methadone may be used for long-term treatment of opioid addictions.

2. The community health nurse makes referrals to clients for medical management of substance abuse. The nurse may also monitor treatment compliance, provide long-term medication in maintenance programs, or advocate for availability of services.

POWERPOINT LECTURE SLIDES

NOTE: The number on each PPT Lecture Slide directly corresponds with the Concepts for Lecture.

1 Treatment Modalities
- Biological methods
  - Medications
  - Physiologically based therapies

1a Treatment Modalities (continued)
- Psychosocial methods
  - Individual/group/family therapy
  - Behavior modification
  - Contracting
  - Aversion or relaxation therapies

1b Treatment Modalities (continued)
- Sociotherapies
  - Therapeutic communities
  - Residential programs
  - Self-help therapies
    – Publications/educational materials
  - Mutual-help groups
    – Individuals with same substance abuse problems

2 Role of Community Health Nurse
- Refer for medical management
- Monitor treatment compliance
- Administer long-term medications
- Advocate for available services

LEARNING OBJECTIVE 11

Analyze the role of the community health nurse in tertiary prevention of substance abuse.

CONCEPTS FOR LECTURE

1. The community health nurse may be tasked with identifying cases of substance abuse and making referrals for individual and families. The nurse must be educated in the signs and symptoms of drug abuse. Once identified, the nurse may monitor the use of medications during the withdrawal period, make appropriate referrals for psychosocial therapy, and be asked to reinforce contracts made with individuals in substance abuse treatment programs.

2. The community health nurse, as an advocate, may initiate support groups or energize community members and professionals to initiate support groups. The nurse may need to become politically active in support of the development of treatment programs and for insurance coverage for treatment.

POWERPOINT LECTURE SLIDES

NOTE: The number on each PPT Lecture Slide directly corresponds with the Concepts for Lecture.

1. Role of Community Health Nurse in Tertiary Prevention
   - Identify cases
   - Referral of individuals and families
   - Education for signs and symptoms
   - Monitor use of medications during withdrawal
   - Psychosocial therapy referral
   - Contract reinforcement

2. Role of Community Health Nurse
   - Initiation of support groups
   - Political activism to support development of treatment programs
   - Political activity and advocacy for insurance coverage for treatment

SUGGESTIONS FOR CLASSROOM ACTIVITIES

Have students prepare and give a 5-minute speech that identifies a community substance abuse problem or concern. Students are to role-play as community health nurses who will be speaking before a community forum or town hall meeting requesting the need for a substance abuse support group. They may select any commonly abused substance and an at-risk group.

SUGGESTIONS FOR CLINICAL ACTIVITIES

Have students attend an AA or other mutual help group meeting to identify strategies for tertiary prevention of substance abuse.

LEARNING OBJECTIVE 12

Discuss harm reduction and its role in control of substance abuse.

CONCEPTS FOR LECTURE

1. Harm reduction is an alternative approach to the control of substance abuse. With the traditional approach to substance abuse being the reduction of actual drug use, harm reduction focuses on moderation of substance use and minimization of its harmful effects. Examples of harm reduction might include a needle exchange program, a methadone program, availability of syringe filters, initiation of outpatient wound clinics for injection abscesses, and wound care programs at needle exchange sites.

POWERPOINT LECTURE SLIDES

NOTE: The number on each PPT Lecture Slide directly corresponds with the Concepts for Lecture.

1. Harm Reduction
   - Moderation of substance use
   - Minimization of harmful effects of substance use
   - Change in approach to problem

SUGGESTIONS FOR CLASSROOM ACTIVITIES

Have students research literature for articles on harm reduction strategies and outcomes. Ask students to present a summary of their article and make recommendations for the local community.

SUGGESTIONS FOR CLINICAL ACTIVITIES

1. Invite a volunteer agency counselor who works with a needle exchange program or other harm reduction programs in the community to discuss the goals of the program, the barriers to success, and funding.
2. Have students identify types of harm reduction programs available in the local area.

32

CHAPTER

Societal Violence

RESOURCE LIBRARY

 COMPANION WEBSITE

Audio Glossary
Exam Review Questions
Case Study: Violence and Teenagers
MediaLink Application: Raising Awareness of
  Domestic Abuse (video)

Media Links
Challenge Your Knowledge
Update *Healthy People 2010*
Advocacy Interviews

LEARNING OBJECTIVE 1

Compare types of societal violence.

CONCEPTS FOR LECTURE

1. Societal violence costs millions of dollars in hospital care and millions of days of lost work productivity. Even though reports of societal violence are increasing, actual violent crime rates are decreasing in the United States. Violence is defined as the intentional use of physical force or power, threatened or actual, against oneself, another person, or a group or community that either results in or has a high likelihood of resulting in injury, death, psychological harm, maldevelopment, or deprivation.

2. Types of societal violence include family violence, assault and homicide, and suicide.

3. Family violence encompasses child and elder maltreatment and intimate partner violence. Child maltreatment involves intentional physical or mental harm to a child by someone responsible for the child's welfare. Types of child abuse include physical abuse, emotional abuse, sexual abuse, and neglect, which is the failure to provide for a child's physical, educational, or emotional needs. Intimate partner violence (IPV) refers to any behavior within an intimate relationship that causes physical, psychological, or sexual harm to those in the relationship. Battering is considered a form of intimate partner violence and is defined as chronic and continuing violence of one partner against another that is characterized by vulnerability, entrapment, and loss of control of one's life on the part of the abused partner. Psychological battering exists when there is no current physical or sexual abuse perpetrated, but fear of potential abuse

POWERPOINT LECTURE SLIDES

NOTE: The number on each PPT Lecture Slide directly corresponds with the Concepts for Lecture.

1 Societal Violence
- Definition
- Trends

2 Types of Societal Violence
- Family violence
- Assault and homicide
- Suicide

3 Family Violence
- Child maltreatment
  - Physical abuse
  - Emotional abuse
  - Sexual abuse
  - Neglect

3a Family Violence (continued)
- Elder maltreatment
  - Types of abuse
- Intimate partner violence
  - Battering
    - Psychological battering

4 Assault and Homicide
- Populations at risk
- School-related fatalities

5 Suicide
- Incidence and prevalence
- Societal impact

keeps the victim subservient. Elder maltreatment is purposeful physical or psychological harm or exploitation of elderly persons occurring within families or in institutional settings. Nearly 700,000 to 1.2 million older adults are abused each year in the United States. Different types of abuse may be encountered by community health nurses, including physical and sexual abuse, neglect, emotional abuse, financial or material exploitation, violation of personal rights, and abandonment.

4. Even with homicide rates declining, 1.6 million people were treated for assault-related injuries in emergency departments. Nearly 64,000 of these were sexual assaults. Assaults and homicides affect all societies. Schools are becoming settings for increased violence, especially involving weapons.

5. Suicide affects the United States with approximately 4.5% of Americans attempting suicide at some point in their lives. Suicide is the third leading cause of death for men ages 15 to 24, and the eighth leading cause for all U.S. men, resulting in great monetary costs to society.

SUGGESTIONS FOR CLASSROOM ACTIVITIES

1. Assign students to small groups: child abuse, elder abuse, IPV, and suicide. Have students locate information or data on local, regional, and state violence statistics. Provide suggestions for data sources: Internet, health department publications, local law enforcement data, and Web sites that document a community's features.

2. Have students collect newspaper reports of societal violence and determine the extent of the focus on different types of violence in the news media.

SUGGESTIONS FOR CLINICAL ACTIVITIES

Invite law enforcement officers to post conference to discuss the types and incidence of violent crimes, domestic violence, homicides, and suicides in the community.

LEARNING OBJECTIVE 2

Analyze the influence of biophysical, psychological, physical environmental, sociocultural, behavioral, and health system factors on societal violence.

CONCEPTS FOR LECTURE

1. Biophysical considerations are factors that contribute to violence and those that arise as a consequence of violence. Age and physiologic status affect susceptibility to violence as evidenced by shaken baby syndrome and pregnancy increasing a woman's vulnerability to IPV. Suicide rates vary according to age and methods used. Children experiencing maltreatment are more prone to physical and functional disabilities and hospitalizations. Racial and ethnic disparities occur in particular forms of societal violence as well as in varying socioeconomic groups.

2. Psychological considerations for family violence include poor coping skills, the emotional climate of

POWERPOINT LECTURE SLIDES

NOTE: The number on each PPT Lecture Slide directly corresponds with the Concepts for Lecture.

1 Biophysical Considerations
- Age and physiologic status
  - Shaken baby syndrome
  - Pregnancy
  - Age and suicide rate differences
  - Age and methods of suicide

1a Biophysical Considerations (continued)
- Gender
  - Child maltreatment
  - Rate differences in gender

the family, personality traits of the abuser or the victim, and presence of psychopathy, which increases a family's susceptibility to violence.

3. Physical environmental considerations note that rural regions are more prone to certain types of violence, possibly due to the effects of isolation, and urban settings have violence that involves forearms, suggestive of accessibility and means of committing crimes involving guns. Workplace violence has been acknowledged as another setting to consider.

4. Sociocultural factors that the community health nurse needs to consider in assessing an individual, family, or community's predisposition to violence are cultural themes; norms that grant financial and physical control of women to men or personal beliefs in strict gender roles; immigrant status for women that because of language barriers, they may not report abuse; and cultural attitudes. Family risk factors include social isolation; parental lack of understanding of child development, which can result in poor discipline judgment; family disorganization; and lack of family cohesion. Other sociocultural factors such as low income, limited resource availability, and social isolation may increase stress and result in violence.

5. Behavioral factors address the relationship between alcohol or drug abuse and IPV, smoking and a risk of suicide, sexual orientation and vulnerability to physical or sexual abuse, workplace homicides and the interrelationship between certain behavioral factors and violence.

6. Health system factors contribute indirectly to violence through providers' hesitancy to report findings or identify clients at risk for suicide, or their lack of understanding between chronic physical illness and suicide and the need for more effective disease management.

- Ethnicity
  - Disparities among groups

 Psychological Considerations
- Family violence
  - Poor coping skills
  - Emotional climate of family
  - Personality traits of abuser or victim
  - Presence of psychopathy

 Physical Environmental Considerations
- Rural regions
  - Isolation
- Urban settings
  - Access to firearms
- Workplace

 Sociocultural Considerations
- Cultural themes
- Norms
- Immigrant status
- Cultural attitudes
- Low income/limited resource availability
- Social isolation

Sociocultural Considerations (continued)
- Family risk factors
  - Social isolation
  - Parental lack of understanding of child development
  - Family disorganization
  - Lack of family cohesion

 Behavioral Considerations
- Alcohol abuse
- Smoking
- Sexual orientation
  - Physical or sexual abuse
- Workplace homicides
- Causal effects of all factors

 Health Care System Considerations
- Providers hesitant to report findings
- Providers failing to identify clients at risk for suicide
  - Relationship between physical illness and suicide
    - Need for better disease management

SUGGESTIONS FOR CLASSROOM ACTIVITIES

Assign small groups to research information about contributing factors in shaken baby syndrome, teen and adult suicide, and elder abuse. Have students present their findings in class by addressing the six dimensions of health.

SUGGESTIONS FOR CLINICAL ACTIVITIES

Invite a pediatrician, social worker, community health nurse, and emergency room nurse to post conference to discuss shaken baby syndrome, incidence, signs and symptoms, and other pertinent social data.

Learning Objective 3

Identify major foci in primary prevention of societal violence.

Concepts for Lecture

1. Primary prevention focuses on three major approaches: increasing personal aversion to violence as a means of resolving conflict, increasing personal abilities to deal with stress, and eliminating or reducing factors that contribute to stress.

2. Eleven primary prevention goals have been identified with respective nursing interventions at both the individual/family and the community level. At the very basic, individual level, the first goals address the development of effective coping skills, the development of self-esteem, the development of realistic expectation of self and others, and the development of effective parenting and interpersonal skills. The next level of goals affects individuals, families and communities through availability of treatment facilities for psychopathology or substance abuse, promotion of nonviolent conflict resolution, providing emotional and material support, and encouraging the reduction of risk behaviors. Finally, primary prevention goals address the broader need for decreased availability of weapons, drugs, and alcohol, changing societal attitudes toward violence, and developing policies that discourage violence.

PowerPoint Lecture Slides

NOTE: The number on each PPT Lecture Slide directly corresponds with the Concepts for Lecture.

1 Primary Prevention
- Increasing personal aversion to violence
  - School-based suicide prevention programs
  - Teaching alternative methods of conflict resolution
- Increasing personal abilities to deal with stress
  - Imposing cultural and social sanctions against violence

1a Primary Prevention (continued)
- Eliminating or reducing factors that contribute to stress
  - Identify needs for special support services
    - Respite care
    - Crisis intervention and hotlines

2 Goals of Primary Prevention
- Develop effective coping skills
- Develop self-esteem
- Develop realistic expectation of self and others
- Develop effective parenting and interpersonal skills

2a Goals of Primary Prevention (continued)
- Treatment of psychopathology or substance abuse
- Promotion of nonviolent conflict resolution
- Provision of emotional and material support
- Reduction of risk behaviors

2b Goals of Primary Prevention (continued)
- Decrease availability of weapons, drugs, and alcohol
- Change in societal attitudes toward violence
- Develop policies that discourage violence

Suggestions for Classroom Activities

Assign small groups with case studies that depict teen depression rates at a local high school, a family with an older parent with Alzheimer's, and a pregnant woman with unexplained bruises. Ask groups to identify risk factors and develop a nursing care plan for their case study.

Suggestions for Clinical Activities

Invite a community health nurse and a school nurse to discuss nursing interventions for teen suicide prevention in local schools. Ask them to discuss community resources and support networks.

LEARNING OBJECTIVE 4

Describe approaches to the secondary prevention of societal violence.

CONCEPTS FOR LECTURE

1. Secondary prevention approaches address the identification of persons at risk for violence through case finding and education of the public about contributing factors.
2. Secondary prevention includes a provision of counseling for persons at risk and for treatment for victims of violence through referral services, advocating for the availability of counseling services and engaging in political activity and advocacy to ensure adequate treatment facilities.
3. Lastly, secondary prevention measures focus on the need to identify episodes of violence, making provisions for safe environments, and providing treatment for violent persons.

POWERPOINT LECTURE SLIDES

NOTE: The number on each PPT Lecture Slide directly corresponds with the Concepts for Lecture.

1. Secondary Prevention: Education and Screening
   - Identify persons at risk for violence
     ○ Case finding
     ○ Education of the public about contributing factors

2. Secondary Prevention: Counseling and Treatment
   - Provide counseling for persons at risk
   - Provide treatment for victims of violence through referral services
   - Advocate for the availability of counseling services
   - Engage in political activity and advocacy to ensure adequate treatment facilities

3. Secondary Prevention Measures: Identification of Violence
   - Identify episodes of violence
   - Make provisions for safe environments
   - Provide treatment for violent persons

SUGGESTIONS FOR CLASSROOM ACTIVITIES

Have students interview various health professionals who may come into contact with victims of domestic violence and inquire about screening protocols, referral processes, and availability of safe environments for victims and treatment facilities for violent persons. Report the results of the interview during a subsequent class.

SUGGESTIONS FOR CLINICAL ACTIVITIES

Ask students to develop a care plan for a client that addresses secondary nursing intervention strategies for violence. Provide an opportunity to discuss at post conference.

LEARNING OBJECTIVE 5

Discuss considerations in tertiary prevention of societal violence.

CONCEPTS FOR LECTURE

1. Tertiary prevention of societal violence addresses four major foci. The first involves the prevention of suicide clusters and copycat murders. Nursing interventions at the community level focus on assisting in the development of community response plans and advocating for control of media exposure to violence.
2. The second addresses a need for providing care to families of homicide and suicide victims. The community health nurse may assist family members to work through feelings of grief and guilt, or to help families find positive ways to cope with loss. The nurse may refer for assistance with legal matters or for counseling.

POWERPOINT LECTURE SLIDES

NOTE: The number on each PPT Lecture Slide directly corresponds with the Concepts for Lecture.

1. Tertiary Prevention: First Focus
   - Prevent suicide clusters and copycat murders
     ○ Assist in the development of community response plans
     ○ Advocate for control of media exposure to violence

2. Tertiary Prevention: Second Focus
   - Provide care to families of homicide and suicide victims

CONCEPTS FOR LECTURE *continued*

There is also a need to advocate for support services for families of victims.

3. The third focus considers the need to treat the consequences of violence through referral for physical and psychological treatment services and advocacy for available services for victims and perpetrators of violence.

4. The fourth focuses on reducing sources of stress through referral, respite care services, expansion of social support networks, and assistance with employment and other social needs. Community health nurses may refer to sources of assistance, develop or expand social support networks, arrange for respite care, or assist with employment and other social needs. At the community level, the nurse may advocate for social changes to minimize sources of stress that contribute to violence or for the need for additional respite care and support services.

POWERPOINT LECTURE SLIDES *continued*

- ○ Assist family members to work through feelings of grief
- ○ Assist families to find positive ways to cope with loss
- ○ Refer for assistance with legal needs
- ○ Refer for counseling
- ○ Advocate for support services for families of victims

3 Tertiary Prevention: Third Focus
- Treat the consequences of violence
  - ○ Refer for physical and psychological treatment services
  - ○ Advocate for available services for victims and perpetrators of violence

4 Tertiary Prevention: Fourth Focus
- Reduce sources of stress
  - ○ Refer to sources of assistance
  - ○ Develop or expand social support networks
  - ○ Arrange for respite care
  - ○ Assist with employment and other social needs
  - ○ Advocate for social changes to minimize sources of stress

SUGGESTIONS FOR CLASSROOM ACTIVITIES

Provide case study scenarios for students to develop tertiary intervention strategies in class.

SUGGESTIONS FOR CLINICAL ACTIVITIES

Arrange for students to observe at a local shelter for battered victims, and other sites, if appropriate, that provide services to families dealing with stressors. Ask students to identify tertiary prevention strategies that may or may not be addressed at the clinical agency.

LEARNING OBJECTIVE 6

Analyze the role of community health nurses with respect to societal violence.

CONCEPTS FOR LECTURE

1. Community health nurses need to have an active role in responding to societal violence by being involved in assessing risk factors, using diagnostic reasoning, and planning and implementing interventions to control the problem.

2. Before interventions can be implemented, community health nurses must assess the community to identify risk factors at the individual, family, or population level by using the six dimensions of health and anticipate situations that may be precursors to violence, such as unemployment or causes of social stress.

3. Diagnostic reasoning results from the community assessment data that identifies increased potentials for violence due to identified risk factors, behaviors, or attitudes.

4. Planning and implementing interventions include the primary, secondary, and tertiary interventions used by community health nurses working with individuals, families, or communities.

POWERPOINT LECTURE SLIDES

NOTE: The number on each PPT Lecture Slide directly corresponds with the Concepts for Lecture.

1 Role of Community Health Nurse
- Active role
- Assess risk factors
- Nursing diagnoses
- Plan/implement interventions

2 Assessment
- Assess community to identify risk factor
  - ○ Use six dimensions of health
- Anticipate situational precursors to violence
  - ○ Unemployment
  - ○ Causes of social stress

3 Nursing Diagnoses
- Assessment data
  - ○ Identify increased potentials for violence
    - Risk factors

POWERPOINT LECTURE SLIDES *continued*
  – Behaviors
  – Attitudes
 Plan/Implement Interventions
  • Primary
  • Secondary
  • Tertiary

SUGGESTIONS FOR CLASSROOM ACTIVITIES

Assign students a case study and ask them to develop three nursing diagnoses and nursing interventions at each of the three prevention levels that address individual, family, and community violence.

SUGGESTIONS FOR CLINICAL ACTIVITIES

Have students develop a nursing diagnosis and nursing interventions at each of the three intervention levels for one of their community experiences that identifies potential areas for violence, such as bullying in schools, or suicide.

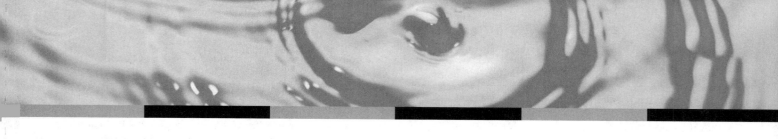

TEST BANK

CHAPTER 1

1.1 The nurse is designing a program for pregnant adolescents in the community. The program will focus on fetal development, appropriate nutrition, developing social support systems, and screening for potential abuse by partners or others. This is an example of: 1. Community based nursing. 2. Community focused care. 3. Community health nursing. 4. Community driven care.	Answer: 3 Rationale: Community health nursing is the practice of promoting and protecting the health of populations using knowledge from nursing, social, and public health sciences. The community will benefit from the program because the adolescents will be healthier and deliver healthier infants, thus saving on health care costs. Community based nursing is nurses providing sick care in community settings. Community focused care is bringing nursing knowledge and expertise to the community, but it does not have a population focus. Community driven care focuses on the needs of the community as a whole and emphasizes community participation in determining those needs. It can limit the focus of practice to health needs identified by the population group, and could thus exclude pregnant adolescents. Step in the Nursing Process: Planning Category of Client Need: Health Promotion and Maintenance Cognitive Level: Application Learning Objective 1-1: Define community health nursing. Test Taking Tip: Review the answer choices and choose that answer which is the least limiting.
1.2 The nurse meets with members of the community in open forums to help determine ways to improve health. The nurse identifies health problems in the community based on the community input and personal community assessment. In this situation, the nurse is practicing: 1. Community focused care. 2. Public health nursing. 3. Community oriented care. 4. Community driven care.	Answer: 1 Rationale: Community focused care brings nursing knowledge and expertise to the community, but may not have a population focus. Public health nursing has a perceived focus of environmental sanitation and controlling communicable diseases. Community driven care focuses on the needs of the community as a whole, but can be limited to only addressing needs identified by community members. Community oriented care is limiting, focusing program development on small aggregates while potentially ignoring health issues affecting larger population groups. Step in Nursing Process: Planning Category of Client Need: Health Promotion and Maintenance Cognitive Level: Application Learning Objective 1-2: Distinguish among community based, community focused, and community driven nursing. Test Taking Tip: Understand the focus of community oriented, public health, community focused, and community driven nursing.
1.3 The nurse holds community forums to gain input in determining health needs for the community. The community input discusses nutrition education, but the nurse notices that many community members are outside smoking before entering the building. The nurse acknowledges the importance of nutrition education, but addresses the community about also incorporating smoking cessation education as part of a total lifestyle choice program. The nurse is practicing: 1. Population focused nursing. 2. Community focused nursing.	Answer: 4 Rationale: The nurse gained input from the community as to their concerns, but also noted that a health concern was smoking. Part of community driven nursing is raising community awareness so community members can acknowledge health needs that were previously ignored. Population focused nursing addresses care toward overall communities and groups, but does not indicate community involvement in this process. Community focused nursing is directed to sick care in community settings. Public health nursing is indicative of governmental or official agency oversight and jurisdiction with a focus on control of communicable diseases and environmental sanitation. Step in Nursing Process: Assessment Category of Client Need: Health Promotion and Maintenance Cognitive Level: Application Learning Objective 1-2: Distinguish among community based, community focused, and community driven nursing and describe their relationship to community health nursing.

3. Public health nursing. 4. Community driven nursing.	Test Taking Tip: Understand community based, community focused, and community driven nursing.
1.4 Following a natural disaster in a community, the community nurse focuses the care given on addressing the mental health needs and assessing stress levels in a community. This is: 1. Public health nursing. 2. Program-focused nursing. 3. Community oriented nursing. 4. Community advocacy.	Answer: 2 Rationale: Program-focused nursing includes activities and efforts that target specifically designated health problems or specific target populations. Public health nursing has its emphasis on environmental aspects and communicable disease. Community oriented nursing can be limiting in that it focuses on program development for small aggregates while potentially ignoring health issues affecting larger groups. Community advocacy is an action taken on behalf of individuals, families, or populations to create or support an environment that promotes health. Advocacy implies arguing on someone else's behalf. Step in Nursing Process: Assessment Category of Client Need: Psychosocial Integrity Cognitive Level: Application Learning Objective1-3: Differentiate between district and program-focused community health nursing. Test Taking Tip: Understand the difference between district and program-focused community health nursing.
1.5 The nurse has developed several programs to address health needs in the community that encompass the lifespan. In addition, the nurse makes regular visits to residents in the community who need additional nursing care. The nurse is practicing: 1. Program-focused nursing. 2. Community oriented nursing. 3. District nursing. 4. Public health nursing.	Answer: 3 Rationale: In district nursing, the community health nurse is responsible for addressing all the health needs of a given population. In district nursing, the nurse also addresses needs of specific individuals, as well as the community as a whole. Program-focused nursing targets a specific health problem or a specific population. Community oriented nursing focuses on program development for small aggregates rather than the community as a whole. Public health nursing emphasizes environmental aspects of a community's health and control of communicable disease. Step in Nursing Process: Implementation Category of Client Need: Health Promotion and Maintenance Cognitive Level: Application Learning Objective1-3: Differentiate between district and program-focused community health nursing. Test Taking Tip: Recognize that the program encompasses several programs over the lifespan, and how this differentiates from program-focused.
1.6 The nurse works with the local recreation department and police department to implement a night basketball program during the summer for adolescents in the community. The goals of the program are to give adolescents an activity for exercise as well as minimize potential for risky behaviors among this population group. What are the attributes of community health nursing that the nurse is using? (Select all that apply) 1. Population consciousness. 2. Creativity. 3. Continuity. 4. Collaboration. 5. Orientation to health.	Answer:1, 2, 4, 5 Rationale: Community health nurses must have an awareness of what is occurring in the population and be aware of interactive factors that influence health and wellbeing. A midnight basketball program recognizes that during the summer, adolescents will have more time available and may not use it productively. A basketball program provides activity and an outlet for socialization within supervised parameters, thus potentially decreasing risky behaviors that could lead to lawbreaking. The nurse is being creative in helping to implement a program that will provide a healthy activity without it being perceived as something structured and "healthful." Collaboration has occurred among the nurse, recreation, and police departments to implement a program with benefits for all the partners concerned. It is an orientation to health with the emphasis being on health promotion rather than disease cure. Step in Nursing Process: Implementation Category of Client Need: Health Promotion and Maintenance Cognitive Level: Application Learning Objective 1-4: Identify at least five attributes of community health nursing. Test Taking Tip: Know the attributes of community health nursing.
1.7 The community health nurse assesses the community for potential health concerns. Based on personal observation and community input, the nurse creates nursing diagnoses for the community and plans programs	Answer: 4 Rationale: The ANA Public Health Nursing: Scope and Standards of Practice utilize the framework of the nursing process and core functions of public health to evaluate the quality of community health nursing care in the practice setting. The Quad Council competencies delineate nursing practice at two levels and do not address standards. The nurse generalist level of practice is one of the levels identified by the Quad

for implementation that address these health concerns. Included in these programs is a method that evaluates outcomes. What method is the nurse utilizing?
1. Quad Council health competencies.
2. Nurse generalist level of practice.
3. Council of Linkages competencies.
4. ANA Public Health Nursing: Scope and Standards of Practice.

Council. The Council of Linkages incorporates competencies of the skills, knowledge, and attitudes required for effective public health practice.
Step in Nursing Process: Planning
Category of Client Need: Health Promotion and Maintenance
Cognitive Level: Application
Learning Objective1-6: Summarize the standards for community health nursing practice.
Test Taking Tip: Recognize the standards of practice that would be used to evaluate quality of care.

1.8 The nurse is working with the local community to establish an immunization program, and is developing a tool to evaluate the quality of the planned nursing care. The tool that the nurse is developing to use in evaluating the quality of the planned nursing care should include standards of care for community health nursing practice. Therefore, the tool would reflect the standards of: (Select all that apply.)
1. Advocacy.
2. Research.
3. Collegiality.
4. Autonomy.
5. Leadership.

Answers: 1, 2, 3, 5
Rationale: The standards of care for community health nursing practice include advocacy, research, collegiality, education, and leadership.
Step in Nursing Process: Planning
Category of Client Need: Safe, Effective Care Environment
Cognitive Level: Application
Learning Objective1-6: Summarize the standards for community health nursing.
Test Taking Tip: Understand the standards for community health nursing.

1.9 The eight domains of competencies for community health nursing:
1. Reflect the practice of the experienced community health nurse at only the specialist level and include cultural competence.
2. Reflect the practice of the experienced community health nurse at the generalist level and exclude communication.
3. Include expectations, which range from awareness through knowledge to proficiency and include financial planning.
4. Must all be incorporated into any particular community health nursing position and include advanced public health practice.

Answer: 3
Rationale: The competencies reflect expectations ranging from awareness to proficiency and the competencies include financial planning. The competencies are developed for two levels of practice, one of which is the specialist, and the competencies include cultural competence. The competencies are developed for two levels of practice, one of which is the generalist, and the competencies include communication. Any community health nursing position may incorporate all or just some of the competencies, and advanced public health practice is not included (basic public health practice).
Step in Nursing Process: Planning
Category of Client Need: Safe, Effective Care Environment
Cognitive Level: Application
Learning Objective 1-7: Identify the eight domains of competency for community health nursing.
Test Taking Tip: Understand the differences between the eight domains of competency for community health nursing.

1.10 The community health nurse is helping the client identify alternative solutions. The best description of the primary focus of nursing and of the nurse's role in this situation is:
1. Client-oriented and educator.
2. Delivery-oriented and case manager.
3. Client-oriented and counselor.
4. Population-oriented and counselor.

Answer: 3
Rationale: This is an example of client oriented community health nursing and of a counselor role. The role of counselor includes helping the client identify alternative solutions. This is an example of a client-oriented focus but not of an educator role. The role of educator is to assess the need for education, develop the education plan, present health education, and evaluate outcome of the health education. This is not an example of a delivery-oriented focus, which are roles designed to enhance the operation of the health care delivery system itself; and the role of case manager does not include identification of alternative solutions. This is not an example of a population-oriented focus, which is directed toward promoting, maintaining and restoring the health of the population. The counselor role is not population oriented.

Step in Nursing Process: Implementation
Category of Client Need: Health Promotion and Maintenance
Cognitive Level: Analysis
Learning Objective 1-8: Distinguish among client-oriented, delivery-oriented, and population-oriented community health nursing roles.
Test Taking Tip: Understand the differences among client-oriented, delivery-oriented, and population-oriented community health nursing roles.

1.11 The community health nurse is demonstrating behavior to be learned by the client and the family. The best description of the primary focus of nursing care and of the nurse's role in this situation is:
1. Client-oriented and role model.
2. Delivery-oriented and educator.
3. Client-oriented and referral resource.
4. Population-oriented and collaborator.

Answer: 1
Rationale: The focus of nursing care in this situation is the client and the behavior is role modeling. Delivery-oriented nursing involves the operation or the health care delivery system, and role model is a better description of this behavior than educator. The focus of nursing care is the client but this is not a referral resource. Population-oriented care involves promotion, maintenance, and restoration of the population. The behavior that the nurse is demonstrating is not collaboration.
Step in Nursing Process: Implementation
Category of Client Need: Safe, Effective Care Environment
Cognitive Level: Analysis
Learning Objective 1-8: Distinguish among client-oriented, delivery-oriented, and population-oriented community health nursing roles.
Test Taking Tip: Know the differences among client-oriented, delivery-oriented, and population-oriented community health nursing roles.

1.12 The roles of the community health nurse are categorized based on the primary focus of nursing care. The difference between delivery-oriented roles as compared to the client-oriented and population-oriented roles is that delivery-oriented roles are:
1. More concerned with developing policies.
2. Designed to enhance operations of the health care delivery system.
3. More involved in provision of services than client- and population-oriented roles.
4. Focused on coalition building and researching.

Answer: 2
Rationale: The delivery-oriented roles are designed to enhance the operation of the health care delivery system. The population-oriented roles are concerned with developing policies. The client-oriented roles involve direct provision of services, moreso than the other two roles. Population-oriented roles include coalition building and researching.
Step in Nursing Process: Implementation
Category of Client Need: Safe, Effective Care Environment
Cognitive Level: Analysis
Learning Objective 1-8: Distinguish among client-oriented, delivery-oriented, and population-oriented community health nursing roles.
Test Taking Tip: Be able to distinguish the differences among client-oriented, delivery-oriented, and population-oriented community health nursing roles.

1.13 The best example of a client-oriented role would be the nurse who:
1. Determines the need for policy development.
2. Determines who is providing care to the client.
3. Assesses the client's health status.
4. Motivates followers to take action.

Answer: 3
Rationale: The caregiver (a client-oriented role) assesses client health status. The policy advocate role (population-oriented) determines the need for policy development. The coordinator role (delivery-oriented) determines who is providing care to the client. The change agent (population-oriented role) motivates followers to take action.
Step in Nursing Process: Implementation
Category of Client Need: Safe, Effective Care Environment
Cognitive Level: Application
Learning Objective 1-9: Describe at least five client-oriented roles performed by community health nurses.
Test Taking Tip: Know the client-oriented roles performed by community health nurses.

1.14 The best description of one of the delivery-oriented roles for the community health nurse working in a local clinic is:
1. Serving as initial point of contact between client and agency.
2. Planning nursing interventions.
3. Identifying the need for action.
4. Initiating and directing change.

Answer: 1
Rationale: The liaison role (delivery-oriented) is one of serving as the initial point of contact between the client and agency. The caregiver role (client-oriented) is one of planning nursing interventions. The leader (population-oriented) is one who identifies the need for action. The change agent (population-oriented) is one who initiates and directs change.
Step in Nursing Process: Implementation
Category of Client Need: Safe, Effective Care Environment
Cognitive Level: Analysis

1.15 Community health nurses are concerned with the health of the population. The best example of a nurse functioning in a population-oriented role is in:
1. Assessing the client's need for education.
2. Advocating for a mother who is being seen in a clinic.
3. Carrying out an investigation of specific cases of meningitis.
4. Developing an educational plan for a group of adolescents.

Answer: 3
Rationale: The case finder role is population-oriented. The role of educator is client-oriented. The role of liaison is delivery-oriented. The educator role is client-oriented.
Step in Nursing Process: Implementation
Category of Client Need: Safe, Effective Care Environment
Cognitive Level: Analysis
Learning Objective 1-11: Describe at least four population-oriented roles performed by community health nurses.
Test Taking Tip: Know the population-oriented roles performed by community health nurses.

CHAPTER 2

2.1 A school health program has been designed for elementary schools in a community. This type of care focuses on the:
1. Neighborhood.
2. Community.
3. Aggregate.
4. Population.

Answer: 3
Rationale: Aggregates are subpopulations within the larger population, possessing some characteristics, such as elementary school-age children. A neighborhood is a smaller homogeneous group with self-defined boundaries. Elementary schools are not considered neighborhoods. A community is a group of people with common interests who function collectively to address common concerns. The health program is specific to elementary school-age children. The program is designed for a specific subset of the population, not the entire population.
Step in Nursing Process: Implementation
Category of Client Need: Health Promotion and Maintenance
Cognitive Level: Analysis
Learning Objective 2-1: Distinguish among neighborhoods, communities, and aggregates as populations served by community health nurses.
Test Taking Tip: Differentiate between the levels of groups served by the community health nurse.

2.2 Community discussion has focused on the effect of diabetes on the population because a predominantly African American area of the city has recorded a higher incidence of diabetes. The focus of the community nurse's efforts should be on the:
1. Aggregate.
2. Neighborhood.
3. Population.
4. Community.

Answer: 2
Rationale: A neighborhood is part of a community and can be defined by heritage or ethnic background. This area of the city is a geographic area with boundaries as well as possessing a common cultural heritage. An aggregate is a subpopulation possessing some common characteristics but not defined by boundaries. Population is incorrect as this is the total community makeup and not just a specific area of the city that possesses the higher incidence. Community addresses the whole community. The problem is focused in one area of the community, not the entire community.
Step in Nursing Process: Implementation
Category of Client Need: Safe, Effective Care Environment
Cognitive Level: Analysis
Learning Objective 2-1: Distinguish among neighborhoods, communities, and aggregates as populations served by community health nurses.
Test Taking Tip: Know the differences in the definitions of communities, neighborhoods, and aggregates.

2.3 One of the highlights of the nurse's practice is participating as a health volunteer for an annual re-enactment of a Civil War battle. The population focus for the nurse in this situation is the:
1. Community.
2. Aggregate.

Answer: 1
Rationale: A community is a group that shares common interests and social interaction. Re-enactments of historical events are an expression of a community's interaction, heritage, and identity. An aggregate is a subpopulation of the community as a whole. A neighborhood is a specific area of a community with self-defined boundaries. Population refers to the entire area but does not necessarily indicate common identity, heritage, or interaction.

| | 3. Neighborhood.
4. Population. | Step in Nursing Process: Implementation
Category of Client Need: Health Promotion and Maintenance
Cognitive Level: Analysis
Learning Objective 2-1: Distinguish among neighborhoods, communities, and aggregates as populations served by community health nurses.
Test Taking Tip: Know the differences in definitions of communities, neighborhoods, and aggregates. |

2.4 The best definition of population health is where the population:
1. Has low rates of illness, and systems to address potential health problems.
2. Displays aggregated indicators of individual well-being.
3. Has a process to improve quality of life.
4. Is capable of attaining the best possible biologic, psychologic, and sociologic outcomes for its members.

Answer: 4
Rationale: The attainment of the greatest possible biologic, psychological, and social well-being of the population as an entity and its individual members is the best definition for population health. Low rate of illness and systems is a limited definition and describes a biomechanical model of health. Aggregated indicators is a holistic model that is more expanded, but focuses on conceptual factors that influence a positive state of health. Process is a dynamic model of health, a process that improves the quality of life.
Step in Nursing Process: Implementation
Category of Client Need: Health Promotion and Maintenance
Cognitive Level: Comprehension
Learning Objective 2-2: Define population health.
Test Taking Tip: Look for the most comprehensive set of indicators as an outcome for health.

2.5 The nurse wants to target care to improve the health status of the community and uses summary indicators of health as a method to measure health status. This approach is:
1. Holistic.
2. Descriptive.
3. Biomechanical.
4. Analytic.

Answer: 2
Rationale: The descriptive approach to population health uses a set of summary indicators to define health, where the distribution of health in the population is noted as its average level of health. Holistic approaches health utilizing multiple factors that influence a positive state of health, rather than concrete indicators that summarize health. The biomechanical approach focuses more on health problems rather than the overall health status. Analytic approaches health from a wider perspective in terms of factors influencing health and interventions to improve health status, not just what the health status is at the moment.
Step in Nursing Process: Assessment
Category of Client Need: Health Promotion and Maintenance
Cognitive Level: Analysis
Learning Objective 2-2: Define population health.
Test Taking Tip: Know the varying levels that address how population health is approached.

2.6 The nurse decides to use an analytic approach to address a community's health status. The analytic approach is best described as:
1. Utilizing health indicators to define population health.
2. Addressing the factors that influence health.
3. Focusing on the community's health problems.
4. Viewing factors that influence health which will direct interventions to improve health status.

Answer: 4
Rationale: The analytic approach is one that views population health in a broader perspective, addressing factors that influence health. This then directs interventions to improve health status. Utilizing health indicators is the descriptive approach for population health status. Addressing factors is the holistic model of addressing population health. Focusing on the community's health problems is the biomechanical model for population health.
Step in Nursing Process: Implementation
Category of Client Need: Safe, Effective Care Environment
Cognitive Level: Application
Learning Objective 2-2: Define population health.
Test Taking Tip: Recognize the different facets to the approaches for defining population health.

2.7 A community forum is held to brainstorm improving the community. The forum chairperson is the nurse, who acts as moderator. Many residents attend and offer suggestions. They identify strengths and weaknesses, and discuss how best to develop a plan of action. They reach a potential consensus on a plan. The forum

Answer: 1, 3, 5
Rationale: As a moderator, the nurse is fostering dialogue among the participants. By meeting, the residents are brought together by the vision of community. Needs and assets are assessed with strengths and weaknesses. The formation of a committee fosters the sense of responsibility and cohesion to continue the process.
Leadership could occur in the meeting, but there is no mention of collaboration and partnerships. There is no mention of diversity among the residents.
Step in Nursing Process: Planning
Category of Client Need: Health Promotion and Maintenance

decides to form a committee to further continue the momentum. Select the characteristics displayed by this forum that are indicative of healthy communities. (Select all that apply.)

1. Foster dialogue among residents to develop a shared vision for the community.
2. Promote community leadership that fosters collaboration and partnerships.
3. Engage in action based on a shared vision of the community.
4. Embrace diversity among residents.
5. Assess both needs and assets.

Cognitive Level: Application
Learning Objective 2-2: Define population health.
Test Taking Tip: Understand characteristics that are indicative of health communities that improve population health.

2.8 While community nurses have always advocated for their clients, the current emphasis for public health practice is:

1. Controlling epidemic diseases such as bird flu.
2. Preventing contagious diseases such as tuberculosis.
3. Improving global sanitation efforts.
4. Advocating for social justice.

Answer: 4
Rationale: Advocating for social justice has become the emphasis on current public health practice. The control of epidemics was the focus of early public health efforts. Disease prevention characterized public health efforts in the mid 1900s. Improving global sanitation efforts is not the current emphasis in public health practice.
Step in Nursing Process: Implementation
Category of Client Need: Safe, Effective Care Environment
Cognitive Level: Analysis
Learning Objective 2-3: Describe changes in approaches to population health.
Test Taking Tip: Distinguish between the eras of public health practice for their respective focus.

2.9 Approaches to population health have been characterized as "public health revolutions." Personal behavior change to promote individual and population health is considered the:

1. First revolution.
2. Second revolution.
3. Third revolution.
4. Fourth revolution.

Answer: 2
Rationale: The second revolution focused on personal behavior changes as a means to approach population health, which reflected the social norms of the time. The first revolution approached population health through sanitation efforts to control communicable diseases. The third revolution emphasizes health as one dimension of quality of life, with building healthy communities and workplaces to help strengthen social networks for health and improving people's capabilities for healthy lives. There is no fourth revolution.
Step in Nursing Process: Evaluation
Category of Client Need: Health Promotion and Maintenance
Cognitive Level: Analysis
Learning Objective 2-3: Describe changes in approaches to population health.
Test Taking Tip: Understand how social changes changed the approaches to public health and created the "revolutions."

2.10 An example of primary prevention is:

1. Advocating for legislation for outpatient mental health services.
2. Developing health programs for treating obesity.
3. Developing nutrition education programs for school-age populations.
4. Screening school-age populations for cholesterol.

Answer: 3
Rationale: Primary prevention is a level that promotes general optimal health or is an action taken prior to the occurrence of health problems or is directed at avoiding them. A nutrition education program for school-age populations promotes health and can educate to prevent future health problems related to inadequate nutrition. Advocating for legislation is an example of tertiary prevention. Developing health programs and screening populations are examples of secondary prevention.
Step in Nursing Process: Planning
Category of Client Need: Health Promotion and Maintenance
Cognitive Level: Application
Learning Objective 2-4: Describe the three levels at which population health occurs.
Test Taking Tip: Differentiate between the levels of prevention and where they are focused for care.

2.11 A secondary prevention activity is:

1. Having a client group participate in grocery shopping for healthy food choices.

Answer: 4
Rationale: Performing glucose screenings is an early identification for a health problem. Secondary prevention focuses on early identification of existing health problems and takes place after the problem occurs. Grocery shopping and

2. Immunizing a client group against hepatitis A.
3. Implementing an exercise program for outpatient stroke clients.
4. Performing glucose screenings for diabetes at a local mall.

immunizations are primary preventions, which are actions taken prior to an occurrence and directed toward their avoidance. Immunization protects against disease and shopping for healthy food choices is health protection. An exercise program for outpatient stroke clients is tertiary prevention.

Step in Nursing Process: Implementation
Category of Client Need: Health Promotion and Maintenance
Cognitive Level: Application
Learning Objective 2-4: Describe the three levels at which population health occurs.
Test Taking Tip: Differentiate between the levels of prevention and where they are focused for care.

2.12 A diabetes client group has successfully lowered their insulin needs through a combination of diet and exercise. The nurse designs an overall group diet plan for the group to follow. This is an example of:
1. Tertiary prevention.
2. Secondary prevention.
3. Primary prevention.
4. Health protection.

Answer: 1
Rationale: Tertiary prevention aims to return the client to optimal functioning and prevent further deterioration. A diet plan implemented after the problem has occurred to prevent further deterioration is tertiary prevention. Secondary prevention identifies and treats existing health problems to help resolve problems and prevent serious consequences. Primary prevention seeks to prevent health problems from occurring. Health protection involves specific activities that are taken to maintain health.

Step in Nursing Process: Evaluation
Category of Client Need: Health Promotion and Maintenance
Cognitive Level: Application
Learning Objective 2-4: Describe the three levels at which population health occurs.
Test Taking Tip: Differentiate between the levels of prevention and where they are focused for care.

2.13 The goal of initial population health objectives formulated by the Department of Health and Human Services (DHHS) in 1980 was to:
1. Identify determinants of health.
2. Eliminate health disparities among the population.
3. Reduce mortality.
4. Increase the span of healthy life.

Answer: 3
Rationale: Preventing mortality was the primary goal of the DHHS document *Promoting Health/Preventing Disease: Objectives for the Nation*. This document was published in 1980, with the target date of 1990. Determinants of health were not examined in the 1980 document. One of the goals of *Healthy People 2010* is to eliminate health disparities. One of the three goals of *Healthy People 2000* was to increase the span of healthy life.

Step in Nursing Process: Assessment
Category of Client Need: Health Promotion and Maintenance
Cognitive Level: Analysis
Learning Objective 2-5: Describe trends in national health objectives for 1990, 2000, and 2010.
Test Taking Tip: Understand how trends in national health objectives refined subsequent national health policies.

2.14 As population health objectives for the United States were refined with the United States Department of Health and Human Services (DHHS) national policies, objectives were based on a systematic approach to health. Select the two best goals that reflect the current DHHS population health objectives.
1. Increase the span of healthy life.
2. Increase the quality and length of healthy life.
3. Achieve access to preventive health services for all.
4. Eliminate health disparities.
5. Provide health insurance for all citizens.

Answer: 2, 4
Rationale: The most recent goals for the United States DHHS *Healthy People 2010* were to increase quality and length of life and eliminate health disparities. These goals have been updated and refined from *Healthy People 2000*. Improving quality of life versus reduced mortality is in the 1990 document. The goal of the 2000 document is to eliminate health disparities by 2010, rather than just reduce disparities. Among the three goals set for *Healthy People 2000* was to increase the span of healthy life and achieve access to preventive services for all. The most current policy from the DHHS aims to have a more systematic approach to achieving national population health objectives. This approach refined these goals into two more overarching goals for the *Healthy People 2010* document. The document does not address providing health insurance for all citizens.

Step in Nursing Process: Evaluation
Category of Client Need: Health Promotion and Maintenance
Cognitive Level: Application
Learning Objective 2-5: Describe trends in national health objectives for 1990, 2000, and 2010.
Test Taking Tip: Understand how trends in national health objectives refined subsequent national health policies.

2.15 The national health objective to improve the health status of the population is generally put on a timetable of:
1. Five years, so that appropriate revisions can be made.
2. Seven years, to allow for sufficient time to assess objective achievement.
3. Ten years, to fully assess the effectiveness of objective achievement.
4. Twelve years, to allow time to develop new objectives.

Answer: 3

Rationale: Ten years has been the hallmark for achieving the objectives of all the national health objective documents, including the 1980 *Promoting Health/Preventing Disease: Objectives for the Nation* document for 1990, the 1990 *Healthy People 2000* document, and the 2000 *Healthy People 2010* document. Five years is too soon to assess full achievement of the objectives, though a preliminary review would be done in that time. Seven years is not mentioned as a possibility for objective assessment. Twelve years is too long for developing new objectives.

Step in Nursing Process: Assessment

Category of Client Need: Health Promotion and Maintenance

Cognitive Level: Analysis

Learning Objective 2-5: Describe trends in national health objectives for 1990, 2000, and 2010.

Test Taking Tip: Understand how trends in national health objectives refined subsequent national health policies.

CHAPTER 3

3.1 The *Report of the Massachusetts Sanitary Commission* drafted by Lemuel Shattuck was notable for its recommendations. The most important effect of this document was:
1. Establishing workhouses for the sick poor.
2. Refuting that poverty was the result of deficiencies in moral character.
3. Mobilizing social reform to sanitary engineering.
4. Establishing state boards of health.

Answer: 4

Rationale: While Shattuck's report called for many far-reaching initiatives to monitor the public's health, the most far-reaching of the effects of the document was the establishments of local and state boards of health to monitor the health of the population. Until the late nineteenth century, it was held that poverty was the result of one's moral character. Workhouses for the poor had been in place since the late eighteenth century. Chadwick's *Inquiry into the Sanitary Conditions of the Labouring Population of Great Britain* shifted the view from social reform to sanitary engineering.

Step in the Nursing Process: Assessment

Category of Client Need: Health Promotion and Maintenance

Cognitive Level: Application

Learning Objective 3-1: Describe the contributions of historical figures who influenced the development of community health nursing.

Test Taking Tip: Differentiate among the various results of nineteenth century historical figures who addressed community health.

3.2 National health care systems were established as early as the 1860s in Europe. National health insurance for the United States was first proposed in the:
1. Mid-nineteenth century.
2. Early twentieth century.
3. Mid-twentieth century.
4. Late twentieth century.

Answer: 2

Rationale: National health insurance was proposed as early as 1912 as an element of Theodore Roosevelt's 1912 election platform. Germany initiated a national health program in the 1860s, as did Great Britain, though the latter was unsuccessful. While efforts to address national health insurance in the United States had been proposed in the mid- and late twentieth century, its earliest origin was at the turn of the century.

Step in the Nursing Process: Assessment

Category of Client Need: Health Promotion and Maintenance

Cognitive Level: Comprehension

Learning Objective 3-1: Describe the contributions of historical figures who influenced the development of community health nursing.

Test Taking Tip: Understand when national health insurance was first proposed in the United States.

3.3 Ancient civilizations understood the importance of clean water. The group most associated with developing systems to ensure water purity were the:
1. Romans.
2. Greeks.
3. Egyptians.
4. Aztecs.

Answer: 1

Rationale: Many ancient civilizations were known for some aspect of protecting their water supplies. The Romans were known for their engineering achievements in developing water purification systems, aqueducts, and other methods of keeping clean water pure and separate from contamination. Other civilizations developed some measures to protect their water supplies, but not quite to the extent of the Romans.

Step in the Nursing Process: Assessment

Category of Client Need: Health Promotion and Maintenance

Cognitive Level: Comprehension

Learning Objective 3-1: Describe the contributions of historical figures who influenced the development of community health nursing.

Test Taking Tip: Be aware of ancient civilizations' contributions to community health.

3.4 The first organized approach to home nursing of the sick was established in 1813 by the Ladies' Benevolent Society of Charleston, South Carolina in response to a yellow fever epidemic. An important aspect of the care provided by this organization was that it was:
1. Restricted to those who were able to pay for services.
2. Nondenominational and nondiscriminatory in an era of racial discrimination.
3. Directed to those residing in the Jewish community.
4. Restricted to women and children.

Answer: 2
Rationale: Though the care was given by upper class women to those who needed nursing care, the Ladies' Benevolent Society of Charleston was notable in that its services were nondenominational and nondiscriminatory in a region and time where racial discrimination was the prevailing behavior. Payment for services was not a hallmark of the Ladies' Benevolent Society. Services to the Jewish Community were organized in Philadelphia in 1819 by Rebecca Gratz. There were no restrictions to whom the Ladies' Benevolent Society nursed.
Step in the Nursing Process: Assessment
Category of Client Need: Health Promotion and Maintenance
Cognitive Level: Application
Learning Objective 3-2: Discuss the contributions of community health nurses to social and health care reform.
Test Taking Tip: Be aware of the early efforts of organized nursing societies and their mission.

3.5 Margaret Sanger combined social activism with nursing to her clients by:
1. Providing education regarding improved nutrition for families.
2. Reducing rural childbirth morbidity and mortality rates.
3. Advocating for better care for the mentally ill.
4. Providing information about contraceptive services to women.

Answer: 4
Rationale: Margaret Sanger combined social activism with nursing by providing contraceptive information to poor women, which was in defiance of the United States laws at the time. She endured many legal battles and her legacy was ultimately the free dissemination of contraceptive information to those who desired it. Among community health nursing care, education was always a component in their early efforts. Reducing rural childbirth mortality and morbidity rates was done by Mary Breckenridge in the Frontier Nursing Service. Dorothea Dix was an early activist for advocating for the mentally ill.
Step in the Nursing Process: Implementation
Category of Client Need: Health Promotion and Maintenance
Cognitive Level: Application
Learning Objective 3-2: Discuss the contributions of community health nurses to social and health care reform.
Test Taking Tip: Know the early pioneers of community health nursing and their efforts toward improving the health of populations.

3.6 Which nurse combined political activism with health promotion and disease prevention to improve individual and societal conditions affecting health?
1. Mary Brewster.
2. Lina Struthers.
3. Lillian Wald.
4. Lavinia Dock.

Answer: 3
Rationale: Lillian Wald is the person most closely aligned with community health nursing and coined the term *public health nurse*. She accomplished many reforms to improve the health of New York and was politically active in lobbying for these improvements in addition to providing nursing care to the immigrant population served by the Henry St. Settlement. All the other nurses worked with Wald at the Henry St. Settlement, but branched out to other aspects of nursing and political activism.
Step in the Nursing Process: Assessment
Category of Client Need: Health Promotion and Maintenance
Cognitive Level: Comprehension
Learning Objective 3-2: Discuss the contributions of community health nurses to social and health care reform.
Test Taking Tip: Be aware of the many accomplishments achieved by early community health nurses.

3.7 Two events that demonstrated the effectiveness of community health nursing in the United States were the: (Select all that apply)
1. Visiting nurse services of Metropolitan Life Insurance Company.
2. School nursing program in New York City.
3. Formation of the Red Cross.
4. Improvement of sanitary conditions in slum areas.

Answer: 1, 2
Rationale: The visiting nurse services of Metropolitan Life Insurance Company were an overwhelming success in decreasing insurance costs for the company. These services were provided on a three month pilot, and because of its success, the Metropolitan Life Insurance Company extended this program until the 1950s. Use of a single school nurse in New York City and the impact of reducing absenteeism resulted in the establishment of school nurses throughout the city. The formation of the Red Cross had no bearing on community health, but was organized primarily to help people in times of war and disaster. While improving sanitary conditions improved overall health, this was an ongoing process and not a discrete event. Benevolent societies preceded the formal development of community health nursing.
Step in the Nursing Process: Assessment

Category of Client Need: Health Promotion and Maintenance
Cognitive Level: Application
Learning Objective 3-3: List significant historical events in the development of community health nursing in the United States.
Test Taking Tip: Understand the impact of selected events on the population's health.

3.8 William Rathbone enlisted Florence Nightingale's assistance to develop a concept of nursing care, which he later adopted in the United States after witnessing its benefits to his dying wife. This aspect of nursing care came to be known as:
1. Parish nursing.
2. Community nursing.
3. District nursing.
4. Home nursing.

Answer: 3
Rationale: After seeing the effectiveness of the nursing care to his wife, Rathbone conceived of district nursing to improve the overall health of set populations in local districts. Early efforts were not successful, however, until Rathbone solicited Nightingale's help. She made this concept successful. Although district nursing evolved into community nursing and later parish nursing, the original idea was for district nursing as conceived by Rathbone. Home nursing was already done by either trained nurses or by family members.
Step in the Nursing Process: Planning
Category of Client Need: Health Promotion and Maintenance
Cognitive Level: Application
Learning Objective 3-3: List significant historical events in the development of community health nursing in the United States.
Test Taking Tip: Recognize the early efforts of health reformers to impact the health of a population.

3.9 Historical events that have shaped and formed the development of community nursing in the United States include the: (Select all that apply)
1. Settlement house movement.
2. Passage of immigration limiting legislation.
3. Passage of legislation specific to community nursing.
4. Standardization of community nursing practice.
5. Creation of district nursing.

Answer: 1, 3, 4
Rationale: The settlement house movement was started in answer to the rise of immigration to the United States to help the immigrants assimilate to United States culture and mores. The immigrant population in the United States drew Lillian Wald and her followers to provide nursing care to this group and thus improve their overall health, which then translated to the overall population. Wald and other nurses then advocated for legislation specific to the population health, most notably with the Sheppard-Towner Act in 1921. Standardization of practice resulted in the formation of the National Organization of Public Health Nurses in 1912. District nursing was a movement primarily located in Great Britain.
Step in the Nursing Process: Evaluation
Category of Client Need: Health Promotion and Maintenance
Cognitive Level: Application
Learning Objective 3-3: List significant historical events in the development of community health nursing in the United States.
Test Taking Tip: Understand how societal events and changes have shaped and influenced community health nursing in the United States.

3.10 Governmental efforts to address health promotion-focused public health began with the passage of which legislation?
1. Sheppard-Towner Act.
2. Social Security Act.
3. Hill-Burton Act.
4. Child Health Act.

Answer: 1
Rationale: The Sheppard-Towner Act represented the first federal legislation that specifically targeted an aspect of community health, most notably maternal-child health. The Social Security Act didn't originally focus on health promotion efforts. The Hill-Burton Act, passed after World War II, focused on the building of hospitals rather than community health. The Child Health Act was not passed until 1967, and did address health promotion, but longer than the first federal legislative efforts in 1921.
Step in the Nursing Process: Implementation
Category of Client Need: Health Promotion and Maintenance
Cognitive Level: Comprehension
Learning Objective 3-4: Describe evidence for a shift in public health policy toward a greater emphasis on health promotion.
Test Taking Tip: Understand how legislation reflected the social shifts in emphasis on community health care.

3.11 The passage of the amended Social Security Act created Medicare and Medicaid, which increased demands for health care services. The National Health Planning and Resources Development Act of 1974

Answer: 2
Rationale: The 1974 Act recognized health practitioner efforts to improve public health status, which was an early legislative shift to recognize health promotion as an effective effort to improve public health status. Increasing funding for health services was not the goal of the 1974 act. Increasing funds to improve indigent health status was not addressed in the 1974 Act, though it was for the 1965 amended Social

attempted to address the demand for health care services by:
1. Increasing funds for more health services to improve public health status.
2. Recognizing the contribution of health practitioners to the public health status.
3. Increasing funds to improve the health status of the indigent poor.
4. Recognizing that increased hospitals improved the public health status.

Security Act. Increased hospital building was not a public policy shift of recognizing an emphasis on health promotion.
Step in the Nursing Process: Implementation
Category of Client Need: Health Promotion and Maintenance
Cognitive Level: Comprehension
Learning Objective 3-4: Describe evidence for a shift in public health policy toward a greater emphasis on health promotion.
Test Taking Tip: Understand how subsequent legislation addressed the shifts in public health policy toward health promotion.

3.12 Insurance expenditures for health spending led to the development of diagnosis-related groups (DRGs) in an effort to control spending. DRGs provided the driving force for health efforts to be directed toward:
1. Emphasizing health promotion to decrease hospitalizations and medical costs.
2. Decreasing length of stays for hospitalizations.
3. Organize services to be more cost-effective.
4. Placing the emphasis on the community to improve population health status.

Answer: 1
Rationale: The effect of DRGs has shifted emphasis to health promotion of populations rather than medical care for conditions preventable by health promotion efforts. DRGs pay a flat fee in advance for client diagnosis which may not benefit the client health status. DRGs have not been proven to make services more cost-effective, though that has been one of its objectives. DRGs have not emphasized the community as a whole to improve a population's health status. That is achieved through a variety of methods, not solely DRGs.
Step in the Nursing Process: Planning
Category of Client Need: Health Promotion and Maintenance
Cognitive Level: Comprehension
Learning Objective 3-4: Describe evidence for a shift in public health policy toward a greater emphasis on health promotion.
Test Taking Tip: Understand the shifts in public policy to emphasize health promotion.

3.13 National health policy in the United States has created several documents that address population health, and targets community health nursing practice. The most current policy promulgated by the United States Department of Health and Human Services is the:
1. Lalonde Report.
2. Future of Public Health.
3. Declaration of Alma Alta.
4. Healthy People 2010.

Answer: 4
Rationale: Healthy People 2010 is the most current policy of the United States government to address improving the population health, and targets community health nursing practice. The Lalonde Report addressed Canadian population health. The Future of Public Health is a document of the Institute of Medicine, which impacts community health but is not the national health policy. The Declaration of Alma Alta is an international document addressing primary health care.
Step in the Nursing Process: Planning
Category of Client Need: Health Promotion and Maintenance
Cognitive Level: Comprehension
Learning Objective 3-5: Describe national and international events that are shaping current and future community health nursing practice.
Test Taking Tip: Become aware of the national and international policies that impact community health nursing practice.

3.14 The *Ottawa Charter for Health Promotion* was significant for community health nursing practice because it:
1. Focused on social, economic, and political reforms as strategies to improve global health.
2. Provided a mechanism for prospective payment for hospital services.
3. Identified assessment, policy formation, and assurance as key indicators for global health.
4. Created specific mechanisms to categorize nursing services.

Answer: 1
Rationale: Inherent in the *Ottawa Charter's* strategies is the emphasis on community health nursing to achieve the goal of improving global health. Prospective payment of services was the feature of DRGs. The Future of Public Health by the Institute of Medicine focused on assessment, policy formation, and assurance as key indicators. The Nursing Interventions Classification (NIC) created a mechanism to categorize nursing services.
Step in the Nursing Process: Diagnosis
Category of Client Need: Health Promotion and Maintenance
Cognitive Level: Comprehension
Learning Objective 3-5: Describe national and international events that are shaping current and future community health nursing practice.
Test Taking Tip: Become aware of the national and international policies that impact community health nursing practice.

3.15 An event that will shape future community health nursing practice is the:

1. Emphasis on prospective payment for nursing services.
2. Threat of terrorism to harm the public's health.
3. Surveillance of the CDC on population health.
4. International effort to eradicate smallpox.

Answer: 2

Rationale: Terrorist threats and governmental focus on terrorism may serve to detract attention to overall population health. Community health nursing efforts will be focused on maintaining a balance between terrorist threats and safeguarding population health. DRGs emphasize prospective payment. Surveillance of the CDC focuses on diseases that affect population health, not community health nursing practice. Smallpox was eradicated in 1977, so international efforts are not geared toward this aspect of global health.

Step in the Nursing Process: Assessment

Category of Client Need: Health Promotion and Maintenance

Cognitive Level: Comprehension

Learning Objective 3-5: Describe national and international events that are shaping current and future community health nursing practice.

Test Taking Tip: Become aware of the national and international policies that impact community health nursing practice.

CHAPTER 4

4.1 Community health nursing utilizes theory to:

1. Provide evaluations for community nursing interventions.
2. Explain community health problems.
3. Evaluate health status and use the nursing process to improve health.
4. Provide statistical data for assessing the health status of a community.

Answer: 3

Rationale: Theoretical models assist community health nurses to evaluate health status and use that assessment information to plan, implement, and evaluate effective nursing care to improve a community's health. Theory can direct attention to relevant aspects of a community's health and which interventions would be most effective. While the other selections are correct, they are not the best use of theory because they only address one aspect of theory for use in community health nursing. A theoretical foundation for community health nursing practice will utilize all aspects of the nursing process, not discrete elements.

Step in Nursing Process: Implementation

Category of Client Need: Health Promotion and Maintenance

Cognitive Level: Application

Learning Objective 4-1: Identify the need for a theoretical foundation for community health nursing.

Test Taking Tip: Understand how theory guides community health nursing practice.

4.2 Various models are used by community health nurses to provide care for the community. The most effective model for community health nurses is the:

1. Epidemiologic model.
2. Nursing model.
3. Conceptual model.
4. Health Belief model.

Answer: 2

Rationale: Nursing models utilize aspects of epidemiologic models but go further to suggest interventions to protect, improve, or restore health. The epidemiologic model examines factors that influence health and illness, but do not suggest interventions for implementation. A conceptual model provides abstract and general concepts and their linkages to a phenomenon of interest, but does not provide interventions to improve health. The Health Belief model is a well-known model that explains behaviors for change, but does not provide nursing interventions to address a community's health.

Step in Nursing Process: Planning

Category of Client Need: Health Promotion and Maintenance

Cognitive Level: Application

Learning Objective 4-1: Identify the need for a theoretical foundation for community health nursing.

Test Taking Tip: Differentiate between the epidemiologic and nursing models used by community health nurses to best address a community's health.

4.3 What is the best explanation for the use of epidemiology as a cornerstone of community health?

1. It provides an overall plan to address a community's health needs.
2. It links cause and effect determinants of a community's health status.

Answer: 4

Rationale: Epidemiology is the study of the distribution of health and illness within a population, factors that determine its health status, and use of the knowledge generated by it to control the development of health problems. Epidemiology does not provide a plan of action to address a community's health needs. While it studies factors that determine a population's health status, it does not necessarily provide the cause and effect linkages. Communicable illnesses comprise part of the aspect of epidemiology in surveillance, but that is not epidemiology's sole function.

Step in Nursing Process: Assessment

Category of Client Need: Health Promotion and Maintenance

3. It monitors communicable illnesses that can affect a community's health. 4. It studies distribution of health and illness and its factors in a population, and uses this knowledge to control development of a community's health problems.	Cognitive Level: Application Learning Objective 4-2: Describe basic principles of epidemiology. Test Taking Tip: Understand the relationship of epidemiology to community health.
4.4 The number of cases of diabetes in the community has remained stable during the last year. In January, ten new diagnoses of diabetes were confirmed in the community. This represents: 1. Morbidity. 2. Case rate. 3. Incidence. 4. Prevalence.	Answer: 3 Rationale: While the number of diabetes cases is stable, new diagnoses identified during a specified period of time represents incidence. Morbidity is described in terms of incidence and prevalence of a condition. Case rate is the percentage of persons with the condition. Prevalence is the total number of people affected by a particular condition. Step in Nursing Process: Assessment Category of Client Need: Health Promotion and Maintenance Cognitive Level: Application Learning Objective 4-2: Describe basic principles of epidemiology. Test Taking Tip: Understand the differences in meaning among the various epidemiologic terms.
4.5 The nurse is compiling childhood illness statistics and finds that the morbidity for chicken pox is higher for the community by comparison to the local county. This means there: 1. Are new cases of chicken pox in the community. 2. Is a large group of children affected by chicken pox in the community. 3. Has been a rise in the number of children with chicken pox during a specified period of time in the community. 4. Is a larger percentage of children with chicken pox in the community.	Answer: 3 Rationale: Morbidity is described in terms of incidence and prevalence. The morbidity for chicken pox indicates the total number and new cases identified during and at a specified period of time. Incidence is the number of new cases alone. Prevalence is the group affected by chicken pox. The percentage with chicken pox represents case rate. Step in Nursing Process: Assessment Category of Client Need: Health Promotion and Maintenance Cognitive Level: Application Learning Objective 4-2: Describe basic principles of epidemiology. Test Taking Tip: Understand the differences in meaning among the various epidemiologic terms.
4.6 Prevalence is: 1. A community of 65,000 with 2500 known cases of asthma. 2. A community of 65,000 with a higher number of cases of asthma than the rest of the state. 3. A community of 65,000 with 15 cases of asthma diagnosed during the summer months. 4. A community of 65,000 with a higher percentage of deaths resulting from asthma than the rest of the state.	Answer: 1 Rationale: Prevalence is the total number of people affected by a particular condition at a specified point of time. A higher number of asthma cases than the rest of the state is morbidity. New cases diagnosed during a specified period of time is incidence. Case fatality rate for a particular condition represents the percentage of persons with the condition who die as a result of it. Step in Nursing Process: Assessment Category of Client Need: Health Promotion and Maintenance Cognitive Level: Application Learning Objective 4-2: Describe basic principles of epidemiology. Test Taking Tip: Understand the differences in meaning among the various epidemiologic terms.
4.7 The nurse is compiling statistics about lung cancer in the community, which has experienced an average of fifteen years from diagnosis to death. This concept of epidemiology is: 1. Mortality rate. 2. Survival time.	Answer: 2 Rationale: The average length of time from diagnosis to death is survival time. Mortality rate is the ratio of the numbers of deaths from a specific condition. Morbidity rate reflects the incidence and prevalence of a specific condition. Survival rate is the proportion of people with a given condition who remain alive after a specific period. Step in Nursing Process: Assessment Category of Client Need: Health Promotion and Maintenance

3. Morbidity rate.
4. Survival rate.

Cognitive Level: Application
Learning Objective 4-2: Describe basic principles of epidemiology.
Test Taking Tip: Understand the differences in meaning among the various epidemiologic terms.

4.8 An example of the epidemiologic triad is:
1. Rural Mississippi, deer, and Lyme disease.
2. Potato salad, outdoor picnic, and food poisoning.
3. Sun, beach, and sunburn.
4. Standing water, mosquitoes, and warm weather.

Answer: 2
Rationale: The epidemiologic triad consists of agent, host, and environment. Potato salad is the agent, the host is food poisoning, and the environment is the outdoor picnic.
Step in Nursing Process: Assessment
Category of Client Need: Health Promotion and Maintenance
Cognitive Level: Application
Learning Objective 4-2: Describe basic principles of epidemiology.
Test Taking Tip: Know how the elements of the epidemiologic triad interact.

4.9 A "web of causation" can be:
1. Access to alcohol, decreased enforcement of minors, and attractive media portrayal of alcohol that contributes to adolescent alcohol usage.
2. Mosquitoes, West Nile virus, and decreased mosquito spraying.
3. Oil refinery, flare emissions, and asthma.
4. Adolescent pregnancy rate, lower socioeconomic status and education, and close friends with infants.

Answer: 1
Rationale: Web of causation explores the influence of multiple factors on a specific health condition. The factors of access to alcohol, decreased enforcement of age checking, and the attractive portrayal of alcohol in the media contributes to adolescent alcohol usage. The other examples are of the epidemiologic triad.
Step in Nursing Process: Evaluation
Category of Client Care: Health Promotion and Maintenance
Cognitive Level: Application
Learning Objective 4-3: Apply selected epidemiological and nursing models to community health nursing practice with individuals, families, and populations.
Test Taking Tip: Know how the web of causation uses multiple factors to explain development of a specific health condition.

4.10 Determinants of health to address the development of cancer in a community could include the: (Select all that apply.)
1. Proximity of the community to chemical plants that have a poor history of regulating emissions.
2. High percentage of tobacco use among the male population.
3. Prevailing diet high in unprocessed foods and low fat.
4. Availability of health facilities.
5. Mean age of the male population.

Answer: 1, 2, 3
Rationale: Determinants of health are broad categories of factors that influence health and illness. Determinants of health to address the development of cancer in a community would be the proximity to chemical plants with emissions, tobacco usage, and diet. Availability of health facilities has no bearing on the development of cancer. Mean age of a population has no bearing on cancer development.
Step in Nursing Process: Assessment
Category of Client Need: Health Promotion and Maintenance
Cognitive Level: Application
Learning Objective 4-3: Apply selected epidemiological and nursing models to community health nursing practice with individuals, families, and populations.
Test Taking Tip: Understand how the various determinants of health can influence a community's health.

4.11 After a disaster has affected a community, recovery efforts are focused on supporting the community's existing strengths to restore it to its best level of optimal functioning. Neumann's nursing model identifies this as:
1. The normal line of defense.
2. The flexible line of defense.
3. The line of resistance.
4. Reconstitution.

Answer: 4
Rationale: This is tertiary prevention, which, in Neumann's model, stabilizes a system and brings it back to the normal line of defense, bringing it to reconstitution. The normal line of defense is the community's normal range of response to stressors. The flexible line of defense provides a protective cushion, preventing stressors from penetrating the normal line of defense. When the flexible line of defense cannot protect the system, penetration of the normal line of defense occurs. Lines of resistance are the internal factors that act to return the community to a normal or improved state, protecting it against stressor penetration of the basic structure. Once stressor penetration occurs (the disaster), the system engages in activities aimed at reconstitution, stabilizing the systems and bringing it back to the normal line of defense.
Step in Nursing Process: Implementation
Category of Client Need: Health Promotion and Maintenance
Cognitive Level: Application
Learning Objective4-3: Apply selected epidemiological and nursing models to community health nursing practice with individuals, families, and populations.
Test Taking Tip: Be aware of how levels of prevention in Neumann's model correlate with the concepts.

4.12 In the community-as-partner model, the nurse assesses the health status of the community core and factors in related subsystems that affect health by:
1. Evaluating the community in terms of its health statistics.
2. Participating with members of the community.
3. Applying the levels of prevention.
4. Using the web of causation.

Answer: 2
Rationale: In the community-as-partner model, the nurse participates with the members of the community to assess the health status of the community and factors that affect health. Evaluating the community in terms of its health status is not working with the community members. The levels of prevention can be used in any model, but this is not a characteristic of community-as-partner. The web of causation is an epidemiologic model and not a nursing model.
Step in Nursing Process: Assessment
Category of Client Need: Health Promotion and Maintenance
Cognitive Level: Application
Learning Objective 4-3: Apply selected epidemiological and nursing models to community health nursing practice with individuals, families, and populations.
Test Taking Tip: Understand how the various nursing models are applied to community health nursing practice.

4.13 The nursing process guides the nurse in community health. Other processes used by community health nurses in their practice include the: (Select all that apply.)
1. Epidemiologic process.
2. Case management process.
3. Illness model process.
4. Health education process.
5. Web of causation process.

Answer: 1, 2, 4
Rationale: The community health nurse uses the epidemiologic, case management, and health education processes in addition to the nursing process to provide care to individuals, families, and population groups. An illness model focuses on the aspects of disease and does not take into consideration the impact on a community's health. Web of causation is a model exploring the influences of factors in the development of a specific health condition.
Step in Nursing Process: Implementation
Category of Client Need: Health Promotion and Maintenance
Cognitive Level: Analysis
Learning Objective 4-3: Apply selected epidemiological and nursing models to community health nursing practice with individuals, families, and populations.
Test Taking Tip: Know the processes the community health nurse utilizes when providing care in the community.

4.14 Based on an assessment of health needs of local musicians in a community, a health clinic recently opened and provided "one-stop" health care to this local population. This innovation in the interventions wheel model would be at the:
1. Individual level.
2. Community level.
3. Systems level.
4. Group level.

Answer: 3
Rationale: The interventions wheel model covers three levels of population-based practice: individual-focused, community-focused and systems-focused practice. Opening a health clinic dedicated to a specific group such as the musicians focuses on organizational change and health care delivery structures. The individual level focuses on change in individual health status, knowledge, or skills. Community-level interventions address change in community norms or behaviors in a community.
Step in Nursing Process: Implementation
Category of Client Care: Health Promotion and Maintenance
Cognitive Level: Application
Learning Objective 4-3: Apply selected epidemiological and nursing models to community health nursing practice with individuals, families, and populations.
Test Taking Tip: Understand epidemiological and nursing models.

4.15 The Los Angeles County Public Health Nursing Practice Model (LAC PHN) links public health nursing with principles of public health practice using the nursing process. Its overall goal is to have healthy people in healthy communities. Health indicators rather than health determinants are used in this model. A concern for this model is that:
1. Community health nurses engage in the interventions described in the intervention wheel.
2. It fails to acknowledge that health system factors may contribute to the existence of health problems.

Answer: 2
Rationale: The LAC PHN uses health indicators, but the model does not acknowledge how health system factors may contribute to health problems, nor does it provide guidance beyond the health indicators listed other than recommending that additional indicators may be used. It also does not provide direction to assess factors that contribute to undesirable health outcomes.
Step in Nursing Process: Evaluation
Category of Client Need: Health Promotion and Maintenance
Cognitive Level: Analysis
Learning Objective 4-3: Apply selected epidemiological and nursing models to community health nursing practice with individuals, families, and populations.
Test Taking Tip: Be aware of the differences among the various nursing models in community health practice.

3. Clients must play an active role in their health.
4. The focus of the evaluation is only on health outcomes.

CHAPTER 5

5.1 The client is experiencing nasal congestion from a cold. The client self-administers an over-the-counter cold product to alleviate symptoms. The best description of the health care system the client is using is:
1. Complementary health care.
2. Scientific health care.
3. Personal health care.
4. Popular health care.

Answer: 4
Rationale: The popular health care subsystem is where care is provided by oneself, family, or friends. Complementary health care consists of providers and practices outside the mainstream health care system. The scientific health subsystem is care based on scientific research-derived evidence. Personal health care is the sector that provides health-related services to individual clients.
Step in Nursing Process: Implementation
Category of Client Care: Health promotion and maintenance
Cognitive Level: Application
Learning Objective 5-1: Describe the popular health care subsystem.
Test Taking Tip: Be aware of the differences in the various health care subsystems in the United States.

5.2 The client is being treated for chronic headache pain in a local clinic. In addition to the medical care the client is receiving, the client also visits an acupuncture clinic and states that both therapies help the headache pain. This type of health care subsystem the client is employing is:
1. Complementary.
2. Personal.
3. Popular.
4. Alternative.

Answer: 1
Rationale: Using acupuncture therapy in conjunction with standardized medical care is an example of complementary therapy. Complementary health care practices are used in conjunction with scientific care to complement and enhance its effects. Personal health care provides health-related services to individual clients. Popular health care is what an individual does for oneself. Alternative health care is used in place of scientific interventions.
Step in Nursing Process: Evaluation
Category of Client Need: Physiological Integrity
Cognitive Level: Application
Learning Objective 5-2: Distinguish between the complementary and alternative subsystems of care.
Test Taking Tip: Know the distinctions between complementary and alternative health care subsystems.

5.3 West Nile virus has been diagnosed in the state. The state health department has ordered mosquito spraying in the affected area and public service announcements are being broadcast in the local media to alert the population to drain water from loose tires and other areas where there may be stagnant water. What obligations are being addressed by the state health department? (Select all that apply.).
1. Prevent epidemics and the spread of disease.
2. Protect the public from environmental hazards.
3. Prevent injury.
4. Promote healthy behavior and good mental health.
5. Respond to disasters and assist.

Answer: 1, 2, 3
Rationale: By ordering the mosquito spraying and using the public service announcements, the state health department is preventing the spread of West Nile virus and protecting the public from environmental hazards, thus also preventing potential further injury. The actions are not geared to promoting healthy behavior and good mental health. This action is not responding to a disaster and assisting with recovery.
Step in Nursing Process: Implementation
Category of Client Care: Safe, Effective Care Environment
Cognitive Level: Application
Learning Objective 5-3: Identify six fundamental obligations of official public health agencies.
Test Taking Tip: Understand how agency obligations can be applied to a situation.

5.4 After a hurricane has devastated an area, the United States Public Health service sends a group of health care workers to open satellite clinics

Answer: 3
Rationale: Sending health care personnel to staff and open clinics is ensuring accessibility of needed health care services to an area that has been devastated by a natural disaster. It is not preventing epidemics and spread of disease as such, nor does

in the area. This action is best considered:
1. Preventing epidemics and the spread of disease.
2. Preventing injury.
3. Ensuring quality and accessibility of needed health care services.
4. Promoting healthy behavior and good mental health.

this action prevent injury. While having accessibility to health care services can promote healthy behavior, this is not the best answer.
Step in Nursing Process: Implementation
Category of Client Care: Safe, Effective Management of Care
Cognitive Level: Analysis
Learning Objective 5-3: Identify six fundamental obligations of official public health agencies.
Test Taking Tip: Know the fundamental obligations of official public health agencies.

5.5 The organizational structure of the United States health care delivery system can best be described by three subsystems:
1. Personal health system, popular health system, and scientific health system.
2. Popular health system, alternative health system, and scientific health system.
3. Scientific health system, complementary health system, and alternative health system.
4. Scientific health system, complementary health system, and popular health system.

Answer: 4
Rationale: There are three health care subsystems that describe the organizational structure for the United States, which are the scientific, complementary/alternative, and popular. Complementary/alternative health system is a combined system, not divided into separate systems. Answers that have one without the other do not describe the full organizational structure of health subsystems in the United States.
Step in Nursing Process: Assessment
Category of Client Need: Health Promotion and Maintenance
Cognitive Level: Analysis
Learning Objective 5-4: Describe the organizational structure of the U.S. health care delivery system
Test Taking Tip: Understand that the three subsystems represent the facets of health care needs in society.

5.6 The March of Dimes has instituted a public awareness campaign to decrease premature births. It has also conducted media campaigns to raise public awareness of this health problem in addition to research about prematurity and government lobbying efforts. Official government efforts to address prematurity include research and public awareness. The March of Dimes is a voluntary agency. The primary emphasis of the March of Dimes campaign is on:
1. Funding, research, and education.
2. Research, education, and policy development.
3. Education, policy development, and funding.
4. Policy development, research, and public health practice.

Answer: 2
Rationale: The primary emphasis of voluntary agencies such as the March of Dimes is on research, education, and policy development, primarily through lobbying. Official health agencies can develop policy independently and do research. Education is one of the components of official health agencies. Voluntary health agencies are accountable to their supporters, whereas official health agencies are accountable to the population.
Step in Nursing Process: Implementation
Category of Client Need: Health Promotion and Maintenance
Cognitive Level: Analysis
Learning Objective 5-5: Compare and contrast official and voluntary health agencies.
Test Taking Tip: Be able to distinguish the differences between official and voluntary agencies.

5.7 The "Tour for Cure" is an annual bike relay sponsored by the Multiple Sclerosis (MS) Society. Entrants are sponsored for each mile by voluntary donations, which go to the MS Society to fund research activities and provide services to those diagnosed with MS. The Tour highlights awareness and public education of the disease. As a voluntary health agency, select two additional functions the MS Society can accomplish.
1. Promote legislation through lobbying.

Answers: 1, 2
Rationale: The bike relay helps to fund research that specifically addresses multiple sclerosis. The mission of the MS Society is to find a cure for this disease. The awareness raised by the bike relay educates the public and health professionals about MS. Clients with MS can receive services funded by the MS Society. Though focused on one disease, lobbying efforts are directed to legislation that addresses those who have MS, which also advocates for the public health and can assist in planning and organization. A voluntary health agency is not responsible for providing sufficient health professionals to care for those diagnosed with this disease, though it can have funds to help train them. A voluntary health agency does not have the authority to enforce laws and regulations.
Step in Nursing Process: Implementation
Category of Client Need: Safe, Effective Care Environment
Cognitive Level: Application

---

2. Health planning and organization.
3. Ensure sufficient health professionals to care for those with MS.
4. Enforce laws and regulations that help to diagnose and treat those with MS.

Learning Objective 5-6: Describe at least five functions performed by voluntary health agencies.
Test Taking Tip: Understand the many functions performed by voluntary health agencies.

5.8 The nurse has been monitoring the community's rates of cardiac disease and sees that they are increasing. The nurse holds a community forum to address the impact of cardiac disease on the community's health. Those attending are given information about cardiac disease including interventions related to diet and exercise to decrease risk. Several church groups who attend the forum offer to host health fairs to provide additional information to the community as well as transportation to physician visits for older community members. Public health services exemplified in this situation include: (Select all that apply.)
1. Monitoring health status to identify health problems.
2. Diagnosing and investigating health problems and hazards.
3. Informing, educating, and empowering people regarding health issues.
4. Mobilizing community partnerships to identify and solve health problems.

Answers: 1, 3, 4
Rationale: While monitoring the community's health, the nurse has identified cardiac disease as a health problem in the community. Convening a community forum is informing, educating, and empowering the community. Community partnerships are mobilized and the church groups are offering to host health fairs and linking people to health services by providing transportation. Diagnosis and investigating health problems and hazards are not services utilized in this forum.
Step in Nursing Process: Planning
Category of Client Need: Health Promotion and Maintenance
Cognitive Level: Application
Learning Objective 5-7: Identify ten essential public health services.
Test Taking Tip: Be able to distinguish how several services can be offered within one example.

5.9 An example of diagnosing and investigating health problems and hazards in the community is:
1. Correlating pediatric asthma visits to the local ED with local emissions from a nearby fuel plant.
2. Providing asthma education programs to local elementary school teachers.
3. Informing the local health department about the increased rise in asthma attacks.
4. Lobbying the local fuel plant to decrease its emissions.

Answer: 1
Rationale: Correlating pediatric asthma visits to the ED with emissions from the local fuel plant is linking health problems and is diagnosing a health problem within the community. Lobbying the fuel plant to decrease emissions is not diagnosing or investigating. Informing the health department is providing information, but not diagnosing or investigating. Providing asthma education programs to elementary school teachers informs and educates them as to asthma in the pediatric population.
Step in Nursing Process: Assessment
Category of Client Need: Health Promotion and Maintenance
Cognitive Level: Application
Learning Objective 5-7: Identify ten essential public health services.
Test Taking Tip: Understand how diagnosis and investigation of health problems are linked together.

5.10 A member of the community with tuberculosis (TB) refuses to be compliant with his/her TB treatment protocol and is sent to a minimum security correctional facility to ensure that the TB medications are done with directly observed therapy (DOT) by the medical personnel there. The client initiates legal action to prevent

Answer: 3
Rationale: Police power is the power to provide for the health, safety, and welfare of the people. The state, not the federal government or local jurisdiction, has primary authority in matters of health. The state government retains the ultimate responsibility for the health of the public and can use police power as an essential power to enforce laws and regulations regarding health.
Step in Nursing Process: Implementation
Category of Client Need: Safe, Effective Care Environment
Cognitive Level: Application

this from happening but is overruled by the judge. Which government level of authority authorizes this power?
1. Local government.
2. County government.
3. State government.
4. Federal government.

Learning Objective 5-8: Discuss the involvement of local, state, and national governments in health care in the United States.
Test Taking Tip: Recognize the governmental authority levels in health care.

5.11 After doing a community assessment, the nurse lobbies for and succeeds in obtaining a government grant to fund an immunization clinic in a community with inadequate well-child care services. This is:
1. Tertiary prevention.
2. Secondary prevention.
3. Primary prevention.
4. Disease prevention.

Answer: 3
Rationale: Outcomes for primary prevention focus on access and the ability of the population to obtain the goods and services necessary to promote health and prevent illness. In a community with inadequate well-child care, an immunization clinic will provide the primary prevention service of immunizations to prevent those illnesses. Tertiary prevention outcomes focus on restoration and optimal functioning after disability occurs, which is not the focus in immunizations. Secondary prevention focuses on early diagnosis and treatment, not a purpose of immunization. Prevention of disease is not solely done through primary prevention.
Step in Nursing Process: Implementation
Category of Client Need: Health Promotion and Maintenance
Cognitive Level: Application
Learning Objective 5-9: Identify outcomes of care at the primary, secondary, and tertiary levels of prevention.
Test Taking Tip: Differentiate between the levels of prevention.

5.12 A secondary prevention outcome in a community would be:
1. Increasing the Emergency Medical Services (EMS) in a community where these services are provided only by the local volunteer fire department.
2. Opening walk-in clinics in a community.
3. Increasing the number of home health physical therapist services in a community.
4. Monitoring the amount of health screening services done in a community.

Answer: 1
Rationale: Secondary prevention outcomes focus on limiting disability when it is identified. Increasing EMS services in a community where services are provided only by a local volunteer fire department will help to improve access to emergency services, which could then translate into better outcomes for those who now have better access to these services. Opening walk-in clinics in a community increases access to services to promote health, which is primary prevention. Increasing home health physical therapist services is tertiary prevention. Monitoring screening services is surveillance, not an outcome of a prevention level.
Step in Nursing Process: Implementation
Category of Client Need: Health Promotion and Maintenance
Cognitive Level: Application
Learning Objective 5-9: Identify outcomes of care at the primary, secondary, and tertiary levels of prevention.
Test Taking Tip: Differentiate between the levels of prevention.

5.13 Increasing rehabilitative services in a community where the population majority is older than 65 involves:
1. Primary prevention level.
2. Secondary prevention level.
3. Tertiary prevention level.
4. Disease prevention level.

Answer: 3
Rationale: Tertiary prevention is directed toward restoring optimal level of function, and an outcome of increasing rehabilitative services for an older population that traditionally has a greater degree of disability from diseases. Primary prevention addresses the ability to access services to promote health and prevent illness. Secondary prevention addresses identification of conditions to halt further progression of disability. Disease prevention addresses preventing diseases, not rehabilitation.
Step in Nursing Process: Implementation
Category of Client Need: Health Promotion and Maintenance
Cognitive Level: Application
Learning Objective 5-9: Identify outcomes of care at the primary, secondary, and tertiary levels of prevention.
Test Taking Tip: Differentiate between the levels of prevention.

5.14 Among the suggestions for health system reform from the Institute of Medicine's Committee on Quality of Health Care in America is:
1. Avoiding waste of resources.
2. Reducing waits and delays in services provided.

Answer: 4
Rationale: Individualizing care based on client needs and values is one of the ten rules the Committee has established to reform health care processes. The Institute of Medicine has six aims for improvement, which include avoiding waste of resources, reducing waits and delays for services, and providing evidence-based services to those who can benefit from them, but also to withhold those services from those who cannot benefit from them. These six aims for improvement do not involve health care reform.

3. Providing evidence-based services to those who can benefit from them and withholding services from those who cannot benefit from them.
4. Individualizing care based on client needs and values.

Step in Nursing Process: Planning
Category of Client Need: Health Promotion and Maintenance
Cognitive Level: Analysis
Learning Objective 5-10: Describe potential approaches to health system reform, including the possibility of a national health care system.
Test Taking Tip: Be aware that suggestions may include either the aims for improvement or the rules for health care reform.

CHAPTER 6

6.1 Among the advantages for the United States involvement in global health initiatives are to: (Select all that apply.)
1. Determine the course of policy decisions in global health.
2. Protect domestic interests from terrorism and communicable diseases.
3. Utilize humanitarian interests to defuse distrust of the United States.
4. Improve the economy by opening markets for United States-produced goods.
5. Enhance United States security by increasing trust and defusing hatred among disadvantaged populations.

Answers: 2, 3, 4, 5
Rationale: Global health initiatives have advantages for United States involvement, among them protecting the country from the threat of communicable diseases that could be used as a terrorism device. Participation in humanitarian interests promotes global health, which benefits the United States both economically and diplomatically, while also helping to defuse distrust. Markets for United States-produced goods can result from involvement in global health initiatives. Determining the course of policy decisions for global health is not an advantage for United States involvement. Participation in global health initiatives can improve international trust, reaping diplomatic benefits for the United States.
Step in Nursing Process: Evaluation
Category of Client Need: Safe, Effective Care Environment
Cognitive Level: Analysis
Learning Objective 6-1: Discuss the advantages of United States involvement in global health initiatives.
Test Taking Tip: Be aware that United States involvement in global health initiatives goes beyond the direct benefit of improving global health.

6.2 A national health service organizes its annual influenza immunization program for its elder population to protect them against pneumonia. However, there is a shortage of the vaccine. The national health system guarantees that all elders will receive this flu protection. The system is experiencing:
1. Balancing individual and population needs with limited resources.
2. Difficulty in reaching hard-to-serve populations.
3. Problems with distributing available resources.
4. Coordination difficulties to meet local health needs.

Answer: 3
Rationale: The shortage of the flu vaccine will most directly impact the distribution of available resources. Balancing individual and population needs with limited resources is not the difficulty in this situation, because this program is directed toward a specific segment. There is no indication that this population is hard to serve, nor is there any indication that there are coordination difficulties to meet local health needs.
Step in Nursing Process: Implementation
Category of Client Need: Health Promotion and Maintenance
Cognitive Level: Application
Learning Objective 6-2: Identify at least five policy dilemmas faced by national health care systems.
Test Taking Tip: Understand how policy dilemmas can affect national health care systems.

6.3 A national health budget is developed to provide preventive health services to all segments of the population. The majority of the population lives in outlying rural areas. A dilemma for this health service is:
1. Reaching hard-to-serve populations.
2. Reconciling individual practice patterns with national standards and systems.
3. Balancing the need for regional and national coordination of health services.
4. Integration of primary care with hospital and specialty services.

Answer: 1
Rationale: A rural population will traditionally be harder to reach than an urban population; therefore, this population's access to preventive services will become an additional concern. Reconciling individual practice patterns to national standards is not addressed, nor is there any indication that coordination is necessary at this time. Primary care integration with hospital and specialty services is not addressed with preventive services.
Step in Nursing Process: Planning
Category of Client Need: Health Promotion and Maintenance
Cognitive Level: Application
Learning Objective 6-2: Identify at least five policy dilemmas faced by national health systems.
Test Taking Tip: Understand how policies can create dilemmas for the national health system in trying to improve the health of its population.

6.4 A centralized system of health is a cornerstone of a national health system. However, there is a long wait for routine health care and many citizens utilize voluntary and private health care services rather than waiting for the government health care system to address their health needs. The dilemma of this centralized system is:
1. Balancing curative technology with allocations for prevention and promotion.
2. Ensuring community participation in policy making.
3. Balancing professional practice autonomy with accountability for population health outcomes.
4. Providing necessary services without impeding the work of the voluntary health sector.

Answer: 4
Rationale: While there is a centralized health system, long waits for service have resulted in many people looking to the private sector for health services. The centralized health system does provide the necessary health services, but the long waits can impact overall health, so citizens using voluntary and private health services can impede this sector. Professional practice autonomy is not applicable in this example. Community participation in policy making is not mentioned. Curative technology is not part of this example.
Step in Nursing Process: Evaluation
Category of Client Need: Health Promotion and Maintenance
Cognitive Level: Application
Learning Objective 6-2: Identify at least five policy dilemmas faced by national health systems.
Test Taking Tip: Understand how the different policy dilemmas can affect national health systems.

6.5 The United States health care system is described as "hyperpluralist", in which health policy is made at the local, state, and national government levels, whereas many other countries have centralized systems of health care. This difference can best be described as:
1. Decentralization.
2. Locus of decision making.
3. Cost containment.
4. Coverage and access.

Answer: 2
Rationale: The locus of decision making is one area where national health care systems differ. Most European countries and Japan have centralized health systems, where health decisions are made at the national level. The United States, by comparison, has a decentralized system where decisions are made at all levels of government, as well as the level of the organization, provider, or client. Cost containment refers to how costs are contained within a certain level, but that is not a government decision process. Coverage and access refers to what degree health services are available to the population and what health services are delivered.
Step in Nursing Process: Assessment
Category of Client Need: Health Promotion and Maintenance
Cognitive Level: Application
Learning Objective 6-3: Compare selected features of national health care systems.
Test Taking Tip: Understand how the locus of decision making reflects national health policy.

6.6 National health systems have limitations or freedom in terms of consumer choice for health care. This reflects:
1. Cost containment.
2. Coverage and access.
3. Health system performance.
4. Professional autonomy.

Answer: 4
Rationale: National health systems vary in the degree of autonomy utilized by both the population and providers within the system. Some national health services provide a large degree of autonomy for citizens and providers to have access to care and diagnostic services, whereas others are constrained by the particular health coverage they have. Cost containment does not address consumer choice in terms of limitations or freedom. Coverage and access describe availability of services for consumers. Health system performance reflects how a system accomplishes its goals compared to a system with similar resources.
Step in Nursing Process: Implementation
Category of Client Need: Safe, Effective Care Environment
Cognitive Level: Application
Learning Objective 6-3: Compare selected features of national health care systems.
Test Taking Tip: Understand how features of national health care systems affect autonomy.

6.7 The Gates Foundation is funding the development of a viable AIDS vaccine and the eradication of child-hood diseases through immunization. Though based in the United States, this foundation is considered a:
1. Bilateral agency.
2. Sector-wide approach to health.

Answer: 4
Rationale: Non-governmental organizations (NGOs) are agencies outside of official government-sponsored agencies that work for the public good. The Gates Foundation has committed its resources and funding to engage in activities that address worldwide health concerns. Examples of NGOs include religious groups, philanthropic foundations, corporations, and other organizations. Bilateral agencies usually involve only two countries on a project. Sector-wide approaches to health focus attention on the resolution of health-related problems by addressing

3. Unilateral agency.
4. Non-governmental organization.

conditions that affect health in a broader social sense. Unilateral agencies represent one country.
Step in Nursing Process: Implementation
Category of Client Need: Health Promotion and Maintenance
Cognitive Level: Analysis
Learning Objective 6-4: Describe two types of international health agencies.
Test Taking Tip: Understand how different organizations have international foci on health.

6.8 The purpose of multilateral health agencies, such as the World Health Organization (WHO), is to:
1. Direct and coordinate global health efforts and work with countries to strengthen their health programs.
2. Work on set programs with selected countries to improve health efforts.
3. Improve health outcomes in Third World countries.
4. Coordinate health programs and efforts with other United Nations Assembly members.

Answer: 1
Rationale: As a multilateral agency, WHO works with many countries in health-related activities. WHO is the primary agency affiliated with the UN that deals with global health issues. It does not restrict its activities to setting programs. While many of its efforts are directed to Third World countries, its focus is health for all people worldwide.
Step in Nursing Process: Implementation
Category of Client Need: Health Promotion and Maintenance
Cognitive Level: Comprehension
Learning Objective 6-4: Describe two types of international health agencies.
Test Taking Tip: Understand the scope of multilateral agencies in health matters.

6.9 As part of the NAFTA trade agreement, sister cities in Mexico and the United States have had cultural exchanges to learn and share health practices and treatments. This could best be described as an effort of:
1. Global health concerns.
2. International health.
3. Bilateral assistance.
4. Border protection.

Answer: 2
Rationale: International health involves health matters that affect two or more countries. Cultural exchanges to learn and share health practices between the United States and Mexican practitioners is an example of international health cooperation. Global health addresses multinational efforts. Cultural exchanges are not bilateral assistance, but mutual learning experiences. Border protection involves actions taken to protect a national border from something occurring in another nation.
Step in Nursing Process: Implementation
Category of Client Need: Health Promotion and Maintenance
Cognitive Level: Application
Learning Objective 6-5: Distinguish between international and global health.
Test Taking Tip: Understand the differences between international and global health efforts.

6.10 Select the best example of global health.
1. Peace Corps volunteers working in a third world country helping to improve water quality in local villages.
2. Rotary volunteers working in Nigeria to immunize children against polio.
3. Doctors without Borders providing health care to war-torn areas in Indonesia.
4. The World Bank providing funding grants to Middle Eastern countries to improve their health infrastructure.

Answer: 4
Rationale: The World Bank is a multilateral agency that provides funding and technical assistance to countries. Improving a region's health infrastructure in individual countries is an example of global health where multi-national efforts address health problems that cross national borders. Peace Corps volunteers working in a third world country are helping a specific country, as are the Rotary volunteers and Doctors without Borders. These are international health efforts.
Step in Nursing Process: Implementation
Category of Client Need: Health Promotion and Maintenance
Cognitive Level: Application
Learning Objective 6-5: Distinguish between international and global health.
Test Taking Tip: Be able to distinguish between international and global health.

6.11 One of the positive aspects of exporting United States technology globally has been to help improve the quality of health care through health innovations and information.

Answer: 3
Rationale: While rapid dissemination of health innovations and information from United States technology has benefited developing nations, it has also opened new markets and exposed these countries to the less desirable aspects of United States businesses, such as marketing by tobacco companies and the expansion of fast food companies. This has resulted in these populations adopting United States practices,

A negative effect of introducing United States technology globally has:
1. Created inequities for health innovations.
2. Increased the spread of communicable diseases.
3. Marketed unhealthful products such as tobacco and fast foods to a new population.
4. Promoted economic growth and created job inequities.

and higher rates of morbidity from cancer and obesity. The introduction of health innovations and information usually decreases communicable diseases, and economic growth increases do not necessarily create job inequities.
Step in Nursing Process: Implementation
Category of Client Need: Health Promotion and Maintenance
Cognitive Level: Application
Learning Objective 6-6: Discuss positive and negative health effects of globalization.
Test Taking Tip: Understand that globalization is a two-sided coin with both positive and negative aspects.

6.12 One of the feared outcomes of NAFTA was job loss within the United States to the other non-United States partners in NAFTA. The argument against this outcome cited the following advantages:
1. Promotion of economic growth through job creation in the other countries, thus improving health.
2. Decreasing the spread of communicable diseases due to improved technology.
3. Developing global health standards.
4. Improving environmental outcomes.

Answer: 1
Rationale: Concerns about United States involvement in NAFTA was related to job loss in the United States. Arguments rebutting this cited that NAFTA would increase economic opportunities for other NAFTA partners, thus increasing employment and income, which in turn would create better financial prosperity and improved health outcomes. Global health standards are not a function of the NAFTA globalization and environmental outcomes have not been addressed. Communicable disease spread was not an outcome addressed with NAFTA participation.
Step in Nursing Process: Implementation
Category of Client Need: Health Promotion and Maintenance
Cognitive Level: Application
Learning Objective 6-6: Discuss positive and negative health effects of globalization.
Test Taking Tip: Understand how creating economic opportunity for one area can mean decreased opportunity for another.

6.13 A global health policy agenda should include which essential element?
1. Primary health care for all.
2. Eliminating all debt for developing countries.
3. Creating a centralized agency for health policy with all nations.
4. Supporting participation by the disadvantaged in health policy development.

Answer: 4
Rationale: A global health policy agenda should include support for participation in health policy development by the disadvantaged, who would benefit the most from having input in this process. Developing primary health care and eliminating debt are not elements of a global health policy agenda, but strategies to improve health. Creating a centralized agency for health policy could be considered a strategy.
Step in Nursing Process: Planning
Category of Client Need: Health Promotion and Maintenance
Cognitive Level: Application
Learning Objective 6-7: Identify elements of a global policy health agenda.
Test Taking Tip: Differentiate between elements and strategies for global health agendas.

6.14 Identify three elements of a global health policy agenda. (Select all that apply.)
1. Sufficient financial aid to improve health and health infrastructure.
2. Coordinate aid to match programs with needs.
3. Create partnerships between government agencies, the private sector, and academia.
4. Represent health interests in other policy-making sectors.
5. Use communication technology to provide information.

Answers: 1, 4, 5
Rationale: A global health policy agenda includes aid to improve health and health infrastructures in all countries, and representation of health interests in other policy-making sectors, such as the economic sector. Using communication technology to provide information is needed for effective policy making. Coordinating aid to match programs and creating partnerships among agencies, the private sector, and academia are strategies to implement a global health policy agenda.
Step in Nursing Process: Planning
Category of Client Need: Health Promotion and Maintenance
Cognitive Level: Analysis
Learning Objective 6-7: Identify elements of a global health policy agenda.
Test Taking Tip: Understand the difference between elements of a health agenda policy and strategies to implement them.

6.15 The community health nurse is considering how best to educate the community about potential threats to health from terrorism. What is the best way to accomplish this? (Select all that apply.)

Answers: 2, 4
Rationale: Holding public forums to educate the community about coping with psychological effects from terrorist threats and raising community awareness about signs and symptoms of potential biologic agents provides information for the community to act if a terrorist attack occurs. Raising community awareness about immigrants in the community is stereotyping.

1. Raise community awareness about increased immigrants to the population.
2. Hold public forums to educate the community about coping with psychological effects.
3. Hold public forums to educate the community about taping windows in the event of a chemical attack.
4. Raise community awareness about the signs and symptoms of potential biologic agents.

Taping windows is not necessarily the most effective method of protection in a chemical attack.
Step in Nursing Process: Planning
Category of Client Need: Health Promotion and Maintenance
Cognitive Level: Application
Learning Objective 6-8: Describe community health nursing involvement with respect to international terrorism.
Test Taking Tip: Understand how disseminating information can be an effective nursing intervention with regard to terrorism.

CHAPTER 7

7.1 After a natural disaster hits the community, a grass-roots organization is formed to improve conditions post recovery. The nurse joins the organization and volunteers to contact public officials about the organization's concerns. This role is best described as:
1. Politician.
2. Activist.
3. Citizen.
4. Researcher.

Answer: 2
Rationale: Though this is a role of citizen, through speaking out on policy issues and becoming acquainted with elected officials, the nurse is displaying the role of activist. Contacting public officials and joining relevant coalitions is a political activist role.
Step in Nursing Process: Planning
Category of Client Need: Health Promotion and Maintenance
Cognitive Level: Application
Learning Objective 7-1: Analyze potential community health nursing roles in policy development.
Test Taking Tip: Be aware of the differences in the roles of a community health nurse in policy development.

7.2 As part of a public hearing on amending health policy in the state, the nurse is asked to present identified health issues that directly impact the community and to assess the current health policy. In this role, the nurse is operating as a:
1. Citizen.
2. Activist.
3. Politician.
4. Researcher.

Answer: 4
Rationale: In this situation, the nurse is acting as a researcher. As a community health expert, the nurse is qualified to publicly address the merits and drawbacks of health issues that affect a community and draw upon current research for presentation. Assessing a proposed health policy change for its effect on the community allows the nurse to assess its quality, integrity, and identification of issues as well as review decisions to ensure they reflect current knowledge. A citizen's role is to stay informed, but by speaking as a community expert, the nurse goes beyond that role. In an activist role, the nurse would work for a specific outcome, but in this situation the nurse has been asked to present and comment on health issues. The nurse is not proposing legislative policy issues, so it is not a politician role.
Step in Nursing Process: Evaluation
Category of Client Need: Health Promotion and Maintenance
Cognitive Level: Application
Learning Objective 7-1: Analyze potential community health nursing roles in policy development.
Test Taking Tip: Understand community health nursing roles and their impact on policy development.

7.3 After working many years as a community nurse, the nurse seeks appointment to a statewide board that is in charge of developing strategies to improve health outcomes in the state. This role is best described as:
1. Citizen.
2. Activist.
3. Politician.
4. Researcher.

Answer: 3
Rationale: The nurse can utilize experience as a community nurse to become a front-line policy maker by seeking appointment to a board that can develop and enforce health policy. This is the role of politician. The citizen role is one of an informed voter. The activist role addresses a role that seeks a definite outcome. The researcher role seeks to identify health policy issues, not policy formation or regulation.
Step in Nursing Process: Planning
Category of Client Need: Health Promotion and Maintenance
Cognitive Level: Application
Learning Objective 7-1: Analyze potential community health nursing roles in policy development.
Test Taking Tip: Understand community health nursing roles and their impact on policy development.

7.4 The nurse stays informed of events that impact the community by going to public forums to learn more about various issues. The nurse also joins the state nursing organization. In this role, the nurse is:
1. Citizen.
2. Activist.
3. Politician.
4. Researcher.

Answer: 1
Rationale: By staying informed and participating in public forums, the nurse is acting in the role of citizen. Joining politically active professional nursing organizations to participate in policy development is another activity of the citizen role. The activist role will consciously seek to ensure a set outcome. The politician role involves greater depth, such as seeking appointment to a regulatory body or seeking office to develop policy on the legislative level. The researcher role identifies issues and reviews decisions for quality, integrity, and objectivity based on the data of the policy decisions.
Step in Nursing Process: Implementation
Category of Client Need: Health Promotion and Maintenance
Cognitive Level: Application
Learning Objective 7-1: Analyze potential community health nursing roles in policy development.
Test Taking Tip: Understand community health nursing roles and their impact on policy development.

7.5 The nurse is a member of the state nursing organization, and is asked to speak before a state senate committee about a proposed bill to increase funding to outpatient mental health clinics to improve health outcomes for the mentally ill. Public policy development by this route is known as:
1. Legislation.
2. Administrative decision.
3. Judicial decision.
4. Regulation.

Answer: 1
Rationale: A bill is proposed as part of the legislative process when a formally worded statement of public policy interest is needed to have legal enforcement behind it. Proposing a bill is an avenue for policy development as pending legislation. The nurse addressing a committee regarding the merits of the proposed legislation is engaging in the legislative process by providing the committee with input as to the respective merits or detractions of the legislation. Decisions, administrative or judicial, are made as additions to legislation either through executive orders or through the courts. Regulation addresses legislation implemented by regulatory agencies.
Step in Nursing Process: Assessment
Category of Client Need: Safe, Effective Care Environment
Cognitive Level: Application
Learning Objective 7-2: Discuss three avenues for public policy development.
Test Taking Tip: Understand the avenues for public policy development.

7.6 Amendments to the Nurse Practice Act in the state where the nurse is licensed now require that Advanced Practice Registered Nurses be board certified through a nationally recognized accrediting agency. Enforcement of this amendment is done through:
1. Administrative decision.
2. Legislation.
3. Judicial decision.
4. Regulation.

Answer: 4
Rationale: Regulation addresses how policies are implemented. Regulatory agencies specify how policies are realized in actual behavior. The amendment to the Nurse Practice Act, while done through legislation, is then implemented through a regulatory agency. Administrative and judicial decisions are done by either an executive or judge.
Step in Nursing Process: Implementation
Category of Client Need: Health Promotion and Maintenance
Cognitive Level: Application
Learning Objective 7-2: Discuss three avenues for public policy development.
Test Taking Tip: Understand the avenues for public policy development.

7.7 An amendment to a state law that bans smoking in local music clubs and bars has generated much opposition from the restaurant industry, which cites that it will decrease their business and reduce a tax income to the state. The legislative session where this amendment was proposed expires and the amendment is dead. However, the governor signs an executive order that puts this ban into effect. The restaurant industry sues the state and the court rules in favor of the governor. In this situation, health policy has been developed through: (Select all that apply.)

Answers: 2, 3
Rationale: Though the amendment was proposed through legislation, when the legislative session ended, it rendered the amendment dead. An executive order, as long as it is not in contradiction to existing law, can be done by an executive office (the governor) to create policy. Judicial decisions reflect the court's interpretation of laws, which in this case upheld the administrative decision made through executive order. Regulation is a rule or order with legal force to uphold a procedure following implementation which has not yet occurred. Special interest lobbying was not used in this process.
Step in Nursing Process: Implementation
Category of Client Need: Health Promotion and Maintenance
Cognitive Level: Application
Learning Objective 7-2: Discuss three avenues for public policy development.
Test Taking Tip: Understand the avenues for public policy development.

1. Legislation.
2. Administrative decision.
3. Judicial decision.
4. Regulation.
5. Special interest lobbying.

7.8 The state medical board has proposed legislation to include physicians on the state board of nursing to interpret the Nurse Practice Act. Local nursing organizations have testified in public hearings opposing this measure. What aspect of policy development is this? 1. Administrative decision. 2. Legislation. 3. Judicial decision. 4. Regulation.	Answer: 4 Rationale: When regulations deal with sensitive areas, the regulatory body involved may hold public hearings to solicit input. Including physicians on the state board of nursing to interpret the Nurse Practice Act would affect how nursing is practiced. Therefore nursing input is necessary to support the nursing position on the proposed regulations. Judicial or administrative decisions are not involved at this level, and while it is proposed legislation, it ultimately comes under the jurisdiction of the regulatory agency. Step in Nursing Process: Assessment Category of Client Need: Safe, Effective Management of Care Cognitive Level: Application Learning Objective 7-2: Discuss three avenues for public policy development. Test Taking Tip: Understand the avenues for public policy development.
7.9 Activities and outcomes related to the evaluation aspect of policy development would include: 1. Direction for future policy decisions based on implementation, performance, and impact from the policy. 2. Impact of program performance with interpretation and resource acquisition. 3. Policy statements with alternative development and coalition building. 4. Policy agenda with support mobilization and problem definition.	Answer: 1 Rationale: Evaluating policy development includes evaluating how well the policy is implemented and its performance and impact. Based on whether the implementation, performance, and impact are appropriate or not, the policy may also provide directions for future policy decision. Program performance with interpretation and resource acquisition is part of program implementation, which is not evaluation. Formulation of goals and programs addresses policy statements with alternative developments and coalition building. Setting the agenda involves defining the problem, which leads to a policy agenda. Step in Nursing Process: Evaluation Category of Client Need: Safe, Effective Care Environment Cognitive Level: Application Learning Objective 7-3: Describe at least four aspects of the policy development process. Test Taking Tip: Understand how evaluation reflects the whole and end result of policy development.
7.10 Compromise, negotiation, networking, and coalition building are essential activities in policy development while: 1. Implementing the program as a result of the developed policy. 2. Evaluating how well the policy has been implemented. 3. Formulating the goals and programs to result from the policy. 4. Setting the agenda to define the problem to be addressed by the policy.	Answer: 3 Rationale: Formulating goals and programs for policy development involve compromise, negotiation, networking, and coalition building to collect the data, analyze it, and disseminate it. It involves groups working together toward a mutually acceptable and beneficial policy statement. Policy evaluation is the end stage of evaluation. Implementing the program occurs after formulating the goals of the program. The initial step in policy development is to set the agenda. Step in Nursing Process: Planning Category of Client Need: Safe, Effective Care Environment Cognitive Level: Application Learning Objective 7-3: Describe at least four aspects of the policy development process. Test Taking Tip: Know how related activities are matched with the respective stages of policy development.
7.11 The rational model of policy development most closely resembles the nursing process in that it: 1. Has similar categories to define, implement, and evaluate health policy concerns. 2. Identifies problems, solutions, participants, and opportunities for choice in health policy. 3. Creates windows of opportunity for nurses to influence health policy development.	Answer: 1 Rationale: The rational model mirrors the nursing process in its categories of assessment (defining a problem based on input), diagnosis (identifying a goal for resolution), implementation (determining, prioritizing, and specifying criteria for problem resolution), and evaluation (examining the outcome). Windows of opportunity for nurses to influence health policy development is a feature of Kingdon's policy stream model, part of the political stream. The "garbage can" model identifies problems, solutions, and opportunities for choice in health policy. Alternatives to what is proposed as policy is a feature of the stage-sequential model. Step in Nursing Process: Planning Category of Client Need: Safe, Effective Care Environment Cognitive Level: Application

4. Provides proposed policy alternatives.	Learning Objective 7-3: Describe at least four aspects of the policy development process. Test Taking Tip: Understand how different aspects of policy can be developed.
7.12 Before creating policy and implementing it in the stage-sequential model, the first stage is to: 1. Formulate goals. 2. Implement the program. 3. Set the agenda. 4. Evaluate the process.	Answer: 3 Rationale: In the stage-sequential model of policy development, agenda setting is the first step. In this step, the problem is perceived and defined, and support is mobilized to set a policy agenda. Program implementation follows formulating goals and programs, which comes after agenda setting. Evaluation is the final step in this model. Step in Nursing Process: Planning Category of Client Need: Safe, Effective Care Environment Cognitive Level: Application Learning Objective 7-3: Describe at least four aspects of the policy development process. Test Taking Tip: Understand the steps of the stage-sequential model.
7.13 A health policy is developed that allows for creating housing for homeless men during adverse weather, but no provision is made for homeless families. The evaluation criteria that would best reflect this policy inequity is: 1. Cost. 2. Equity. 3. Feasibility. 4. Appropriateness.	Answer: 2 Rationale: The primary issue with creating homeless accommodations that serve only a male population is that of equity. Health policy needs to reflect equitable distribution of resources. While cost, feasibility, and appropriateness may factor into this, equity is the primary concern. Step in Nursing Process: Evaluation Category of Client Need: Safe, Effective Care Environment Cognitive Level: Analysis Learning Objective 7-4: Identify criteria for health policy evaluation. Test Taking Tip: Be aware of criteria that are used to determine effectiveness of health policy.
7.14 A health policy proposed by the state Department of Health and Human Services addresses creating a charity health system in which all citizens can receive comprehensive preventive health care. While the health system is being debated in the legislature, which criteria for evaluation should be used to assess its potential effectiveness? (Select all that apply.) 1. Cost. 2. Feasibility. 3. Resource needs. 4. Location. 5. Reimbursement guarantees from private insurance.	Answer: 1, 2, 3 Rationale: Cost, feasibility, and resource needs are all evaluation criteria for health policy. Location is not an evaluation criteria for health policy. Reimbursement guarantees do not enter evaluation criteria when developing health policy. Step in Nursing Process: Evaluation Category of Client Need: Health Promotion and Maintenance Cognitive Level: Analysis Learning Objective 7-4: Apply criteria for health policy evaluation. Test Taking Tip: Understand how evaluation criteria are applied to policy.
7.15 The local homeless shelter has a policy that requires that residents have documentation regarding their tuberculosis exposure. A member of the community states that this violates an individual's right to privacy. What evaluation criteria would address this? 1. Resource needs. 2. Equity. 3. Quality. 4. Feasibility.	Answer: 3 Rationale: Health care policies must safeguard individual rights and be capable of implementation or enforcement. Requiring a homeless shelter resident to provide proof of TB status safeguards the other residents and is a measure of the quality of the policy. Resource needs, equity, and feasibility are not addressed by this criterion. Step in Nursing Process: Evaluation Category of Client Need: Safe, Effective Care Environment Cognitive Level: Analysis Learning Objective 7-4: Apply criteria for health policy evaluation. Test Taking Tip: Understand how evaluation criteria can be applied to specific policy situations.
7.16 The most important criterion in evaluating health policy is its: 1. Ability to be implemented. 2. Ability to achieve the desired outcome on the target population.	Answer: 2 Rationale: While all criteria listed are important, the most important is the ability for the policy to have the desired outcome on the target population. If the policy does not have the desired outcome, none of the other criteria listed have any importance. Step in Nursing Process: Evaluation

| 3. Equitable distribution of the health care resources.
4. Effect on the target population. | Category of Client Need: Health Promotion and Maintenance
Cognitive Level: Application
Learning Objective 7-4: Apply criteria for health policy evaluation.
Test Taking Tip: Be able to determine the most important criteria for health policy evaluation. |

CHAPTER 8

8.1 Which of these options is a true statement? (Select all that apply.) 1. Lost productivity from illness has minimal effect on societal outcomes. 2. Educational level is associated with health outcomes. 3. Society benefits from an employed and healthy workforce. 4. Chronic illness in a stable workforce does not impact productivity. 5. Health insurance guarantees a healthy workforce.	Answer: 2, 3 Rationale: The higher the educational level, the higher the societal productivity, which leads to better health outcomes through informed health choices. Health affects the national economic welfare, so an employed and healthy workforce is necessary for an economically healthy society. Chronic illness in a stable workforce impacts productivity, as people with chronic diseases may take more time off for the chronic illness. Lost productivity from illness has a direct effect on societal outcomes, as indicated by WHO statistics that use AIDS as an example. Health insurance does not guarantee a healthy workforce as the insurance may be limiting in coverage or expensive to purchase. Step in Nursing Process: Evaluation Category of Client Need: Health Promotion and Maintenance Cognitive Level: Analysis Learning Objective 8-1: Analyze interrelationships among economic conditions, health care services, and health status. Test Taking Tip: Know the interrelationships between economic conditions and health status.
8.2 In an attempt for economic health reform, block grants are given to states to address health problems. An example of a good use of a block grant to a state would be: 1. Opening statewide immunization centers to provide childhood immunization coverage. 2. Developing a research program to address causes of poverty. 3. Increasing Medicaid coverage for those meeting its qualifications. 4. Developing public education programs to address smoking.	Answer: 1 Rationale: A block grant is a sum of money given to states by the federal government, intended to be used by each state as it sees fit, but within broadly defined parameters. All selections would be potential uses for a block grant. Opening statewide immunization centers to provide immunization coverage is the better choice because it represents a primary prevention mechanism that will protect the population from communicable diseases and improve health status. It will also not use additional health care services. Conducting research and developing education programs are appropriate, but the immunization program is an active direct-services approach. Increasing Medicaid coverage is not an appropriate use for a block grant because federal and state guidelines address Medicaid eligibility. Step in Nursing Process: Assessment Category of Client Need: Health Promotion and Maintenance Cognitive Level: Application Learning Objective 8-1: Analyze interrelationships among economic conditions, health care services, and health status. Test Taking Tip: Discern the best use of a block grant.
8.3 Social instability is a concern for societal health because it can lead to: 1. Poverty. 2. Ill health that results from disruptive economic conditions. 3. Developing alternative methods of health care. 4. Social conflict.	Answer: 2 Rationale: While poverty can impact health, it is not a necessary outcome of social instability. Economic conditions can be disrupted as a result of social instability which can lead to ill health because economic conditions and access to health care services can be affected. Alternative methods to health care are not dependent on social instability and can be developed at any time. Social conflict is not necessarily a result of social instability. Step in Nursing Process: Evaluation Category of Client Need: Health Promotion and Maintenance Cognitive Level: Analysis Learning Objective 8-1: Analyze interrelationships among economic conditions, health care services, and health status. Test Taking Tip: Understand the far-reaching effects of societal conditions on health status.

8.4 One of the biggest concerns influencing the economic health status of the United States now is the:
1. Rise in asthma among children.
2. Baby boom generation.
3. Declining birth rate.
4. Rise of adolescent mental health problems.

Answer: 2
Rationale: As the baby boom generation is aging, they represent a concern to the United States economic health status. They are the largest generation in population size, and are projected to live longer and consume more health resources than any other population group to date. The birth rate in the United States is not declining, and while there are concerns about adolescent mental health problems and the rise of childhood asthma, these do not represent immediate priority concerns regarding the economic health status.
Step in Nursing Process: Assessment
Category of Client Need: Safe, Effective Care Environment
Cognitive Level: Application
Learning Objective 8-2: Discuss factors contributing to escalating health care costs.
Test Taking Tip: Be aware of the ramifications of an aging population.

8.5 The number of physicians in the United States nationwide is sufficient to meet health care needs, but this number has contributed to escalating health care costs due to:
1. Increased numbers of uninsured citizens.
2. Decreased hospital beds nationwide.
3. The higher number of specialists than generalists.
4. More expensive prescription medications being prescribed.

Answer: 3
Rationale: Specialists have higher reimbursements and fees, and represent two-thirds of the physician workforce in the United States; as such, specialists contribute to escalating health care costs. Nationwide hospital beds have not decreased. While there is a large segment of the population who is uninsured, this is not reflected in the number of physicians and there is no evidence that physicians are necessarily prescribing more expensive medications.
Step in Nursing Process: Planning
Category of Client Need: Safe, Effective Care Environment
Cognitive Level: Comprehension
Learning Objective 8-2: Discuss factors contributing to escalating health care costs.
Test Taking Tip: Understand factors that increase health care costs.

8.6 In an economically disadvantaged city, many people receive their health care through charity systems that are set up by local physicians. This can contribute to rising health care costs by:
1. Affecting the consumer price index.
2. Increased use of technology in diagnostic tests.
3. Utilizing hospital beds.
4. Uncompensated care which can lead to cost shifting.

Answer: 4
Rationale: Reimbursement is limited or nonexistent in charity care, so people who utilize this system tend to be uninsured or underinsured. Uncompensated care can lead to cost shifting, where these costs are passed along to those who are able to pay, either out of pocket or through insurance. The consumer price index is not dependent on uncompensated care. Traditionally there is decreased use of technology for underinsured and uninsured populations. There is a finite number of hospital beds, which is unaffected through utilization.
Step in Nursing Process: Evaluation
Category of Client Need: Health Promotion and Maintenance
Cognitive Level: Analysis
Learning Objective 8-2: Discuss factors contributing to escalating health care costs.
Test Taking Tip: Notice how intangibles can affect the rise in health care costs.

8.7 Welfare reform was a needed answer to public demand to curtail costs. One result of welfare reform that has placed a burden on the health sector is:
1. The increase in Medicaid assistance.
2. Prohibiting or restricting immigrants' access to public assistance, thus overburdening uncompensated care.
3. Mandating that all women enter the workforce.
4. Limitation of prenatal care access.

Answer: 2
Rationale: The welfare reform process was designed to encourage welfare-to-work participation among its participants. If anything, the change from the welfare Aid to Families with Dependent Children (AFDC) to the Temporary Assistance for Needy Families (TANF) reduced the numbers of people using Medicaid. Research has indicated that welfare reform had little effect on access to prenatal care. However, welfare reform prohibited immigrants' access to public assistance, thereby increasing the burden of uncompensated care on the health sector.
Step in Nursing Process: Implementation
Category of Client Need: Safe, Effective Care Environment
Cognitive Level: Application
Learning Objective 8-3: Discuss the effects of economic factors on the provision of public health services.
Test Taking Tip: Understand how welfare reform has affected health care access.

8.8 The ability to have health insurance is associated with: (Select all that apply.)
1. Eliminating health disparities.
2. A greater likelihood of receiving health promotive services.

Answers: 2, 3
Rationale: Health disparities address the differences in measures of health status or access to health services, which have been associated with insurance status as well as other factors. Having health insurance does not lessen the difficulty in obtaining health care because there may be restrictions on the type of health insurance a person has. Having health insurance is associated with having a regular source of

3. Having a regular source of care.
4. No difficulty in obtaining health care.
5. Having full-time employment.

care and a greater likelihood of receiving health promotive services. Not all who are employed full-time can afford health insurance as their incomes may be within the gap that is between federal coverage, but too expensive to purchase privately.
Step in Nursing Process: Assessment
Category of Client Need: Health Promotion and Maintenance
Cognitive Level: Application
Learning Objective 8-3: Discuss the effects of economic factors on the provision of public health services.
Test Taking Tip: Recognize that health insurance is not without its limitations.

8.9 As a factor, income inequity has been linked to poorer health status due to:
1. Increased incidence and prevalence of acute and chronic diseases.
2. Numbers of public health clinics.
3. Receiving governmental assistance.
4. The changeover from Aid to Families with Dependent Children (AFDC) to Temporary Assistance for Needy Families (TANF).

Answer: 1
Rationale: Income inequities are linked to increased incidence and prevalence of acute and chronic diseases. People with limited income may not have health insurance or may not be able to access health care services in addition to economic hardships. Allocation of income typically goes to higher priorities, and health care needs usually suffer, which can increase the incidence of chronic and acute conditions. Public health clinics do not enter this equation, nor does the receipt of government assistance, even with the change from AFDC to TANF.
Step in Nursing Process: Evaluation
Category of Client Need: Health Promotion and Maintenance
Cognitive Level: Application
Learning Objective 8-3: Discuss the effects of economic factors on the provision of public health services.
Test Taking Tip: Understand how income inequities exacerbate health problems.

8.10 Public health agencies have traditionally relied on financing health care services for uninsured populations through:
1. Managed care organizations.
2. Private-sector market approaches.
3. Out-of-pocket payment.
4. Government funding.

Answer: 4
Rationale: Public health services provided through public health agencies have relied on government funding. This has led to an underfunding of these services, because government directions have been diverted to homeland security concerns. Public health agencies do not receive funding from managed care organizations or the private sector. They do receive payment from out-of-pocket payments from its users, but this is not their major source of funding.
Step in Nursing Process: Assessment
Category of Client Need: Health Promotion and Maintenance
Cognitive Level: Analysis
Learning Objective 8-4: Distinguish among selected approaches to financing health care services.
Test Taking Tip: Understand the connection between public health care services and government funding of them.

8.11 One of the biggest concerns among the older population in recent years has been the increasing cost of prescription medications. Medicare has addressed this aspect in which section?
1. Part A
2. Part B
3. Part C
4. Part D

Answer: 4
Rationale: Part D is the Medicare Prescription Drug Plan, which was designed to provide drug subsidization for those enrolled in Medicare. Part C, which is the Medicare + Choice, permits Medicare enrollees to exercise similar health care options as others in the population. Part B covers medically necessary provider services not covered under Part A. Part B coverage is optional and requires an additional payment premium. Part A covers medically necessary hospitalization, skilled nursing facility SNF care, some home health care, hospice, and blood products administered in in-patient facilities.
Step in Nursing Process: Implementation
Category of Client Need: Safe, Effective Management of Care
Cognitive Level: Comprehension
Learning Objective 8-4: Distinguish among selected approaches to financing health care services.
Test Taking Tip: Understand what the various parts of Medicare entail.

8.12 There is common confusion about the differences between Medicare and Medicaid among those who are not recipients. What are the differences?
1. Medicare only covers health care services for people over age 65,

Answer: 2
Rationale: As originally legislated, Medicare provided partial coverage of health services to the population who reached the age for receiving Social Security benefits at age 65. Medicaid was established to provide health services to the medically needy, categorically needy, and certain special groups who fell outside of the mainstream for any health care services. Medicare does not cover all health care services, nor does Medicaid. While Medicare traditionally does not cover preventive care, it has started

2. Medicare provides partial coverage for health services when eligible for Social Security benefits and Medicaid provides health services to the indigent.
3. Medicare does not cover preventive services, but Medicaid provides such coverage.
4. Medicare funding is solely on the federal level and Medicaid has no federal funding.

to provide limited coverage of preventive services, as does Medicaid in such services as immunizations. Funding for Medicare comes from the federal level. Medicaid funding is administered by the states, but with block grants given by the federal government.
Step in Nursing Process: Implementation
Category of Client Need: Safe, Effective Care Environment
Cognitive Level: Comprehension
Learning Objective 8-4: Distinguish among selected approaches to financing health care services.
Test Taking Tip: Understand the differences in Medicare and Medicaid.

8.13 The State Children's Health Insurance Program (SCHIP) was established by Congress to provide health insurance coverage for low-income children whose parents did not have insurance coverage or who did not qualify for Medicaid benefits. Transfer of federal oversight and responsibility to the states for this program is a process known as:
1. Shared responsibility.
2. Block grant funding.
3. Devolution.
4. Health care innovation.

Answer: 3
Rationale: The establishment of the SCHIP programs was an attempt by the federal government to provide for health services for low-income children. The federal government gave the states the option of expanding existing Medicaid programs or creating separate CHIP programs. This is devolution, the transfer of responsibility for an area from federal to state government. It is not shared responsibility, block grant funding, or health care innovation.
Step in Nursing Process: Implementation
Category of Client Need: Health Promotion and Maintenance
Cognitive Level: Application
Learning Objective 8-4: Distinguish among selected approaches to financing health care services.
Test Taking Tip: Know how the SCHIP programs differ from Medicaid.

8.14 When health services are paid for by a third party such as private health insurance, the payment is usually called:
1. Retrospective reimbursement.
2. Deductible payment.
3. Prospective reimbursement.
4. Capitation payment.

Answer: 3
Rationale: Third party payment is made through reimbursement for services rendered. Prospective payment is most commonly utilized today, with payment given at a predetermined fixed rate for a specific set of services. Retrospective reimbursement was formerly the primary form of third party payment for services rendered based on the cost of the services. Rising health prices and spiraling insurance health care costs now limit this form of reimbursement because some services were given solely for reimbursement purposes and not for health reasons. Deductible payments are those payments the person makes out of pocket until a limit is reached where the insurance company will take over responsibility for payment. Capitation refers to a prospective payment system that pays health plans or providers a fixed amount per enrollee per month for providing a defined set of health needs.
Step in Nursing Process: Implementation
Category of Client Need: Health Promotion and Maintenance
Cognitive Level: Application
Learning Objective 8-5: Analyze the effects of selected health care reimbursement mechanisms.
Test Taking Tip: Understand the different types of reimbursement.

8.15 It is now rare for an insurance plan to not require some cost sharing with enrollees. Deductible payments are one form of cost sharing. Another form of cost sharing is the:
1. Co-payment made with each health service rendered.
2. Out-of-pocket payment for services not covered by the insurance plan.
3. Current Procedural Terminology (CPT) code utilized by the health service provider.
4. Capitation system.

Answer: 1
Rationale: Co-payments are out-of-pocket payments that the insured has agreed to pay as part of the contract with the insurance provider. Typically, co-payments are made with each health service visit. Out-of-pocket payments as complete payment are made for services not covered under an insurance plan. CPT codes refer to health services coded for billing purposes and reimbursement by providers and do not involve direct payment from the insured person. Capitation does not require co-payment.
Step in Nursing Process: Implementation
Category of Client Need: Safe, Effective Care Environment
Cognitive Level: Application
Learning Objective 8-5: Analyze the effects of selected health care reimbursement mechanisms.
Test Taking Tip: Understand the different ways in which those who have insurance still need to share costs with the insurance provider.

9.1 The American work ethic is considered to be one that is hard-working and individualistic. The work ethic of a population is designated as part of its:
1. Nationality.
2. Ethnicity.
3. Acculturation.
4. Culture.

Answer: 4
Rationale: Culture is a universal experience and can transcend ethnic lines. Ethnicity can be part of culture. In culture, people act in prescribed behavior patterns, though the patterns may have variations from group to group. The American work ethic is considered a cultural characteristic of its citizens. Nationality is the country of birth. Ethnicity is an aggregate of cultural practices and social influences that shape a community's distinct identity. Acculturation is the process of becoming cultured into a group.
Step in Nursing Process: Assessment
Category of Client Need: Health Promotion and Maintenance
Cognitive Level: Analysis
Learning Objective 9-1: Differentiate among culture, race, nationality, and ethnicity.
Test Taking Tip: Understand that culture encompasses different aspects of its citizenry.

9.2 Nursing students from various backgrounds enroll in a university's nursing curriculum. The process by which they become nurses includes aspects of:
1. Worldview.
2. Ethnicity.
3. Acculturation.
4. Culture.

Answer: 3
Rationale: Acculturation is cultural assimilation, where there is acquisition of some beliefs, values, and behaviors of another culture, in this case, nursing. While the students ultimately become part of the nursing culture, they have to be assimilated or undergo acculturation to become part of that culture. Ethnicity is an aggregate of cultural practices, social influences, and racial characteristics which is not part of entering the nursing culture. Worldview refers to how a cultural group views the universe and their relationship to it.
Step in Nursing Process: Implementation
Category of Client Need: Health Promotion and Maintenance
Cognitive Level: Application
Learning Objective 9-1: Differentiate among culture, race, nationality, and ethnicity.
Test Taking Tip: Know how acculturation is distinct from culture.

9.3 While people in the United States are Americans, many citizens may refer to themselves as a hyphenated American, i.e., "Irish-American," "African-American," etc. This term would refer to one's:
1. Ethnicity.
2. Race.
3. Nationality.
4. Culture.

Answer: 1
Rationale: Referring to oneself as a "hyphen-American" is ethnicity, which is an aggregate of cultural practices, social influences, and racial characteristics that shape a distinct identity. Many Americans of different national origins celebrate and practice customs that originated in their ancestors' countries of birth. Nationality is the country of birth. Race is an artificial categorization based on genetic inheritance and appearance. Culture is the sum of the ways of thinking and acting within a group that defines the group. Ethnicity can be present in culture.
Step in Nursing Process: Assessment
Category of Client Need: Health Promotion and Maintenance
Cognitive Level: Application
Learning Objective 9-1: Differentiate among culture, race, nationality, and ethnicity.
Test Taking Tip: Understand the distinct differences among culture, race, nationality, and ethnicity.

9.4 The African-American population of the United States has a higher incidence of cardiovascular disease and diabetes. There is evidence that this could be related to a diet that is:
1. High in fat and sugars.
2. High in starchy vegetables and sugars.
3. Low in fiber-rich foods and exercise.
4. Low in processed foods and fat.

Answer: 1
Rationale: The traditional African-American diet that relies on foods high in fat and sugars is connected to the high rates of cardiovascular disease and diabetes in the United States. It also has historical roots in foods that were affordable on very limited incomes, which tended to be the fattier meats and foods with sugar. A diet low in processed food and fats helps to eliminate these risk factors. Fiber-rich foods in addition to exercise contribute to cardiovascular and diabetes prevention. While starchy vegetables and sugars can contribute to diabetes, the fat content is a determinant in cardiovascular disease.
Step in Nursing Process: Evaluation
Category of Client Need: Health Promotion and Maintenance
Cognitive Level: Application
Learning Objective 9-2: Discuss direct and indirect influences of culture on health and health care.
Test Taking Tip: Understand how traditional patterns of eating can influence health.

9.5 It is not uncommon when conducting health teaching to an older person of Asian background for that person to agree to questions posed by the nurse. What would be a more reliable method to determine that person's understanding of the health teaching?

1. Have another member of the person's family do the teaching.
2. Ask the person to give an explanation, in their own words, of the health teaching.
3. Ensure that there is an interpreter nearby while doing the health teaching.
4. Use simple language that the person can understand.

Answer: 2

Rationale: There is a great respect for authority among older people of Asian background. As such, they tend to agree with what is being said or done rather than question it, even if only for clarity of understanding. It would be considered disrespectful to question authority. The nurse could elicit understanding of the person by asking them to explain what was taught—essentially a "return demonstration". There is no indication that the person does not understand English; therefore an interpreter may not be necessary. A family member might wish to be present, but it is not necessary to the success of the health teaching. Using simple language is not the most reliable method to determine the person's understanding of the health teaching; it would be best to elicit understanding of the person by asking them to explain what was taught.

Step in Nursing Process: Evaluation
Category of Client Need: Health Promotion and Maintenance
Cognitive Level: Application
Learning Objective 9-2: Discuss direct and indirect influences of culture on health and health care.
Test Taking Tip: Be aware of cultural influences on the perception of health providers.

9.6 The nurse performs a home visit for a client who is originally from Mexico. The nurse notices that the client seems somewhat passive during the health teaching and when questions are asked about the client's home treatment course. Based on the nurse's assessment, which of the following is the most accurate reason for the client's behavior?

1. The client is not interested in what the nurse is doing.
2. The client probably does not understand English.
3. There may be cultural factors that explain the client's behavior.
4. The client may be uncomfortable with having the nurse in the home.

Answer: 3

Rationale: The client's cultural background may influence how the client responds to questions and teaching. In the Mexican culture, it is expected that the nurse, as the authority figure, will take care of all the client's needs. The nurse may perceive this as disinterest. The client assumes a dependent position in healthcare. There is no indication that the client is not fluent in English, or that there is discomfort in having the nurse perform a home visit.

Step in Nursing Process: Assessment
Category of Client Need: Health Promotion and Maintenance
Cognitive Level: Application
Learning Objective 9-2: Discuss direct and indirect influences of culture on health and health care.
Test Taking Tip: Understand how different ethnic groups can perceive health care.

9.7 The most important facet to developing cultural competence is for the nurse to:

1. Gain proficiency in another language beyond English.
2. Identify the goals for culturally competent care.
3. Understand the culture of the client.
4. Understand and recognize the nurse's own cultural background.

Answer: 4

Rationale: Until the nurse can understand and acknowledge the cultural background from which the nurse operates, it will be very difficult to develop cultural competence. Gaining proficiency in another language and understanding the client's culture is important to developing cultural competence as well as understanding the goals of culturally competent care, but less important than the nurse understanding and recognizing his or her own cultural background.

Step in Nursing Process: Assessment
Category of Client Need: Health Promotion and Maintenance
Cognitive Level: Application
Learning Objective 9-3: Describe cultural competence.
Test Taking Tip: Understand the ways in which the nurse can become the most culturally competent.

9.8 Steps to developing cultural competence in the community include which of the following? (Select all that apply)

1. Maintaining an up-to-date demographic, cultural, and epidemiologic community profile.
2. Ensuring that health clinics employ minority staff to deliver care.

Answer: 1, 3, 5

Rationale: Maintaining an up-to-date community demographic profile and engaging in partnerships to help design relevant services are two measures to help develop culturally competent care. Employing minority staff and treating all clients the same way does not indicate cultural competence and could actually be offensive to the clients. It is important to recognize that differences within subgroups of a particular culture may exist.

Step in Nursing Process: Implementation
Category of Client Need: Health Promotion and Maintenance

3. Engaging in community partnerships to help design culturally relevant services. 4. Ensuring that all clients are treated in the same manner. 5. Recognizing subgroup differences within cultural groups.	Cognitive Level: Application Learning Objective 9-3: Describe cultural competence. Test Taking Tip: Know that cultural competence has several steps and layers.
9.9 A community has had an influx of immigrant workers due to the new construction in the community. The staff of the local public health clinic know the level of their care meets and exceeds standards set and do not see a need to change. The staff could be displaying: 1. Cultural competence. 2. Cultural proficiency. 3. Cultural blindness. 4. Cultural destructiveness.	Answer: 3 Rationale: Treating everyone alike and ignoring cultural differences such as this example, with an influx of an immigrant population, is cultural blindness. Cultural destructiveness happens when the dominant culture in the organization believes other cultures are inferior. Cultural proficiency occurs when the organization is proactive with diversity and seeks to incorporate it. Cultural competence is the result of the products of developing culturally sensitive care. Step in Nursing Process: Implementation Category of Client Need: Health Promotion and Maintenance Cognitive Level: Application Learning Objective 9-4: Identify barriers to cultural competence. Test Taking Tip: Understand how barriers to cultural competence can impede care.
9.10 The local clinic employs a Hispanic receptionist, who is also used as an interpreter for the many non-English speaking Latino clients who utilize the clinic. Members of the staff believe the clients should learn English, and they have refused offers from the receptionist to learn some basic phrases. They are hindering culturally competent care through: 1. Cultural destructiveness. 2. Cultural blindness. 3. Cultural pre-competence. 4. Cultural incapacity.	Answer: 4 Rationale: A token minority staff is employed to aid clients who cannot speak English and the staff feels no need to change. This is cultural incapacity. Cultural destructiveness occurs when organization members believe others are inferior to the dominant culture and no attempt is made to promote cultural diversity in the workforce. Cultural blindness fails to recognize the differences among cultures and the influence of culture on health and health care. Cultural pre-competence has the organization planning to be culturally competent, but displays complacence based on minimal effort toward that goal. Step in Nursing Process: Implementation Category of Client Need: Health Promotion and Maintenance Cognitive Level: Application Learning Objective 9-4: Identify barriers to cultural competence. Test Taking Tip: Understand how cultural destructiveness and cultural incapacity differ.
9.11 A local hospital has established outreach clinics in the community to provide health care. Several staff members within the clinic component refuse to go to some of the outreach clinics claiming that the clinics are in a bad section of the community and the residents there are not interested in health promotion. These staff members are displaying: 1. Cultural destructiveness. 2. Cultural blindness. 3. Cultural incapacity. 4. Cultural pre-competence.	Answer: 1 Rationale: Cultural destructiveness occurs when members of the organization lack cultural knowledge. Linking an area of a community with a preconceived idea of its residents contributes to cultural destructiveness. Cultural incapacity occurs when there is token minority representation with no attempt to engage in any cross-cultural training. Cultural blindness is where the organization treats everyone the same way. Cultural pre-competence is where the organization makes plans for cultural competence, but is complacent about its efforts toward it. Step in Nursing Process: Implementation Category of Client Need: Health Promotion and Maintenance Cognitive Level: Application Learning Objective 9-4: Identify barriers to cultural competence. Test Taking Tip: Know the differences among the barriers to cultural competence.
9.12 An important component in a cultural assessment of a group is to: (Select all that apply.) 1. Come prepared with prior research done on the group. 2. Talk and interview members of the group. 3. Look for similarities in one's own group. 4. Ask personal questions about the group.	Answer: 2, 3 Rationale: Talking with members of the group can provide insights into the group's culture. Looking for similarities in the group with one's own group can help the nurse understand the group culture. While doing prior research on a group is acceptable, it could also cause the nurse to have pre-conceived ideas. Asking personal questions may be resented by group members, so this should be ascertained before asking such questions. Acknowledging the group's reliance on alternative therapies implies stereotyping a group and is not part of a cultural assessment process. Step in Nursing Process: Assessment Category of Client Need: Health Promotion and Maintenance Cognitive Level: Application

5. Acknowledge the group's reliance on alternative therapies.

Learning Objective 9-5: Conduct a cultural assessment of an individual, family, group, or health system.
Test Taking Tip: Understand basic concepts to a cultural assessment of a group.

9.13 A nurse's client sees a physician for his health needs as well as a practitioner of Chinese medicine. The client states that both therapies are beneficial for maintaining the client's level of health. The nurse supports the client's choice after being reassured that the Chinese practitioner has met standards for: (Select all that apply.)
1. Safety, efficacy, and quality in the Chinese medicine practice.
2. USDA standards in the herbal preparations used.
3. No adverse interactions between herbal preparations used and any prescription medications the client might be on.
4. Causing no additional stress on the client.
5. Nationwide certification in Chinese medicine.

Answers: 1, 3, 4
Rationale: The client is utilizing complementary alternative therapy (CAT) with the combination of Western and Chinese medicine. The World Health Organization (WHO) has identified safety, efficacy, and quality as a consideration for CAT. CAT should put no additional stress on the client, nor should the Chinese herbal preparations used have any adverse interaction with any prescribed medication. While the USDA has some regulatory control with herbal preparations, it cannot set standards for their usage, because herbal preparations are considered supplements and not medication. Nationwide certification in Chinese medicine is not required for the practice of Chinese medicine.
Step in Nursing Process: Evaluation
Category of Client Need: Health Promotion and Maintenance
Cognitive Level: Application
Learning Objective 9-5: Conduct a cultural assessment of an individual, family, group, or health system.
Test Taking Tip: Understand how CAT can be utilized in a cultural assessment.

9.14 An organization that is delivering culturally competent care is characterized by:
1. Treating all who utilize its services in the same manner.
2. Providing services that are accepting and respectful of diverse populations.
3. Having conscious adaptation of care to the cultural context.
4. Being aware of personal perspectives.

Answer: 2
Rationale: An organization that is culturally competent displays acceptance and respect for other cultures. Its mission and policies support services for diverse populations and adherence to this is monitored. Treating all clients in the same manner is closer to cultural blindness. Conscious adaptation of care to the cultural context and awareness of personal perspectives are characteristics of individual cultural competence.
Step in Nursing Process: Evaluation
Category of Client Need: Health Promotion and Maintenance
Cognitive Level: Comprehension
Learning Objective 9-6: Design, implement, and evaluate culturally competent care and health care delivery systems.
Test Taking Tip: Know the differences in cultural competence in individuals versus organizations.

9.15 The health clinic staff is working on becoming culturally competent. Strategies for attempting to develop this competence might include: (Select all that apply.)
1. Increasing the diversity of the staff providing care.
2. Soliciting input from various cultural organizations.
3. Concluding that their current method of care delivery needs little modification.
4. Holding cultural training sessions for its staff members.
5. Developing a competence in the languages spoken by the client population.

Answers: 1, 2, 4, 5
Rationale: Developing culturally competent care includes additional staff from diverse cultures, soliciting input from community cultural organizations and holding training sessions for staff members, among other strategies. Developing culturally competent care would also involve analyzing their current care delivery for cultural appropriateness; it would still need modification in order to become truly culturally competent. Developing a competence in the languages spoken by the client population would allow for better communication and understanding between the health clinic staff and the clients seen.
Step in Nursing Process: Implementation
Category of Client Need: Health Promotion and Maintenance
Cognitive Level: Application
Learning Objective 9-6: Design, implement, and evaluate culturally competent care and health care delivery systems.
Test Taking Tip: Know the various methods and strategies to design culturally competent care.

CHAPTER 10

10.1 Global warming is affecting human health by increasing the:
1. Temperature of the Gulf of Mexico, resulting in more intense hurricanes that have increased loss of human life.
2. Amount of air pollution from burning fossil fuels, leading to increased respiratory diseases.
3. Environmental radiation exposure from nuclear power plants.
4. Numbers of children affected by lead paint exposure.

Answer: 1
Rationale: Global warming has increased ocean and Gulf water temperatures that increase the depth and severity of hurricanes, which has led to increased loss of life. Air pollution from fossil fuels is not an effect of global warming, nor is radiation exposure from nuclear power plants. Lead exposure from paint has no relation to global warming.
Step in Nursing Process: Evaluation
Category of Client Need: Health Promotion and Maintenance
Cognitive Level: Application
Learning Objective 10-1: Analyze the interrelationships among environmental factors and human health.
Test Taking Tip: Know the effects from increased water temperature.

10.2 An oil storage tank has leaked and the surrounding residential area has been saturated with the leaked oil. Among the health precautions the homeowner should take are:
1. Use a strong detergent to clean their yards.
2. Avoid planting vegetables in the contaminated soil.
3. Install smoke detectors in the homes as a fire precaution.
4. Inform the local media regarding the contaminant spill.

Answer: 2
Rationale: Planting vegetables in the soil should be avoided until the soil can be certified as safe. Growing and consuming food grown in contaminated soil can lead to illness from the contaminants. While detergents can be used to clean the yards, these detergents need to be appropriate to avoid further soil contamination. Installing smoke detectors as a fire precaution is unnecessary because the oil-saturated soil will not burn. Informing the local media is not going to protect health.
Step in Nursing Process: Implementation
Category of Client Need: Safe, Effective Management of Care
Cognitive Level: Application
Learning Objective 10-1: Analyze the interrelationships among environmental factors and human health.
Test Taking Tip: Connect how soil contaminants can impact health.

10.3 The local community has no zoning plan and as such, the community has a coal-fired energy plant located next to a residential area. There is a higher rate of respiratory disease among the residents who are in closer proximity to the plant. This phenomenon could be explained by:
1. Urban sprawl.
2. The community ecological footprint.
3. Poor land use mix.
4. The built environment.

Answer: 3
Rationale: Land use mix refers to an environment that has a mix of residential, commercial, and non-commercial uses. In a community with no zoning regulations, the land use mix is haphazard, resulting in a fuel plant that is located next to a residential area. A coal-fired fuel plant will have emissions that can lead to respiratory conditions. The built environment includes buildings and spaces, but is not the appropriate answer. Urban sprawl refers to communities that are built beyond set geographic limits. The ecological footprint refers to the area of biologically productive space required for a person.
Step in Nursing Process: Assessment
Category of Client Need: Health Promotion and Maintenance
Cognitive Level: Application
Learning Objective 10-2: Discuss elements of the natural, built, and social environments that affect population health.
Test Taking Tip: Understand how elements of the environment can affect population health.

10.4 A once prosperous and thriving neighborhood has become run down and its residents have a lower socioeconomic status. There is greater unemployment in this neighborhood and the police have seen a rise in crime in unemployed young adults. This is an effect of a declining:
1. Built environment.
2. Natural environment.
3. Social environment.
4. Ecological environment.

Answer: 3
Rationale: A once thriving neighborhood that is now run down, with a higher amount of lower socioeconomic residents and higher unemployment, will see an effect on health through the decreasing of the neighborhood quality. A variety of factors will impact health, from a rise in crime to other factors that include potentially more environmental toxins, crowding, etc. than more affluent areas. Natural environment refers to the flora and fauna of an area. Built environment refers to buildings and spaces created by people. Ecologic environment is the interaction of the natural, built, and social environments.
Step in Nursing Process: Evaluation
Category of Client Need: Health Promotion and Maintenance
Cognitive Level: Application

10.5 The nurse is working with local schools on an asthma program for its students. The nurse performs home visits to students who are diagnosed with asthma. One of the factors assessed in the home environment is the presence of:
1. Pesticides.
2. Peeling paint.
3. A fuel source for cooking.
4. Secondhand smoke.

Answer: 4
Rationale: Exposure to secondhand smoke can lead to exacerbations of asthma in children. The nurse is using the role of surveillance to determine factors in the home environment that could trigger asthma attacks. While pesticides could present a factor, secondhand smoke is a more indicative factor. Peeling paint and fuel source for cooking are not factors in asthma attacks.
Step in Nursing Process: Assessment
Category of Client Need: Health Promotion and Maintenance
Cognitive Level: Application
Learning Objective 10-3: Analyze the roles of the community health nurse with respect to environmental health issues at the individual, family, and population levels, and the role of the community health nurse in this implementation.
Test Taking Tip: Understand the role of the nurse in linking environment to health.

10.6 After a series of heavy rains, the nurse in the local health department increases the water monitoring of the local beach because several upstream creeks flow into it. Which of the following is the most accurate reason for the monitoring?
1. To make sure that tidal currents are safe for swimming.
2. To monitor the water for potential microorganisms that could prevent safe swimming.
3. To monitor the water purity of the creek flow.
4. To make sure that no debris is swept into the water.

Answer: 2
Rationale: After heavy rains, water is stirred up, especially when other water sources drain into the water, such as from upstream creeks. This can impair the water quality, making it unsafe for swimming due to a potential increase in microorganisms. Tidal currents do not require water monitoring. Routine monitoring of the creek's water purity is important, but it is more of a priority after heavy rains, which can stir up the bottom when the water level rises. Monitoring water quality has no bearing on whether debris is swept into the water.
Step in Nursing Process: Evaluation
Category of Client Need: Health Promotion and Maintenance
Cognitive Level: Application
Learning Objective 10-3: Analyze the role of the community health nurse with respect to environmental health issues at the individual/family and population levels.
Test Taking Tip: Understand the population impact of water quality on recreation.

10.7 A section of the community has flooded over the past several years after heavy rains. This section of the community never previously flooded, but has undergone tremendous development within the past five years. Which of the following would be the most accurate explanation for the standing water?
1. The drainage system has not been inspected regularly.
2. There are insufficient storm sewers to handle the increased development.
3. The development has increased the amount of impervious surfaces that do not absorb the rain water.
4. There has been an overall change in the precipitation patterns in the region.

Answer: 3
Rationale: Increased development can result in paving land, which creates impervious surfaces that would otherwise be able to absorb rainwater. This leads to increased standing water after heavy rains. There is no indication that weather patterns have changed, or that the drainage system or storm sewers are involved or are inadequate.
Step in Nursing Process: Assessment
Category of Client Need: Health Promotion and Maintenance
Cognitive Level: Application
Learning Objective 10-4: Identify factors in the natural, built, and social environments that influence the health of an individual/family or a selected population group.
Test Taking Tip: Understand how factors in the environment can impact a community's living conditions.

10.8 Due to budget cuts, the community has reduced its garbage pickup frequency from twice a week to once a week. However, residents complain to the local government

Answer: 1
Rationale: A cutback in the collection of garbage can allow it to pile up, which increases the potential for animal pests around the garbage and to potentially spread disease. Despite making the area look unsightly, this does not have the potential to affect health, nor do weeds from uncollected grass clippings. The amount of trash

because they fear this could lead to an increase in:
1. Animal pests that could spread disease.
2. Making the area look unsightly.
3. Spreading weeds from uncollected grass clippings.
4. The amount of trash generated per household.

generated per household is not likely to increase; it will only accumulate from it being collected less frequently.
Step in Nursing Process: Evaluation
Category of Client Need: Health Promotion and Maintenance
Cognitive Level: Application
Learning Objective 10-4: Identify factors in the natural, built, and social environments that influence the health of an individual/family or a selected population.
Test Taking Tip: Understand how social factors can have a potential impact on health.

10.9 Environmental factors that negatively influence health include: (Select all that apply)
1. Green space in communities.
2. Urban sprawl.
3. Disparities in socioeconomic status.
4. Gang violence.
5. Organized recreation programs.

Answers: 2, 3, 4
Rationale: All answers influence health. Urban sprawl, disparities in socioeconomic status and gang violence have negative impacts on health. Green space in communities can contribute to exercise and mental relaxation, which improve health. Organized recreation programs can provide creative outlets for the community members, which improves health.
Step in Nursing Process: Evaluation
Category of Client Need: Health Promotion and Maintenance
Cognitive Level: Comprehension
Learning Objective 10-4: Identify factors in the natural, built, and social environments that influence the health of an individual/family or a selected population group.
Test Taking Tip: Understand how positive and negative environmental factors influence health.

10.10 The nurse is aware that the poison control hotline has received an increase in calls. Based on this information, the nurse should:
1. Target homes for poisons contained in household cleaning agents.
2. Enforce local ordinances for selling household chemical agents.
3. Promote legislation for restricting hazardous materials in the home.
4. Educate the public about the hazards of household chemicals and medications and their proper storage.

Answer: 4
Rationale: Educating the public about the hazards of household chemicals and medications and appropriate storage is a primary prevention intervention the nurse should use for poison control. Targeting homes for poisons does not represent an intervention. Enforcing local ordinances is not a realistic responsibility of the nurse. Promoting legislation is an appropriate action, but will not necessarily result in a decrease in hotline calls.
Step in Nursing Process: Planning
Category of Client Need: Health Promotion and Maintenance
Cognitive Level: Application
Learning Objective 10-5: Analyze the role of the community health nurse in primary prevention measures for environmental issues that affect population health.
Test Taking Tip: Understand primary prevention strategies for environmental health.

10.11 The amount of trash collected in the community is overwhelming local resources to collect and store it. The best approach the nurse can take to aid in helping decrease the amount of generated trash is:
1. Educating the community about overbuying household products.
2. Discouraging overuse of materials that generate trash.
3. Promoting recycling efforts in the community.
4. Encouraging use of fewer polluting products.

Answer: 3
Rationale: Promoting recycling efforts can decrease the garbage stream, the amount of trash generated, and landfill space. In addition, recycling can promote energy conservation, which reduces use of fossil fuels. Educating the community about overbuying household products does not necessarily mean that garbage generation would decrease. Educating about the use of fewer polluting products or discouraging use of trash-generating materials also does not mean that garbage generation would decrease.
Step in Nursing Process: Implementation
Category of Client Need: Health Promotion and Maintenance
Cognitive Level: Application
Learning Objective 10-5: Analyze the role of community health nurses in primary prevention measures for environmental issues that affect population health.
Test Taking Tip: Understand how promoting one aspect of environmental health can have far-reaching effects.

10.12 In a community known for its older homes, many young couples are renovating houses. A prevention measure to ensure the safety of these families would be to:
1. Encourage the safe removal of lead-based paint in the homes.

Answer: 1
Rationale: A primary prevention measure for an older home would be to encourage the removal of any lead-based paint. Screening and monitoring lead levels are secondary prevention measures. Chelation therapy is a tertiary prevention measure.
Step in Nursing Process: Implementation
Category of Client Need: Health Promotion and Maintenance
Cognitive Level: Application

2. Screen all members for lead levels.
3. Monitor lead levels in the family members.
4. Institute chelating measures for lead removal in the family members.

Learning Objective 10-5: Analyze the role of community health nurses in primary prevention measures for environmental issues that affect population health.
Test Taking Tip: Distinguish among primary, secondary, and tertiary prevention measures for environmental issues that affect population health.

10.13 The nurse notices that a child in the neighborhood does not play as energetically as before. Knowing that the parents are renovating their older house, the nurse encourages the parents to:
1. Have the child go to bed earlier.
2. Eat more foods with protein.
3. Screen the child for serum lead levels.
4. Screen the child for hearing difficulties.

Answer: 3
Rationale: During a house renovation, particularly in a house built before 1970, there is a possibility that the house may have lead paint. Children should be screened for lead levels if there has been a change in activity or affect. Having an earlier bedtime or eating a protein-rich diet will have no effect if lead levels are high. Screening for hearing difficulties is not an appropriate intervention if lead exposure is suspected.
Step in Nursing Process: Implementation
Category of Client Need: Safe, Effective Care Environment
Cognitive Level: Application
Learning Objective 10-6: Identify secondary and tertiary prevention measures for individuals or populations affected by environmental health problems and the role of the community health nurse in their implementation.
Test Taking Tip: Understand the role of screening as an effective secondary prevention measure.

10.14 Mosquito control services have been reduced in the community and the nurse is concerned about the rise of mosquito-borne diseases. Effective secondary prevention community intervention measures would include: (Select all that apply.)
1. Promoting accessibility of diagnostic and treatment services for diseases caused by mosquitoes.
2. Monitoring the incidence of diseases caused by mosquitoes.
3. Promoting ordinances that control insect breeding areas.
4. Instituting an education program about insect control.
5. Installing sentinel chicken monitoring stations in local firehouses.

Answer: 1, 2, 5
Rationale: Promoting accessibility and treatment services and monitoring incidence of diseases caused by mosquitoes, including the installation of sentinel chicken monitoring stations in local firehouses, are secondary prevention measures that are aimed at protecting the population. Promoting ordinances and instituting an education program about insect control are examples of primary prevention.
Step in Nursing Process: Implementation
Category of Client Need: Safe, Effective Care Environment
Cognitive Level: Application
Learning Objective 10-6: Identify secondary and tertiary prevention measures for individuals or populations affected by environmental health problems.
Test Taking Tip: Differentiate between primary and secondary prevention measures.

10.15 After a hurricane has devastated the community, the nurse becomes involved in local recovery efforts. An effective tertiary prevention measure to aid in the recovery would be to:
1. Promote environmental policies to prevent recurrence of problems that result from environmental changes caused by the hurricane.
2. Promote legislation to reduce pollutant emissions.
3. Promote replacement of hazard-producing industrial processes.
4. Screen for the effects of environmental changes that result from the hurricane.

Answer: 1
Rationale: Promoting environmental policies to prevent recurrence is a tertiary measure. Damage has already occurred and the objective is to restore capability to its optimal level. Promoting legislation and screening are secondary measures. Promoting replacement of hazard-producing processes is a primary measure.
Step in Nursing Process: Implementation
Category of Client Need: Safe Effective Care Environment
Cognitive Level: Application
Learning Objective 10-6: Identify secondary and tertiary prevention measures for individuals or populations affected by environmental health problems and the role of the community health nurse in their implementation.
Test Taking Tip: Understand where tertiary prevention measures fit within environmental health.

CHAPTER 11

11.1 Health promotion involves:
1. Education about healthy behavior, which leads to behavioral change.
2. Behavior manipulation through transfer of knowledge.
3. Informing the client about the nature and causes of illness.
4. Enabling clients and reforming social structures.

Answer: 4
Rationale: Health promotion enables clients, empowers them, and also reforms social structures. Knowledge of healthy behavior does not lead to behavioral change. Health promotion rejects manipulation of behavior but focuses on increasing one's capacity to act rather than be acted upon. Health education includes informing the client about the nature and causes of illness.
Step in Nursing Process: Implementation
Category of Client Need: Health Promotion and Maintenance
Cognitive Level: Comprehension
Learning Objective 11-3: Define health promotion.
Test Taking Tip: Review the definition of health promotion.

11.2 The nurse is comparing and contrasting examples of health promotion and health education to a group of student nurses. Which of the following topics is most appropriate to include in health education?
1. Political lobbying.
2. Raising critical consciousness.
3. Developing self-care skills.
4. Developing public policy.

Answer: 3
Rationale: Health education includes development of self-care skills. Political lobbying, raising critical consciousness, and developing public policy are part of health promotion, not health education.
Step in Nursing Process: Assessment
Category of Client Need: Safe Effective Care Environment
Cognitive Level: Analysis
Learning Objective 11-2: Distinguish health promotion from health education.
Test Taking Tip: Recognize the differences between health promotion and health education.

11.3 There has been an outbreak of measles at a local high school. The nurse is encouraging students to take the measles immunization. Those who are susceptible are reminded of the serious consequences of measles. The nurse educates the students on the benefits of the immunization. Most students decide the benefits outweigh the barriers to the immunization. The model used to guide health promotion in this situation is the:
1. Precaution Adoption Process model.
2. Health Belief model.
3. Precede-Proceed model.
4. Theory of Reasoned Action model.

Answer: 2
Rationale: The Health Belief model includes individual perceptions of susceptibility and seriousness, modifying factors, perceptions of benefits and barriers to action, and cues to action. The Precaution Adoption Process model describes the stages that occur in decisions to adopt or not adopt a health-related behavior. The Precede-Proceed model reflects diagnostic activities that take place prior to planning health promotion activities. The Theory of Reasoned Action model is based on the premises that attitudes to a health-related behavior reflect a person's attitudes to the expected consequences of the behavior, and attitudes are the product of subjective norms influenced by others.
Step in Nursing Process: Implementation
Category of Client Need: Health Promotion and Maintenance
Cognitive Level: Analysis
Learning Objective 11-3: Describe selected models for health promotion practice.
Test Taking Tip: Differentiate between the various health promotion models.

11.4 The nurse is using the premise that attitudes to a health-related behavior reflect a person's attitudes to the expected consequences of the behavior. The nurse is using the:
1. Theory of Reasoned Action model.
2. Pender Health Promotion model.
3. Precaution Adoption Process model.
4. Health Belief model.

Answer: 1
Rationale: The Theory of Reasoned Action model is based on two premises. The first premise is that attitudes to a health-related behavior reflect a person's attitudes to the expected consequences; the second premise is that attitudes are the product of subjective norms influenced by others. Pender's Health Promotion model directs nursing interventions for health promotion. Pender's model describes behavior being influenced by attitudes and behavior-specific cognitions and affect that result in a commitment to action. The Precaution Adoption Process model describes the stages that occur in decisions to adopt or not adopt a health-related behavior. The Health Belief model includes individual perceptions of susceptibility and seriousness, modifying factors, perceptions of benefits and barriers to actions, and cues to action.
Step in Nursing Process: Planning
Category of Client Need: Health Promotion and Maintenance
Cognitive Level: Analysis
Learning Objective 11-3: Describe selected models for health promotion practice.
Test Taking Tip: Differentiate between the various health promotion models.

11.5 The health promotion strategy that emphasizes enhancing people's motivation to act and that reflects the view of personal agency is:
  1. Empowerment.
  2. Social marketing.
  3. Health education.
  4. Manipulation.

Answer: 2
Rationale: Social marketing emphasizes enhancing people's motivation to act and reflects the view of personal agency. Empowerment focuses on the environmental conditions that affect people's abilities to act in ways that promote health. Health education provides the information and skills that are part of the strategies of empowerment and social marketing. Manipulation is not a health promotion strategy.
Step in Nursing Process: Implementation
Category of Client Need: Health Promotion and Maintenance
Cognitive Level: Application
Learning Objective 11-4: Identify three strategies for health promotion.
Test Taking Tip: Differentiate among the various health promotion strategies.

11.6 A group of community leaders is using radio and television messages to try to educate high school students about the consequences of smoking. The social marketing "P" that the radio and television messages represent is:
  1. Product.
  2. Price.
  3. Place.
  4. Promotion.

Answer: 4
Rationale: Promotion refers to the communication strategies used, which in this situation is educating students about the consequences of smoking. The product is the need or service that the target audience is being asked to adopt, in this case not smoking. Price reflects the cost of or barriers to giving up an unhealthy behavior (e.g., weight gain, not seeming "cool"). The place is the location where the product or service can be obtained (e.g., location of smoking cessation services).
Step in Nursing Process: Implementation
Category of Client Need: Health Promotion and Maintenance
Cognitive Level: Application
Learning Objective11- 5: Describe the four Ps of social marketing.
Test Taking Tip: Know how the four Ps are used in social marketing.

11.7 A group of community leaders is using radio and television messages to try to educate high school students about the consequences of smoking. The social marketing "P" represented by not smoking is:
  1. Product.
  2. Price.
  3. Place.
  4. Promotion.

Answer: 1
Rationale: The product is the need or service that the target audience is being asked to adopt; in this case not smoking. Price reflects the cost of or barriers to giving up an unhealthy behavior; in this case the price or barrier could be peer pressure. The place is the location where the product or service can be obtained. Promotion refers to the communication strategies used, in this case radio and television messages but this does not reflect the specific desired outcome of not smoking. Policy refers to laws and regulations that influence the behavior at issue, such as high school policies regarding the students smoking.
Step in Nursing Process: Implementation
Category of Client Need: Health Promotion and Maintenance
Cognitive Level: Application
Learning Objective 10-5: Describe the four Ps of social marketing.
Test Taking Tip: Know how the four Ps are used in social marketing.

11.8 Giving residents a voice in designing communities to promote healthy living is an example of:
  1. Health education.
  2. Empowerment.
  3. Social marketing.
  4. Health learning.

Answer: 2
Rationale: Empowerment focuses on the environmental conditionals that affect people's abilities to act in ways that promote health. Health education provides the information and skills that are a part of empowerment and social marketing. Social marketing emphasizes enhancing people's motivation to act and reflects the view of personal agency. Health learning is a type of learning that is a desired result of the health education encounter.
Step in Nursing Process: Implementation
Category of Client Need: Health Promotion and Maintenance
Cognitive Level: Application
Learning Objective 11-6: Analyze the significance of empowerment for health promotion.
Test Taking Tip: Understand empowerment.

11.9 The goals of health education, according to the Joint Commission on Accreditation of HealthCare Organizations (JCAHO), include: (Select all that apply.)
  1. Client participation in health decision making.
  2. Increased potential to comply with health recommendations.

Answers: 1, 2, 4
Rationale: The Joint Commission on Accreditation of HealthCare Organizations (JCAHO) has identified six goals of health education in the acute care setting. The six goals include: client participation in health decision making; increased potential to comply with health recommendations; development of self-care skills; improved client and family coping; increased participation in continuing care for specific conditions; and adoption of healthier lifestyles. Dependence on the health care system is not one of the goals of health education in the acute care setting, and lack of reliance on the health care system is not one of the goals.

3. Dependence on the health care system. 4. Adoption of healthier lifestyles. 5. Lack of reliance on the health care system.	Step in Nursing Process: Assessment Category of Client Need: Health Promotion and Maintenance Cognitive Level: Comprehension Learning Objective 11-7: Describe the health education process. Test Taking Tip: Understand the health education process.
11.10 The nurse is designing a health education program for the community. The initial step should be to: 1. Prioritize learning needs. 2. Write specific outcomes. 3. Assess the community. 4. Select teaching strategies.	Answer: 3 Rationale: The health education program begins with assessing the community. Prioritizing learning needs would follow the assessment. Writing specific outcomes would follow and then teaching strategies would be selected. Step in Nursing Process: Assessment Category of Client Need: Health Promotion and Maintenance Cognitive Level: Comprehension Learning Objective 11-8: Design and implement a health education program for a selected population. Test Taking Tip: Be able to explain the steps in designing a health education program.
11.11 The best definition of health literacy is the ability to 1. Use the information and services to enhance health. 2. Read and explain the health information. 3. Read, write, and interpret the health information. 4. Understand and act on health instructions.	Answer: 1 Rationale: The best definition includes the ability to use the health information and services in ways that enhance health. The ability to use the information is critical to identifying the best definition. Step in Nursing Process: Assessment Category of Client Need: Health Promotion and Maintenance Cognitive Level: Application Learning Objective 11-9: Analyze the implications of language and health literacy for health promotion. Test Taking Tip: Understand health literacy.
11.12 The nurse is writing an evaluating tool for the use of the Internet for health-related information. Elements that should be included in the evaluation are: (Select all that apply.) 1. Currency of information. 2. Purpose of the site. 3. Sources of financial support. 4. Owner of the site. 5. Popularity of the site.	Answers: 1, 2, 3, 4 Rationale: Evaluative elements should include the currency of information, the purpose of the site, sources of financial support for the site, and the owner of the site and their reputability. Popularity of the site is not one of the evaluative elements. Step in Nursing Process: Evaluation Category of Client Need: Safe Effective Care Environment Cognitive Level: Application Learning Objective 11-10: Identify criteria for evaluating health information on the Internet. Test Taking Tip: Recognize the elements of an effective evaluation tool for the Internet.
11.13 It is most important for health promotion programs to be evaluated for how: 1. Holistic the program was for the beneficiaries. 2. Costly the program was to the beneficiaries. 3. Many participants were involved in the program. 4. Empowering the program was for the beneficiaries.	Answer: 4 Rationale: Even though all selections could be evaluated, the most important criterion is how empowering the program was, that is, whether it allowed beneficiaries to assume control of the program. Step in Nursing Process: Evaluation Category of Client Need: Safe, Effective Care Environment Cognitive Level: Comprehension Learning Objective 11-11: Discuss criteria for evaluating health promotion programs. Test Taking Tip: Recognize the most important aspect that should be evaluated in a health promotion program.
11.14 The nurse is teaching a group of high school students the most common risk factors that contribute to the burden of disease in a country such as the United States. Topics should include: 1. Unsafe sex, alcohol use, and indoor air pollution. 2. Iron deficiency, obesity, and poor hygiene.	Answer: 3 Rationale: In developed countries such as the United States, the risk factors include obesity, tobacco use, alcohol use, high blood pressure, and high cholesterol. Indoor air pollution is not a common risk factor in the United States. Poor hygiene is not a common risk factor in the United States. Sanitation is not a common risk factor in the United States. Step in Nursing Process: Assessment Category of Client Need: Health Promotion and Maintenance Cognitive Level: Application

3. High cholesterol, tobacco use, and high blood pressure.
4. Obesity, sanitation, and high blood pressure.

Learning Objective 11-8: Design and implement a health education program for a selected population.
Test Taking Tip: Know how to design and implement a health education program for a group of high school students.

11.15 The best example of how the nurse can create a climate in which clients do not feel threatened is the nurse teaching a class about:
1. Exercise, where the nurse begins the first session with a description of the difficulties the nurse sometimes finds in trying to exercise.
2. Stress, where the nurse plays soft music throughout the first session.
3. Good nutrition, where the nurse provides a meal for the first session.
4. Diabetes, where the nurse asks a group of diabetics to talk to the class during the first session.

Answer: 1
Rationale: The nurse who teaches a class about exercise, and shares his or her own personal experience, is creating a climate in which the clients do not feel threatened and in which the nurse educator is seen as a source of support rather than a threat. The other choices do not achieve this result as well.
Step in Nursing Process: Implementation
Category of Client Need: Health Promotion and Maintenance
Cognitive Level: Application
Learning Objective 11-11: Discuss criteria for evaluating health promotion programs.
Test Taking Tip: Be able to evaluate the teaching environment.

CHAPTER 12

12.1 A client-centered goal of case management is:
1. Cost containment and cost-efficiency
2. Improved quality of life.
3. Decreased paperwork.
4. Financial viability.

Answer: 2
Rationale: Improved quality of life is a client-centered goal or benefit of case management. Cost containment and cost-efficiency, decreased paperwork, and financial viability are system-centered goals or benefits of case management.
Step in Nursing Process: Planning
Category of Client Need: Safe, Effective Care Environment
Cognitive Level: Comprehension
Learning Objective 12-1: Identify client-centered and system-centered goals of case management.
Test Taking Tip: Know the differences between the goals of client-centered and system-centered case management.

12.2 The best example of a system-centered goal or benefit of case management is:
1. Reduced duplication of services.
2. Better coordination of care.
3. Increased access to services.
4. Ability to function independently.

Answer: 3
Rationale: Increased access to services is the best example of a system-centered goal or benefit of case management. Reduced duplication of services, better coordination of care, and the ability to function independently are examples of client-centered goals or benefits of case management.
Step in Nursing Process: Planning
Category of Client Need: Safe, Effective Care Environment
Cognitive Level: Comprehension
Learning Objective 12-1: Identify client-centered and system-centered goals of case management.
Test Taking Tip: Distinguish client-centered and system-centered goals of case management.

12.3 The most correct statement regarding case management is that:
1. Clients need to be "case managed."
2. The best case managers refer clients to community resources for assistance.
3. Institutional settings provide the most effective case management setting.
4. The case manager should have primary responsibility for services provided.

Answer: 4
Rationale: In case management, the case managers should have primary responsibility for services provided to clients. Clients do not need to be case managed; the services and resources the clients receive are the object of the case management. Case managers should provide services themselves rather than refer clients to other sources. Effective case management activity occurs in a variety of settings, not just in the acute care setting.
Step in Nursing Process: Assessment
Category of Client Need: Safe, Effective Care Environment
Cognitive Level: Analysis
Learning Objective 12-2: Discuss standards and principles of case management practice.
Test Taking Tip: Understand case management.

12.4 The nurse is concerned about providing the client with choices related to health care. This is an example of a/an:
1. Equity-related concern.
2. Non-maleficence-related concern.
3. Beneficence–related concern.
4. Autonomy-related concern.

Answer: 2
Rationale: Non-maleficence related concerns center around the need to provide clients with choices and the need to prevent harm to clients. Equity-related concerns involve the fair allocation of resources based on elements such as age, gender, socioeconomic status, and so on. Beneficence-related concerns include issues related to providing care over an appropriate timeframe. Autonomy-related concerns relate to the need for balance between the client's autonomy with the case manager's responsibility to provide services appropriate to client needs, given resource constraints.
Step in Nursing Process: Implementation
Category of Client Need: Safe, Effective Care Environment
Cognitive Level: Comprehension
Learning Objective 12-3: Analyze legal and ethical issues related to case management.
Test Taking Tip: Know the differences among the various types of legal and ethical concerns related to case management.

12.5 The local health department has been criticized for not providing effective communicable disease control programs. This best describes:
1. Negligence at the population level.
2. Breach of contract at the population level.
3. Abandonment at the individual level.
4. Variance of care at the individual level.

Answer: 1
Rationale: Negligence is the failure to act in a situation as a reasonably prudent nurse would if faced with the same situation. Failure of a local health department to provide effective communicable disease control programs could be considered an example of negligence at the population level. Breach of contract occurs when a managed care organization drops a client from the plan without adequate justification or when the system fails to pay for care that should be covered by the plan. Abandonment occurs when the case manager terminates services to a client with continuing needs without notifying the client or arranging for services from another provider. Variances are deviations from the typical path, which is not the best description of this situation.
Step in Nursing Process: Implementation
Category of Client Need: Health Promotion and Maintenance
Cognitive Level: Application
Learning Objective 12-3: Analyze legal and ethical issues related to case management.
Test Taking Tip: Recognize the different types of legal and ethical issues related to case management.

12.6 The blueprint that guides the clinician in the provision of care is the:
1. Referral.
2. Utilization review.
3. Resource file.
4. Clinical pathway.

Answer: 4
Rationale: The clinical pathway is a blueprint that guides the clinician in the provision of care. Referral is the process of directing a client to another source of information or assistance. The resource file organizes and stores information on area resources. Utilization review is a process of monitoring the necessity of care and the resources used and may involve preadmission review, concurrent review, retrospective review, or telephonics.
Step in Nursing Process: Planning
Category of Client Need: Safe, Effective Care Environment
Cognitive Level: Application
Learning Objective 12-4: Identify criteria for selecting clients in need of case management.
Test Taking Tip: Understand clinical pathways and their role in case management.

12.7 Social indicators that show the need for case management include: (Select all that apply.)
1. History of drug abuse.
2. Homelessness.
3. Lack of insurance.
4. History of family violence.
5. Single parenthood.

Answers: 2, 3, 4, 5
Rationale: Social indicators that show a need for case management include homelessness or an unhealthy home environment, being uninsured, evidence of family violence, and single parenthood. History of drug abuse is a personal indicator, not a social indicator.
Step in Nursing Process: Assessment
Category of Client Need: Health Promotion and Maintenance
Cognitive Level: Application
Learning Objective 12-5: Assess the need for case management and factors influencing the case management situation.
Test Taking Tip: Distinguish among the categories of indicators for case management.

12.8 A client who has asthma is being assisted by the case manager to achieve control of the disease. This is an example of:
1. Case management.
2. Disease management.
3. A multidisciplinary plan.
4. Risk management.

Answer: 2
Rationale: Disease management is the process of intensively managing a particular disease across different care settings. Case management is assisting the same client to meet a wide variety of health and social needs. Clinical pathways are multidisciplinary plans for use with specific groups of clients with specific health problems. The case manager might use a clinical pathway to promote asthma control, but this is only one aspect of disease management. Although the disease management plan might include assessment of risk factors that trigger asthma attacks, this is only one aspect of control of the disease.
Step in Nursing Process: Planning
Category of Client Need: Health Promotion and Maintenance
Cognitive Level: Analysis
Learning Objective 12-6: Discuss aspects of developing a case management plan.
Test Taking Tip: Understand the differences among the aspects of developing a case management plan.

12.9 Effective case management plans are:
1. Generic.
2. Static.
3. Time-limited.
4. Outcomes-based.

Answer: 4
Rationale: Effective case management plans are interdisciplinary, outcomes-based, clinically-specific, flexible (not static), and include avenues for provider documentation. The plans are not generic and they are not time-limited, if needed.
Step in Nursing Process: Planning
Category of Client Need: Safe, Effective Care Environment
Cognitive Level: Comprehension
Learning Objective 12-6: Discuss aspects of developing a case management plan.
Test Taking Tip: Recognize the aspects of effective case management plans.

12.10 Why are clinical pathways beneficial? They are:
1. Multidisciplinary plans that incorporate best practices.
2. Involve primarily nursing.
3. Only used for health promotion.
4. Intended to not require written documentation.

Answer: 1
Rationale: Clinical pathways are multidisciplinary plans that incorporate best practices for use with specific groups of clients. They do not primarily involve nursing and they are used for health promotion and disease management. Use of pathways requires documentation, although documentation may be streamlined by the use of a pathway.
Step in Nursing Process: Planning
Category of Client Need: Health Promotion and Maintenance
Cognitive Level: Analysis
Learning Objective 12-7: Identify advantages and disadvantages of clinical pathways.
Test Taking Tip: Explain the benefits of clinical pathways.

12.11 The client has become unstable. The case manager should:
1. Delegate the care to an assistive personnel.
2. Refuse to continue care.
3. Retain care of the client.
4. Make an automatic referral.

Answer: 3
Rationale: Care of unstable clients should not be delegated to unlicensed assistive personnel or automatically referred, but should be retained by the case manager or other qualified personnel. After assessment the client might be referred to the primary care provider.
Step in Nursing Process: Implementation.
Category of Client Need: Safe, Effective Care Environment
Cognitive Level: Analysis
Learning Objective 12-8: Describe at least three considerations in delegation.
Test Taking Tip: Understand delegation.

12.12 Among the following choices, what is the best example of a consideration for the nurse manager in making delegation decisions? The client's
1. Age.
2. Education.
3. Ability for self-care.
4. Ability to pay for services.

Answer: 3
Rationale: The nurse manager is guided by the following decisions when making delegation decisions: stability of the client; competence of the person to whom the task is being delegated; level of decision making and problem solving required; ability of the client for self-care; and the predictability of the outcome of the task. None of the other choices are appropriate considerations for making delegation decisions.
Step in Nursing Process: Implementation
Category of Client Need: Safe, Effective Care Environment
Cognitive Level: Comprehension
Learning Objective 12-8: Describe at least three considerations in delegation.
Test Taking Tip: Understand delegation.

12.13 The nurse is making a referral for the client. The first consideration for the nurse should be the:
1. Factors that might prevent the client from following through with the referral.
2. Client's eligibility for the service.
3. Cost of the referral services.
4. Acceptability of the referral to the client.

Answer: 4
Rationale: The first consideration in making a referral is the acceptability of the referral to the client. The second consideration is the client's eligibility for the service provided. The presence of situational constraints or factors in the client's situation that would prevent him or her from following through with the referral is the third consideration.
Step in Nursing Process: Assessment
Category of Client Need: Safe, Effective Care Environment
Cognitive Level: Analysis
Learning Objective 12-5: Assess the need for case management and factors influencing the case management situation.
Test Taking Tip: Know the considerations the nurse must consider when making a referral for a client.

12.14 The case manager arranges for the transfer of the client's records from the primary care provider to the home health agency. This best describes what role function of the case manager?
1. Clinical expert.
2. Consultant.
3. Coordinator of care.
4. Change agent.

Answer: 3
Rationale: The coordinator of care arranges seamless care across systems and agencies to meet client needs. An example of the coordinator of care's role function is arranging for transfer of client records from the primary care provider to the home health agency. The consultant provides assistance to clients and other health care professionals regarding client needs and available services. The clinical expert is knowledgeable regarding clinical conditions and best, evidence-based practice. The change agent promotes change in client behaviors and/or health care delivery systems.
Step in Nursing Process: Implementation.
Category of Client Need: Health Promotion and Maintenance
Cognitive Level: Application
Learning Objective 12-6: Discuss aspects of developing a case management plan.
Test Taking Tip: Recognize the role functions of the case manager.

12.15 The process of _____ compares processes and outcomes among competing organizations to identify performance levels that a particular agency wants to exceed.
1. Assessing.
2. Screening.
3. Delegation.
4. Benchmarking.
5. Diagnosing.

Answers: 4
Rationale: Benchmarking is a process of comparing processes and outcomes among competing organizations to identify performance levels that a particular agency wants to exceed. Assessment involves identification of the need for case management services. Screening involves risk identification. Delegation involves transferring authority to a competent individual. Diagnosing involves identifying needs.
Step in Nursing Process: Implementation
Category of Client Need: Health Promotion and Maintenance
Cognitive Level: Comprehension
Learning Objective 12-9: Describe the benchmarking process and its use in case management.
Test Taking Tip: Understand how benchmarking is used in case management.

CHAPTER 13

13.1 A small community is attempting to rejuvenate itself through housing and business development. This best describes the concept of community:
1. Mobilization.
2. Organization.
3. Competence.
4. Development.

Answer: 4
Rationale: Community development is often the term used to refer to the rejuvenation of communities through housing and business development. Community mobilization is a similar concept that involves working with individuals and groups to provide population-based community driven assessments, interventions, and evaluations. Community organization is a process by which community groups are helped to identify common problems or goals, mobilize resources, and develop and implement strategies for reaching the goals they have collectively set. Community competence is defined as the ability of the community to engage in effective problem solving.
Step in Nursing Process: Assessment
Category of Client Need: Health Promotion and Maintenance
Cognitive Level: Comprehension
Learning Objective 13-1: Discuss the relationship of community empowerment to other similar concepts.
Test Taking Tip: Differentiate community concepts.

13.2 The community has identified strategies for reaching the goals that were collectively set. This best describes the concept of community:
1. Organization.
2. Development.
3. Building.
4. Goal setting.

Answer: 1

Rationale: Community organization is the process by which community groups are helped to identify common problems or goals, mobilize resources, and develop and implement strategies for reaching the goals they have collectively set. Community development is often the term used to refer to the rejuvenation of communities through housing and business development. Community building is defined as continuous, self-renewing efforts by residents and professionals to engage in collective action, aimed at problem-solving and enrichment, that creates new or strengthened social networks, new capacities for group action and support, and new standards and expectations for the life of the community. Community goal setting is not a community concept.

Step in Nursing Process: Planning
Category of Client Need: Health Promotion and Maintenance
Cognitive Level: Application
Learning Objective 13-1: Discuss the relationship of community empowerment to other similar concepts.
Test Taking Tip: Differentiate community concepts.

13.3 The nurse assists residents to collect information about pollution and to present a petition to the City Council requesting greater accountability from local businesses regarding pollution. This best describes:
1. Individual empowerment.
2. Community empowerment.
3. Community competence.
4. Individual accountability.

Answer: 2

Rationale: Community empowerment focuses on increased civic participation and preparation for collective action to address common concerns or achieve common goals. Individual empowerment focuses on improving individual skills and self-esteem as a precursor to taking control of one's own life. Community competence is defined as the ability of the community to engage in effective problem solving. Even though one might think the situation involves community competence, the best description is community empowerment. Individual accountability is not an applicable description of this situation.

Step in Nursing Process: Implementation
Category of Client Need: Health Promotion and Maintenance
Cognitive Level: Application
Learning Objective 13-2: Identify levels of community empowerment.
Test Taking Tip: Differentiate community concepts.

13.4 The community health nurse assists neighborhood residents to form a neighborhood watch to help control gang crimes. This best describes:
1. Vertical empowerment.
2. Internal empowerment.
3. Horizontal empowerment.
4. External empowerment.

Answer: 3

Rationale: Horizontal empowerment is internal to the community and is reflected in the community's ability to solve problems by mobilizing its own resources. Vertical empowerment involves efforts to change power structures outside the community and to leverage outside power and resources to address community concerns and may involve organizing marginalized groups to make demands on the larger society. Horizontal is the best description. Internal and external are not terms used to describe empowerment in this description.

Step in Nursing Process: Implementation
Category of Client Need: Health Promotion and Maintenance
Cognitive Level: Application
Learning Objective 13-2: Identify levels of community empowerment.
Test Taking Tip: Differentiate levels of community empowerment.

13.5 The community health nurse assists a homeless adolescent with a substance abuse problem to enroll in school, to find work, and to enroll in a recovery program. Recognizing that empowerment may occur at a variety of levels, what best describes the higher end of the continuum in relation to this scenario? The nurse assists:
1. A community organization to link with legal advocates and others to promote legislation to protect the civil rights of homeless adolescents.

Answer: 1

Rationale: Empowerment may occur at a variety of levels. Community empowerment may be conceived as occurring along a continuum from personal empowerment to the creation of coalitions and linking with outside resources to address concerns. The community organization linking with legal advocates and others to promote legislation to protect the homeless adolescents' civil rights is the higher end of the continuum. At the level of personal empowerment, a community health nurse might help a homeless adolescent find work and enroll in a recovery program. At the next level, the nurse might assist a group of homeless adolescents to find a support group that permits them to share knowledge of resources. Helping to create an organization composed of homeless adolescents and members of the social services community to address the health care needs of the homeless adolescents would be an example of the third level of empowerment. At the fourth level, the community health nurse might assist the community organization to link with legal advocates and others to promote legislation to protect the civil rights of homeless adolescents.

2. A group of homeless adolescents to form a support group.
3. In creating an organization composed of homeless adolescents and members of the social services community to address the health care needs of homeless adolescents.
4. In organizing local housing for homeless adolescents.

Step in Nursing Process: Evaluation
Category of Client Need: Health Promotion and Maintenance
Cognitive Level: Application
Learning Objective 13-2: Identify levels of community empowerment.
Test Taking Tip: Analyze empowerment.

13.6 The community health nurse is focusing on the use of families, friends, and neighbors within the community to help in resolving community problems. This best describes the:
1. Community Organization model.
2. Natural Helpers model.
3. Community Action model.
4. Planned Approach to Community Health model.

Answer: 2
Rationale: The Natural Helpers Model is not a process model, but focuses on the use of natural helpers within the community to promote community empowerment. The community organization model is a process model that is involved in community analysis and initiative design. The community action model is involved with identifying community members for training. The Planned Approach to Community Health model is involved with mobilizing community members and developing a comprehensive intervention plan with multisectoral collaboration.
Step in Nursing Process: Assessment
Category of Client Need: Health Promotion and Maintenance
Cognitive Level: Application
Learning Objective 13-3: Apply selected models for community empowerment.
Test Taking Tip: Review selected community empowerment models.

13.7 The group of community activists is selecting its members, and identifying goals and purposes. These group tasks are congruent with which stages of the nursing process? (Select all that apply.)
1. Assessment.
2. Diagnosis.
3. Planning.
4. Implementation.
5. Evaluation.

Answers: 1, 2
Rationale: Selecting its members and identifying goals and purposes relates to the assessment and diagnosis steps of the nursing process. The assessment and diagnosis component of the nursing process relates to the orientation stage of group development, which relates to group tasks of selection of group members, training for group participation, and identification of goals and purposes. Planning involves establishment of modes of decision making, development of mechanisms for conflict resolution, development of communication networks and development of a climate conducive to group collaboration. Evaluation involves planning of evaluative mechanisms for outcomes of action taken, assignment of member roles and tasks in evaluation, data collection, analysis or evaluative findings and possible group dissolution.
Step in Nursing Process: Assessment
Category of Client Need: Health Promotion and Maintenance
Cognitive Level: Application
Learning Objective 13-4: Describe the process of community empowerment.
Test Taking Tip: Review the steps of the nursing process.

13.8 Community assessment in relation to community empowerment has two general purposes. The second general purpose is to provide:
1. Information for change.
2. Stimulus for change.
3. Data needed for the change.
4. Information for empowerment.

Answer: 4
Rationale: Community assessment, in the context of community empowerment, has two general purposes. The first is to provide information for change and the second is to provide information for empowerment. A stimulus for change and information for empowerment are not general purposes of community assessment in relation to community empowerment.
Step in Nursing Process: Assessment
Category of Client Need: Health Promotion and Maintenance
Cognitive Level: Comprehension
Learning Objective 13-4: Describe the process of community empowerment.
Test Taking Tip: Review the two general purposes of community assessment in relation to community empowerment.

13.9 Community members must have confidence in each other and yet demand that persons responsible for action on behalf of the community also be responsible for their actions. This best describes what

Answer: 2, 5
Rationale: The challenge of reconciling trust and accountability is illustrated by the example of community members trusting each other yet demanding that persons responsible for action on behalf of the community also be responsible for their own actions. Reconciling individual and community needs involves creating common purposes, values, and complementary roles. Reconciling people and place involves

challenges to community empowerment planning?

1. Reconciling individual and community needs.
2. Reconciling trust.
3. Reconciling people and place.
4. Reconciling idealism and practicality.
5. Reconciling accountability.

recognizing and addressing diversity among community members whose needs may not all be the same despite their residence in the same community. Reconciling idealism and practicality involves supporting the core values of the community in the context of the constraints imposed by the reality of the situation.
Step in Nursing Process: Assessment
Category of Client Need: Health Promotion and Maintenance
Cognitive Level: Comprehension
Learning Objective 13-5: Apply criteria to evaluate community empowerment.
Test Taking Tip: Review the challenges involved with community empowerment.

13.10 The community is a passive target of interventions without having input into decisions regarding those interventions. This best describes which level of community participation?

1. Partnership.
2. Manipulation.
3. Consulting.
4. Delegation.

Answer: 2
Rationale: The first two levels of community participation, manipulation and therapy, actually reflect non-participation, in which clients and communities are passive targets of interventions without having input into decisions regarding those interventions. The next three levels reflect token participation: informing the community regarding potential actions or interventions, consulting with members of the community in designing actions, and placating community members by listening to their input but not necessarily incorporating it into decisions. The last three levels of participation are considered true participation and reflect reallocation of power to community members. The first level of participation is partnership, in which community members and decision makers have joint authority for decisions and action. The second level of participation is delegated power, in which the decision-making authority has delegated power for certain decisions to community members. At the highest level of participation, citizen power, community members have control over the issue and all decisions or intervention programs related to it.
Step in Nursing Process: Assessment
Category of Client Need: Health Promotion and Maintenance
Cognitive Level: Comprehension
Learning Objective 13-5: Apply criteria to evaluate community empowerment.
Test Taking Tip: Study the levels of community participation.

13.11 The community health nurse is working with a group trying to determine the best location for a new community center. The elderly representatives in the group are not participating in the discussions. The nurse should:

1. Respect their right to be silent and not encourage discussion from them.
2. Manipulate the discussion so that they must contribute.
3. Comment on the fact that they have not participated in the discussion and ask why.
4. Encourage more discussion from the younger representatives, as that will encourage the elderly to join in the discussion.

Answer: 3
Rationale: In this situation the nurse should comment on the fact that the elderly have not participated and ask them why. The ensuing discussion may expose the conflict and the group can start to work on it. Recognizing the existence of conflict and identifying its sources and possible solutions are strategies for constructive use of conflict. A conflict that is ignored in the hope that it will resolve itself is likely to become worse.
Step in Nursing Process: Implementation
Category of Client Need: Health Promotion and Maintenance
Cognitive Level: Analysis
Learning Objective 13-6: Analyze the role of community health nurses in community empowerment.
Test Taking Tip: Review the process of community empowerment.

13.12 A community group is meeting to discuss the most critical issues related to the community's health care delivery system. The nurse in charge of the meeting is encouraging all group members to participate and is trying to provide positive reinforcement for all group contributions. The nurse is most likely trying to:

1. Establish a climate in which group members feel respected.

Answer: 1
Rationale: Establishing a climate in which group members feel respected and in which differences are accepted contributes to an effective network. This means that all group members should be encouraged to participate and should receive positive reinforcement for their contributions. The nurse is not manipulating the discussion. Encouraging participation does not prevent conflict. Even though more discussion might be encouraged by the nurse's actions, the nurse's actions most likely will establish a climate in which group members feel respected.
Step in Nursing Process: Implementation
Category of Client Need: Health Promotion and Maintenance
Cognitive Level: Analysis

2. Manipulate the discussion so that all must participate.
3. Resolve conflict before it can occur.
4. Encourage more discussion.

Learning Objective 13-6: Analyze the role of community health nurses in community empowerment.

Test Taking Tip: Review the process of community empowerment.

13.13 The operation stage of group development is analogous to what stage of the nursing process?
1. Assessment.
2. Planning.
3. Implementation.
4. Evaluation.

Answer: 3

Rationale: The operation stage of group development is analogous to the implementation stage of the nursing process. It is during this stage that the group assigns and performs specific roles and tasks to achieve group-designated goals and objectives. The orientation stage of group development is analogous to the assessment stage of the nursing process, as is the accommodation stage to planning and the dissolution stage to evaluation.

Step in Nursing Process: Implementation

Category of Client Need: Health Promotion and Maintenance

Cognitive Level: Application

Learning Objective 13-6: Analyze the role of community health nurses in community empowerment.

Test Taking Tip: Review the tasks of group development by stage and the related nursing process component.

13.14 The best answer to the final measure of the effectiveness of community empowerment efforts would be the extent to which the:
1. Budget was not overspent.
2. Community members were included in policy making.
3. Initial data was shown to be reliable.
4. Time schedules were met.

Answer: 2

Rationale: A final measure of the effectiveness of community empowerment efforts would be the extent to which community members are included in policy making. The ultimate goal of effective community organizing and empowerment should be the inclusion of community members in every aspect of policy making. The issue regarding the budget not being overspent, initial data being reliable and time schedules being met are not the best answers to the final measure of the effectiveness of community empowerment.

Step in Nursing Process: Assessment

Category of Client Need: Health Promotion and Maintenance

Cognitive Level: Analysis

Learning Objective 13-6: Analyze the role of community health nurses in community empowerment.

Test Taking Tip: Review the effectiveness of community empowerment.

13.15 The influence of community health nurses in community empowerment lies in enactment of three roles. Those three roles are discovery, decision, and:
1. Discussion.
2. Planning.
3. Drive.
4. Evaluation.

Answer: 3

Rationale: The third role is drive. In the drive role, community health nurses assist in mobilizing the community for change. The discovery role involves making community members aware of the need for empowerment and building a compelling case for change in the status quo. In the decision role, community health nurses assist community members to determine potential alternative strategies, to evaluate them, and to select the strategies most likely to contribute to achievement of community-identified goals.

Step in Nursing Process: Assessment

Category of Client Need: Health Promotion and Maintenance

Cognitive Level: Comprehension

Learning Objective 13-6: Analyze the role of community health nurses in community empowerment.

Test Taking Tip: Review the three roles of the community health nurse in influencing community empowerment.

CHAPTER 14

14.1 The nurse is completing an assessment on a five-year-old child. One of the questions the nurse asks the mother is how many people live together in the house. The mother states that the father, two aunts, one uncle, three children, and she live

Answer: 2

Rationale: The extended family includes family members other than spouses and children, such as grandparents, aunts, uncles, and cousins. The nuclear conjugal family is composed of husband, wife, and children. A cohabiting family consists of a man and a woman living together without being married. A stepfamily is composed of two adults, at least one of whom has remarried following divorce or the death of a spouse.

together in the house. On the basis of the mother's answer, which of the following would be the most appropriate description of the family type?
1. Nuclear conjugal family.
2. Extended family.
3. Stepfamily.
4. Cohabiting family.

Step in Nursing Process: Assessment
Category of Client Need: Health Promotion and Maintenance
Cognitive Level: Application
Learning Objective 14-1: Describe at least five family types and their characteristic features.
Test Taking Tip: Understand the different family types.

14.2 Forty percent of families in the United States are married couples without children under 18 years of age living in the home. Based on this statistic, which description does this statistic most accurately reflect?
1. Extended families.
2. Binuclear families.
3. Nuclear dyads.
4. Cohabiting families.

Answer: 3
Rationale: Forty percent of families in the United States are nuclear dyads, married couples without children under 18 years of age living in the home. Extended families include family members other than spouses and children such as grandparents, aunts, uncles, and cousins. A cohabiting family consists of a man and a woman living together without being married. A binuclear family is a family in which a child is a member of two nuclear households.
Step in Nursing Process: Assessment
Category of Client Need: Health Promotion and Maintenance
Cognitive Level: Analysis
Learning Objective 14-1: Describe at least five family types and their characteristic features.
Test Taking Tip: Understand the different family types.

14.3 An adolescent tells the nurse that she lives with her mother from Monday to Friday each week and then she lives with her father on Saturday and Sunday. This family constellation is best described as a/an:
1. Binuclear family.
2. Stepfamily.
3. Extended family.
4. Nuclear conjugal family.

Answer: 1
Rationale: The existence of stepfamilies may contribute to the creation of a binuclear family in which a child is a member of two nuclear households as a result of joint-custody visitation rights. A stepfamily is composed of two adults, at least one of whom has remarried following divorce or the death of a spouse. Extended families include family members other than spouses and children such as grandparents, aunts, uncles, and cousins. The nuclear conjugal family is composed of husband, wife, and children.
Step in Nursing Process: Assessment
Category of Client Need: Health Promotion and Maintenance
Cognitive Level: Application
Learning Objective14-1: Describe at least five family types and their characteristic features.
Test Taking Tip: Understand the different family types.

14.4 Research demonstrates that foster children have a higher incidence of _____ than other children receiving public assistance. (Select all that apply.)
1. Mental disorders.
2. Educational success.
3. Attention deficit hyperactivity disorder.
4. Depression.
5. Economic prosperity.

Answer: 1, 3, 4
Rationale: Studies indicate that foster children have a higher incidence of mental disorders (57%) than other children receiving public assistance (4%). Common diagnoses include attention deficit hyperactivity disorder, depression, and developmental disorders. Studies do not indicate a higher incidence of economic prosperity.
Step in Nursing Process: Assessment
Category of Client Need: Health Promotion and Maintenance
Cognitive Level: Comprehension
Learning Objective 14-1: Describe at least five family types and their characteristic features.
Test Taking Tip: Understand the different family types.

14.5 The nurse explains that families pass through predictive stages. This explanation is based on:
1. Structural-functional models.
2. Systems models.
3. Developmental models.
4. Focal models.

Answer: 3
Rationale: Developmental models are based on the supposition that human beings and social units, such as families, develop in a logical fashion with predictable stages or milestones during their development. Systems models conceive of families as open systems in which the whole of the system is more than the sum of its component parts or members but also includes the interactions among them. A structural-functional approach to family is based on the principle that all families possess structure designed to allow them to perform specific functions. The focal model is used to describe families.
Step in Nursing Process: Assessment.
Category of Client Need: Health Promotion and Maintenance

Cognitive Level: Comprehension
Learning Objective 14-2: Describe elements of at least one theoretical model applied to families.
Test Taking Tip: Explain the developmental model.

14.6 The nurse is assessing a family dealing with the stress of unemployment and the stress of a child with chronic asthma. The assessment reveals that the family is attending to only those aspects of the situation that do not cause distress or pain. Which of the following best describes the assessment?
1. Denial.
2. Selective inattention.
3. Isolation.
4. Rationalization.

Answer: 2
Rationale: Selective inattention is described as attending to only those aspects of the situation that do not cause distress or pain. Denial is ignoring threat-provoking aspects of a situation or changing the meaning of the situation to make it less threatening. Isolation is separating emotion from content in a situation so one can deal objectively with otherwise threatening or emotionally overwhelming conditions. Rationalization is giving a "good" or rational excuse, but is not the real reason for responding to a situation with a particular behavior.
Step in Nursing Process: Assessment
Category of Client Need: Health Promotion and Maintenance
Cognitive Level: Analysis
Learning Objective 14-3: Identify family assessment considerations in the biophysical, psychological, physical, environmental, sociocultural, behavioral, and health system dimensions.
Test Taking Tip: Understand family coping.

14.7 The nurse assesses the father's role within the family to be primarily formal. Which of the following might the father use to describe formal roles? (Select all that apply.)
1. Comforter.
2. Chauffeur.
3. Financial manager.
4. Caregiver.
5. Confidant.

Answer: 2, 3
Rationale: Formal roles are expected sets of behaviors associated with family positions such as breadwinner, homemaker, house repairman, chauffeur, child caretaker, financial manager, and cook. Informal roles influence the psychological dimension within the family by determining whether, how, and by whom emotional needs are met; examples include comforter, caregiver and confidant.
Step in Nursing Process: Assessment
Category of Client Need: Health Promotion and Maintenance
Cognitive Level: Application
Learning Objective 14-4: Differentiate between formal and informal family roles.
Test Taking Tip: Distinguish among the various family roles.

14.8 Which of the following would best indicate a maturational crisis?
1. Marriage.
2. Illness.
3. Death.
4. Natural disasters.

Answer: 1
Rationale: A maturational crisis is viewed as a normal transition point where old patterns of communication and old roles must be exchanged for new patterns and roles. Examples of transition periods when maturational crises may occur are adolescence, marriage, parenthood, and one's first job. Examples of situational crises (when the family experiences an event that is sudden, unexpected, and unpredictable) are illness, accidents, death, and natural disasters.
Step in Nursing Process: Assessment
Category of Client Need: Health Promotion and Maintenance
Cognitive Level: Application
Learning Objective 14-5: Differentiate between situational and maturational crises.
Test Taking Tip: Distinguish between maturational and situational crises, noting that one is a normal transition point.

14.9 The nurse is educating the family regarding general needs for adequate nutrition, rest, and physical activity. Which level of prevention does this describe?
1. Primary prevention.
2. Secondary prevention.
3. Tertiary prevention.
4. Health maintenance.

Answer: 1
Rationale: Primary prevention involves health promotion (not health maintenance) and protection or illness prevention. Examples include education regarding adequate nutrition, rest, and physical activity. Secondary prevention may be aimed at assisting families to obtain needed care for existing health problems or helping families to deal with these problems. Tertiary prevention involves assisting families to cope with long-term health problems or to deal with the consequences of those problems.
Step in Nursing Process: Planning
Category of Client Need: Health Promotion and Maintenance
Cognitive Level: Application
Learning Objective 14-6: Discuss family-focused intervention at the primary, secondary, and tertiary levels of prevention.
Test Taking Tip: Understand the differences among primary, secondary, and tertiary prevention.

14.10 The community health nurse is advocating with local police for adequate protection for a woman and her children. Which level of prevention is reflective of this?
1. Primary prevention.
2. Secondary prevention.
3. Tertiary prevention.
4. Health promotion.

Answer: 2
Rationale: Secondary prevention may be aimed at assisting families to obtain needed care for existing health problems or helping families to deal with these problems. Primary prevention involves health promotion and protection or illness prevention. Examples include education regarding adequate nutrition, rest, and physical activity. Tertiary prevention involves assisting families to cope with long-term health problems or to deal with the consequences of those problems.
Step in Nursing Process: Implementation
Category of Client Need: Health Promotion and Maintenance
Cognitive Level: Analysis
Learning Objective 14-6: Discuss family-focused intervention at the primary, secondary, and tertiary levels of prevention.
Test Taking Tip: Distinguish secondary prevention from primary and tertiary levels.

14.11 Crisis intervention is an important part of:
1. Primary prevention.
2. Secondary prevention.
3. Tertiary prevention.
4. Health promotion.

Answer: 2
Rationale: Crisis intervention is an important element of secondary prevention in the care of families. Crisis intervention focuses on secondary prevention and is directed toward helping members to discuss and define the problem and to express their feelings concerning the crisis situation. Primary prevention involves health promotion and protection or illness prevention. With respect to tertiary prevention, community health nurses may assist families to cope with long-term health problems or to deal with the consequences of those problems.
Step in Nursing Process: Assessment
Category of Client Need: Health Promotion and Maintenance
Cognitive Level: Application.
Learning Objective 14-6: Discuss family-focused intervention at the primary, secondary, and tertiary levels of prevention.
Test Taking Tip: Understand family-focused intervention.

14.12 The community health nurse is making a home visit with a family who has a child who recently became a paraplegic. The nurse suggests some home modifications to accommodate the child's disability. Which of the following levels of prevention does this example most appropriately describe?
1. Primary prevention.
2. Secondary prevention.
3. Tertiary prevention.
4. Health maintenance.

Answer: 3
Rationale: Tertiary prevention involves assisting families to cope with long-term health problems or to deal with the consequences of those problems. Primary prevention involves health promotion and protection or illness prevention. Examples include education regarding adequate nutrition, rest, and physical activity. Secondary prevention may be aimed at assisting families to obtain needed care for existing health problems or helping families to deal with these problems.
Step in Nursing Process: Planning
Category of Client Need: Health Promotion and Maintenance
Cognitive Level: Analysis
Learning Objective 14-6: Discuss family-focused intervention at the primary, secondary, and tertiary levels of prevention.
Test Taking Tip: Distinguish tertiary prevention measures from primary and secondary measures.

14.13 Which of the following is the most appropriate related goal for the affective family function?
1. Regulate sexual activity.
2. Meet the emotional needs of family members.
3. Provide financial resources.
4. Meet the family members' needs for food.

Answer: 2
Rationale: A goal related to the affective function would be to meet the emotional needs of family members. A goal related to the reproductive function would be to regulate sexual activity. A goal for the economic function would be related to providing financial resources. A goal for provision of needs would be to meet the family members' needs for food.
Step in Nursing Process: Planning
Category of Client Need: Health Promotion and Maintenance
Cognitive Level: Analysis
Learning Objective 14-2: Describe elements of at least one theoretical model applied to families.
Test Taking Tip: Understand family functions and related goals.

14.14 The nurse has drawn an ecomap to assist the family who is experiencing some relationship difficulties. The ecomap:
1. Is a diagram of a family tree.

Answer: 4
Rationale: An ecomap is a visual representation depicting relationships of family members with each other and with outside forces. A genogram, not an ecomap, is a diagram of a family tree. An ecomap does not demonstrate health and does not prioritize family relationships.

2. Demonstrates how healthy the family is.
3. Prioritizes family relationships.
4. Depicts the relationships within and outside the family.

Step in Nursing Process: Assessment
Category of Client Need: Health Promotion and Maintenance
Cognitive Level: Application
Learning Objective 14-3: Identify family assessment considerations in the biophysical, psychological, physical environmental, sociocultural, behavioral, and health system dimensions.
Test Taking Tip: Understand the different family assessment tools.

14.15 The nurse observes that the family is exhibiting strengths in the face of the adversity they are facing. The best description of the strengths the nurse is observing is:
1. Faith.
2. Resilience.
3. Projection.
4. Intellectualization.

Answer: 2
Rationale: Resilience is the phenomenon of doing well in the face of diversity. Projection is attributing one's own motivation to other people. Intellectualization is focusing on abstract, technical, or logical aspects of a threatening situation to insulate oneself from painful emotions generated. Faith is not the best description in this situation.
Step in Nursing Process: Assessment
Category of Client Need: Health Promotion and Maintenance
Cognitive Level: Application
Learning Objective 14-3: Identify family assessment considerations in the biophysical, psychological, physical, environmental, sociocultural, behavioral, and health system dimensions.
Test Taking Tip: Understand the differences between faith, resilience, projection, and intellectualization.

CHAPTER 15

15.1 A student asks an instructor to explain population health management. The best answer is that population health management:
1. Focuses on health promotion.
2. Is designed to improve overall population health status.
3. Is designed to identify particular health risk groups.
4. Identifies illness prevention strategies.

Answer: 2
Rationale: Even though the other choices may be correct, the most complete answer is that population health management is designed to improve overall population health status. It involves health promotion and it involves illness prevention strategies.
Step in Nursing Process: Assessment
Category of Client Need: Health Promotion and Maintenance
Cognitive Level: Application
Learning Objective 15-1: Discuss the rationale for including members of the population in every phase of population health assessment and health program planning.
Test Taking Tip: Understand population health management.

15.2 The nurse is discussing factors affecting the health of population groups. The nurse discusses the shorter life spans of Native Americans as compared to the rest of the population. This is an example of a:
1. Sociocultural consideration.
2. Behavioral consideration.
3. Biophysical consideration.
4. Health system consideration.

Answer: 3
Rationale: Human biological factors influencing a population's health reflect specific physical attributes of its members. Native Americans have shorter expected life spans than the rest of the population because of the higher incidence of some chronic diseases, alcoholism, and homicide. Considerations in assessing the sociocultural dimension include information about community government and leadership, language, income and education levels, employment levels and occupations, marital status and family composition, and religion. Behavioral areas to be considered include consumption patterns, leisure pursuits, and other health-related behaviors. Health system considerations include existing services, level of performance of the services and areas in which services are lacking.
Step in Nursing Process: Assessment
Category of Client Need: Health Promotion and Maintenance
Cognitive Level: Application
Learning Objective 15-2: Describe factors in each of the six dimensions of health to be considered in assessing the health of a population.
Test Taking Tip: Understand the factors of health that need to be considered when assessing the health of a population.

15.3 Twelve new cases of the measles have been diagnosed last week in a particular county. In that same county, twenty children are currently under treatment for the measles. The incidence of measles is:
1. Eight.
2. Twelve.
3. Twenty.
4. Unknown.

Answer: 2
Rationale: Incidence rates indicate the number of new cases of the condition identified over a period. Prevalence rates indicate the total number of cases of a particular condition at any given time.
Step in Nursing Process: Evaluation
Category of Client Need: Health Promotion and Maintenance
Cognitive Level: Analysis
Learning Objective 15-2: Describe factors in each of the six dimensions of health to be considered in assessing the health of a population.
Test Taking Tip: Distinguish prevalence from incidence in relation to morbidity.

15.4 After studying the community, the nurse reports widespread unemployment, lack of housing and crowded living conditions as being major factors influencing community health. These factors are related to which dimension of health?
1. Physical environmental dimension.
2. Biophysical dimension.
3. Psychological dimension.
4. Behavioral dimension.

Answer: 3
Rationale: The psychological environment influences the health of the population by increasing or mediating exposure to stress and affects the ability of the population to function effectively. Widespread unemployment, lack of housing, and crowded living conditions are sources of stress and will create a psychological environment that is not conducive to health.
Step in Nursing Process: Assessment
Category of Client Need: Health Promotion and Maintenance
Cognitive Level: Assessment
Learning Objective 15-2: Describe factors in each of the six dimensions of health to be considered in assessing the health of a population.
Test Taking Tip: Distinguish among the different psychological considerations.

15.5 All of the following are factors that affect the health of a population. The sociocultural dimension factors include: (Select all that apply.)
1. Language.
2. Annual birth rate.
3. Family composition.
4. Population density.
5. Transportation accessibility.

Answer: 1, 3, 5
Rationale: Considerations in assessing the sociocultural dimension include information about community government and leadership, language, income and education levels, employment levels and occupations, marital status and family composition, and religion. Transportation is included as a sociocultural dimension. Population density relates to physical environmental considerations. Annual birth rate relates to biophysical considerations.
Step in Nursing Process: Assessment
Category of Client Need: Health Promotion and Maintenance
Cognitive Level: Comprehension
Learning Objective 15-2: Describe factors in each of the six dimensions of health to be considered in assessing the health of a population.
Test Taking Tip: Distinguish among the different sociocultural considerations.

15.6 The best description of a population nursing diagnosis includes: (Select all that apply.)
1. Existing threats to health.
2. Potential threats to health.
3. Emerging threats to health.
4. Population strengths.
5. Population competencies.

Answer: 1, 2, 3, 4, 5
Rationale: Population nursing diagnoses provide a comprehensive picture of the population's health. They may be negative or positive. Population nursing diagnoses should reflect existing, emerging, and potential threats to health, as well as strengths or competencies.
Step in Nursing Process: Planning
Category of Client Need: Health Promotion and Maintenance
Cognitive Level: Analysis
Learning Objective 15-3: Describe the components of a population nursing diagnosis.
Test Taking Tip: Understand the components of population nursing diagnoses.

15.7 The nurse is planning a health program for a community. The first task the nurse should consider in planning for the program is:
1. Analyze the issue.
2. Create the planning group.
3. Define and prioritize the issue.
4. Set the stage for evaluation.

Answer: 3
Rationale: The first step in the program planning process is defining and prioritizing the issue to be addressed. Then the planning group is created, the issue is analyzed, the program is developed, and the stage is set for the evaluation.
Step in Nursing Process: Planning.
Category of Client Need: Health Promotion and Maintenance
Cognitive Level: Comprehension
Learning Objective 15-4: Identify at least five tasks in planning health programs to meet the needs of populations.
Test Taking Tip: Explain the steps in planning a health program.

15.8 The nurse determined the members of the planning group for the community health program. The next step the nurse should take is to:
1. Prioritize the issues.
2. Analyze the issue.
3. Develop the program.
4. Start the evaluation.

Answer: 2
Rationale: After the planning group is identified, the issue is analyzed. Then the program is developed and the stage is set for the evaluation. Prioritization does not occur until the development has started.
Step in Nursing Process: Planning.
Category of Client Need: Health Promotion and Maintenance
Cognitive Level: Comprehension
Learning Objective 15-4: Identify at least five tasks in planning health programs to meet the needs of populations.
Test Taking Tip: Explain the steps in planning a health program.

15.9 The objective that best reflects the characteristics of an effective program objective is:
1. Seventy-five percent of program participants will lose weight.
2. Thirty-two percent of program participants will demonstrate how to administer insulin by the end of the third week.
3. One-hundred percent of program participants will understand the new food pyramid by the end of the second week.
4. Fifty percent of program participants will quit smoking.

Answer: 2
Rationale: Effective program objectives must be measurable, precise, time-specific, reasonable, within group capability, legal, congruent with community morals and values, carry minimal side effects, and fit budget limitations. The objective which states seventy-five percent of program participants will lose weight is not precise and is not time-specific. The objective that states one-hundred percent of program participants will understand the new food pyramid by the end of the second week is not measurable; it does not state how one would measure the understanding. The objective that states fifty percent of program participants will quit smoking is not time-specific.
Step in Nursing Process: Planning
Category of Client Need: Health Promotion and Maintenance
Cognitive Level: Application
Learning Objective 15-4: Identify at least five tasks in planning health programs to meet the needs of populations.
Test Taking Tip: Be able to write a program objective.

15.10 The nurse is working in a weight control program and realizes that most of the participants want to lose weight, but they are unable to because of the difficulties involved in stopping an addictive behavior. This best demonstrates the theory of:
1. Processing.
2. Delineation.
3. Implementation.
4. Cause and effect.

Answer: 4
Rationale: The theory of cause and effect suggests that although many participants wish to lose weight, they are unable to do so because of the difficulties involved in stopping an addictive behavior. The theory of implementation describes the strategies for implementing the program in a real-life situation. Processing and delineation are not program theories.
Step in Nursing Process: Implementation
Category of Client Need: Health Promotion and Maintenance
Cognitive Level: Analysis
Learning Objective 15-5: Analyze the elements of a program theory or logic model and its usefulness in health program planning.
Test Taking Tip: Recognize program theory.

15.11 All of these questions can guide the program evaluation. Which question addresses analysis and use of evaluative data?
1. What will be evaluated?
2. What standards will be used to judge the program's performance?
3. What conclusions can be drawn from comparing program data with the standards selected?
4. What evidence will be used to compare program performance with the standards selected?

Answer: 3
Rationale: The question that asks what conclusions can be drawn from comparing program data with the standards selected addresses analysis and use of evaluative data. The other questions guide the development of the evaluation plan.
Step in Nursing Process: Evaluation
Category of Client Need: Health Promotion and Maintenance
Cognitive Level: Analysis
Learning Objective 15-5: Analyze the elements of a program theory or logic model and its usefulness in health program planning.
Test Taking Tip: Understand program evaluation.

15.12 The students ask the instructor to explain empowerment evaluation. The best answer is that empowerment evaluation assists communities to:
1. Improve their quality of life.
2. Delay decisions about a program.

Answer: 1
Rationale: The best answer to this question is that empowerment evaluation assists communities to develop the skills to assess and improve their own quality of life. Even though delaying decisions about a program, calling for a discontinuation of a program, and increasing the resources in a program might be a benefit of empowerment evaluation, they are not the best answers.
Step in Nursing Process: Evaluation

3. Call for a discontinuation of a program.
4. Increase the resources in a program.

Category of Client Need: Health Promotion and Maintenance
Cognitive Level: Analysis
Learning Objective 15-5: Analyze the elements of a program theory or logic model and its usefulness in health program planning.
Test Taking Tip: Understand program evaluation.

15.13 A community health nurse is asked to assist in an evaluation of an existing program for which evaluative mechanisms were not established during the program planning. This best describes the:
1. Prospective evaluation.
2. Outcome evaluation.
3. Retrospective evaluation.
4. Process evaluation.

Answer: 3
Rationale: Retrospective evaluation is designed after the program is completed, or at least in the process of being implemented. Prospective evaluation is planned and criteria are determined prior to program implementation. Process evaluation is one concerned with the quality of interactions between program staff and recipients. Outcome evaluation focuses on the consequences of the program for the health and welfare of the population.
Step in Nursing Process: Evaluation
Category of Client Need: Health Promotion and Maintenance
Cognitive Level: Analysis
Learning Objective 15-5: Analyze the elements of a program theory or logic model and its usefulness in health program planning.
Test Taking Tip: Understand program evaluation.

15.14 The nurse is planning a program to encourage exercise among high school students. Teachers and parents will be involved in implementing the program. The activity that best describes the third level of acceptance of this health care program is:
1. Marketing the program to the high school students.
2. Convincing the principal of the benefits of the program.
3. Meeting with the teachers to explain the program.
4. Encouraging parents to promote the program.

Answer: 1
Rationale: Marketing the program to the high school students is the third level of acceptance. Convincing the principal of the benefits of the program would be an example of the first level of acceptance. Meeting with the teachers and encouraging parents to promote the program would be the second level of acceptance, which involves convincing those who are to carry out the plan to implement it as designed.
Step in Nursing Process: Implementation
Category of Client Need: Health Promotion and Maintenance
Cognitive Level: Analysis
Learning Objective 15-6: Describe the four levels of acceptance of a health care program.
Test Taking Tip: Be able to recognize the four levels of acceptance of a health care program.

15.15 There are a number of considerations to be made when designing a program evaluation. The consideration that influences all other aspects of the process is:
1. Who should conduct the evaluation.
2. The type of evaluation to be conducted.
3. What design will be utilized.
4. The purpose of the evaluation.

Answer: 4
Rationale: Who should conduct the evaluation, the type of evaluation, and the design of the evaluation are all considerations to be made in designing a program evaluation; however, the purpose of the evaluation is the only consideration that influences all other aspects of the process.
Step in Nursing Process: Evaluation
Category of Client Need: Health Promotion and Maintenance
Cognitive Level: Application
Learning Objective 15-7: Describe three types of considerations in evaluating a health care program.
Test Taking Tip: Understand the types of considerations in evaluating a health care program.

CHAPTER 16

16.1 The nurse is working with a three-year-old child who is demonstrating difficulty with several developmental milestones. The nurse plans to assess the child's age-specific development in the areas of fine motor, gross motor, personal-social interaction, and language. An

Answer: 2
Rationale: Development from birth to six years of age is assessed by means of the Denver Developmental Screening Test, which is a test of age-specific development in the areas of fine motor, gross motor, personal-social interaction, and language.
Step in the Nursing Process: Assessment
Category of Client Need: Health Promotion and Maintenance
Cognitive Level: Application

appropriate test for the nurse to use would be the:
1. Goodenough Draw-a-Man Test.
2. Denver Developmental Screening Test.
3. Preschool Developmental Test.
4. Developmental Milestone Inventory.

Learning Objective 16-1: Identify factors affecting the health of children and adolescents.
Test Taking Tip: Understand when it is appropriate to use screening tests.

16.2 The nurse is teaching a class to recent nursing graduates who have decided to work in the area of pediatrics. The nurse explains that the most common cause of delayed development is:
1. Lead poisoning.
2. Physical abuse.
3. Mental retardation.
4. Alcohol use during the third trimester.

Answer: 3
Rationale: The most common cause of delayed development is mental retardation.
Step in the Nursing Process: Assessment
Category of Client Need: Health Promotion and Maintenance
Cognitive Level: Application
Learning Objective 16-1: Identify factors affecting the health of children and adolescents.
Test Taking Tip: Know the common reasons for delayed development.

16.3 The community health nurse is designing a program to educate parents of twelve-year-old children. The nurse plans to explain the usual behavioral expectations of most twelve-year-olds. The best description of this teaching would be that it involves:
1. Anticipatory guidance.
2. Behavior-focused teaching.
3. Developmental psychology.
4. Community-driven teaching.

Answer: 1
Rationale: Anticipatory guidance involves providing information to parents and others regarding behavioral expectations of children and adolescents at a specific age, before they reach that age.
Step in the Nursing Process: Implementation
Category of Client Need: Health Promotion and Maintenance
Cognitive Level: Analysis
Learning Objective 16-1: Identify factors affecting the health of children and adolescents.
Test Taking Tip: Understand anticipatory guidance.

16.4 The nurse is explaining how maintaining high rates of immunization among children not only protects individual children from disease, but also serves to protect other members of the population. This best describes:
1. Active immunity.
2. Passive immunity.
3. Acquired immunity.
4. Herd immunity.

Answer: 4
Rationale: Herd immunity is the level of protection provided to unimmunized people when immunization rates are high among the rest of the population. Active immunity is the immunity resulting from the development of antibodies within the body that neutralize or destroy the infective agent. Passive immunity is immunity acquired by the introduction of preformed antibodies into an unprotected individual. Acquired immunity is immunity resulting from the development of active or passive immunity.
Step in the Nursing Process: Planning
Category of Client Need: Health Promotion and Maintenance.
Cognitive Level: Analysis
Learning Objective 16-1: Identify factors affecting the health of children and adolescents.
Test Taking Tip: Know how to explain immunity.

16.5 The nurse is working with a family of five: the mother, father, and three children. The children are constantly exposed to hostility and aggressive behaviors by both parents. The nurse knows that these children will be more likely to:
1. Run away from home at the time of adolescence.
2. Commit suicide.
3. Display these same behaviors themselves.
4. Become submissive adults.

Answer: 3
Rationale: Research has shown consistently that children exposed to hostility and aggressive behaviors by other family members are more likely to display these same behaviors themselves.
Step in the Nursing Process: Assessment.
Category of Client Need: Health Promotion and Maintenance
Cognitive Level: Application
Learning Objective 16-1: Identify factors affecting the health of children and adolescents.
Test Taking Tip: Understand effects of certain behaviors on child development.

16.6 The nurse is teaching a class on the effects of maternal alcohol consumption during pregnancy. The nurse explains that the effects can include: (Select all that apply.)
1. Low birth weight.
2. Central nervous system dysfunctions.
3. Placenta previa.
4. Spontaneous abortion.
5. Fetal death.

Answers: 1, 2, 3, 4, 5
Rationale: Fetal alcohol syndrome (FAS) is a condition that results from maternal alcohol consumption during pregnancy and is characterized by growth retardation, facial malformations, and central nervous system dysfunctions that may include mental retardation. It is also associated with spontaneous abortion. Other potential effects include placenta previa and fetal death.
Step in the Nursing Process: Implementation
Category of Client Need: Health Promotion and Maintenance
Cognitive Level: Application
Learning Objective 16-1: Identify factors affecting the health of children and adolescents.
Test Taking Tip: Understand the effects of fetal alcohol syndrome.

16.7 An example of an intervention that reflects primary prevention is:
1. Screening for sickle cell anemia.
2. Referring a child with asthma.
3. Dental care.
4. Educating the parents of an AIDS infant on the disposal of bodily fluids.

Answer: 3
Rationale: Primary prevention interventions promote the health of children and adolescents. Some categories of intervention that reflect primary prevention include: reducing prematurity, low birth weight, and infant mortality; promoting growth and development; providing adequate nutrition; promoting safety; preventing communicable diseases; dental care; support for effective parenting; and other primary prevention activities. Secondary prevention is geared toward resolution of health problems currently experienced by children, and tertiary prevention is geared toward the particular health problems experienced by children. Screening for sickle cell anemia would be secondary prevention as would care of the child with asthma. Tertiary prevention for an infant with AIDS may entail educating parents on the disposal of bodily fluids.
Step in the Nursing Process: Implementation
Category of Client Need: Health Promotion and Maintenance
Cognitive Level: Application
Learning Objective 16-2: Describe at least five primary prevention measures appropriate to the care of children and adolescents and analyze the role of the community health nurse with respect to each.
Test Taking Tip: Understand primary prevention measures.

16.8 The nurse is planning to teach an educational program on child and adolescent safety. Facts that the nurse should include are:
1. Most incidents of poisoning occur outside of the home.
2. The use of appropriate child safety restraints decreases the risk of death by 10%.
3. Most playground fatalities occur at school.
4. Among adolescents, half of the poisoning incidents were intentional suicide attempts.

Answer: 4
Rationale: Among adolescents, half of the poisoning incidents were intentional suicide attempts. Most poisoning incidents (90%) occur in the home. The use of appropriate child safety restraints decreases the risk of death by 50%. Seventy percent of playground fatalities occur at home.
Step in the Nursing Process: Implementation
Category of Client Need: Health Promotion and Maintenance
Cognitive Level: Application
Learning Objective 16-2: Describe at least five primary prevention measures appropriate to the care of children and adolescents and analyze the role of the community health nurse with respect to each.
Test Taking Tip: Understand statistics about child and adolescent safety.

16.9 The mother of a one-year-old child is asking the nurse how many immunizations her child will receive by the time her child is two. The nurse explains that a two-year-old child should have received approximately _____ doses of vaccine.
1. 10.
2. 12.
3. 15.
4. 23.
5. 25.

Answer: 4
Rationale: By two years of age, children in the United States should have received as many as 23 doses of vaccine to protect them against 12 communicable diseases.
Step in the Nursing Process: Planning
Category of Client Need: Health Promotion and Maintenance
Cognitive Level: Comprehension
Learning Objective 16-2: Describe at least five primary prevention measures appropriate to the care of children and adolescents and analyze the role of the community health nurse with respect to each.
Test Taking Tip: Know how many vaccinations a child receives by age two.

16.10 The nurse is planning to teach a class about dental care to a group of expectant women. The nurse should teach that dental hygiene should begin:
1. At birth.
2. When the first tooth erupts.
3. When the child can hold a toothbrush.
4. When the child starts solid food.

Answer: 2
Rationale: Dental hygiene should begin as soon as the child's first tooth erupts. At this time, parents can be encouraged to rub teeth briskly with a dry washcloth.
Step in the Nursing Process: Intervention
Category of Client Need: Health Promotion and Maintenance
Cognitive Level: Comprehension
Learning Objective 16-2: Describe at least five primary prevention measures appropriate to the care of children and adolescents and analyze the role of the community health nurse with respect to each.
Test Taking Tip: Understand dental hygiene measures.

16.11 Four factors that contribute to parental efficacy include positive mastery experiences in past care of infants, vicarious experience obtained through parent training programs, verbal persuasion by significant others of one's capabilities, and:
1. An appropriate physical and affective state.
2. A higher income and a higher educational level.
3. A two-parent home.
4. An extended family.

Answer: 1
Rationale: In a review of related literature, the authors of this book found four factors that contributed to efficacy: positive mastery experiences in past care of infants; vicarious experience obtained through parent training programs; verbal persuasion by significant others of one's capabilities; and an appropriate physical and affective state.
Step in the Nursing Process: Assessment
Category of Client Need: Health Promotion and Maintenance
Cognitive Level: Application
Learning Objective 16-2: Describe at least five primary prevention measures appropriate to the care of children and adolescents and analyze the role of the community health nurse with respect to each.
Test Taking Tip: Understand the factors that contribute to parental efficacy.

16.12 The mother asks the nurse when her infant should be screened for tuberculosis (TB). The nurse explains that routine screening for TB usually occurs initially:
1. At birth.
2. At nine months of age.
3. At three years of age.
4. When the child starts school.

Answer: 2
Rationale: The tuberculin skin test is usually performed as routine screening at the age of 9 months.
Step in the Nursing Process: Intervention
Category of Client Need: Health Promotion and Maintenance
Cognitive Level: Analysis
Learning Objective 16-3: Identify at least three approaches to providing secondary preventive care for children and adolescents and give examples of community health nurse interventions related to each.
Test Taking Tip: Know when a child is first screened for tuberculosis.

16.13 The nurse is working with two parents who have a child who was diagnosed with leukemia. The parents seem to adapt, but do not accept the illness. The model that would best explain the parents' reaction is the:
1. Time-bound model.
2. Integrated model.
3. Chronic sorrow model.
4. Non-acceptance model.

Answer: 3
Rationale: In the chronic sorrow model, parents adapt, but may never accept the illness and experience continuing sorrow that fades and burgeons based on circumstances in the life of the child and the family. In the time-bound model parents adapt over time to the presence of the disease. The integrated model is one that integrates both perspectives: parents and families do adapt, but are apt to experience periods in which adaptation is more or less difficult. In the non-acceptance model the parents do not adapt to or accept the illness.
Step in the Nursing Process: Assessment
Category of Client Need: Health Promotion and Maintenance
Cognitive Level: Analysis
Learning Objective 16-3: Identify at least three approaches to providing secondary preventive care for children and adolescents and give examples of community health nursing interventions related to each.
Test Taking Tip: Distinguish secondary prevention measures.

16.14 There are usually three aspects to tertiary prevention with children and adolescents with a chronic illness or disability. Two of the aspects include preventing recurrence of problems and preventing further consequences. The third is:
1. Promoting adjustment.
2. Referring for other medical opinions.

Answer: 1
Rationale: Tertiary prevention is geared toward the particular health problems experienced by children or adolescents. Generally there are three aspects to tertiary prevention with children and adolescents. The three aspects are preventing recurrence of problems, preventing further consequences, and in the case of chronic illness or disability, promoting adjustment.
Step in the Nursing Process: Intervention
Category of Client Need: Health Promotion and Maintenance
Cognitive Level: Application

3. Providing palliative care.
4. Diagnosing secondary problems.

Learning Objective 16-3: Describe three tertiary preventive considerations in the care of children and adolescents and analyze the role of the community health nurse with respect to each.
Test Taking Tip: Distinguish tertiary prevention measures.

16.15 A mother frequently brings her six-month-old to the clinic with a complaint of diaper rash. The nurse plans to teach the mother ways to prevent the diaper rash from recurring. This would be an example of:
  1. Primary prevention.
  2. Secondary prevention.
  3. Tertiary prevention.
  4. Protective promotion.

Answer: 3
Rationale: Educating parents to prevent the recurrence of a health problem is an example of preventing problem recurrence, which is tertiary prevention. Secondary prevention is geared toward resolution of health problems currently experienced by children, and tertiary prevention is geared toward the particular health problems experienced by children.
Step in the Nursing Process: Intervention
Category of Client Need: Health Promotion and Maintenance
Cognitive Level: Analysis
Learning Objective 16-4: Describe three tertiary preventive considerations in the care of children and adolescents and analyze the role of the community health nurse with respect to each.
Test Taking Tip: Distinguish tertiary prevention measures.

CHAPTER 17

17.1 The nurse is planning a class to promote women's health. It would be appropriate to include:
  1. The leading cause of death among women in the United States is diabetes.
  2. Approximately 20% of women will receive a diagnosis of cancer during their lifetime.
  3. Rheumatoid arthritis is the most common chronic condition in women.
  4. Women with disabilities report fewer symptoms than men with disabilities.

Answer: 3
Rationale: Rheumatoid arthritis is the most common chronic condition in women. The leading cause of death among women is heart disease. Approximately one-third of women will receive a diagnosis of cancer at some time in their lives. Women with disabilities report more symptoms than men with disabilities.
Step in the Nursing Process: Assessment
Category of Client Need: Health Promotion and Maintenance
Cognitive Level: Application
Learning Objective 17-1: Identify at least two factors in each of the dimensions of health as they relate to the health of women.
Test Taking Tip: Recognize factors that relate to women's health.

17.2 A woman, age 22, is admitted to the hospital in labor. She admits to having no prenatal care. She is among what percentage of pregnancies in the United States that have late or no prenatal care?
  1. 4%.
  2. 10%.
  3. 15%.
  4. 20%.

Answer: 1
Rationale: In 2002, nearly 4% of pregnancies in the United States received late or no prenatal care.
Step in the Nursing Process: Assessment
Category of Client Need: Health Promotion and Maintenance
Cognitive Level: Comprehension
Learning Objective 17-1: Identify at least two factors in each of the dimensions of health as they relate to the health of women.
Test Taking Tip: Recognize factors that relate to women's health.

17.3 The nurse is interviewing a female client who admits to having poor coping skills, drug abuse, and a recent divorce with loss of child custody. The nurse knows the client is most at risk for:
  1. Self-mutilation.
  2. Bulimia.
  3. Chronic fatigue syndrome.
  4. Depression.

Answer: 4
Rationale: General risk factors for depression include poor coping skills, negative life events, and substance abuse. Chronic fatigue syndrome may result in changes in self-concept, alienation, and decreased quality of interpersonal interactions. Women with bulimia tend to isolate themselves in order to disguise their pattern of binge eating.
Step in the Nursing Process: Assessment
Category of Client Need: Health Promotion and Maintenance
Cognitive Level: Analysis
Learning Objective 17-2: Identify health problems common to women.
Test Taking Tip: Recognize common health problems in women.

17.4 During an interview, the client admits to the nurse that she self-induces vomiting after every meal and that she uses laxatives daily. The nurse recognizes that these symptoms best describe:
1. A binge eating disorder.
2. A post-traumatic stress disorder.
3. Bulimia.
4. Anorexia nervosa.

Answer: 3
Rationale: Bulimia is characterized by recurrent episodes of binge eating followed by compensatory mechanisms such as purging by means of self-induced vomiting or use of laxatives, diuretics, or emetics. Bingeing disorders are characterized by uncontrollable eating for a period of time. These symptoms are not typical of a post traumatic stress disorder. Anorexia is characterized by active resistance to maintaining a minimal body weight, usually by not eating.
Step in the Nursing Process: Assessment
Category of Client Need: Health Promotion and Maintenance
Cognitive Level: Application
Learning Objective 17-2: Identify health problems common to women.
Test Taking Tip: Be familiar with eating disorders in women.

17.5 The nurse is working on a psychiatric unit in a large hospital and encounters a female client with a history of being abused. What client statement best supports the belief that this client is at risk for more violence?
1. "I am financially independent."
2. "My partner is enrolled in Alcoholics Anonymous."
3. "I only finished the eighth grade and then I quit school."
4. "My partner encourages me to use condoms."

Answer: 3
Rationale: Women's risk of violence is increased by financial dependence, their partners' association with other women, an inability to negotiate condom use, their partners' use of alcohol, and low educational level. Other risks are lower household income and drug use.
Step in the Nursing Process: Evaluation
Category of Client Need: Health Promotion and Maintenance
Cognitive Level: Analysis
Learning Objective 17-2: Identify health problems common to women.
Test Taking Tip: Understand violence as it relates to women's health.

17.6 The nurse is interviewing a client who states that she is a lesbian. What statement by the client indicates the need for more education?
1. "Since I only have sex with females I am at a lower risk for some sexually transmitted diseases."
2. "I have less risk factors for breast cancer than a heterosexual."
3. "I do need to have routine Pap smears."
4. "I have an increased risk of heart disease."

Answer: 2
Rationale: There is a higher prevalence of certain risk factors for breast cancer among lesbian women. Women who engage in sexual activity exclusively with other women seem to be at lower risk for some sexually transmitted diseases. Routine Pap smears are as important for lesbians as for heterosexuals. There is an increased risk for heart disease among lesbians, perhaps because lesbians smoke more than their heterosexual sisters and tend to have a higher body mass index.
Step in the Nursing Process: Evaluation
Category of Client Need: Health Promotion and Maintenance
Cognitive Level: Application
Learning Objective 17-3: Describe at least three unique considerations in assessing the health needs of lesbian, bisexual, and transgender clients.
Test Taking Tip: Understand health needs of lesbians.

17.7 The most accurate description the nurse could give a colleague about homophobia is that it:
1. Is prohibited in more than 75% of the United States.
2. Encompasses a belief system that is used to justify discrimination against lesbians.
3. Is an intolerance of all homosexuals.
4. Has led to homosexual activity being criminalized in all states.

Answer: 3
Rationale: Homophobia encompasses a belief system that is believed to justify discrimination against gays and lesbians. Homosexual activity is criminalized in 16 states. As of 2004, only 15 states had strong laws that prohibit discrimination based on sexual orientation.
Step in the Nursing Process: Assessment
Category of Client Need: Health Promotion and Maintenance
Cognitive Level: Application
Learning Objective 17-3: Describe at least three unique considerations in assessing the health needs of lesbian, bisexual, and transgender clients.
Test Taking Tip: Understand homophobia.

17.8 The nurse is working with a female client, trying to assist her in balancing personal needs with those of other family members. What is the goal that this intervention best relates to?
1. Maintaining balance, perspective, and priorities in life.

Answer: 1
Rationale: An intervention related to the goal of maintaining balance, perspective, and priorities could best be demonstrated by the intervention of helping clients learn to balance personal needs with those of other family members.
Step in the Nursing Process: Implementation
Category of Client Need: Health Promotion and Maintenance
Cognitive Level: Analysis

2. Developing and maintaining healthy relationships.
3. Developing and maintaining a healthy sense of self.
4. Developing and maintaining a physically healthy body and preventing acute and chronic illness.

Learning Objective 17-4: Identify concerns in primary prevention for women and analyze the role of the community health nurse with respect to each.
Test Taking Tip: Distinguish among primary prevention measures for women.

17.9 The nurse is working with a group of abused women, trying to assist them in developing a sense of self so that they will avoid blaming themselves for the abuse. What is the goal that this intervention best relates to?
1. Maintaining balance, perspective, and priorities in life.
2. Developing and maintaining healthy relationships.
3. Developing and maintaining a healthy sense of self.
4. Developing and maintaining a physically healthy body and preventing acute and chronic illness.

Answer: 3
Rationale: An intervention related to the goal developing and maintaining a healthy sense of self could best be demonstrated by the intervention of helping the abused women to develop a strong sense of self in order to avoid blaming themselves for the abuse.
Step in the Nursing Process: Implementation
Category of Client Need: Health Promotion and Maintenance
Cognitive Level: Analysis
Learning Objective 17-4: Identify concerns in primary prevention for women and analyze the role of the community health nurse with respect to each.
Test Taking Tip: Distinguish among primary prevention measures in women.

17.10 Which statement by the nurse correctly describes some health promotion needs of the perimenopausal and postmenopausal years?
1. Calcium supplementation does not affect risk of fractures.
2. Dietary vitamin D supplementation is discouraged among this population.
3. Women should be encouraged to limit alcohol intake because it increases calcium excretion.
4. Smoking decreases calcium excretion.

Answer: 3
Rationale: Women should be encouraged to limit alcohol intake because it increases calcium excretion. Long-term calcium supplementation has been shown to reduce risks of fractures. Vitamin D supplementation promotes calcium absorption and should be encouraged in this population. Smoking increases calcium excretion.
Step in the Nursing Process: Intervention
Category of Client Need: Health Promotion and Maintenance
Cognitive Level: Analysis
Learning Objective 17-4: Identify concerns in primary prevention in women and analyze the role of the community health nurse with respect to each.
Test Taking Tip: Distinguish among primary prevention measures in women.

17.11 Secondary prevention focuses on _____ for existing health problems. (Select all that apply.)
1. Screening.
2. Diagnosis.
3. Treatment.
4. Rehabilitation.
5. Prevention.

Answer: 1, 2, 3
Rationale: Secondary prevention focuses on screening and diagnosis and treatment for existing health problems. Tertiary prevention focuses on rehabilitation and preventing the recurrence of health problems.
Step in the Nursing Process: Assessment
Category of Client Need: Health Promotion and Maintenance
Cognitive Level: Application
Learning Objective 17-5: Describe areas of secondary prevention activity with women and design community health nurse interventions related to each.
Test Taking Tip: Distinguish among secondary prevention measures.

17.12 The community health nurse is working with a 17-year-old mother of two. Evidence of spousal abuse is confirmed. The nurse knows that:
1. It is unethical to confirm the diagnosis with the client.
2. Part of the primary goal is to assist the woman to feel empowered.

Answer: 2
Rationale: If there is evidence of abuse, it is unethical for the nurse not to confirm this diagnosis with the client. Part of the primary goal is to empower the client to change the situation. The nurse should not become a source of control for the client but the nurse should assist the woman to reestablish a feeling of control herself. The client should be assisted and encouraged to make her own decisions.
Step in the Nursing Process: Intervention
Category of Client Need: Health Promotion and Maintenance
Cognitive Level: Analysis

---

3. The nurse should become a source of control in the client's life. 4. The nurse should make immediate decisions for the client.	Learning Objective 17-6: Describe two elements of secondary prevention of physical abuse of women and analyze the role of the community health nurse in addressing abuse. Test Taking Tip: Understand how the nurse can help the abused female client.
17.13 The nurse is working with a pregnant client who has six children. The ages of the children range from six months to twelve years of age. An example of tertiary prevention in working with this client would include education regarding: 1. Prenatal care. 2. Appropriate nutrition. 3. Dental hygiene. 4. Effective contraception to prevent subsequent pregnancies.	Answer: 4 Rationale: Tertiary prevention with respect to this client involves the use of an effective contraceptive to prevent subsequent pregnancies. Tertiary prevention focuses on rehabilitation and preventing the recurrence of health problems. Areas in which tertiary prevention are particularly warranted include pregnancy, abuse, and STDs. Appropriate nutrition would be primary prevention. Dental hygiene would be primary prevention. Prenatal care would be primary prevention. Step in the Nursing Process: Intervention Category of Client Need: Health Promotion and Maintenance Cognitive Level: Analysis Learning Objective 17-1: Identify at least two factors in each of the dimensions of health as they relate to the health of women. Test Taking Tip: Distinguish tertiary prevention measures in women's health care.
17.14 Which statement by the client indicates that she has correctly understood the nurse's teaching? 1. "Perimenopause occurs after menopause." 2. "Menopause typically occurs after the third pregnancy." 3. "The potential for childbearing is high during premenopause." 4. "Postmenopause occurs over a period of approximately three years."	Answer: 3 Rationale: Premenopuase includes the reproductive years; there is great potential for childbearing. Perimenopause is a transitional period three to nine years prior to menopause. Menopause occurs after 12 months without menstruation, typically around age 50. Postmenopause is the period from menopause to death (may be as much as a third of life). Step in the Nursing Process: Assessment Category of Client Need: Health Promotion and Maintenance Cognitive Level: Application Learning Objective 17-1: Identify at least two factors in each of the dimensions of health as they relate to the health of women. Test Taking Tip: Distinguish among premenopause, perimenopause, menopause, and postmenopause.
17.15 The nurse is working with a group of lesbian, bisexual, and transgender women. What statements should the nurse be most concerned about regarding psychological considerations in working this group of clients? (Select all that apply.) 1. "I do not live my life openly, but I never fear someone will find out I am a lesbian." 2. "I constantly monitor everything I say and do for fear my mother will find out I am a lesbian." 3. "I constantly feel negative feelings about my sexual preference." 4. "I am coming out and sometimes I have contradictory feelings of excitement and relief." 5. "The excitement of coming out is overwhelming."	Answer: 1, 2 Rationale: The lesbian, bisexual, or transgender woman who does not live her identity openly must deal with the fear that someone will discover who she really is. Although these women grieve the loss of hiding who they are, the grief is not sanctioned by society and is another source of hidden stress. Lesbians or bisexual women may internalize negative social attitudes to their sexual identities, leading to greater risk of suicide. Coming out causes contradictory feelings of excitement and relief. Step in the Nursing Process: Intervention Category of Client Need: Health Promotion and Maintenance Cognitive Level: Analysis Learning Objective 17-7: Describe at least two actions that the community health nurse can take to provide more sensitive and effective care to lesbian, bisexual, and transgender clients. Test Taking Tip: Understand the psychological needs of the lesbian, bisexual, and transgender client.

CHAPTER 18

18.1 Men are _____ as likely as women to die from heart disease and _____ times more likely to commit suicide.	Answer: 3 Rationale: Men are twice as likely as women to die from heart disease and three times more likely to commit suicide. Step in the Nursing Process: Assessment Category of Client Need: Health Promotion and Maintenance

1. Three times, four. 2. Four times, two. 3. Twice, three. 4. Twice, six.	Cognitive Level: Comprehension Learning Objective 18-1: Describe major considerations in assessing the biophysical, psychological, physical environmental, sociocultural, behavioral, and health care system factors affecting men's health. Test Taking Tip: Understand some of the major issues in men's health.
18.2 The community is devoting a month to men's health. Which of the following would be appropriate information to advertise? 1. Men have lower rates of sexually transmitted diseases as compared to women. 2. Men are less likely to die from cancer as are women. 3. Men develop heart disease earlier and die more frequently than do women. 4. Worldwide, the most frequent cause of death in young and middle adult men is prostate cancer.	Answer: 3 Rationale: Men develop heart disease at earlier ages and they die earlier than women. Men have higher rates of sexually transmitted diseases as compared to women. Men are more likely to die from cancer than women. Worldwide, the most frequent cause of death in young and middle adult men is traffic accidents. Step in the Nursing Process: Assessment Category of Client Need: Health Promotion and Maintenance Cognitive Level: Application Learning Objective 18-1: Describe major considerations in assessing the biophysical, psychological, physical environmental, sociocultural, behavioral, and health care system factors affecting men's health. Test Taking Tip: Describe biophysical considerations that influence the health of men.
18.3 Society has socialized men to accept a stereotypical male role, which makes it difficult for men to meet their basic psychological needs. General dimensions of this stereotyped role include a need to: 1. Freely demonstrate affection. 2. Be more reliant on others. 3. Participate in routine health care screenings. 4. View oneself as superior to others.	Answer: 4 Rationale: General dimensions of this stereotyped role include a need to refrain from behaviors ascribed to women as freely demonstrating affection, a need to be self-reliant, and a need to be powerful and superior. Internalization of the typical male gender role has been shown to be associated with less attention to routine health care screenings. Step in the Nursing Process: Evaluation Category of Client Need: Health Promotion and Maintenance Cognitive Level: Application Learning Objective 18-1: Describe major considerations in assessing the biophysical, psychological, physical environmental, sociocultural, behavioral, and health care system factors affecting men's health. Test Taking Tip: Understand psychological considerations in men's healthcare.
18.4 The nurse is working in a small rural community. The community has had a very high rate of suicide among its male population. The nurse decides to screen the male population for the presence of suicide risks. Those risks are high rates of: (Select all that apply.) 1. Depression. 2. Progressively debilitating disorders. 3. Divorce. 4. Substance abuse. 5. High stress occupations.	Answer: 1, 2, 4 Rationale: Suicide risk factors include high rates of depression, high rates of progressively debilitating disorders, and high rates of substance abuse. High rates of divorce and high stress jobs are not included as risks for suicide. Step in the Nursing Process: Assessment Category of Client Need: Health Promotion and Maintenance Cognitive Level: Application Learning Objective 18-1: Describe major considerations in assessing the biophysical, psychological, physical environmental, sociocultural, behavioral, and health care system factors affecting men's health. Test Taking Tip: Distinguish among the psychological considerations in men's health care.
18.5 The male client is complaining of not being able to achieve and maintain an erection sufficient for sexual activity. This is characteristic of: 1. Erectile dysfunction. 2. Prostatitis. 3. Testicular cancer. 4. A psychological issue.	Answer: 1 Rationale: Erectile dysfunction occurs when a man cannot achieve or maintain an erection sufficient for satisfactory sexual activity. Age and atherosclerosis contribute to the development of erectile dysfunction. Step in the Nursing Process: Assessment Category of Client Need: Health Promotion and Maintenance Cognitive Level: Application Learning Objective 18-1: Describe major considerations in assessing the biophysical, psychological, physical environmental, sociocultural, behavioral, and health care system factors affecting men's health. Test Taking Tip: Review major considerations that affect men's health.

18.6 The nurse is caring for a bisexual male client. In addition to routine adult immunizations, the nurse is aware that the client needs to receive the:
1. Meningococcal vaccine.
2. Hepatitis A and B vaccine.
3. Hepatitis B vaccine.
4. Pneumococcal vaccine.

Answer: 2

Rationale: In addition to the routine adult immunizations, gay, bisexual, and transgender men should receive immunization for hepatitis A and B. Routine immunizations for the bisexual male client would not include meningococcal and pneumococcal vaccinations. Hepatitis B is not correct as the client needs to receive both the hepatitis A and B series.

Step in the Nursing Process: Implementation

Category of Client Need: Health Promotion and Maintenance

Cognitive Level: Analysis

Learning Objective 18-2: Describe factors that contribute to adverse health effects for gay, bisexual, and transgender men.

Test Taking Tip: Know the health needs for gay, bisexual, and transgender men.

18.7 An adolescent shares with the nurse that he is gay and that he is going to tell his parents. The nurse knows that parental response to the disclosure of homosexuality is strongly influenced by the: (Select all that apply.)
1. Strength of traditional gender role conceptions.
2. Perceptions of the probable attitudes of significant others in the family's network.
3. Parental age.
4. Parental education.
5. Parental race.

Answer: 1, 2, 3, 4

Rationale: The parental response to the disclosure of homosexuality is strongly influenced by a variety of factors, which include: the strength of traditional gender role conceptions; perceptions of the probable attitudes of significant others in the family's social network; and parental age and education level. The younger and better educated parents tend to be more accepting. Race is not an influencing factor.

Step in the Nursing Process: Assessment.

Category of Client Need: Health Promotion and Maintenance

Cognitive Level: Application

Learning Objective 18-2: Describe factors that contribute to adverse health effects for gay, bisexual, and transgender men.

Test Taking Tip: Understand issues in caring for gay, bisexual, and transgender men.

18.8 A therapist who works primarily with gay and lesbian couples is aware that the same kinds of stress that affect heterosexual relationships also affect gay and lesbian relationships. But the therapist knows that the stress is different with respect to:
1. Extended family involvement.
2. Inequalities of power.
3. Disparity in income.
4. Coming out.

Answer: 4

Rationale: With the exception of the stage of coming out, most issues that affect the stability or relationships among heterosexual and non heterosexual couples are the same. Extended family involvement, inequalities of power, and disparity in income tend to have the same affect on gay and lesbian relationships.

Step in the Nursing Process: Assessment.

Category of Client Need: Health Promotion and Maintenance

Cognitive Level: Application

Learning Objective 18-2: Describe factors that contribute to adverse health effects for gay, bisexual, and transgender men.

Test Taking Tip: Understand the stressors for gay, bisexual, and transgender men.

18.9 A nurse is working with a group of elderly men in a community health clinic. Even though the nurse might need to discuss each of these statements, which statement should the nurse address first?
1. "I know I can eat this fried chicken every day because I exercise a lot."
2. "I cannot eat as much as I used to."
3. "My sleep patterns have changed."
4. "I have to turn the volume up on the television these days."

Answer: 1

Rationale: There are some commonly encountered patterns of health behavior among men. One such behavior is a tendency to view exercise as sufficient to compensate for unhealthy behaviors such as a high intake of dietary fats. The statements regarding eating patterns, sleep patterns and hearing changes could be addressed after addressing the statement regarding exercise and a high intake of dietary fats.

Step in the Nursing Process: Implementation

Category of Client Need: Health Promotion and Maintenance

Cognitive Level: Analysis

Learning Objective 18-3: Identify major considerations in primary prevention for men and analyze the role of the community health nurse with respect to each.

Test Taking Tip: Review primary prevention and male health care.

18.10 The nurse is trying to help the male client see the same situation in a different light. The best description of this technique is:
1. Processing.
2. Reframing.
3. Acknowledgement.
4. Cause and effect.

Answer: 2

Rationale: Reframing, which focuses on helping men to see the same situation in a different light, is one technique that can be used to promote positive behavioral change.

Step in the Nursing Process: Implementation

Category of Client Need: Health Promotion and Maintenance

Cognitive Level: Application

Learning Objective 18-3: Identify major considerations in primary prevention for men and analyze the role of the community health nurse with respect to each.

Test Taking Tip: Recognize some behavioral change strategies in working with men.

18.11 A six-point program intended to facilitate creation of health care services that better meet the health promotion needs of men is called HEALTH. The T in this acronym stands for:
1. Typical.
2. Transfer.
3. Tailor.
4. Temperature.

Answer: 3
Rationale: The T in HEALTH stands for Tailor. Health care services for men should be tailored to their specific needs with input from those involved.
Step in the Nursing Process: Implementation
Category of Client Need: Health Promotion and Maintenance
Cognitive Level: Application
Learning Objective 18-3: Identify major considerations in primary prevention for men and analyze the role of the community health nurse with respect to each.
Test Taking Tip: Know the acronym HEALTH in relation to men's health promotion.

18.12 The nurse is working in a community health clinic and is planning a secondary prevention program. One such example could be a program:
1. That eliminates high-risk behaviors.
2. Related to diabetes prevention.
3. That encourages blood pressure screening.
4. That explains adult immunizations.

Answer: 3
Rationale: Primary prevention for health concerns specific to men focuses on increasing their use of health-promoting behaviors in the areas of chronic disease prevention, coping, immunization, safety practices, and elimination of high-risk behaviors. Secondary prevention involves the earliest possible detection of health needs through effective screening such as blood pressure screening. It also encompasses the actual treatment of the health needs of disorders themselves.
Step in the Nursing Process: Planning
Category of Client Need: Health Promotion and Maintenance
Cognitive Level: Application
Learning Objective 18-4: Describe secondary prevention considerations for men and related community health nursing roles.
Test Taking Tip: Understand secondary prevention as compared to primary prevention for men.

18.13 The nurse is talking with a male client who is on a regimen of antihypertensive medications. The nurse knows that there are side effects that affect masculine roles associated with these medications. Those side effects include:
1. Impotence and hyperglycemia.
2. Impotence and dizziness.
3. Decreased tolerance for physical activity and tremors.
4. Erectile dysfunction and hoarseness.

Answer: 2
Rationale: Examples of side effects associated with antihypertensive medications include impotence, dizziness, and decreased tolerance for physical activity. Hyperglycemia, decreased tolerance for physical activity, tremors, erectile dysfunction and hoarseness are not side effects of antihypertensive medications that affect the masculine role.
Step in the Nursing Process: Assessment
Category of Client Need: Health Promotion and Maintenance
Cognitive Level: Application
Learning Objective 18-5: Identify areas of emphasis in tertiary prevention for men and analyze the role of the community health nurse in each.
Test Taking Tip: Know the medications that affect masculine roles.

18.14 The nurse is working with a client who had his testes surgically removed as part of treatment for testicular cancer. The treatment had a profound impact on his self-image. An important area of tertiary prevention for this client would be:
1. Encouraging him to join a support group.
2. Referring him to a marriage counselor.
3. Hormone therapy.
4. Antidepressant medications.

Answer: 1
Rationale: Tertiary prevention for men is directed at those disorders that influence men's health in some ongoing manner or that have a likelihood of recurrence. The goals of tertiary prevention are to assist men in coping with the continuing manifestations of illness and to reduce the likelihood of future episodes of an illness. An important area of tertiary prevention involves encouraging men to join support groups.
Step in the Nursing Process: Implementation
Category of Client Need: Health Promotion and Maintenance
Cognitive Level: Analysis
Learning Objective 18-5: Identify areas of emphasis in tertiary prevention for men and analyze the role of the community health nurse in each.
Test Taking Tip: Review tertiary prevention measures for men's health.

18.15 Behavioral factors seem to make a greater contribution to men's health status as compared to women. This is most likely because:
1. Men are more apt to perform healthful behaviors.
2. Men are more reliant on others.

Answer: 4
Rationale: Men are generally more likely than women to engage in high-risk behaviors. Because of their gender socialization, men are more inclined to engage in high-risk behaviors and less apt to perform healthful behaviors.
Step in the Nursing Process: Assessment
Category of Client Need: Health Promotion and Maintenance
Cognitive Level: Application

3. Men are more educated about health issues.
4. Men are generally more likely to engage in high-risk behaviors.

Learning Objective 18-1: Describe major considerations in assessing the biophysical, psychological, physical environmental, sociocultural, behavioral, and health care system factors affecting men's health.
Test Taking Tip: Review behavioral considerations in men's health.

CHAPTER 19

19.1 The nurse is presenting a workshop about aging. The nurse is including information about longevity and declining endocrine and immune function. In what theory category does this information belong?
1. Psychological.
2. Biological.
3. Sociological.
4. Individualism.

Answer: 2
Rationale: In general there are three categories of theories that explain how and why aging occurs. Biological theories include specific programmed aging theories that address longevity, and declining endocrine and immune function. Psychological theories focus on psychological changes that occur with age. Sociological theories focus on changes in roles and relationships that occur with advancing aging. Individualism is not a theory category for aging.
Step in the Nursing Process: Assessment
Category of Client Need: Health Promotion and Maintenance
Cognitive Level: Application
Learning Objective 19-1: Describe three categories of theories of aging.
Test Taking Tip: Know the three categories of aging.

19.2 The nurse is comparing and contrasting examples from the psychological and sociological theories. Which of the following would be included in the examples from psychological theories?
1. Error theories.
2. Mutually exclusive theories.
3. Jung's theory.
4. Disengagement theory.

Answer: 3
Rationale: Psychological theories include Jung's theory of individualism, in which the individual's mental focus changes from the external to the internal world, and the developmental theories. Error theories are biological theories. Theories in the sociological category tend to be mutually exclusive. Disengagement theory is a sociological theory.
Step in the Nursing Process: Assessment
Category of Client Need: Health Promotion and Maintenance
Cognitive Level: Application
Learning Objective 19-1: Describe three categories of theories of aging.
Test Taking Tip: Recognize the theories within the three main categories of aging.

19.3 A student is developing a poster for a class presentation. The purpose of the poster is to explain aging. Part of the information on the poster demonstrates how the elderly withdraw from life as a means of making way for a younger generation in preparation for death. The theory that the student is using is:
1. Disengagement theory.
2. Erikson's theory.
3. Programmed theory.
4. Jung's theory.

Answer: 1
Rationale: Disengagement theory proposes that individuals withdraw themselves from life as a means of making way for a younger generation in preparation for death. Erikson's theory focuses on psychological/developmental stages. Programmed theories address longevity, and declining endocrine and immune function. Jung's theory involves individualism, in which the individual's mental focus changes from the external to the internal world.
Step in the Nursing Process: Assessment
Category of Client Need: Health Promotion and Maintenance
Cognitive Level: Application
Learning Objective 19-1: Describe three categories of theories of aging.
Test Taking Tip: Understand the various aging theories.

19.4 The client is complaining of signs and symptoms related to the major changes involved in aging, which is loss of physical reserve capacity. Those signs and symptoms would include:
1. Loss of verbal ability and increased urine flow.
2. Decreased walking speed and increase in verbal memory.
3. Increased reaction times and declining strength.
4. Slowed reaction time and loss of skeletal muscle.

Answer: 4
Rationale: The major change involved in aging is loss of physical reserve capacity, which results in slowed reaction times, decreased psychomotor and walking speed, loss of verbal memory, declining strength, decreased urine flow, and loss of skeletal muscle.
Step in the Nursing Process: Assessment
Category of Client Need: Health Promotion and Maintenance
Cognitive Level: Application
Learning Objective 19-2: Describe biophysical, psychological, physical environmental, sociocultural, behavioral, and health system factors influencing the health of the elderly population.
Test Taking Tip: Recognize the signs and symptoms associated with loss of physical reserve capacity.

19.5 Which of the following is the best example that the nurse could use to explain comorbidity?
1. The 65-year-old client and his spouse both have diabetes mellitus.
2. The 72-year-old client is taking an antihypertensive medication that interferes with his asthma.
3. The 86-year-old client is the primary caregiver for his 90-year-old spouse.
4. The 67-year-old client does not experience the usual symptoms that are associated with emphysema.

Answer: 2
Rationale: Comorbidity is the coexistence of more than one chronic physical and/or mental illness in the same person at the same time. This complicates diagnosis and treatment of illness in older adults. The best example would be the 72-year-old who has hypertension and asthma.
Step in the Nursing Process: Assessment
Category of Client Need: Health Promotion and Maintenance
Cognitive Level: Analysis
Learning Objective 19-2: Describe biophysical, psychological, physical environmental, sociocultural, behavioral, and health system factors influencing the health of the elderly population.
Test Taking Tip: Understand comorbidity.

19.6 The nurse is assessing a 72-year-old client. The nurse is gathering data as to the client's ability to perform the basic activities of daily living (BADLs). Those activities include the ability to: (Select all that apply.)
1. Walk at least 12 steps.
2. Dress oneself.
3. Bathe oneself.
4. Feed oneself.
5. Use the telephone.

Answer: 2, 3, 4
Rationale: Basic activities of daily living are personal care activities and include the ability to feed, bathe, and dress oneself, plus toileting and transfer skills (getting in or out of a chair or bed). Use of the telephone is an intermediate of instrumental activity of daily living. Walking at least 12 steps is not a basic activity of daily living.
Step in the Nursing Process: Assessment
Category of Client Need: Health Promotion and Maintenance
Cognitive Level: Comprehension
Learning Objective 19-2: Describe biophysical, psychological, physical environmental, sociocultural, behavioral, and health system factors influencing the health of the elderly population.
Test Taking Tip: Understand the basic activities of daily living.

19.7 The intervention that would be most appropriate for the client with functional incontinence would be to encourage the client:
1. To empty his/her bladder every two hours while awake.
2. Not to drink any liquids after 5:00 PM each evening.
3. To call for assistance when the urge to urinate is felt.
4. To wear an adult-type diaper during the daytime hours.

Answer: 3
Rationale: Functional incontinence is the inability to reach the toilet in time due to impaired mobility or decreased manual dexterity in undressing. The most appropriate intervention would be to encourage the client to call for assistance when the urge to urinate is felt.
Step in the Nursing Process: Intervention
Category of Client Need: Health Promotion and Maintenance
Cognitive Level: Analysis
Learning Objective 19-2: Describe the biophysical, psychological, physical environmental, sociocultural, behavioral, and health system factors influencing the health of the elderly population.
Test Taking Tip: Understand the various types of elderly incontinence.

19.8 The nurse explains that the reason that primary prevention among the elderly is important is because they are the:
1. Group that has more acute illness.
2. Fastest-growing segment of the population.
3. Most politically-involved group of the population.
4. Group that is the most health-conscious.

Answer: 2
Rationale: The elderly population is the fastest growing segment of the population. They exhibit the highest prevalence of chronic (not acute) illness. They are not the most politically involved or the most health-conscious.
Step in the Nursing Process: Assessment
Category of Client Need: Health Promotion and Maintenance
Cognitive Level: Application
Learning Objective 19-3: Identify major considerations in primary prevention in the care of the older adults and analyze community health nursing roles related to each.
Test Taking Tip: Understand primary prevention in the care of the older adult.

19.9 The nurse is teaching a class about nutrition to a group of elderly clients. The nurse knows that the elderly client is at risk for fat-soluble vitamin toxicity due to:
1. Decreased renal function.
2. Increased protein binding.

Answer: 3
Rationale: Care should be taken in the use of fat-soluble vitamins (A, D, E, and K), which are stored in the body more readily than water-soluble vitamins and may lead to vitamin toxicity in the elderly due to diminished metabolism.
Step in the Nursing Process: Implementation
Category of Client Need: Health Promotion and Maintenance
Cognitive Level: Application

3. Diminished metabolism.
4. Decreased liver function.

Learning Objective 19-3: Identify major considerations in primary prevention in the care of older adults and analyze community health nursing roles related to each.
Test Taking Tip: Understand the nutritional needs of the elderly.

19.10 The community health nurse is advocating for a screening service for older adults. This is an example of:
1. Primary prevention.
2. Secondary prevention.
3. Tertiary prevention.
4. Self-management.

Answer: 2
Rationale: Secondary prevention with older adults focuses on screening and treatment of disease. Primary prevention focuses on health promotion. Tertiary prevention activities focus on preventing complications of existing conditions and preventing their recurrence.
Step in the Nursing Process: Planning
Category of Client Need: Health Promotion and Maintenance
Cognitive Level: Application
Learning Objective 19-4: Describe secondary preventive measures for at least four health problems common among older clients.
Test Taking Tip: Understand secondary prevention and the elderly client.

19.11 The nurse is talking with a 78-year-old client who has chronic obstructive pulmonary disorder (COPD) and has described excessive use of cough medicine. The nurse should teach the client that this excessive use can make him more susceptible to respiratory infections by:
1. Decreasing clearance of secretions.
2. Decreasing his immunity.
3. Causing less fluid intake.
4. Decreasing nutritional intake.

Answer: 1
Rationale: Community health nurses can suggest that the client with COPD refrain from excessive use of cough medicines because they decrease clearance of secretions and make clients more susceptible to respiratory infection. The excessive use will not affect his immunity, cause less fluid intake or cause a decrease in his nutritional intake.
Step in the Nursing Process: Implementation
Category of Client Need: Health Promotion and Maintenance
Cognitive Level: Application
Learning Objective 19-4: Describe secondary prevention measures for at least four health problems common among older clients.
Test Taking Tip: Understand common secondary prevention needs of elderly clients.

19.12 Specific areas of tertiary prevention in the care of older populations include: (Select all that apply.)
1. Monitoring health status.
2. Palliative care.
3. End-of-life care.
4. Caring for caregivers.
5. Providing rehabilitation.

Answer: 1, 2, 3, 4
Rationale: Four specific areas of tertiary prevention in the care of older populations include monitoring health status, palliative care, end-of-life care, and caring for caregivers. Rehabilitation would not be an area of tertiary prevention.
Step in the Nursing Process: Assessment
Category of Client Need: Health Promotion and Maintenance
Cognitive Level: Comprehension
Learning Objective 19-5: Identify at least three foci for tertiary prevention with older clients and give examples of related community health nursing interventions.
Test Taking Tip: Understand tertiary prevention in the older client.

19.13 The nurse is teaching a group of elderly clients. The nurse should try to circumvent hearing loss by:
1. Using a higher-pitched voice.
2. Employing verbal teaching techniques.
3. Facing the listener while speaking.
4. Using background music.

Answer: 3
Rationale: Strategies to circumvent hearing loss include using a lower-pitched voice; facing the listener while speaking; employing nonverbal teaching techniques; using clear, concise terminology; and having the client use a hearing aid if needed. Background noise should be limited.
Step in the Nursing Process: Implementation
Category of Client Need: Health Promotion and Maintenance
Cognitive Level: Application
Learning Objective 19-6: Identify considerations that may influence the community health nurse's approach to health education for older clients.
Test Taking Tip: Understand the considerations when teaching the elderly client.

19.14 The nurse is writing a pamphlet to be used by graduate students as they plan health promotion classes for elderly clients. Which of the following should be included in the pamphlet?
1. Teaching sessions should be at least 30 minutes.
2. Teaching sessions should occur prior to a mealtime.

Answer: 4
Rationale: Lessons should proceed at a slower pace as the elderly client is more accepting of that pace. Teaching sessions should be kept short (10 to 15 minutes) because endurance may be limited. Lessons should occur at times when learners are rested and comfortable. Older clients do retain material as well as younger clients once material is learned.
Step in the Nursing Process: Implementation
Category of Client Need: Health Promotion and Maintenance
Cognitive Level: Application

3. Older clients do not retain material as well as younger clients.
4. Lessons should proceed at a slower pace.

Learning Objective 19-6: Identify considerations that may influence the community health nurse's approach to health education for older clients.
Test Taking Tip: Understand teaching/learning strategies that should be utilized with elderly clients.

19.15 The nurse is working with a 76-year-old client who has recently moved in with his daughter and her family. The most appropriate intervention to foster independence in the client would be to encourage the client to:
1. Exercise several times a week.
2. Move into an assisted living facility.
3. Purchase a cellular phone.
4. Assume specific roles within the household.

Answer: 4
Rationale: When older persons are living with family members, the nurse can encourage family members to foster independence in the client. This may include encouraging them to assign specific roles within the household to the older family member.
Step in the Nursing Process: Implementation
Category of Client Need: Health Promotion and Maintenance
Cognitive Level: Analysis
Learning Objective 19-7: Analyze the influence of factors unique to older clients on evaluation of nursing care.
Test Taking Tip: Understand the unique needs of the elderly client.

CHAPTER 20

20.1 The nurse is aware that many members of the community, though they are employed, need to obtain additional foodstuffs every month from the local community food bank. The nurse knows that this indicates that:
1. There are insufficient employment opportunities in the community.
2. Poverty is increasing in the community.
3. Better information about food economy should be disseminated in the community.
4. The local grocery stores do not carry sufficient supplies.

Answer: 2
Rationale: Poverty can be defined in terms of the amount of income spent on essential goods and services, such as food. If employed community residents are not able to obtain sufficient food with their paychecks and need to utilize local food bank supplies, this is an indication that there is poverty in the community. There is no indication that there are insufficient employment opportunities in the community, nor does it indicate that better information about food economy would stretch the food bought from the income. There is no indication that local grocery stores have insufficient supplies.
Step in the Nursing Process: Planning
Category of Client Need: Health Promotion and Maintenance
Cognitive Level: Application
Learning Objective 20-1: Analyze the effects of factors contributing to poverty and homelessness.
Test Taking Tip: Understand how having an insufficient food supply could be an indicator of poverty.

20.2 There is a low unemployment rate in a community that has experienced a large growth in gentrification. Yet, many community residents live in motels and campgrounds because there is a lack of affordable housing for lower-income residents. These residents could be considered:
1. To be very close to poverty.
2. To have problems with substance abuse.
3. Homeless due to their transitory lodgings.
4. An easily mobile workforce.

Answer: 3
Rationale: Homelessness can include those who lack a fixed, regular residence. Those living in motels and campgrounds are not living in a dwelling with a fixed address. Gentrification develops existing homes in the community, but displaces low-income housing with higher-income housing. This creates a lack of affordable housing for those who earn lower wages, which increases the threat of homelessness among the population, even those who are employed. There is no indication that substance abuse is involved nor does it indicate poverty. Living in motels or campgrounds does not imply a mobile workforce.
Step in the Nursing Process: Assessment
Category of Client Need: Health Promotion and Maintenance
Cognitive Level: Application
Learning Objective 20-1: Analyze the effects of factors contributing to poverty and homelessness.
Test Taking Tip: Understand that the stereotypical picture of homelessness may not always apply.

20.3 The nurse realizes that many of the young adult members of the community have poor nutrition habits and knows that these are risk factors for obesity, diabetes, and cardiovascular disease. These risk factors can affect their:
1. Future income and health potential.

Answer: 1
Rationale: While these risk factors may not manifest themselves in obvious health problems, these biophysical factors can influence future income and health potential. Development of chronic diseases can impact quality of employment in terms of absence that can result in decreased income, which affects overall earnings potential and can affect ability to have appropriate and effective health care. The ability to obtain health care, to develop social support system networks, and to change dietary habits are not impaired by having risk factors.
Step in the Nursing Process: Assessment

2. Ability to obtain health care.
3. Ability to network social support systems.
4. Future potential to change their dietary habits.

Category of Client Need: Health Promotion and Maintenance
Cognitive Level: Application
Learning Objective 20-2: Identify biophysical, psychological, physical environmental, sociocultural, behavioral, and health system factors that influence the health of poor and homeless clients.
Test Taking Tip: Understand the risk factors that influence the health of poor and homeless clients.

20.4 The nurse investigates a local park where several complaints have been lodged against people who sleep there at night and rummage through the trash cans. The nurse sees several inappropriately overdressed people sitting on the benches with many worn shopping bags clustered around them. After speaking with these people, the nurse contacts a local mental health agency to refer them for services. What is the best rationale for this intervention?
1. Mental health agencies are the best source for homeless referrals.
2. Shelters and shower facilities are easily obtained through mental health agencies.
3. Homeless funding is best found in mental health agencies.
4. Many homeless people have concurrent mental health illness.

Answer: 4
Rationale: Mental illness is a psychological factor that contributes to homelessness. While not every person has mental illness, the nurse's intervention to contact a local mental health agency comes after speaking with the homeless people in the park. Sleeping on the benches, rummaging through trash, and inappropriately overdressing in clothes are indications that the people in the park are homeless. Approximately 25% of homeless people have mental illness. Mental health agencies are not the best source for homeless referrals, but are the best source for a homeless person who has mental illness. Mental health agencies are not source facilities for shelters or shower facilities. Mental health agencies are not the best source for homeless funding.
Step in the Nursing Process: Implementation
Category of Client Need: Psychosocial Integrity
Cognitive Level: Application
Learning Objective 20-2: Identify biophysical, psychological, physical environmental, sociocultural, behavioral, and health system factors that influence the health of poor and homeless clients.
Test Taking Tip: Understand the statistics of homelessness.

20.5 In addressing factors that contribute to poverty, homelessness, and the health of the community, the nurse should assess:
1. Employment and home environment.
2. Lack of affordable housing and social support.
3. Mental illness and social support.
4. Mobility and age of client.

Answer: 2
Rationale: Sociocultural dimensions play a role in poverty, homelessness, and their effects on health. Lack of affordable housing, social support and welfare reform, mobility, and employment are societal conditions that contribute to poverty and homelessness. Home environment is a physical environment factor. Mental illness is a psychological factor. Age is a biophysical factor.
Step in the Nursing Process: Assessment
Category of Client Need: Health Promotion and Maintenance
Cognitive Level: Application
Learning Objective 20-2: Identify biophysical, psychological, physical environmental, sociocultural, behavioral, and health system factors that influence the health of poor and homeless clients.
Test Taking Tip: Understand that sociocultural factors are those that a community can address.

20.6 An example of a primary prevention approach to homelessness that the nurse can incorporate into practice is to:
1. Assess and diagnose community factors that lead to homelessness.
2. Diagnose and implement community programs that address homelessness.
3. Implement and evaluate community programs that address homelessness.
4. Assess and evaluate community factors that lead to homelessness.

Answer: 1
Rationale: Before homelessness can be addressed, an assessment must be done to address what factors are involved in homelessness. Diagnosis of the factors follows next. Diagnosis and implementation of programs cannot occur without assessment. Implementation and evaluation of programs cannot occur without the previous steps. Assessment and evaluation of homelessness factors are the beginning and end step of the process.
Step in the Nursing Process: Assessment
Category of Client Need: Health Promotion and Maintenance
Cognitive Level: Analysis
Learning Objective 20-3: Describe approaches to primary prevention of homelessness and analyze related roles of community health nurses with respect to each.
Test Taking Tip: Understand the steps to preventing homelessness.

20.7 The major emphasis in primary prevention that relates to the health of the poor and homeless in a community is to:
1. Have appropriate support services in place to address the health needs of these aggregates.
2. Ensure health services in the schools to keep children healthy.
3. Mitigate or prevent the factors that cause homelessness and poverty.
4. Ensure sufficient employment opportunities are available for all adults.

Answer: 3
Rationale: In order to prevent health problems from arising due to homelessness or poverty, the primary prevention emphasis is to eliminate or prevent them. Mitigation may be the best, and most realistic, approach for this. Having appropriate support services in place to address health needs is a primary approach, but it does not address the underlying cause. Ensuring appropriate school health services will keep students healthy, but it is not the major emphasis in addressing the roots of homelessness and poverty. Employment alone is insufficient if adults are working in low-paying jobs and cannot afford housing.
Step in the Nursing Process: Implementation
Category of Client Need: Health Promotion and Maintenance
Cognitive Level: Application
Learning Objective 20-4: Identify major areas of emphasis in primary prevention of health problems in poor and homeless clients.
Test Taking Tip: Understand primary prevention that relates to the health of the poor and homeless.

20.8 The nurse visits a family in the community and becomes aware that the family is facing the loss of their house because of the primary income earner's recent illness, which depleted the household income. The nurse should intervene to aid the family by:
1. Referring them to their local church.
2. Contacting local social service agencies for emergency housing funds.
3. Finding employment for other family members.
4. Arranging for home health services for the primary income earner.

Answer: 2
Rationale: When faced with a financial crisis, the nurse can help the family by contacting social service agencies about emergency funds for the family during this time. This is primary prevention. Referring to the local church does not indicate that financial help is available. Finding employment for other family members may not be appropriate because ages are not given. Arranging for home health does not address the financial crisis.
Step in the Nursing Process: Implementation
Category of Client Need: Health Promotion and Maintenance
Cognitive Level: Application
Learning Objective 20-4: Identify major areas of emphasis in primary prevention of health problems in poor and homeless clients.
Test Taking Tip: Understand that primary prevention seeks to address the most important issue first to avoid further crises.

20.9 The nurse notices that the population in the homeless shelters has increased, with a noticeable rise of pregnant women. The nurse coordinates with the shelter to provide meals that are more nutritionally adequate than the usual bologna sandwich, chips, and soda that are provided. This is considered:
1. Primary prevention.
2. Secondary prevention.
3. Tertiary prevention.
4. Health promotion.

Answer: 2
Rationale: Secondary prevention efforts seek to alleviate the health effects that result from homelessness. The nutritional needs of pregnant women must be addressed in order to ensure a healthy infant, so working with the shelter to provide more appropriate, nutritionally-sound food will improve nutrition for this population. Primary prevention would address efforts to reduce or eliminate pregnant women from needing the shelter. Tertiary prevention would address efforts to prevent the pregnant women from needing to use the shelter in the future. Health promotion directs efforts toward ensuring the overall health of the women during their pregnancy.
Step in the Nursing Process: Implementation
Category of Client Need: Health Promotion and Maintenance
Cognitive Level: Application
Learning Objective 20-5: Identify areas in which secondary preventive interventions may be required in the care of poor and homeless individuals and analyze the role of the community health nurse in these interventions.
Test Taking Tip: Understand which area of prevention aims to alleviate health effects that result from homelessness and poverty.

20.10 The nurse is working with a runaway adolescent who has been living in a local shelter. The nurse and the adolescent have explored the possibility of the adolescent returning home, and the adolescent is amenable. The most appropriate nursing intervention is to:
1. Contact the family and arrange for a time when the adolescent can return.

Answer: 4
Rationale: When an adolescent runs away, it is important to ascertain the reasons for running away. Interventions are then directed to modifying factors that led to the adolescent running away. Counseling can be arranged for the adolescent and family to explore and help ameliorate the factors contributing to the adolescent running away. Contacting the family and arranging for the return does not address what caused the adolescent to run away in the first place. Working with the shelter to improve conditions for adolescent residents and working with the community to improve programs are appropriate secondary prevention interventions but are not the most appropriate in this situation.
Step in the Nursing Process: Implementation

2. Work with the shelter to improve conditions for adolescent residents.
3. Work with the community to improve programs that address adolescent concerns.
4. Arrange for counseling for the adolescent and family before and after the adolescent returns.

Category of Client Need: Psychosocial Integrity
Cognitive Level: Application
Learning Objective 20-5: Identify areas in which secondary preventive interventions may be required in the care of poor and homeless individuals and analyze the role of the community health nurse in these interventions.
Test Taking Tip: Understand that referral for services can be a secondary prevention intervention.

20.11 The nurse becomes politically involved in supporting a bill that is being debated in the state legislature. This bill would raise the minimum wage in the state and offer programs for re-employment in other job sectors. This is considered:
1. Primary prevention.
2. Secondary prevention.
3. Tertiary prevention.
4. Health promotion.

Answer: 3
Rationale: Tertiary prevention aims to prevent a recurrence of a problem. Advocating politically to increase the minimum wage and having a program for re-employment in other job sectors can help those who are at the poverty level and work in minimum wage jobs. It can also help reduce homelessness by offering job training, which could lead to employment and increasing income and relief from poverty and homelessness. Primary prevention seeks to prevent a problem. Secondary prevention improves the client's status after a problem has been identified. Health promotion seeks to maintain an overall good level of health.
Step in the Nursing Process: Implementation
Category of Client Need: Health Promotion and Maintenance
Cognitive Level: Application
Learning Objective 20-6: Identify strategies for tertiary prevention of poverty and homelessness.
Test Taking Tip: Understand which level of prevention addresses poverty and homelessness.

20.12 A family has been able to earn enough money to raise their overall income level from the federal poverty guidelines. A tertiary prevention strategy to maintain their income at this level would be to: (Select all that apply.)
1. Assist the family in making and adhering to a budget.
2. Explore the factors that led to the family earning less money before.
3. Join a local cooperative to help buying efforts to stretch their income farther.
4. Refer the family to a local social service agency for emergency funds should they need them.
5. Encourage family members to seek higher income employment.

Answer: 1, 3
Rationale: Once the family has increased their income, tertiary prevention strategies would be geared to helping them maintain their income at this level. Making and adhering to a budget would assist the family in knowing where their money goes and how to spend it wisely. Another strategy would be to have them join a cooperative where people who join can increase their spending power without increasing their costs. Exploring factors and referring the family are examples of secondary and primary prevention strategies. Encouraging the family to seek higher income employment is an intrusive intervention and may not be relevant to this situation.
Step in the Nursing Process: Implementation
Category of Client Need: Health Promotion and Maintenance
Cognitive Level: Application
Learning Objective 20-6: Identify strategies for tertiary prevention of poverty and homelessness.
Test Taking Tip: Understand how tertiary prevention strategies can prevent the return to a previous level of poverty.

20.13 A consideration for planning health services for homeless and poor clients could be: (Select all that apply.)
1. An integrated clinic that provides social services in addition to health services.
2. A location that is easily accessible to the population served.
3. Specific health clinics held on specific days.
4. Flexible hours.
5. Including activities that educate and encourage self-care.

Answer: 1, 2, 4, 5
Rationale: Planning health services for the poor and homeless should include integration of services to allow all needs to be met. Location is paramount, because transportation needs may interfere with delivery of health services if the location is not close to where the population lives. Flexible hours can help with those who work in low-paying jobs but who work eight or more hours per day and cannot access health services during traditional hours. Specific clinics held on specific days may be more of a deterrent than a help in providing health services to the homeless and poor. Educating and encouraging self-care activities for the homeless and poor may result in a decrease in the need of utilization of services, which can indicate an improved health status.
Step in the Nursing Process: Implementation
Category of Client Need: Health Promotion and Maintenance
Cognitive Level: Application
Learning Objective 20-7: Describe considerations in implementing care for poor and homeless individuals.
Test Taking Tip: Understand how health care needs of the poor and homeless may differ from the rest of the population.

20.14 Families who are living in a local shelter state that they fear their children may be subject to abuse from other residents in the shelter. A solution for this would be to:
1. Restrict who uses the shelter.
2. Have a separate family area in the shelter.
3. Search everyone who uses the shelter prior to entering.
4. Force the children to stay with their parents at all times.

Answer: 2
Rationale: Families with children residing in shelters are vulnerable to be preyed upon by other subgroups. Having an area in the shelter reserved just for families can help alleviate this concern. Restricting use of the shelter is possible, but not realistic. Searching everyone prior to using the shelter can raise civil rights concerns. Forcing the children to stay with their parents at all times is possible, but is probably not a realistic outcome.
Step in the Nursing Process: Implementation
Category of Client Need: Health Promotion and Maintenance
Cognitive Level: Application
Learning Objective 20-7: Describe considerations in implementing care for poor and homeless individuals.
Test Taking Tip: Understand the needs of special populations who use shelters.

20.15 The primary focus for evaluating care for the poor and homeless includes how well:
1. Training programs employ the homeless.
2. Systems-level outcomes are met.
3. Client-level outcomes are met.
4. Individual and population intervention objectives are met.

Answer: 4
Rationale: The best answer is to evaluate how individual level and population level nursing intervention objectives are met. Training programs are a criterion but may not address how successful they have been utilized. Systems-level outcomes address ease of access of programs but do not necessarily evaluate care. Client-level outcomes include client involvement but do not indicate an evaluation. Training programs are a criterion but may not address how successfully they have been utilized.
Step in the Nursing Process: Evaluation
Category of Client Need: Health Promotion and Maintenance
Cognitive Level: Analysis
Learning Objective 20-8: Identify the primary focus of evaluation in care of poor and homeless clients.
Test Taking Tip: Understand the primary focus of evaluation in care of poor and homeless clients.

CHAPTER 21

21.1 The nurse does postpartal home visits to check on the mother and infant. During the visit, the nurse and mother discuss how the postpartal course is going and how the infant is doing with feeding and sleeping. The nurse provides information and answers any questions the mother may have and performs teaching as needed. This nursing role is considered:
1. Case finding and referral.
2. Care of the sick.
3. Health promotion and illness prevention.
4. Home health nursing.

Answer: 3
Rationale: Promoting maternal and child health is health promotion. The nurse visits the postpartal mother to answer questions, assess how the mother is recuperating, and how the infant is progressing. The nurse performs teaching as needed, which is health promotion and illness prevention. It is not case finding and referral, or care of the sick. Home health nursing is a specific type of home nursing that addresses an illness event.
Step in the Nursing Process: Evaluation
Category of Client Need: Health Promotion and Maintenance
Cognitive Level: Analysis
Learning Objective 21-1: Describe the advantages of a home visit as a means of providing nursing care.
Test Taking Tip: Understand how a home visit can provide the nurse with an opportunity to evaluate and teach as needed.

21.2 The nurse receives a referral to visit a client whose neighbors fear is being abused by a spouse. The client allows the nurse inside, but is obviously reluctant to have the nurse in the home. The nurse could best address the client's concerns by: (Select all that apply.)
1. Tactfully communicating the reason for the visit.
2. Establishing appropriate expectations for the visit for the client and nurse.

Answer: 1, 2, 3
Rationale: Initiating a home visit can present challenges to the nurse and create uncertainty and fear in the client. It is important for the nurse to state the reason for the visit and establish expectations from both perspectives. This allows the start of building a relationship with the client and establishes rapport. Revealing that the neighbors made the referral could be negative and the nurse needs to respect this as a confidential source. Informing the client that her name has been given to a local women's shelter could irreparably damage any relationship the nurse has with the client and halt any progress the nurse may have made in making the client feel sufficiently at ease to speak of any potential abuse.
Step in the Nursing Process: Assessment
Category of Client Need: Health Promotion and Maintenance
Cognitive Level: Application

3. Starting to establish a rapport with the client.
4. Stating that the neighbors made the referral.
5. Informing the client that her name has been given to a local women's shelter.

Learning Objective 21-2: Analyze challenges encountered by community health nurses making home visits.
Test Taking Tip: Understand the client perspective when a home visit is made and how this can be challenging for the nurse.

21.3 The local school reports a high degree of absence from a particular neighborhood. The nurse makes home visits to the neighborhood as part of:
1. Case finding and referral.
2. Health promotion and illness prevention.
3. Tertiary prevention.
4. Health maintenance.

Answer: 1
Rationale: The nurse is investigating a possible cause for school absence from a particular neighborhood, which is case finding and referral. The nurse is seeking to identify the source of the absences and, in doing so, may identify clients who are in need of services which can be provided as referrals. Health promotion and illness prevention are activities directed toward maintaining an optimal level of health. Tertiary prevention addresses optimal return to functioning in the face of disability. Health maintenance is maintaining the current level of health.
Step in the Nursing Process: Assessment
Category of Client Need: Health Promotion and Maintenance
Cognitive Level: Application
Learning Objective 21-3: Identify the major purposes of home visiting programs.
Test Taking Tip: Understand the major purposes of home visiting programs.

21.4 The community has a large number of immigrants. The nurse organizes a home visiting program to this community area to address family health concerns and provide health information. This is considered:
1. Care of the sick.
2. Case finding and referral.
3. Health promotion and illness prevention.
4. Health protection.

Answer: 3
Rationale: Visiting the homes of this population to address health concerns is an aspect of health promotion and illness prevention. The client is in a familiar environment and is more comfortable, which makes teaching easier for the nurse. The population is not indicated as sick. Case finding and referral would apply if the nurse was seeking something specific among this population. Health protection is part of health promotion, but is more of a broad-scale activity done to maintain health.
Step in the Nursing Process: Implementation
Category of Client Need: Health Promotion and Maintenance
Cognitive Level: Analysis
Learning Objective 21-3: Identify the major purposes of home visiting programs.
Test Taking Tip: Understand how special populations benefit from home visits.

21.5 In planning the home visit, the nurse should take into consideration the: (Select all that apply.)
1. Reason for the visit and age of the client.
2. Surrounding neighborhood.
3. Support systems employed by the client.
4. Client's ability to pay for services.
5. Preliminary client treatment goals.

Answer: 1, 2, 3, 5
Rationale: The reason for the visit, age of the client, neighborhood, and client's support systems are all considerations in planning a home visit. The reason for the visit sets the tone for the home visit and the age of the client allows the nurse to perform any health teaching and intervention at an appropriate level. Knowing the surrounding neighborhood for safety allows the nurse to plan an appropriate time for the home visit. In the planning phase, the nurse needs to have some preliminary treatment goals in mind for the client based on the information received prior to the visit, but remain aware that these may be modified or amended when the assessment is completed. The ability of the client to pay for services is important, but is not a necessary step for planning the visit.
Step in the Nursing Process: Planning
Category of Client Need: Health Promotion and Maintenance
Cognitive Level: Application
Learning Objective 21-4: Describe major considerations in planning a home visit.
Test Taking Tip: Understand the process of the home visit.

21.6 Knowing that the home visit is to an older person's home, the nurse should plan to:
1. Speak slowly and loudly to the client to ensure understanding.
2. Be alert to potential safety hazards in the home, such as throw rugs on hard floors.
3. Spend a longer time with the client than with a younger client.

Answer: 2
Rationale: An older client may be more vulnerable to physical hazards in the home, such as throw rugs on hard floors, which could cause the client to trip and fall. In planning a home visit, the nurse should take into consideration the client's age and what factors and risks could pose concerns to the client's health. Speaking slowly and loudly assumes that an older client has hearing deficits, which is a false assumption. Spending additional time with an older client assumes that an older client has fewer interactions with others. All clients' spiritual concerns should be assessed, not just those of the older client.
Step in the Nursing Process: Planning

<table>
<tr><td>

4. Assess the client's spiritual concerns.

</td><td>

Category of Client Need: Safe, Effective Care Environment
Cognitive Level: Application
Learning Objective 21-4: Describe major considerations in planning a home visit.
Test Taking Tip: Understand areas of concern and priority in planning a visit to the home of an elderly client.

</td></tr>
<tr><td>

21.7 After several home visits, the nurse and the client have agreed to improve the client's overall nutritional status. In order to achieve this outcome, the nurse should:
1. Assess the client's food preferences and methods of food preparation.
2. Plan menus for the client to prepare.
3. Accompany the client when food shopping.
4. Refer the client to a Meals-on-Wheels program.

</td><td>

Answer: 1
Rationale: In implementing a home visit, goals are agreed upon for the overall health of the client. In this instance, the improvement of the client's overall nutritional status cannot be achieved unless the nurse assesses the client's food preferences and methods of food preparation. Otherwise, if the nurse plans meals without these considerations, the outcome will not be achieved. Accompanying the client when food shopping will not necessarily guarantee this outcome, nor will a referral to a Meals-on-Wheels program.
Step in the Nursing Process: Implementation
Category of Client Need: Health Promotion and Maintenance
Cognitive Level: Application
Learning Objective 21-5: Identify tasks involved in implementing a home visit.
Test Taking Tip: Understand what is involved with a home visit.

</td></tr>
<tr><td>

21.8 During a home visit, the nurse should:
1. Continue to validate the accuracy of the assessment and resulting diagnosis.
2. Focus on the plan of care as it is written.
3. Concentrate on the already-identified needs.
4. Plan to write an evaluation.

</td><td>

Answer: 1
Rationale: The validity and accuracy of the assessment and resulting diagnosis should always be a factor in the home visit implementation. Additional needs can be added to modify the plan of care, so focusing solely on the plan of care as it is written may not meet the client's needs. Concentrating only on the identified needs may ignore other issues that arise in subsequent home visits. The evaluation is part of every visit and is not something that is done at another time.
Step in the Nursing Process: Implementation
Category of Client Need: Health Promotion and Maintenance
Cognitive Level: Analysis
Learning Objective 21-5: Identify tasks involved in implementing a home visit.
Test Taking Tip: Understand that implementation is an ongoing process in a home visit.

</td></tr>
<tr><td>

21.9 The nurse is making a home visit to a new client. The client is very friendly and welcomes the nurse into the home where the nurse sees that the client has a gun on the coffee table. The nurse hurriedly goes through the visit and leaves. What should the nurse do prior to the next visit?
1. Call the police prior to making the visit.
2. Call the client prior to the visit and state that there cannot be a visible firearm present during the visit.
3. Cancel future visits to this client.
4. Refer the client to another agency for visitation.

</td><td>

Answer: 2
Rationale: The distraction the nurse encountered was both environmental and behavioral. Presence of a firearm is an environmental concern and the nurse's reaction of hurrying through the visit indicates a level of discomfort with the presence of the firearm. Notifying the client prior to the next visit about the presence of the firearm addresses the nurse's concern and lets the client know that this is not acceptable. There is nothing to indicate that the client is creating a distraction. Calling the police is not a necessary step prior to the next visit. Cancelling future visits could impair the client's overall health. Referring the client to another agency is not solving this concern.
Step in the Nursing Process: Implementation
Category of Client Need: Safe, Effective Management of Care
Cognitive Level: Application
Learning Objective 21-6: Analyze the effects of potential distractions during a home visit.
Test Taking Tip: Understand that distractions can originate with the nurse as well as other sources.

</td></tr>
<tr><td>

21.10 During a visit to provide diabetic teaching to a newly-diagnosed client, the client constantly answers the cell phone and has conversations with those callers. The client apologizes after each call. The best intervention that the nurse could do at this time is to:
1. Request that the client not answer the cell phone.

</td><td>

Answer: 4
Rationale: Asking the client if there is a better time to do this teaching subtly conveys to the client that the calls are distracting and also gives the client control over the timing of the teaching. Distractions such as continuous calls can be frustrating to the nurse and can impede teaching. Requesting the client not to answer the cell phone is appropriate but may anger the client, which will impede any learning. Leaving pamphlets for the client to read may not impart the necessary information the client needs to understand diabetes. Having the client repeat back the information the nurse has given would provide an understanding to the nurse of what has been taught, but may also give the impression to the client that the nurse feels the client has not understood the teaching.

</td></tr>
</table>

312

2. Leave some pamphlets for the client to read.
3. Have the client repeat back the information the nurse has given.
4. Ask the client if another time would be better to complete this teaching.

Step in the Nursing Process: Evaluation
Category of Client Need: Health Promotion and Maintenance
Cognitive Level: Application
Learning Objective 21-6: Analyze the effects of potential distractions during a home visit.
Test Taking Tip: Understand alternative solutions to provide when distractions threaten a home visit.

21.11 Evaluation of long-term and short-term criteria for a home visit is important because it:
1. Indicates whether reimbursement will be provided to the agency.
2. Allows for tracking utilization of supplies for home visits.
3. Determines the effectiveness and appropriateness of the interventions and the client's response.
4. Determines whether the interventions are at the primary, secondary, or tertiary level.

Answer: 3
Rationale: Unless there are evaluative criteria, the client's response cannot be determined nor whether the interventions were effective and appropriate. Evaluative criteria can be used for reimbursement and supplies can be tracked with such criteria, but effectiveness of the visit cannot be determined without evaluative criteria. Evaluative criteria can be at any level of prevention.
Step in the Nursing Process: Evaluation
Category of Client Need: Health Promotion and Maintenance
Cognitive Level: Analysis
Learning Objective 21-7: Discuss the need for both long-term and short-term evaluative criteria for the effectiveness of a home visit.
Test Taking Tip: Understand how evaluative criteria need to be both long-term and short-term.

21.12 Home health nursing is considered a subspecialty of community health nursing. How do home health and community health nursing differ?
1. Home health nursing is reimbursable, whereas community health nursing is not.
2. Community health nursing deals only with the health of aggregates.
3. The focus of community health nursing is health promotion, and the focus of home health nursing is health restoration from a state of illness.
4. Home health nursing focuses on the individual and community health nursing focuses on systems.

Answer: 3
Rationale: Home health nursing is a subspecialty of community health nursing. The focus of home health nursing addresses care of those who are ill and in need of nursing services for health restoration from illness. Community health addresses promoting and maintaining the health of the population. As an individual nursing function, community health nursing services are not an insurance reimbursable service, as is home health nursing. Home health nursing provides services to the individual in the home, while community health nursing addresses the health of the population or aggregates within a system.
Step in the Nursing Process: Assessment
Category of Client Need: Health Promotion and Maintenance
Cognitive Level: Analysis
Learning Objective 21-8: Describe the relationship between home health nursing and community health nursing.
Test Taking Tip: Understand the differences and similarities between home health and community heath nursing.

21.13 Important considerations in hospice care include collaborating among healthcare team members in which of the following aspects? (Select all that apply.)
1. Management of pain control.
2. Assisting the family in adjusting to the eventual death of the client.
3. Ensuring that all services provided are able to be reimbursed.
4. Obtaining additional services for identified client needs.
5. Ensuring the client has arrangements made for burial.

Answer: 1, 2, 4
Rationale: Collaboration among healthcare team members in hospice care addresses effective pain management control, assisting the family as needed in adjusting to the eventual outcome of the client, and obtaining additional services for identified client needs. Hospice care is reimbursable, but not all services provided in hospice care may be reimbursed. Ensuring the client has arrangements made for burial is a consideration, but does not necessarily entail collaboration among the healthcare team members.
Step in the Nursing Process: Implementation
Category of Client Need: Psychosocial Integrity
Cognitive Level: Analysis
Learning Objective 21-9: Discuss the need for collaboration in home health and hospice nursing.
Test Taking Tip: Understand the similarities in home health and hospice nursing.

21.14 The home health nurse is making the initial assessment visit to a new client. After doing the assessment for treatment, the nurse completes an

Answer: 3
Rationale: The OASIS assessment form is used when the home health agency is seeing clients who can have their services reimbursed by Medicare. DRGs are not utilized in the OASIS form. Certified home health agencies will be able to receive

OASIS assessment form, which is utilized:

1. To ensure that the appropriate diagnosis related group (DRG) is used for payment.
2. By home health agencies who have certification.
3. For reimbursement purposes in home health agencies with Medicare clients.
4. As a requirement for all home health and hospice agencies.

Medicare and third party reimbursement, but third party reimbursement does not require use of the OASIS. OASIS is not a requirement for all home health and hospice agencies.
Step in the Nursing Process: Evaluation
Category of Client Need: Safe, Effective Care Environment
Cognitive Level: Analysis
Learning Objective 21-10: Discuss funding sources for home health and hospice care.
Test Taking Tip: Understand how the OASIS form is used for reimbursement.

21.15 The OASIS assessment form and the HEDIS (Health Plan Employer Data and Information Set) have evaluative criteria for home health and hospice care that address effectiveness of care and improvement in condition. The most important criteria in evaluating home health and hospice care services are:

1. Client satisfaction with the care provided.
2. Access and availability of the care provided.
3. Effectiveness in maintaining functional ability.
4. Cost of the services provided.

Answer: 1
Rationale: The most important criteria for evaluating home health and hospice care are client satisfaction. Access, availability, effectiveness in maintaining functional ability, and cost all are secondary to client satisfaction.
Step in the Nursing Process: Evaluation
Category of Client Need: Safe, Effective Care Environment
Cognitive Level: Application
Learning Objective 21-11: Apply evaluative criteria for home health and hospice care services.
Test Taking Tip: Understand the most important evaluative criteria for home health and hospice care services.

CHAPTER 22

22.1 The nurse works for the city public health department. While investigating a restaurant that has had several food poisoning complaints lodged against it, the nurse finds that the food preparation area is not within code. It is within the purview of the nurse to:

1. Require the restaurant to stop serving certain items.
2. Have the restaurant shut down until the problems are corrected.
3. Order the restaurant to limit its business hours.
4. Post a notice on the restaurant entrance warning clients of a problem.

Answer: 2
Rationale: To maintain the public health, the nurse working in an official health agency has the force of local ordinances or legislative mandates to reinforce actions taken, in this case, closing the restaurant until the food preparation area problems are corrected. It is not in the public health interest to have the restaurant stop serving certain items or restrict business hours. Posting a notice does not address the food preparation area problems.
Step in the Nursing Process: Implementation
Category of Client Need: Health Promotion and Maintenance
Cognitive Level: Application
Learning Objective 22-1: Discuss the legal and regulatory parameters of nursing in official health agencies.
Test Taking Tip: Understand the force of mandate that the nurse has to enforce measures to address the public health.

22.2 The core functions of public health are assessment, policy development, and assurance. The best example of assurance is being able to:

1. Link people to needed health care services.
2. Investigate health problems and hazards in the community.

Answer: 1
Rationale: Linking people to needed health care services is an assurance function. Investigating health problems and hazards is assessment. Policy development helps to mobilize partnerships to identify health problems and empower the community about health concerns.
Step in the Nursing Process: Implementation
Category of Client Need: Health Promotion and Maintenance
Cognitive Level: Application

3. Mobilize partnerships to identify health problems.
4. Empower the community about health concerns.

Learning Objective 22-2: Describe the core functions and essential services of local health departments.

Test Taking Tip: Understand the many aspects of assurance as a core function of a local health department.

22.3 An essential service related to the assessment core function of public health is:
1. Organizing the community to repair local community playground equipment.
2. Presenting information to the local community government about playground conditions.
3. Investigating alternative designs for safer playgrounds.
4. Compiling statistics about playground injuries in the local community.

Answer: 4
Rationale: Compiling statistics about injuries incurred in local playgrounds is monitoring the health status to identify community health problems, and is a core assessment function. Presenting information to the local city government and organizing the community to repair local playground equipment is a policy development function. Investigating alternative designs for safer playgrounds is an assurance function.
Step in the Nursing Process: Assessment
Category of Client Need: Health Promotion and Maintenance
Cognitive Level: Application
Learning Objective 22-2: Describe the core functions and essential services of local health departments.
Test Taking Tip: Understand how assessment as a core function is expressed as an essential service.

22.4 While all registered nurses are eligible to work in official health agencies, nurses with which levels of education are prepared for public health nursing roles? (Select all that apply.)
1. Diploma level of education.
2. Associate degree level of education.
3. Baccalaureate level of education.
4. Master's level of education.
5. Doctoral level of education.

Answer: 3, 4, 5
Rationale: Baccalaureate education incorporates public health education into its curriculum. Graduate education (Master's and Doctoral) can also focus on public health. Diploma and associate degree levels of education address elements of public health, but are not required components of this curriculum.
Step in the Nursing Process: Evaluation
Category of Client Need: Health Promotion and Maintenance
Cognitive Level: Analysis
Learning Objective 22-3: Discuss educational preparation for nursing in official health agencies.
Test Taking Tip: Understand how specialized courses in a curriculum are necessary for public health nurses to work in official health agencies.

22.5 A priority skill for the nurse who works in the community in an official health agency is:
1. Outcomes identification.
2. Coordinating programs and services.
3. Cultural competence and sensitivity skills.
4. Setting priorities for developing evaluation criteria.

Answer: 3
Rationale: All the skills are necessary for the community nurse to possess. However, the nurse in a public health agency needs to have cultural skills related to cultural competence and cultural sensitivity.
Step in the Nursing Process: Implementation
Category of Client Need: Health Promotion and Maintenance
Cognitive Level: Analysis
Learning Objective 22-4: Analyze the core competencies of the public health workforce as they relate to nursing in official health agencies.
Test Taking Tip: Understand the priority skill necessary for the nurse who works in the community in an official health agency.

22.6 According to the Public Health Nursing Competencies document, to function effectively as a member of an official public health agency, the nurse must be able to:
1. Research, collect, analyze and interpret community health data.
2. Develop collegial collaborative roles with others in the community.
3. Develop health education programs for the community.
4. Consult with other agencies when problem solving.

Answer: 1
Rationale: All the answers are functions of the community health nurse. Functioning as a member of an official public health agency, the nurse must be able to possess and utilize the skills of researching, collecting, analyzing, and interpreting community health data to carry out the core functions of public health. Developing collegial collaborative roles with others in the community can assist the nurse's role as a member of an official public health agency but is not a critical function of this role. The nurse is expected to have planning skills but does not have to develop health education programs for the community. Consulting with other agencies to problem solve is collegiality but not necessarily a role for the nurse in an official agency.
Step in the Nursing Process: Implementation
Category of Client Need: Health Promotion and Maintenance
Cognitive Level: Analysis
Learning Objective 22-4: Analyze the core competencies of the public health workforce as they relate to nursing in official health agencies.
Test Taking Tip: Understand how the nurse must possess the skills to fulfill core functions of public health when employed in an official agency.

22.7 When the nurse has made a community diagnosis of "community risk control: lead exposure," appropriate nursing actions would be:
1. Monitor playgrounds for children eating dirt.
2. Investigate older homes that are being sanded and repainted.
3. Check water quality at various locations in the community.
4. Monitor air quality on days with high smog levels.

Answer: 2
Rationale: Older homes that are being sanded may have been painted with lead paint. The sanding will release the fine paint dust in the air, which can pose a health threat. Eating dirt may not pose a lead hazard unless there is evidence that the dirt contains bits of lead from paint chips. A water quality analysis could show lead levels, but is only required if there is indication that there is a problem with lead solder leaking from older residential plumbing pipes. Monitoring air quality on high smog level days will give data regarding pollutants in the air, but this relates to respiratory issues, which are not affected by lead.
Step in the Nursing Process: Implementation
Category of Client Need: Health Promotion and Maintenance
Cognitive Level: Application
Learning Objective 22-5: Analyze community nursing diagnoses as they relate to nursing in official health agencies.
Test Taking Tip: Understand how lead exposure can be detected in a community.

22.8 Which activities are community health nursing functions when mobilizing community partnerships to identify and solve health problems? (Select all that apply.)
1. Identify key community members.
2. Identify community assets and needs.
3. Assist community members to articulate needs.
4. Identify potential coalition members to address particular health issues.
5. Identify violations of health-related regulations.

Answer: 1, 3, and 4
Rationale: The community health nurse, when mobilizing community partnerships to identify and solve health problems, will identify key members of the community and identify potential coalition members to address particular health issues. The nurse will assist community members to articulate those needs. Identifying community assets and needs is diagnosing and investigating health problems and hazards in the community, and is not an activity when mobilizing community partnerships. Identifying violations of health-related regulations is enforcing laws and regulations protecting health and safety and not an activity in mobilizing community partnerships.
Step in the Nursing Process: Implementation
Category of Client Need: Health Promotion and Maintenance
Cognitive Level: Comprehension
Learning Objective 22-6: Analyze the role of the community health nurse in carrying out the core functions and essential services in local health departments.
Test Taking Tip: Understand how community health nurses can work with local health departments to mobilize partnerships.

22.9 Promoting the community's health within the framework of a voluntary agency while emphasizing spirituality as a component of health is considered:
1. District nursing.
2. Holistic nursing.
3. Faith community nursing.
4. Spiritual nursing.

Answer: 3
Rationale: Faith community nursing is a health promotion, disease prevention role that contains a professional model of health ministry using a registered nurse. Faith community nurses have a significant personal religious history and administer nursing care within a framework of a voluntary agency. District nursing is where the nurse is responsible for the nursing care of a set geographic area. Spiritual nursing is not a recognized nursing role. Holistic nursing treats the whole person, which nursing does, but faith community nursing operates within a model that directs nursing care.
Step in the Nursing Process: Assessment
Category of Client Need: Health Promotion and Maintenance
Cognitive Level: Analysis
Learning Objective 22-7: Define faith community nursing.
Test Taking Tip: Understand the distinctions in the various community nursing roles.

22.10 The client expresses to the nurse a deep conviction of the power of meditation and prayer on the client's overall health status. The nurse suggests to the client that they spend a moment in quiet reflection during the day. This intervention addresses the nurse's understanding of the:
1. Link between personal spirituality and healing.
2. Necessity for the client to have time for personal meditation.

Answer: 1
Rationale: The interrelationship between healing and faith is becoming increasingly explored in health and has applicability in community health. The client acknowledges the importance of personal meditation, but the intervention of meditating at that moment may not meet the client's needs at that time. It may be the nurse's attempt to force meditation, meeting the nurse's need more than the client's. Acknowledging the client's concerns is an important nursing intervention, but is not necessarily met through meditation. It does not imply that the client needs spiritual direction.
Step in the Nursing Process: Implementation
Category of Client Need: Psychosocial Integrity
Cognitive Level: Application

3. Acknowledgment of the client's concerns.
4. Need for spiritual direction in the client's life.

Learning Objective 22-8: Describe the philosophy of nursing in a faith-based community.
Test Taking Tip: Understand the importance of spirituality on health.

22.11 Nursing scope and standards address the competencies that the nurse possesses to provide effective care. A competency that is expected for a faith community nurse would be:
1. Working collaboratively with other health care members.
2. Providing client-focused care.
3. Fostering quality improvement measures in care.
4. Providing care that holistically combines spiritual and emotional components.

Answer: 4
Rationale: A competency of the faith community nurse is to intervene effectively in holistic care of the body, mind, and spirit. While all nursing care addresses the holistic aspect of care, the faith community nurse brings to this care a spiritual dimension of personal self and beliefs that effectively integrates these concepts. All nursing standards address the ability to work collaboratively, provide client-focused care, and foster quality improvement.
Step in the Nursing Process: Implementation
Category of Client Need: Psychosocial Integrity
Cognitive Level: Analysis
Learning Objective 22-9: Describe the scope and standards of nursing in a faith-based community.
Test Taking Tip: Understand how the spiritual aspect of self is important in the scope and standards of faith community nursing.

22.12 A local religious organization opens a clinic to provide comprehensive health care services to the community. While the mission of the clinic and faith organization is to address the needs of the medically underserved and has a sliding scale for payment, anyone in the community can utilize the clinic, including those with health insurance. This faith-based nursing example is best described as:
1. An access model.
2. A mission-ministry model.
3. A paid employee model.
4. A marketplace model.

Answer: 4
Rationale: Scope and standards of nursing of the marketplace model for faith-based nursing are defined by the employing agency and will often focus on interventions for a specific problem or issue; in this case, that specific issue is medically underserved populations. Care is driven by economic values, but has a faith component. The access model focuses on advocacy for underserved populations. The mission-ministry model focuses on reconciliation, health, healing, wholeness, and discipleship. There is no paid employee model of faith-based nursing.
Step in the Nursing Process: Implementation
Category of Client Need: Health Promotion and Maintenance
Cognitive Level: Analysis
Learning Objective 22-10: Differentiate among models for nursing in a faith-based community.
Test Taking Tip: Understand which models of faith-based nursing incorporate a spiritual dimension in addition to an economic dimension.

22.13 A local church employs a member of its congregation to visit its members. This member is a community health nurse. The nurse assesses the health status of the members and plans interventions and evaluates the effectiveness of the care given. Reconciliation and spiritual healing are an important component of the nurse's care and is part of the mission of this church. Which model does this example best describe?
1. Mission-ministry.
2. Access.
3. Marketplace.
4. Voluntary.

Answer: 1
Rationale: A mission-ministry model of faith-based nursing is usually administered to members of a congregation, and the nurse's practice is determined by the congregation. The nurse may be paid or may be a volunteer, but the focus of this model includes reconciliation, healing, wholeness, and discipleship. The access model for faith-based nursing focuses on advocacy. The marketplace model addresses economic factors. The voluntary component of faith-based nursing addresses the nurse who does not receive paid compensation for nursing services performed.
Step in the Nursing Process: Implementation
Category of Client Need: Psychosocial Integrity
Cognitive Level: Analysis
Learning Objective 22-10: Differentiate among models for nursing in a faith-based community.
Test Taking Tip: Know the various models of faith-based nursing.

22.14 The faith-based nurse works with members of the congregation who are dying. In doing so, the nurse provides the dying person and their family with end-of-life care. What is the nurse's role in this example?
1. Health advocate.
2. Personal health counselor.

Answer: 3
Rationale: When working with dying members of a congregation and their family, the faith-based nurse assumes the palliative care role. In this role, the nurse affirms life, but accepts death as a normal part of life. The nurse provides care as necessary and supports families during this time. Health advocate, personal health counselor, and referral agent could be roles in caring for the dying client, but these roles are not as specifically addressing death as a part of life, as the palliative care role does.
Step in the Nursing Process: Implementation

---

3. Palliative care.
4. Referral agent.

Category of Client Need: Psychosocial Integrity
Cognitive Level: Analysis
Learning Objective 22-11: Describe the roles and functions of community health nurses in a faith-based community.
Test Taking Tip: Understand the different roles of the faith-based community nurse.

22.15 The faith-based community nurse recognizes that the faith community has a great need among its older members for daily monitoring and "checking in" to assess their status. The best method for the nurse to ensure this is to:

1. Start a phone tree among the members to call one another on a daily basis.
2. Develop a schedule where the nurse will be able to quickly check in on each member at least twice a week.
3. Organize a volunteer group within the faith community and train them to visit the members.
4. Pair each member with another member of the congregation and assign them the responsibility for checking on that member.

Answer: 3
Rationale: Effective faith-based community nursing makes appropriate use of volunteer members of the congregation. Organizing a phone tree places the burden on the nurse and the older members to check in on one another. Developing a schedule where the nurse can visit at least twice a week will not solve the daily need for monitoring status. Pairing each member with another member is not volunteerism and may be resented if the nurse forces it upon them.
Step in the Nursing Process: Planning
Category of Client Need: Health Promotion and Maintenance
Cognitive Level: Application
Learning Objective 22-11: Describe the roles and functions of community health nurses in a faith-based community.
Test Taking Tip: Understand how the nurse can best utilize other members of the congregation to achieve health goals.

CHAPTER 23

23.1 The nurse at an elementary school in the community has developed an integrated program of health promotion and health surveillance, which has resulted in much lower rates of student absence than other similar schools in the community. What is the best conclusion to draw from this?

1. Students are living in a healthier neighborhood in this school district.
2. This student body has more effectively learned about healthy lifestyles.
3. Lower absenteeism may result in a better academic achievement.
4. Good parental involvement has contributed to this success of this program.

Answer: 3
Rationale: A school health program that reduces school absenteeism could lead to better academic outcomes because the students are in the classroom more. While the students will probably learn healthy lifestyles, it does not necessarily result in better academic outcomes. There is no indication that the student body lives in an area that has a better health profile. There is also no indication of parental involvement in this program.
Step in the Nursing Process: Evaluation
Category of Client Need: Health Promotion and Maintenance
Cognitive Level: Application
Learning Objective 23-1: Identify the overall goal of a school health program.
Test Taking Tip: Understand the link between absenteeism with academic outcomes.

23.2 In the program that the school nurse developed to teach children about health, the teachers assume responsibility for teaching the health principles. The nurse becomes aware that program outcomes are not being achieved. What should the nurse do to resolve this?

1. Reinforce to the teachers the importance of teaching health concepts.

Answer: 4
Rationale: In order for a school health program to succeed, there needs to be involvement on all levels: in the classroom, in the home, and in the community. One person cannot hold the responsibility for teaching and reinforcing health concepts. Reinforcing to the teachers the importance of teaching health creates another burden upon them. For the school nurse to assume all teaching responsibilities will quickly create burnout, and may create a neglect of other school nurse responsibilities. Asking for parental involvement to teach health concepts is a partial solution, but the better solution is an integrated approach.
Step in the Nursing Process: Evaluation
Category of Client Need: Health Promotion and Maintenance

---

2. Plan to assume all teaching responsibilities for health in the school.	Cognitive Level: Application
	Learning Objective 23-2: Describe the components of a coordinated school health program.
3. Ask for parental involvement to help teach health concepts.	Test Taking Tip: Understand how to ensure success for a health program.
4. Modify the program to include strategies to teach health in the classroom and the home.	
23.3 A nurse is being interviewed for a position at a local school. The nurse enters the interview expecting that the position responsibilities will entail screening, monitoring immunization status, and performing minor first-aid duties. The nurse is surprised to learn that other duties include: (Select all that apply.) 1. Case finding and case management. 2. Counseling and referrals to other services. 3. Staff health promotion. 4. Parental, student, and community involvement in school activities. 5. Reviewing health policies in the community.	Answer: 1, 2, 3, 4 Rationale: An integrated school health program involves case finding and case management, counseling and referrals to other services, staff health promotion, and parental, student, and community involvement in school activities in addition to monitoring physical education activities at the school and the nutrition of the meals provided there. Reviewing community health policies is not a school nurse responsibility. Step in the Nursing Process: Planning Category of Client Need: Health Promotion and Maintenance Cognitive Level: Application Learning Objective 22-2: Describe the components of a coordinated school health program. Test Taking Tip: Know the many responsibilities of the school nurse.
23.4 The majority of the student population at the school is African-American. The nurse should be alert to the number of students: 1. With sickle cell disease. 2. With asthma. 3. Who are overweight. 4. Who come from single parent homes.	Answer: 1 Rationale: Sickle cell disease primarily affects African Americans. The nurse should be attentive to members of the student population who may be affected by this, because this can affect school attendance if students experience pain crises. While asthma is rising in the United States, the nurse should not assume that the student population has a disproportionate number of asthma cases. Being overweight is not solely a concern related to racial background. Many children in society today live in single parent homes. There is no indication that this is particularly true of this school population. Step in the Nursing Process: Assessment Category of Client Need: Health Promotion and Maintenance Cognitive Level: Application Learning Objective 23-3: Describe considerations in assessing biophysical, psychological, physical, environmental, sociocultural, behavioral, and health system factors influencing the health of the school population. Test Taking Tip: Understand how cultural and racial backgrounds can influence health factors that can impact a student's ability to attend school regularly.
23.5 The local school board has allowed students with certain chronic conditions to have their medications with them at all times. Which situation should the nurse be particularly alert to? 1. The child with ADHD should take the appropriate medication at the appropriate time. 2. The child with diabetes has a tube of glucagon in his or her backpack. 3. The child with asthma knows how to correctly use the inhaler. 4. The child with a neurogenic bladder is able to self-catheterize.	Answer: 3 Rationale: The child with asthma needs to have access to an inhaler when an attack occurs. Mitigating the effects of an asthma attack includes correct usage of the inhaler, so the nurse would need to assess the child's ability to correctly use the inhaler. ADHD medications are Schedule II medications and, as such, are not allowed to be carried by the child during school hours. A child with diabetes may not be able to use the glucagon in time should he or she become hypoglycemic, so the teacher should be able to know how to apply it. A child with a neurogenic bladder does not need medication to self-catheterize. Step in the Nursing Process: Assessment Category of Client Need: Health Promotion and Maintenance Cognitive Level: Application Learning Objective 23-3: Describe considerations in assessing biophysical, psychological, physical, environmental, sociocultural, behavioral, and health system factors influencing the health of the school population. Test Taking Tip: Understand which medications a student is capable of using appropriately.

23.6 The nurse works in a school that is designated for students with special needs in the district. An important consideration specific to this population is to ensure that these students:
1. Receive an annual flu immunization.
2. Are able to have sufficient time at lunch to eat.
3. Have physical education activities like all students.
4. Have personal care attendants.

Answer: 1
Rationale: Students with special needs generally have conditions that make them vulnerable to illness, so an important consideration is that this population receives annual flu immunizations to protect them. All students should have sufficient time at lunch to eat and all students are to have time for physical activity. Personal care attendants are not always necessary for children with special needs.
Step in the Nursing Process: Implementation
Category of Client Need: Health Promotion and Maintenance
Cognitive Level: Application
Learning Objective 23-3: Describe considerations in assessing biophysical, psychological, physical, environmental, sociocultural, behavioral, and health system factors influencing the health of the school population.
Test Taking Tip: Be aware of the specific needs of special needs children, and how they differ from the needs of any student.

23.7 A local nursing program has contracted with an elementary school to conduct health teaching. As the school year closes, the nursing students plan to do one last health teaching program. What would be the most appropriate topic the nursing students could choose?
1. Alcohol and nutritional supplements.
2. Handwashing and hygiene.
3. Sun, bike, and outdoor safety.
4. Sexually transmitted diseases.

Answer: 3
Rationale: As the school year closes, the students will be out of school for the summer, so safety topics such as sun safety, bike safety, and other outdoor safety tips should be emphasized. The other topics are very appropriate, but can be done at any time during the school year; however, the timing of the safety topic is relevant to the upcoming vacation time.
Step in the Nursing Process: Implementation
Category of Client Need: Health Promotion and Maintenance
Cognitive Level: Application
Learning Objective 23-4: Identify areas of emphasis in primary prevention in the school setting and analyze the role of the community health nurse in each.
Test Taking Tip: Link relevance and timing of topics to primary prevention.

23.8 The nurse at the local high school is aware that students are particularly vulnerable during this developmental stage to many health challenges. What is an appropriate priority topic to support student self-development?
1. Educate about sexually transmitted diseases.
2. Provide strategies to minimize stress and promote self-esteem.
3. Hold in-service programs for teachers to identify students at risk.
4. Collaborate with the local mental health agency to refer students at risk.

Answer: 2
Rationale: All of the topics presented are appropriate to this age level. A priority topic, however, is how to minimize stress and promote self-esteem. High school is a developmental time where students undergo many challenges to their identity and have the pressures of academic achievement and other societal pressures and expectations placed upon them. These challenges can lead to ineffective management and coping. Providing strategies to minimize stress and promote self-esteem can help to educate students about stress management and coping.
Step in the Nursing Process: Implementation
Category of Client Need: Health Promotion and Maintenance
Cognitive Level: Application
Learning Objective 23-4: Identify areas of emphasis in primary prevention in the school setting and analyze the role of the community health nurse in each.
Test Taking Tip: Understand developmental level with regard to the appropriate primary prevention intervention.

23.9 The nurse is aware that most of the students prefer the fried food choices in the school cafeteria and that many of the students are considered overweight by body mass index (BMI) standards. Strategies that the nurse can employ to ameliorate this concern include: (Select all that apply.)
1. Demanding that the food staff eliminate all fried foods.
2. Working with the food staff on menu planning and including healthier choices.
3. Presenting programs to the students about nutrition and healthy choices.

Answer: 2, 3, 4
Rationale: Working with the food staff on menu planning can allow input about healthier choices to be given to the students for food selections. Presenting programs to students and families about nutrition, healthy choices, and school nutrition will allow all parties to become more aware of how nutritional choices affect overall health. Demanding that the food staff eliminate all fried foods is an unrealistic strategy, and will only alienate important members of the school team. Assigning mandatory exercise programs to students with overweight BMIs stigmatizes and targets them as well as displays insensitivity to their self-esteem.
Step in the Nursing Process: Implementation
Category of Client Need: Health Promotion and Maintenance
Cognitive Level: Application
Learning Objective 23-4: Identify areas of emphasis in primary prevention in the school setting and analyze the role of the community health nurse in each.
Test Taking Tip: Understand how working with members of the school team, including students and parents, can result in a better outcome.

4. Allow students to make their own food choices

5. Mandate that teachers provide instruction on nutrition

4. Presenting programs to families at parent-teaching association (PTA) meetings about school nutrition.
5. Assigning mandatory exercise programs to all students whose BMIs are considered overweight.

23.10 The nurse performs vision and hearing screening at the school to identify students who may need referrals for further testing. A responsibility of the nurse in screening is to:
1. Monitor that students who need glasses wear them.
2. Send letters home to parents reminding the students to wear the glasses.
3. Follow up on referrals made to determine outcomes for those students with vision or hearing problems.
4. Ask the teachers if they are aware of any other problems with students in the classroom.

Answer: 3
Rationale: A responsibility of the nurse in the screening category of secondary prevention is to follow up on referrals that result from screening in order to determine the outcome and ensure appropriate care results. Sending letters home to parents reminding the students to wear glasses may not translate to the classroom setting. It is not realistic to monitor students who wear glasses to ensure that this is done. It is appropriate to ask the teachers if they are aware of other problems, but this does not fall within the screening category. It falls within the counseling category.
Step in the Nursing Process: Evaluation
Category of Client Need: Health Promotion and Maintenance
Cognitive Level: Application
Learning Objective 23-5: Describe the facets of secondary prevention in the school setting and analyze related community health nursing roles.
Test Taking Tip: Be aware of the nursing responsibilities that are appropriate to screening.

23.11 After receiving a report from a teacher regarding a student who was previously outgoing and doing well in the classroom but is now appearing withdrawn, the nurse assesses the student. The nurse becomes aware that there is a possibility that abuse is happening in the home and notifies the appropriate agencies. In this example, the nurse is:
1. Making an appropriate referral to ensure the health and safety of the student.
2. Refusing to become involved in a domestic affair.
3. Acting outside of the scope of practice.
4. Releasing any further obligation to the student.

Answer: 1
Rationale: Referral in the presence of an identified problem is secondary prevention. The student that has a dramatic change in appearance and classroom behavior warrants further investigation and appropriate referrals for help, which is done in this situation. The nurse is not refusing to become involved in a domestic situation, as is evident in the referral that was made. The nurse is acting within the scope of practice and is legally obligated to report conditions that can threaten the health and safety of the student. The nurse remains obligated to help the student in this situation.
Step in the Nursing Process: Implementation
Category of Client Need: Safe, Effective Care Environment
Cognitive Level: Application
Learning Objective 23-6: Describe facets of secondary prevention in the school setting and analyze related community health nursing roles.
Test Taking Tip: Understand the legal responsibilities of the nurse in school health.

23.12 A ventilator-dependent student joins the school and does not need a personal care attendant. Before providing care to the student, the nurse should:
1. Research tracheostomy-suctioning procedures.
2. Teach the teacher how to provide appropriate tracheostomy care.
3. Review the student's Individualized Health Care Plan (IHP) for other aspects of care that the student may need in addition to tracheostomy care.
4. Ask to have a joint conference with the parents, teachers, and school administrators about caring for this student.

Answer: 3
Rationale: When a student with special needs attends a school, the student should have an Individualized Health Care Plan (IHP), which details the student's health history, identification of special needs, an overview of the student's basic health status, and information about any medications the student receives, including their administration, timing, dosage, etc. Other needs that are identified in the IHP include nutritional needs, activities with a care plan, and strategies for intervention. The teacher may become involved in the care of the student, but this is not the immediate priority nor is reviewing suctioning procedures. A joint conference may be called, but the IHP should be reviewed first by the nurse to determine its plan, complexity, and completeness.
Step in the Nursing Process: Assessment
Category of Client Need: Safe, Effective Care Environment
Cognitive Level: Application
Learning Objective 23-5: Describe the facets of secondary prevention in the school setting and analyze related community health nursing roles.
Test Taking Tip: Understand the complexity of a special needs student in an academic environment.

23.13 Many of the students at the school have sickle cell disease. An important intervention by the nurse for this population is to:
1. Restrict their activity during physical education time.
2. Ensure that these students receive adequate hydration.
3. Ensure that the room temperatures are warmer than normal.
4. Monitor the students for any bruising.

Answer: 2
Rationale: Ensuring that students with sickle cell disease receive adequate hydration is important because that can ameliorate and prevent the onset of pain crises when they occur, which is preventing recurrence of acute conditions. These students do not need restriction of physical activities. It is important for the students to stay warm, as cold can trigger pain crises, but students can wear appropriate clothing. It is not necessary to have the room warmer because other students may become uncomfortable. It is not necessary to monitor students for bruising.
Step in the Nursing Process: Implementation
Category of Client Need: Health Promotion and Maintenance
Cognitive Level: Application
Learning Objective 23-6: Describe areas of emphasis in tertiary prevention in the school setting and analyze the role of the community health nurse with respect to each.
Test Taking Tip: Understand the interventions that can prevent exacerbations of chronic conditions.

23.14 A student has been diagnosed with a pulmonary condition that necessitates the use of continuous oxygen. The student's family has limited means and expresses concerns about being able to pay for the use of the oxygen. An important action the nurse can take is to:
1. Listen to the parents and express concern.
2. Educate the teachers about positioning the student for the most effective oxygen consumption.
3. Educate the school staff about the student's condition.
4. Refer the parents to the American Lung Association for possible financial help.

Answer: 4
Rationale: Referring the parents for financial aid for this condition helps to prevent complications and promote adjustment of the student and family to this condition, which is an area of emphasis in tertiary prevention. Listening to the parents and expressing concern is an important nursing intervention, but will not actively help the parents at this point. Educating the teachers about positioning and the school staff about the condition will help them understand and assist the student, but is not related to relieving parental fears about the costs associated with this condition.
Step in the Nursing Process: Implementation
Category of Client Need: Safe, Effective Care Environment
Cognitive Level: Application
Learning Objective 23-6: Describe areas of emphasis in tertiary prevention in the school setting and analyze the role of the community health nurse with respect to each.
Test Taking Tip: Understand how parental concerns can affect the overall condition of the student.

23.15 A student joins the school and the parent tells the nurse that the child has a learning disability. The nurse should ask the parent if the child has:
1. Other conditions that the nurse should be aware of.
2. An Individualized Education Plan (IEP).
3. Difficulty in making new friends.
4. Special equipment needs.

Answer: 2
Rationale: An emphasis in tertiary prevention is to prevent adverse effects of learning disabilities, so a new student with diagnosed learning disabilities should have an individualized education plan (IEP) to help the teacher plan appropriate teaching strategies. This will help the student learn as easily as possible. The nurse should be alert to any other conditions the student may have and any special equipment needs, but this is related to preventing complications and promoting adjustment. Information about the ability to make friends in a new environment is related to promoting adjustment, and is not a focus of tertiary prevention.
Step in the Nursing Process: Planning
Category of Client Need: Safe, Effective Care Environment
Cognitive Level: Application
Learning Objective 23-6: Describe areas of emphasis in tertiary prevention in the school setting and analyze the role of the community health nurse with respect to each.
Test Taking Tip: Be aware that learning disabilities can impact the overall health of the child and the ability learn in school.

Chapter 24

24.1 The nurse organizes a fitness program at the workplace in which a dedicated parking spot will be awarded as the prize to the employee who becomes the "most fit" in terms of body mass index (BMI) at the end

Answer: 3
Rationale: Employees are a somewhat "captive audience" in the workplace and can be subject to subtle pressures, both positive and negative. In this instance, this is a positive pressure; because managers have joined, that could be interpreted as a subtle pressure to join. There is no indication that the employees have become

of six months. Many of the top managers join the program and the nurse is surprised at the number of employees who also join. A reason for this response could be that the employees:

1. Really want the dedicated parking spot.
2. Are self-motivated to become more fit.
3. Are responding to subtle pressure to become more fit.
4. Are competing with management as to who is more fit.

self-motivated to fitness, nor is there an indication that the employees have become competitive to win the parking spot.
Step in the Nursing Process: Implementation
Category of Client Need: Health Promotion and Maintenance
Cognitive Level: Application
Learning Objective 24-1: Describe the advantages of providing health care in work settings.
Test Taking Tip: Understand how subtle pressure can be a positive force for health.

24.2 The nurse who monitors the health of employees in a modern office building will need to be alert to what issue?

1. Air quality from the ventilation system.
2. Noise levels from the outside.
3. Injuries sustained from weekend activities.
4. The distance employees walk from the parking area to the building.

Answer: 1
Rationale: A potential health and safety hazard in a modern office building can be the air quality. Many modern office buildings have windows that cannot be opened and the air quality is dependent upon the cleanliness and quality of the ventilation system. Issues such as the number of air exchanges per minute and how often fresh air is taken into the system can impact the overall health of employees in the building. Poor air quality due to mold and inadequate fresh air intake can pose a health hazard. Outside noise level is not necessarily a health hazard unless the noise levels exceed safe standards. Injuries sustained from weekend activities can impact work performance, but may not be a priority of the nurse. The distance that employees walk can possibly pose a health or safety hazard if there are obstacles present, but this is not indicated.
Step in the Nursing Process: Assessment
Category of Client Need: Health Promotion and Maintenance
Cognitive Level: Analysis
Learning Objective 24-2: Identify types of health and safety hazards encountered in work settings.
Test Taking Tip: Understand that health hazards may be subtle.

24.3 The nurse is employed by a white collar business in which the majority of the work is done on computers. Potential health and safety hazards include:

1. Computers that are obsolete in their design and function.
2. Workers who sit all day and become overweight.
3. Poor ergonomic designs of workspace leading to back and carpal tunnel injuries.
4. Insufficient break times that create pressure in employees and lead to stress.

Answer: 3
Rationale: A business that is dependent on employees performing computer work has the potential of creating back and carpal tunnel injuries. Back injuries could result from poorly-designed ergonomic workspaces where the employees have poor spine posture while sitting, which causes hunching, shoulder strain, and possible back strain. Insufficient resting space for wrists or excessive use of the mouse can lead to carpal tunnel injuries. Obsolete computers do not contribute to potential workplace hazards unless there is an electrical problem. Sitting all day does not necessarily translate to someone becoming overweight. Insufficient break times can contribute to stress, but this is not a definitive cause of workplace stress.
Step in the Nursing Process: Evaluation
Category of Client Need: Health Promotion and Maintenance
Cognitive Level: Application
Learning Objective 24-2: Identify types of health and safety hazards encountered in work settings.
Test Taking Tip: Understand how a less physically active work environment can have health and safety hazards.

24.4 The nurse visits the company warehouse and notices that the majority of the forklift operators appear to be between the ages of 18 and 21. What issues should the nurse be alert to?

1. The younger forklift operators have better control of the machine.

Answer: 3
Rationale: Age is a consideration that must be addressed in operating some types of machinery, as well as the maturity to operate the machinery. Younger workers are more likely to be injured on the job than older workers, so the nurse should be alert that the younger forklift operators could be at risk. Age does not impair the ability to operate the forklift, so older operators remain capable of doing this. While the reflexes of the younger operators may be sharper than those of the older operators, it does not mean that they have better control of the machine. There is no indication that the younger operators are not wearing their helmets.

2. The younger forklift operators should wear their helmets. 3. The younger forklift operators may be more likely to be injured. 4. Older forklift operators are not as capable of maneuvering the machines as the younger operators.	Step in the Nursing Process: Assessment Category of Client Need: Safe, Effective Care Environment Cognitive Level: Application Learning Objective 24-3: Identify biophysical, psychological, physical environmental, sociocultural, behavioral, and health system factors that influence health in work settings. Test Taking Tip: Understand the factors that influence health in work settings.
24.5 After a competing business opened a successful branch in the community, absenteeism has increased in the workplace where the nurse is employed. Management has increased work hours and instituted mandatory overtime. The nurse could conclude that: 1. Workplace stress is affecting the employees and manifesting itself in absenteeism. 2. The employees are taking time off to investigate working for the other business. 3. Increased working hours are making the employees ill. 4. Workers are showing increased productivity as a result of these changes.	Answer: 1 Rationale: Stress in the workplace can manifest itself in many ways, and one of them is increased absenteeism. Competition from a rival business can create demands on employees from employers in order to counteract this success. This can create pressure, job strain, and occupational stress. There is no indication that this absenteeism is being used to investigate changing employment to the other business. The increased work hours are possibly making the employees ill, but the job strain pressures may cause them to take illness days for a psychological respite from a stressful workplace. Increased productivity as a result of the changes in hours and overtime is not indicated. Step in the Nursing Process: Evaluation Category of Client Need: Psychosocial Integrity Cognitive Level: Application Learning Objective 24-3: Identify biophysical, psychological, physical environmental, sociocultural, behavioral, and health system factors that influence health in work settings. Test Taking Tip: Understand the link between job stress and absenteeism.
24.6 The nurse has been able to have management institute a family-friendly policy for employees with small children or older parents, which allows them some latitude in job hours in order to attend to these needs. Productivity among the employees has actually risen and absenteeism has decreased. What conclusion can be drawn from this? 1. Having small children or older parents motivates an employee to work more productively. 2. As long as the work gets done, it does not matter what hours are put in by the employees. 3. Relieving the burden of caregiving stress on an employee can create a work climate that becomes more productive. 4. The productivity and decreased absenteeism is due to employees without small children or older parents.	Answer: 3 Rationale: The interrelationship between work and family obligations can impact the health of an employee or the health of the employee's family, which can lead to employee absenteeism and result in decreased productivity. Family-friendly policies that allow for flexible work hours for employees to handle family health concerns with small children or older parents can result in more productive employees, because it relieves a stressor on the employee. Small children or responsibility for older parents is not a motivating force for increased work productivity. Employers are conscious of hours worked so it is not appropriate if employees do not fulfill their job obligations. It cannot be assumed that the productivity and absenteeism is from employees without children or older parents. Step in the Nursing Process: Evaluation Category of Client Need: Health Promotion and Maintenance Cognitive Level: Application Learning Objective 24-4: Analyze spheres of social influence and their effect on the health of employees. Test Taking Tip: Be aware of the demands made upon employees who have small children or who care for older parents.
24.7 A new employee joins the workgroup and comes to the nurse to complain about one of the coworkers who makes inappropriate comments that make the employee feel uncomfortable. The other employees in the group identify this person to the nurse. What should the nurse tell the employee who made the complaint?	Answer: 3 Rationale: Making inappropriate comments that cause someone to feel uncomfortable is a form of harassment, which creates a hostile environment that can affect an employee's physical and/or emotional health. Though the other coworkers state that this is how this person is, it does not excuse the behavior and the group is unlikely to tell this coworker to cease the comments. Ignoring the coworker will not alleviate or remove the problem. Filing a complaint may ultimately happen, but before this, the employee and nurse should speak to the management. The nurse has an ethical obligation to report such behavior to management.

1. Ignore this coworker.
2. File a complaint against the coworker.
3. Go with the nurse to discuss this with the management.
4. Talk to the group to tell this coworker to cease making these comments.

Step in the Nursing Process: Assessment
Category of Client Need: Psychosocial Integrity
Cognitive Level: Application
Learning Objective 24-4: Analyze spheres of social influence and their effect on the health of employees.
Test Taking Tip: Understand how harassment can impact the overall health of the workplace.

24.8 A local company is attempting to decrease its insurance costs and embarks on several changes in its corporate attitude about health. It institutes low fat, heart-healthy food selections in the cafeteria, employs a fitness consultant for the workforce, and encourages the staff to use the stairs rather than the elevators for anything less than two floors. The scope of the company's changes are considered:
1. Health promotion.
2. Eliminating hazardous conditions.
3. Comprehensive.
4. Family-oriented.

Answer: 3
Rationale: An occupational health program that uses wellness as an approach to improve the health of employees through awareness, lifestyle change, and a change in environmental conditions is considered comprehensive in scope. Employing a fitness consultant helps to develop awareness in the employees to create lifestyle changes. Lifestyle changes and changing environmental conditions such as instituting dietary changes in the cafeteria and encouraging the use of stairs is indicative of a comprehensive program. The measures described are not eliminating hazardous conditions. While these measures are considered health promotion, health promotion is just one aspect of this program. It is not definitively family-oriented, because these changes are targeted toward the employee only.
Step in the Nursing Process: Implementation
Category of Client Need: Health Promotion and Maintenance
Cognitive Level: Analysis
Learning Objective 24-5: Describe types of health care programs in work settings.
Test Taking Tip: Understand the different types of health care programs in work settings.

24.9 A local company has set a standard within the community by establishing a child care facility on its premises, which enrolls children from six weeks of age to school age. The facility has a sick care area where children with non-infectious illnesses can come to so their parents do not have to call in sick. The company is considering establishing an adult day care center in addition to its childcare facilities. What could be a reason for this company's innovations?
1. The company wants to be recognized for its family-friendly policies.
2. The company wants to be a family-friendly employer.
3. The company is aware of the correlation between family influences on employee performance and that addressing these concerns helps both the employee and company.
4. The company realizes that it is important to have healthy children and healthy older adults in society.

Answer: 3
Rationale: There is an increasing awareness among some companies about the influence of family on job performance. Most family responsibilities fall on women, who will take sick time or vacation time to address family needs, and this can ultimately impact job performance. Instituting child care services, and possibly elder care services, on its premises helps to address this concern and helps its employees decrease the stressors these employees can face. Being recognized for family-friendly policies does not necessarily address employee health. Being a family-friendly employer does not address or impact employee health. Recognizing the importance of healthy children and older adults does not address employee job productivity.
Step in the Nursing Process: Implementation
Category of Client Need: Health Promotion and Maintenance
Cognitive Level: Application
Learning Objective 24-5: Describe types of health care programs in work settings.
Test Taking Tip: Understand the correlation between the responsibilities of employees with children and older parents on the employee's health and job productivity.

24.10 Providing immunization services, postexposure prophylaxis for communicable disease exposures, modifying or eliminating risk factors in the work environment, and having stress reduction/management

Answer: 2
Rationale: Illness prevention consists of providing immunizations to prevent specific illnesses, modifying or eliminating risk factors in the environment that can develop into a specific health problem, and creating programs to prevent illness or providing postexposure prophylaxis to prevent illness. Health promotion includes activities that are directed toward behavior change to create healthy behaviors that can maintain

---

education for employees is considered:
1. Health promotion.
2. Illness prevention.
3. Injury prevention.
4. Violence prevention.

health. Injury prevention activities safeguard employees from accidents. Violence prevention activities seek to prevent violence from impacting the workplace.
Step in the Nursing Process: Implementation
Category of Client Need: Health Promotion and Maintenance
Cognitive Level: Analysis
Learning Objective 24-6: Describe areas of emphasis in primary prevention in work settings and analyze the role of the community health nurse with respect to each.
Test Taking Tip: Understand the various areas of emphasis of primary prevention in the workplace.

24.11 In order to address the potential for violence on its grounds, a company institutes a violence prevention program. Important elements of this program should include: (Select all that apply.)
1. Developing reporting procedures for employees who suspect violence from others in the workplace.
2. Educating employees about healthy behaviors.
3. Developing worksite policies that promote health.
4. Educating employees about violence prevention, anger management, and recognizing potentially violent situations.
5. Monitoring effective use of equipment.

Answer: 1, 4
Rationale: Educating employees about violence prevention and anger management, recognizing potentially violent situations, and developing reporting procedures for employees who suspect violence are all aspects of a violence prevention program. Educating employees about healthy behaviors could be incorporated into violence prevention, but this is part of health promotion. Developing worksite policies that promote health are also aspects of health promotion. Monitoring effective use of equipment is an aspect of injury prevention from equipment, not violence in the workplace.
Step in the Nursing Process: Planning
Category of Client Need: Safe, Effective Care Environment
Cognitive Level: Application
Learning Objective 24-6: Describe areas of emphasis in primary prevention in work settings and analyze the role of the community health nurse with respect to each.
Test Taking Tip: Understand what is involved with violence prevention in work settings.

24.12 Screening is an important component of secondary prevention. In the workplace, screening is performed to:
1. Determine what first aid should be given.
2. Advocate for adequate health insurance.
3. Report and interpret findings for making referrals.
4. Develop disaster emergency response plans.

Answer: 3
Rationale: Screening in work settings is aimed at recognizing and resolving existing health problems. Reporting and interpreting findings from screenings are used for making referrals. Determining the level of first aid and advocating for adequate health insurance addresses the secondary prevention aspect of treating existing conditions. Developing disaster emergency response plans addresses the aspect of emergency response in secondary prevention.
Step in the Nursing Process: Planning
Category of Client Need: Health Promotion and Maintenance
Cognitive Level: Application
Learning Objective 24-7: Describe major considerations in secondary prevention in work settings and analyze the contribution of community health nursing in each.
Test Taking Tip: Understand what is involved in screening in secondary prevention.

24.13 What interventions should be considered in the secondary prevention aspect of emergency response? (Select all that apply.)
1. Refer to outside medical assistance as needed.
2. Provide immediate first aid as needed.
3. Respond to individual physical or emotional emergencies.
4. Evaluate the health effects of occupational disasters.
5. Refer to continued treatment as needed.

Answer: 3, 4, 5
Rationale: Responding to individual physical or emotional emergencies and evaluating the health effects of occupational disasters is within the aspect of emergency response. Responding to emergency situations is an aspect of secondary prevention in work settings. Referral for continued treatment as needed is part of the emergency response for secondary prevention in work settings. Referring to outside medical assistance as needed and providing first aid as needed are part of treating existing conditions.
Step in the Nursing Process: Evaluation
Category of Client Need: Safe, Effective Care Environment
Cognitive Level: Application
Learning Objective 24-7: Describe major considerations in secondary prevention in work settings and analyze the contribution of community health nursing in each.
Test Taking Tip: Understand what is involved in emergency response in secondary prevention.

24.14 What is an important consideration when assessing an employee's fitness to return to work?
1. Modify the work environment to promote a return to work.
2. Advocate for environmental modifications to prevent recurrent problems.
3. Modify the work environment to accommodate limitations due to disability.
4. Monitor treatment effects and disease status.

Answer: 1
Rationale: An aspect of tertiary prevention is assessing an employee's fitness to return to work after an illness or injury. Modifying the work environment as needed to promote the employee's return to work is in the employer's interest as well as the employee's. Advocating for environmental modifications to prevent recurrent problems addresses the tertiary prevention emphasis of preventing the recurrence of other acute conditions. Modifying the work environment to accommodate limitations due to disability is a tertiary prevention aspect of preventing complications of chronic conditions. Monitoring treatment effects and disease status addresses preventing complications of chronic conditions.
Step in the Nursing Process: Implementation
Category of Client Need: Safe, Effective Care Environment
Cognitive Level: Application
Learning Objective 24-8: Describe emphases in tertiary prevention in work settings and analyze the role of the community health nurse with respect to each.
Test Taking Tip: Understand the emphases in tertiary prevention and the related interventions.

24.15 Which area of tertiary prevention does educating employees about infection control procedures in the work setting address?
1. Assess fitness to return to work.
2. Prevent the recurrence of other acute conditions.
3. Prevent complications of chronic conditions.
4. Prevent the spread of communicable diseases.

Answer: 4
Rationale: Tertiary prevention is geared toward preventing the spread of communicable diseases and this is addressed by the intervention of educating employees about infection control procedures. Assessing fitness to work is not accomplished through education about infection control. Preventing the recurrence of other acute conditions is not addressed in preventing communicable disease spread. Education about infection control does not address preventing complications of chronic conditions.
Step in the Nursing Process: Implementation
Category of Client Need: Health Promotion and Maintenance
Cognitive Level: Application
Learning Objective 24-8: Describe emphases in tertiary prevention in work settings and analyze the role of the community health nurse with respect to each.
Test Taking Tip: Understand the emphases in tertiary prevention and the resulting interventions.

CHAPTER 25

25.1 The community has a population of approximately 15,000 residents. According to the United States Census Bureau, this community is considered:
1. Rural.
2. Urban.
3. Metropolitan.
4. Nonmetropolitan.

Answer: 2
Rationale: Though small, this community is considered urban by United States Census Bureau standards. A core population of 2,500 to 49,999, according to the Census Bureau standards, is an urban cluster. Rural is a population of less than 2,500. Metropolitan refers to the Office of Budget and Management (OMB) designation for metropolitan counties, those that have a population of 250,000 to 1 million. An OMB population that has an urban cluster of 10,000 to 49,000 is a nonmetropolitan micropolitan county.
Step in the Nursing Process: Assessment
Category of Client Need: Health Promotion and Maintenance
Cognitive Level: Analysis
Learning Objective 25-1: Describe various approaches to defining rural and urban.
Test Taking Tip: Understand the population size of each community type.

25.2 The community that has an urban population of 2,500 to 19,999 and is adjacent to a metropolitan area is considered by the United States Department of Agriculture (USDA) to be:
1. Rural.
2. Urban.
3. Metropolitan.
4. Micropolitan.

Answer: 1
Rationale: The United States Department of Agriculture (USDA) classification of rural communities addresses populations that live in nonmetroplitan counties, and can be adjacent or not adjacent to metropolitan areas. Urban communities, per the USDA, are populations that live in metropolitan counties with populations of 250,000 or greater. Metropolitan is a designation for urban areas that is used in other approaches for distinguishing between rural and urban. Micropolitan is an approach used by the Office of Budget and Management (OMB).
Step in the Nursing Process: Assessment

Category of Client Need: Health Promotion and Maintenance
Cognitive Level: Comprehension
Learning Objective 25-1: Describe various approaches to defining rural and urban.
Test Taking Tip: Understand the different definitions of each approach.

25.3 Many rural residents may delay seeking health care until a condition worsens to an extent that more intensive treatment is needed, or a condition that could have been prevented is now chronic. One explanation for this is that rural residents:
1. Do not like to access health care services.
2. Are not knowledgeable of basic health care they should receive.
3. Equate health with the ability to work and the inability to work may trigger seeking needed health care.
4. Are not willing to pay for health services.

Answer: 3
Rationale: For rural residents, the ability to work is equated with health, and they will work with chronic conditions or will only seek health attention when the condition impacts the ability to work. This is a barrier to health care. Many rural residents have limited incomes and little or no health insurance, so accessing care is difficult, but this is not an indication that they are unwilling to pay for health services or dislike accessing them. While some deficits may exist in the rural population regarding health care knowledge, it is a false assumption that rural residents are not knowledgeable regarding the health care they need.
Step in the Nursing Process: Assessment
Category of Client Need: Health Promotion and Maintenance
Cognitive Level: Application
Learning Objective 25-2: Analyze barriers to effective health care in urban and rural areas.
Test Taking Tip: Understand how people define health according to roles in their life.

25.4 A metropolitan area has developed a state-of-the-art, comprehensive public health clinic in the next county that is easily accessible off the local expressway; however, the number of inner-city urban residents who access the services is low. A possible reason for this lower number could be:
1. The inner city urban residents do not like to travel that distance.
2. There may be no public transportation service to the area where the clinic is located.
3. The services provided at the clinic are not needed by the inner city urban population.
4. There are sufficient health clinics located in the inner city.

Answer: 2
Rationale: Many inner city urban residents are dependent upon public transportation for travel because they may not have their own private transportation. No matter how state-of-the-art the facility is, building a clinic for a population that cannot access it becomes a barrier to health. There is no indication that the residents do not like to travel, nor is there any indication that there are sufficient services already present in the urban area or that the services provided are not the ones needed by this population.
Step in the Nursing Process: Evaluation
Category of Client Need: Health Promotion and Maintenance
Cognitive Level: Application
Learning Objective 25-2: Analyze barriers to effective health care in urban and rural areas.
Test Taking Tip: Understand that barriers to health care can be basic.

25.5 A concern for the overall health of residents in rural areas is the number who are overweight. A reason for this is:
1. Rural residents like more high-fat diets.
2. Urban residents traditionally eat healthier.
3. Access to variety in food choices, which defines dietary choices, may be limited in rural areas.
4. Rural residents grow most of their produce, which contributes to them becoming overweight.

Answer: 3
Rationale: Rural residents are more likely than their urban counterparts to be overweight and rural diets tend to contain more fat and calories that those of more urban populations. Local grocery stores may have limited offerings, which can influence dietary food choices. While cultural influences can determine dietary preference, there is no indication that rural residents like high fat diets and that urban residents traditionally eat a healthier diet. Rural residents may grow more of what they eat, but that does not contribute to them being overweight.
Step in the Nursing Process: Assessment
Category of Client Need: Health Promotion and Maintenance
Cognitive Level: Application
Learning Objective 25-3: Identify differences in biophysical, psychological, physical environmental, sociocultural, behavioral, and health system factors as they affect health in urban and rural areas.
Test Taking Tip: Understand the health concerns of individuals living in rural areas.

25.6 Mental health services in rural areas are less adequate than in urban areas. One of the most important

Answer: 4
Rationale: Mental health services are less available in rural areas than urban areas. There is a greater stigma attached to mental illness in rural cultures, which value

aspects that compounds this deficit is the:

1. Type and location of services offered.
2. Lack of funding for additional mental health services.
3. Failure of rural health providers to provide information to the community about mental health services.
4. Underdiagnosis and stigma of mental health problems in rural areas.

self-reliance. The social stigma and lack of anonymity in rural areas has been suggested as a reason for underdiagnosis in these areas. It is the health providers' responsibility to provide information about available mental health services in the area. Type, location, and funding can be concerns for accessing mental health, but the primary reason for not accessing mental health services is its stigma in the rural community.
Step in the Nursing Process: Assessment
Category of Client Need: Psychosocial Integrity
Cognitive Level: Comprehension
Learning Objective 25-3: Identify differences in biophysical, psychological, physical environmental, sociocultural, behavioral, and health system factors as they affect health in urban and rural areas.
Test Taking Tip: Understand how perceptions of mental health can prevent accessing health care services.

25.7 Rural communities are sustained by informal support networks and decreased mobility; whereas, in urban communities:

1. Informal support networks sustain the neighborhoods in communities.
2. Mobility of populations and complex interpersonal interactions can lead to decreased social support.
3. Fear of becoming close to neighbors inhibits development of support systems.
4. Diversity of populations encourages close interpersonal interactions.

Answer: 2
Rationale: Rural communities are characterized by a lack of anonymity among the residents, which contributes to the development of informal support systems that provide social support and trust. In urban communities, there is greater mobility of populations, which can inhibit the development of close relationships for social support. Diversity of populations can encourage or discourage interpersonal relations, depending on how different cultural groups are perceived. Fear of different groups can also inhibit the development of closer interactions that lead to social support.
Step in the Nursing Process: Evaluation
Category of Client Need: Psychosocial Integrity
Cognitive Level: Application
Learning Objective 25-3: Identify differences in biophysical, psychological, physical environmental, sociocultural, behavioral, and health system factors as they affect health in urban and rural areas.
Test Taking Tip: Understand that even in densely populated areas, residents may not have social support systems.

25.8 While rural health departments provide a broader array of services than urban health departments, what is also true of rural health departments?

1. There are better immunization rates among rural residents than urban residents.
2. Rural health care providers do not have as much specialized community health education as their urban counterparts.
3. Rural health departments generally are more poorly funded and have fewer medical specialists than their urban counterparts.
4. The scope of care is more comprehensive in rural health departments than urban health departments.

Answer: 3
Rationale: While rural health services provide the bulk of health care services to this population and have more personnel who specialize in community health, rural health services have lower funding levels and fewer medical specialists, among other deficiencies in rural health services. Lower funding and fewer clinics limit the ability of rural populations to access immunization services. The scope of care is more comprehensive in urban health departments than rural health departments.
Step in the Nursing Process: Evaluation
Category of Client Need: Health Promotion and Maintenance
Cognitive Level: Application
Learning Objective 25-4: Analyze differential effects of government policy on urban and rural health.
Test Taking Tip: Understand how government health policies are not equal in scope for rural and urban areas.

25.9 A positive aspect of government funding for medically underserved areas, both rural and urban, has been to:

1. Provide better accessibility to health services in both areas.
2. Increase Medicaid eligibility for access to services.

Answer: 3
Rationale: Government health policies that address rural areas have focused on improving accessibility and increasing services. Funding has allowed more nurse practitioners to deliver care in underserved areas. Policies have not generally provided better accessibility at this time, because funding may be appropriated, but not utilized. Medicaid eligibility is fixed and is not dependent on specific government policies. Emergency medical services (EMS) have not been shortened as a result of

3. Increase the use of nurse practitioners as providers of care.
4. Shorten the response times for emergency medical services (EMS).

government policies, and EMS response time remains a concern in rural, and some urban, areas.
Step in the Nursing Process: Implementation
Category of Client Need: Safe, Effective Care Environment
Cognitive Level: Application
Learning Objective 25-4: Analyze differential effects of government policy on urban and rural community health.
Test Taking Tip: Understand that funding policies will not always positively impact health services to all.

25.10 The nurse is conducting an assessment of health needs for the rural community. Considering that many residents own firearms, an important aspect of assessment should be to: (Select all that apply.)
1. Educate residents about firearm safety.
2. Collect hunting statistics from the local fish and game department.
3. Collect statistics from the local sheriff regarding crimes that involve firearms.
4. Determine how many of the firearms are registered.
5. Enforce hunting and fishing regulations.

Answer: 2, 3, 4
Rationale: Many rural residents own firearms because hunting is a traditional rural activity, which would be shown in statistics from the local fish and game department. Collecting hunting statistics, which is part of assessment, would give the nurse an indication about how many residents own firearms. Educating the residents about firearm safety is not part of an assessment, but an intervention. Collecting statistics from the local sheriff and determining how many of the firearms are registered is part of assessment, because the local residents may need education about gun safety, as well as potential interventions to decrease use of firearms if they are used in crime. Enforcement of hunting and fishing regulations is not a function of the nurse.
Step in the Nursing Process: Assessment
Category of Client Need: Safe, Effective Care Environment
Cognitive Level: Application
Learning Objective 25-5: Discuss assessment of health needs in urban and rural settings.
Test Taking Tip: Understand how assessment covers potential impacts on health, such as violence and criminal activity.

25.11 The nurse is going door-to-door in the neighborhood to speak with residents about their health concerns. An important result from this action is that the nurse: (Select all that apply.)
1. Becomes aware of the neighborhood demographics first-hand.
2. Becomes friendly with everyone in the neighborhood.
3. Can determine health interventions that directly affect this area.
4. Learns what support systems the neighborhood uses.
5. Learns what areas to avoid for the future.

Answer: 1, 3
Rationale: Going door-to-door in a neighborhood can be time-consuming and lengthy, and demographics can alternatively be obtained through local statistics. But becoming aware of the neighborhood demographics first-hand by meeting with neighborhood residents allows the nurse and the neighborhood residents to become familiar with each other so that trust can be established. In addition, this survey of residents will allow the nurse to get first-hand knowledge of what is needed in the neighborhood for health interventions. Meeting with residents does not guarantee friendship with them, and while the nurse could be learning what support systems are used in the neighborhood, it is not evident that this happened. Avoiding areas could result in the nurse not fully being able to serve the population health needs.
Step in the Nursing Process: Assessment
Category of Client Need: Health Promotion and Maintenance
Cognitive Level: Application
Learning Objective 25-5: Discuss assessment of health needs in urban and rural areas.
Test Taking Tip: Understand that lengthy assessment time in meeting residents may be more effective later on when planning interventions.

25.12 The best strategy for the nurse to achieve a positive intervention outcome to improve lower income housing conditions in the community is to partner with:
1. The Urban League.
2. Habitat for Humanity.
3. Local home builders.
4. The Department of Housing and Urban Development (HUD).

Answer: 2
Rationale: Improving housing conditions correlates with health because better housing leads to better environmental conditions, which in turn leads to better health. Habitat for Humanity addresses improving home conditions in rural and urban areas and partners with people and groups to build houses specifically for lower-income people. In addition, it can provide jobs in an area to improve incomes, which can benefit health outcomes. The community can either be local or rural, so the Urban League will not address conditions in either area. Local home builders are a possibility, but may not be able to provide adequate lower income housing and make a profit. The Department of Housing and Urban Development (HUD) primarily addresses urban housing conditions.
Step in the Nursing Process: Planning
Category of Client Need: Health Promotion and Maintenance
Cognitive Level: Application

25.13 The local health unit in a rural county has operation hours from 9 AM to 5 PM Monday though Friday. County health statistics reveal that health indicators for this population lag behind the state mean. Strategies to improve these health indicators could involve:

1. Having a publicity campaign to make the population aware of the services that are provided at the health unit.
2. Combining the health unit services with another county's health unit.
3. Having flexible hours of operation and providing care in mobile health units throughout the county.
4. Coordinating health services with national health awareness months.

Answer: 3

Rationale: Having set hours of operation may be a barrier for the successful use of a health unit for services. Plus, in a rural area, transportation can also be an issue and potential barrier. Having flexible hours of operation and a mobile health unit can eliminate the barriers of time constraint and transportation, and increases the accessibility of services to a population that needs them. Having a publicity campaign heightens awareness but has no effect on outcome if the services cannot be accessed. Combining services with another county's health unit will increase the problems of accessibility. Coordinating health services with national health awareness months may not necessarily result in increased usage and does nothing to address access.

Step in the Nursing Process: Planning
Category of Client Need: Health Promotion and Maintenance
Cognitive Level: Application
Learning Objective 25-6: Describe goals for intervention in urban and rural settings.
Test Taking Tip: Understand how flexibility and creativity can improve health outcomes.

25.14 After implementing a comprehensive, grant-funded, after-hours health clinic in the community, the nurse evaluates the effectiveness of the clinic. While all residents who use the clinic are very positive about the clinic being in the community, the nurse realizes that it is not as cost-effective as originally hoped. What approaches could the nurse take to make the clinic more cost-effective?

1. Limit the hours of operation.
2. Require clients to pay more up-front.
3. Request more funding from the granting agency.
4. Assess which services are the ones most utilized and concentrate on providing those services.

Answer: 4

Rationale: Operating a comprehensive health services clinic means that some services will be more utilized than others. Assessing which services are the ones most utilized will give an overall picture of how the clinic is best operating. Concentrating on those services may be a better way to run a clinic that can still provide some comprehensive services, but not as all-encompassing as originally planned. This can lead to a more cost-effective use of the funds that are used to run the clinic. In addition, this assessment is part of the evaluation process of determining effectiveness of the health care outcomes. Limiting the hours of operation could be considered, but this may work against the reason the after-hours clinic was initially opened. Requiring clients to pay more up-front is possible, but only if the clients who utilize the clinic have the funds to do so. Requesting more funding from the granting agency is a possibility, but grants usually have a set award amount and it may not be feasible to request more funding.

Step in the Nursing Process: Evaluation
Category of Client Need: Health Promotion and Maintenance
Cognitive Level: Application
Learning Objective 25-7: Analyze approaches to evaluating the effectiveness of health care in rural and urban settings.
Test Taking Tip: Understand how assessment is part of the evaluation process.

25.15 Changing the hours of operation and providing health care services to a rural population using mobile health vans instead of a fixed clinic meets the *Healthy People 2010* core objective of:

1. Eliminating health disparities.
2. Achieving health for all.
3. Increasing accessibility to care.
4. Decreasing medically underserved areas.

Answer: 3

Rationale: The two primary objectives of *Healthy People 2010* are eliminating health disparities and increasing accessibility to care. Providing creative and flexible health services in a rural area with flexible health hours and use of mobile health services meets the goal of increasing accessibility to care. It does not eliminate health disparities. Achieving health for all is from the United Nations' Declaration of Alma Alta. Decreasing medically underserved areas is not one of the *Healthy People 2010* core objectives.

Step in the Nursing Process: Evaluation
Category of Client Need: Health Promotion and Maintenance
Cognitive Level: Application
Learning Objective 25-7: Analyze approaches to evaluating the effectiveness of health care in rural and urban settings.
Test Taking Tip: Be aware of approaches in evaluation that meet national health objectives.

26.1 Clients in correctional settings have unique considerations for care. Providing care in a correctional setting has implications for the client population health as environmental conditions and behaviors in correctional facilities:

1. Can spread communicable diseases.
2. Are well-suited for health promotion interventions.
3. Decrease the potential for communicable disease transmission.
4. Eliminate unhealthy lifestyle behaviors.

Answer: 1

Rationale: Many correctional facilities are overcrowded and essentially unhealthy environments. Such places can spread communicable diseases among the inmate population and potentially provide a cause of spread in the general population when an inmate is released. Health promotion can occur in correctional facilities but the environment is not well-suited for this given its purpose and nature. Conditions and behaviors in correctional facilities contribute to potential communicable disease transmission; they do not decrease it. Lifestyle behaviors can be curtailed to a degree within correctional facilities, but unhealthy lifestyle behaviors are not totally eliminated.

Step in the Nursing Process: Assessment

Category of Client Need: Safe, Effective Care Environment

Cognitive Level: Application

Learning Objective 26-1: Discuss the impetus for providing health care in correctional settings.

Test Taking Tip: Understand the health conditions in correctional facilities and the potential risks they introduce.

26.2 Providing health care to inmates in correctional facilities protects constitutional rights of inmates and:

1. Saves taxpayer monies as compared to providing transportation to healthcare services outside the facility.
2. Ensures the inmate population is at its highest level of health.
3. Allows health problems to be diagnosed earlier.
4. Educates the inmate population about healthy behaviors.

Answer: 1

Rationale: Providing health care within a correctional facility to the inmate population saves taxpayer funds that would be otherwise spent transporting inmates and using taxpayer monies for healthcare in outside facilities. While care can be delivered in correctional facilities, it is not guaranteed that the inmate population will get to its highest level of health, nor does it guarantee that health problems can be diagnosed earlier. There is a potential for educating the inmate population about healthy behaviors but it is not an expectation of healthcare in such a facility.

Step in the Nursing Process: Evaluation

Category of Client Need: Safe, Effective Care Environment

Cognitive Level: Comprehension

Learning Objective 26-1: Discuss the impetus for providing health care in correctional settings.

Test Taking Tip: Understand the benefits of providing healthcare within correctional facilities vs. in outside healthcare facilities.

26.3 An advanced community health nurse in a correctional setting can best utilize this role to:

1. Provide basic care to inmates.
2. Counsel inmates about health promotion activities.
3. Formulate healthcare policy for inmates and evaluate the effects of the facility healthcare program.
4. Treat disease and injuries that occur in this setting.

Answer: 3

Rationale: The advanced practice role of nurse practitioner goes beyond the basic role in the ability to formulate healthcare policy and evaluate the effectiveness of the facility's healthcare program. Providing care to inmates, treating disease and injuries, and counseling about health promotion are all activities of basic nursing practice in correctional facilities.

Step in the Nursing Process: Implementation

Category of Client Need: Health Promotion and Maintenance

Cognitive Level: Application

Learning Objective 26-2: Differentiate between basic and advanced nursing practice in correctional settings.

Test Taking Tip: Understand the differences in the basic and advanced nursing roles.

26.4 Inmates who are admitted to a long-term correctional facility should be:

1. Tested for hepatitis B.
2. Screened for mental health problems.
3. Assessed for HIV symptomatology.
4. Screened and tested for tuberculosis (TB).

Answer: 4

Rationale: Tuberculosis (TB) incidence is highest in correctional facilities, and multidrug-resistant TB occurs in some facilities. TB assessment and screening should be done on all inmates, because the conditions of overcrowding, overall poor health status of some inmates, and the failure to complete the full course of treatment can contribute to spreading the disease among the unaffected population. Inmates do not need to be tested for hepatitis B, HIV symptomatology, or screened for mental health problems unless there are background indicators present.

Step in the Nursing Process: Assessment

Category of Client Need: Health Promotion and Maintenance

Cognitive Level: Application

26.5 Upon incarceration, female inmates should be asked for:
1. Their gynecologic history.
2. The names of their children.
3. The date of their last menstrual period.
4. The date of their last mammogram.

Answer: 3
Rationale: As female incarceration rates rise, their health needs must be considered. Asking the date of the last menstrual period will give an indication of whether or not the female inmate is pregnant, as this poses special health concerns in a correctional facility. Asking for a gynecologic history is important as well as the date of their last mammogram, but this assumes that female inmates have had regular access to these health services, which may not be the case. Asking for the names of their children assumes that all female inmates are mothers.
Step in the Nursing Process: Assessment
Category of Client Need: Safe, Effective Care Environment
Cognitive Level: Application
Learning Objective 26-3: Describe biophysical, psychological, physical environmental, sociocultural, behavioral, and health system factors that influence health in correctional settings.
Test Taking Tip: Understand why female inmates may have special health considerations.

26.6 A dilemma for the nurse in correctional facilities is to:
1. Administer care to a large, diverse population.
2. Provide a therapeutic environment for health within an institutional framework that emphasizes punishment and security concerns.
3. Limit the amount of time for providing care to inmates.
4. Set priorities for the care of inmates.

Answer: 2
Rationale: The correctional facility culture is one of punishment and security. The nurse who provides care for these inmates must balance the role of advocate and creating a therapeutic environment for health amid this institutional culture. Populations in correctional settings are diverse. Care provided in correctional settings is limited. Setting priorities for care is not a dilemma because the nurse is aware of the limitations of the setting where care is being given.
Step in the Nursing Process: Implementation
Category of Client Need: Safe, Effective Care Environment
Cognitive Level: Application
Learning Objective 26-3: Describe biophysical, psychological, physical environmental, sociocultural, behavioral, and health system factors that influence health in correctional settings.
Test Taking Tip: Understand the balance the nurse in a correctional facility faces between being a nurse and also a member of a correctional facility organizational structure.

26.7 Many inmates in correctional facilities have communicable diseases. The most important consideration for the nurse who works in a correctional facility is to:
1. Control the spread of communicable diseases through client education.
2. Advocate for programs that decrease the spread of communicable disease.
3. Use universal precautions when handling blood and body fluids.
4. Ensure that inmate immunizations are current.

Answer: 3
Rationale: A primary prevention intervention, and the most important consideration for the nurse, is to use universal precautions. Communicable disease rates are higher in correctional settings and it is important for the nurse to prevent the spread of these diseases as well as self-protection against those diseases. Advocating for programs and providing client education and immunization are primary prevention strategies, but are not the most important considerations for the nurse. Immunization records, while important, may not be obtainable or known for the inmate population.
Step in the Nursing Process: Implementation
Category of Client Need: Safe, Effective Care Environment
Cognitive Level: Application
Learning Objective 26-4: Identify major aspects of primary prevention in correctional settings and analyze the role of the community health nurse in each.
Test Taking Tip: Understand the primary aspect of prevention for the nurse in administering care.

26.8 Ensuring that the facility has adequate nutrition for its inmates, providing opportunities for rest and exercise, and controlling communicable diseases address:
1. The individual inmate's health.
2. Protecting the health of the whole rather than enhancing the health of the one.

Answer: 2
Rationale: Health promotion is a major aspect of primary prevention. The general purpose of health promotion in a correctional setting is to protect the health of the correctional population rather than enhancing the health of the particular inmate. Promoting health may require the nurse to have an advocacy role. Adequate nutrition, rest and exercise, and control of communicable diseases are all health promotion activities that address the whole. While female inmates have some unique health needs, the above activities address both male and female inmates. The population in correctional facilities is not predominantly female.

3. Aspects of advocacy for the nurse in the correctional setting.
4. Needed aspects of care for a predominantly female inmate population.

Step in the Nursing Process: Implementation
Category of Client Need: Health Promotion and Maintenance
Cognitive Level: Application
Learning Objective 26-4: Identify major aspects of primary prevention in correctional settings and analyze the role of the community health nurse in each.
Test Taking Tip: Understand the goal of health promotion in a correctional setting.

26.9 An inmate has threatened suicide and is put at a level-three observation. This is:
1. Continuous observation.
2. Observation every 5 to 15 minutes with placement in a safe room.
3. Observation every 10 minutes while the inmate is awake and every 30 minutes while asleep.
4. Observation every 30 minutes awake or asleep.

Answer: 3
Rationale: Level-three observation is for inmates who have a moderate risk of suicide. This observation is done every 10 minutes while awake and every 30 minutes while asleep. Continuous observation is done for an inmate who has made a recent suicide attempt. This is level-one observation. Level-two observation is for an inmate who is at high risk for suicide, and observation is done every 5 to 15 minutes while the inmate is in a safe room. Level-four observation is for inmates who have a significant risk history but are not actively suicidal and consists of observation every 30 minutes while awake or asleep.
Step in the Nursing Process: Implementation
Category of Client Need: Psychosocial Integrity
Cognitive Level: Application
Learning Objective 26-4: Identify major aspects of primary prevention in correctional settings and analyze the role of the community health nurse in each.
Test Taking Tip: Understand each degree of observation for inmates at risk for suicide.

26.10 Screening activities in a correctional facility can include screening for: (Select all that apply.)
1. Communicable diseases.
2. Treatment motivation.
3. Chronic conditions.
4. Diagnostic services.
5. Emergency care.

Answer: 1, 2, 3
Rationale: Screening is secondary prevention and identifies health needs of inmates for early identification and treatment. Communicable diseases and chronic conditions such as hypertension or cancers can be determined through screening measures. Treatment motivation is another aspect of screening to determine whether the inmate will adhere to a treatment regimen. Diagnostic services address the diagnosis and treatment aspect of secondary prevention. Emergency care is considered part of diagnosis and treatment as secondary prevention, not screening.
Step in the Nursing Process: Implementation
Category of Client Need: Health Promotion and Maintenance
Cognitive Level: Analysis
Learning Objective 26-5: Describe approaches to secondary prevention in correctional settings and analyze community health nursing roles with respect to each.
Test Taking Tip: Understand the various levels of screening in secondary prevention.

26.11 Diagnosis and treatment in a correctional setting can pose a challenge to the nurse because treatment considerations such as medication distribution must be balanced with the institution's security safeguards. Strategies to ensure success of medication administration include: (Select all that apply.)
1. Directly-observed therapy.
2. Give the inmate a day's worth of medication to self-administer.
3. Place the inmate who will receive medication in the hospital wing of the facility.
4. Combine or simplify medication regimens for fewer doses.
5. Partner an inmate with another inmate receiving medication to ensure monitoring and compliance of medication administration.

Answer: 1, 4
Rationale: Medication administration in correctional facilities is done through directly-observed therapy. Combining or simplifying the medication regimen for fewer doses or fewer medications can promote administration success. Giving an inmate a day's worth of medication can promote hoarding for selling later, as well as not completing the treatment regimen. It is unrealistic to place an inmate in the hospital wing of the facility for medication administration. Partnering an inmate with another inmate receiving medication for monitoring and compliance violates an institution's security safeguards and creates a potentially hazardous environment where medications could be hoarded or illegally distributed to those who do not need them.
Step in the Nursing Process: Planning
Category of Client Need: Safe, Effective Care Environment
Cognitive Level: Application
Learning Objective 26-5: Describe approaches to secondary prevention in correctional settings and analyze community health nursing roles with respect to each.
Test Taking Tip: Realize how medication administration in a correctional facility can present unique challenges for compliance and completion of a treatment regimen.

26.12 As an inmate population ages, a consideration must be made for long-term care planning. One intervention for long-term care would be to:
1. Arrange for Medicare coverage for the inmate.
2. Have the inmate plan advance directives.
3. Provide symptom control.
4. Arrange for use of assistive devices as needed.

Answer: 4
Rationale: An activity related to long-term care planning for an aging inmate population would be to assess their ability to carry out their activities of daily living within the confines of the correctional facility. Assistive devices may be needed in order for the inmate to remain independent; this is tertiary prevention. Inmates' health care is covered under the state or federal correctional codes, so these inmates do not require Medicare coverage. Planning advance directives and providing symptom control are aspects of end-of-life care.
Step in the Nursing Process: Planning
Category of Client Need: Health Promotion and Maintenance
Cognitive Level: Application
Learning Objective 26-6: Discuss considerations in tertiary prevention in correctional settings and analyze related community health nursing roles.
Test Taking Tip: Understand the needs for long-term care planning in correctional facilities.

26.13 A tertiary prevention intervention the nurse can implement at a correctional setting is advocacy for:
1. Long-term care for inmates when discharged.
2. Effective pre-release planning for all inmates.
3. Medical parole and arrange for follow-up care.
4. Use of advance directives when discharged.

Answer: 2
Rationale: Reentry back into society for inmates should include planning pre-release so that the inmate is capable of reentering society with a minimum amount of difficulty. If the inmate has health problems, it is important that the public health be protected and that the inmate receive sufficient health services upon reentry. Long-term care addresses those inmates who will spend almost all or all their lives incarcerated. Medical parole and advance directives address end-of-life planning.
Step in the Nursing Process: Planning
Category of Client Need: Safe, Effective Care Environment
Cognitive Level: Application
Learning Objective 26-6: Discuss considerations in tertiary prevention in correctional settings and analyze related community health nursing roles.
Test Taking Tip: Understand the ramifications of reentry in terms of inmate health.

26.14 Inmates can develop terminal illnesses while incarcerated and medical parole may not be indicated. Tertiary prevention interventions for this population include:
1. Assistance from a personal care attendant.
2. Monitor for adverse effects of treatment.
3. Provide emotional and spiritual support.
4. Monitor treatment compliance.

Answer: 3
Rationale: As with all end-of-life care, inmates need the emotional and spiritual support as their terminal illness progresses. Assistance from a personal care attendant, and monitoring treatment compliance and adverse effects reflect the long-term care planning aspect of tertiary care, not end-of-life care.
Step in the Nursing Process: Implementation
Category of Client Need: Safe, Effective Care Environment
Cognitive Level: Application
Learning Objective 26-6: Discuss considerations in tertiary prevention in correctional settings and analyze related community health nursing roles.
Test Taking Tip: Understand the needs for end-of-life care for inmates in correctional facilities.

CHAPTER 27

27.1 Earthquakes occur periodically on the west coast, so residents in that area are encouraged to be prepared in the event of a large quake. What disaster characteristic does this best relate to?
1. Frequency.
2. Preventability.
3. Imminence.
4. Duration.

Answer: 1
Rationale: Some disasters occur relatively frequently in certain parts of the world. People who live in those areas have some knowledge of what to expect and how to be prepared. Frequency best describes the characteristic in this scenario. Preventability relates to prevention measures that could be taken in relationship to the impending disaster. Imminence relates to the speed and onset of the impending disaster. Duration relates to the length of time involved in the disaster.
Step in the Nursing Process: Assessment
Category of Client Need: Safe, Effective Care Environment
Cognitive Level: Application
Learning Objective 27-1: Describe ways in which disaster events may vary.
Test Taking Tip: Understand the characteristics of a disaster.

27.2 The nurse is preparing a presentation on the roles of the public health care system in preparing for a disaster. The best example of one of these roles would be to:
1. Inspect shelters.
2. Identify disaster risks.
3. Assist in the prevention of injury.
4. Coordinate the provision of emergency health care.

Answer: 2
Rationale: Before a disaster, members of the public health care system should be involved in identifying disaster risks. During a disaster, members should be involved in inspecting shelter sites for health risks, assisting in the prevention of injury, and coordinating the provision of emergency health care.
Step in the Nursing Process: Implementation
Category of Client Need: Safe, Effective Care Environment
Cognitive Level: Application
Learning Objective 27-2: Describe the elements of a disaster.
Test Taking Tip: Recognize the role of the health care system prior to and during a disaster.

27.3 The community is conducting a planning session to identify potential disaster risks and to map potential disaster locations in the community. This period of planning and preparation is best described as the:
1. Pre-disaster stage.
2. Impact stage.
3. Non-disaster stage.
4. Recovery stage.

Answer: 3
Rationale: In the non-disaster stage, planning and preparation occurs by identifying potential disaster risks and mapping their locations in the community. The pre-disaster stage occurs when a disaster event is imminent but has not yet occurred. During this stage, warning, pre-impact mobilization, and evacuation could occur. In the impact stage, the disaster has occurred and the community experiences its immediate effects. During the recovery stage, the focus is on returning the community to equilibrium.
Step in the Nursing Process: Assessment
Category of Client Need: Safe, Effective Care Environment
Cognitive Level: Application
Learning Objective 27-2: Describe the elements of a disaster.
Test Taking Tip: Understand the stages of disaster response.

27.4 The family is listening to the storm warning on the television. There is a strong potential for a severe storm. The family decides not to go to the storm cellar but to continue listening to the broadcasts. This stage of the disaster is best described as the:
1. Non-disaster stage.
2. Pre-disaster stage.
3. Impact stage.
4. Emergency stage.

Answer: 2
Rationale: In the pre-disaster stage, a disaster event is imminent but has not yet occurred. This stage may also be referred to as the warning or threat stage. This is the stage that is best described by the scenario. The non-disaster stage is the period of time before the threat materializes. The disaster has occurred in the impact stage. The emergency stages involves saving lives through rescue efforts for those involved in the disaster.
Step in the Nursing Process: Assessment
Category of Client Need: Safe, Effective Care Environment
Cognitive Level: Application
Learning Objective 27-2: Describe the elements of a disaster.
Test Taking Tip: Understand the stages of disaster response.

27.5 The nurse is using a map to show a group that several pockets of vulnerable populations are located in areas that are likely to be affected by the flooding. This type of map is called a community:
1. Resource map.
2. Disaster map.
3. Population map.
4. Risk map.

Answer: 4
Rationale: A community risk map pinpoints locations of disaster risks within the community and indicates pockets of particularly vulnerable populations in areas that are likely to be affected by disasters. The community resource map indicates locations of resources that are likely to be needed in the event of each of the types of disasters for which the community is at risk. A community disaster map and community population map are not descriptions of hazard maps.
Step in the Nursing Process: Assessment
Category of Client Need: Safe, Effective Care Environment
Cognitive Level: Application
Learning Objective 27-2: Describe elements of a disaster.
Test Taking Tip: Understand the use of maps to delineate spatial dimensions of disaster planning.

27.6 The nurse is determining the extent of the damage caused by a huge tornado. The number of deaths and injuries caused by the tornado is included in the assessment. What type of assessment does this best describe?
1. Pre-disaster assessment.
2. Rapid post-disaster assessment.
3. Post-disaster assessment.
4. Disaster assessment.

Answer: 2
Rationale: Following the occurrence of an actual disaster event, community health nurses will be actively involved in rapid assessment of disaster effects. Rapid assessment involves determining the extent of damage caused by the disaster as well as the number of deaths and injuries. Pre-disaster assessment involves assessing the potential for disaster and response capabilities within a specific community. Assessment during a disaster focuses on identification of disaster effects and related health needs.
Step in the Nursing Process: Assessment
Category of Client Need: Safe, Effective Care Environment

Cognitive Level: Application
Learning Objective 27-3: Describe two aspects of disaster-related assessment.
Test Taking Tip: Understand disaster-related assessments.

27.7 The nurse was caring for a client who had a significant cardiac history. The client died from a myocardial infarction during a hurricane. This is an example of what type of disaster death? 1. Direct. 2. Indirect. 3. Disaster-related natural. 4. Coincidental.	Answer: 3 Rationale: Disaster-related natural deaths are the result of existing conditions that are exacerbated by the disaster, such as this client who died from a myocardial infarction. Direct deaths are those caused by the disaster itself. Indirect deaths are due to circumstances caused by the disaster. Coincidental is not a term that is used to describe disaster deaths. Step in the Nursing Process: Intervention Category of Client Need: Physiological Integrity Cognitive Level: Application Learning Objective 27-4: Identify biophysical, psychological, physical environmental, sociocultural, behavioral, and health system considerations to be assessed in relation to a disaster. Test Taking Tip: Understand the various types of disaster-related deaths.
27.8 The client lost all personal possessions in the fire. The nurse should assist the client to find meaning in the event and address perceptions of personal guilt. What client question related to these issues should the nurse anticipate? 1. "Why did it happen to me?" 2. "What happened?" 3. "What did I do during and right after the fire?" 4. "Why have I acted as I have since the fire?"	Answer: 1 Rationale: Discussing why the fire happened to the client may assist the client to find meaning in the event and address perceptions of personal guilt. Discussing what happened helps the client verbalize experiences and discharge some of the fear and anxiety. Discussing what the client did during and right after the fire helps the client examine his/her behavior and the circumstances and emotions that motivated that behavior. Discussing the reasons for the client's actions and emotions since the fire may help the client identify areas where help is needed to deal with the psychological effects of the fire. Step in the Nursing Process: Assessment Category of Client Need: Psychosocial Integrity Cognitive Level: Application Learning Objective 27-4: Identify biophysical, psychological, physical environmental, sociocultural, behavioral, and health system considerations to be assessed in relation to a disaster. Test Taking Tip: Understand the assessment of psychological considerations in a disaster.
27.9 The nurse is working with a group of elderly clients who were affected by the largest hurricane on record. The clients admit to many psychological responses, from confusion to hysteria. The nurse informs the group that the number of months it takes most people to psychologically recover from a disaster is: 1. Two to three. 2. Four to six. 3. Six to eight. 4. Six to twelve.	Answer: 4 Rationale: Psychological recovery occurs for most people within six to twelve months of the disaster. Psychological recovery occurs for most people within six to twelve months of the disaster, not two to three months. Psychological recovery occurs for most people within six to twelve months of the disaster, not four to six months. Psychological recovery occurs for most people within six to twelve months of the disaster, not six to eight months. Step in the Nursing Process: Implementation Category of Client Need: Psychosocial Integrity Cognitive Level: Comprehension Learning Objective 27-4: Identify biophysical, psychological, physical environmental, sociocultural, behavioral, and health system considerations to be assessed in relation to a disaster. Test Taking Tip: Understand psychological responses related to a disaster.
27.10 The community health nurse lives in an area that is at great risk for hurricanes. The nurse is advocating for stricter building codes and for barriers such as sea walls or dams. What type of prevention does this best describe? 1. Primary. 2. Secondary. 3. Tertiary. 4. Advocacy.	Answer: 1 Rationale: The nursing actions described in this scenario are prevention and minimization of adverse effects, which involve primary prevention. The actual emergency response reflects secondary prevention, whereas recovery involves tertiary prevention. Advocacy is not a term used to describe a type of prevention. Step in the Nursing Process: Planning Category of Client Need: Health Promotion and Maintenance Cognitive Level: Application Learning Objective 27-5: Describe two aspects of primary prevention related to disasters. Test Taking Tip: Review primary prevention as it relates to disasters.

27.11 A group of community leaders is meeting to plan for the upcoming hurricane season. The leader reminds the group that the general intent of disaster preparedness is to:
1. Limit the morbidity and mortality that results from a disaster.
2. Decrease the cost of the disaster to the community.
3. Prepare the community for the impending effects.
4. Increase public awareness of the potential for the disaster.

Answer: 1
Rationale: The general intent of disaster preparedness is to limit the morbidity and mortality that results from a disaster. Decreasing the cost, preparing the community, and increasing public awareness are not the best descriptions of the general intent of disaster preparedness.
Step in the Nursing Process: Planning
Category of Client Need: Safe, Effective Care Environment
Cognitive Level: Application
Learning Objective 27-6: Discuss the principles of community disaster preparedness.
Test Taking Tip: Review the purposes of disaster preparedness.

27.12 Effective disaster planning is based on certain principles. These principles include the requirement that response plans should: (Select all that apply.)
1. Be written so specifically that they are not easily changed.
2. Be based on knowledge about how people generally behave in emergency situations.
3. Enlist the support and coordinate the efforts of the entire community.
4. Account primarily for the physical health needs of victims and helpers.
5. Be kept confidential until executed.

Answer: 2, 3
Rationale: Response plans should be based on knowledge about how people generally behave in emergency situations. They should enlist the support and coordinate the efforts of the entire community. Response plans should be flexible enough to fit the needs of a given disaster situation and they need to be easy to change. They should account for mental and physical health needs of victims and helpers. They should be well known to all involved.
Step in the Nursing Process: Planning
Category of Client Need: Safe, Effective Care Environment
Cognitive Level: Comprehension
Learning Objective 27-6: Discuss the principles of community disaster preparedness.
Test Taking Tip: Understand the requirements of disaster response plans.

27.13 The community has brought in an expert on disaster planning. One of the expert's responsibilities is to evaluate the community's current disaster plan. The expert knows that a comprehensive disaster plan should address: (Select all that apply.)
1. Notification.
2. Warning.
3. Control.
4. Rescue.
5. Evacuation.

Answer: 1, 2, 3, 4, 5.
Rationale: A comprehensive disaster plan should address notification, warning, control, coordination, evacuation and rescue.
Step in the Nursing Process: Planning.
Category of Client Need: Safe, Effective Care Environment
Cognitive Level: Application
Learning Objective 27-7: Identify the component elements of an effective disaster response plan.
Test Taking Tip: Review the elements of a comprehensive disaster plan.

27.14 The nurse is working at a shelter for hurricane victims. The nurse has been assigned to triaging. Two of the clients the nurse first assesses need green tags. Green tags usually indicate victims:
1. With local injuries without immediate systemic complications who can wait several hours for treatment.
2. Who have life-threatening injuries but who can be stabilized and who have a probability of survival.
3. Who have died.
4. With systemic complications that are not yet life-threatening and who can wait 45 to 60 minutes for medical attention.

Answer: 1
Rationale: Green tags indicate victims with local injuries without immediate systemic complications who can wait several hours for treatment. Black tags are attached to victims who are already dead. Red tags are attached to victims who have life-threatening injuries but who can be stabilized and who have a high probability of survival. Yellow tags are assigned to victims who have injuries with systemic complications that are not yet life-threatening and who are able to withstand a wait of 45 to 60 minutes for medical attention.
Step in the Nursing Process: Implementation
Category of Client Need: Safe, Effective Care Environment
Cognitive Level: Analysis
Learning Objective 27-8: Analyze the role of community health nurses in primary, secondary, and tertiary prevention related to disaster situations.
Test Taking Tip: Understand triaging.

27.15 The nurse is working in a clinic that provides counseling for victims of a recent flood. This is an example of:
1. Primary prevention.
2. Secondary prevention.
3. Tertiary prevention.
4. Mental health care.

Answer: 3

Rationale: Examples of tertiary prevention activities include providing follow-up care for psychological problems that result from a disaster. Secondary prevention activities involve immediate and supportive care. Primary prevention involves disaster prevention and minimizing disaster effects. This is not an example of mental health care.

Step in the Nursing Process: Implementation

Category of Client Need: Psychosocial Integrity

Cognitive Level: Analysis

Learning Objective 27-8: Analyze the role of community health nurses in primary, secondary, and tertiary prevention related to disaster situations.

Test Taking Tip: Review what comprises tertiary prevention in a disaster.

CHAPTER 28

28.1 The student is preparing a poster for a presentation in a community health class. The poster discusses one communicable disease that has been completely eradicated from the world. What is that communicable disease?
1. Poliomyelitis
2. Smallpox
3. Rubella
4. Tetanus
5. Mumps

Answer: 2

Rationale: Smallpox is one communicable disease that has been completely eradicated from the world. Poliomyelitis has been targeted for eradication, but there are still cases reported. Rubella has been slated for eradication but there are still cases reported. There are still reported cases of tetanus and mumps each year.

Step in the Nursing Process: Assessment

Category of Client Need: Health Promotion and Maintenance

Cognitive Level: Comprehension

Learning Objective 28-1: Analyze major trends in the incidence of communicable diseases.

Test Taking Tip: Understand incidence of the major communicable diseases.

28.2 The nurse is working in a small rural community. For the last 12 months the community's population has experienced outbreaks of various gastrointestinal diseases. This example best describes a/an:
1. Epidemic.
2. Endemic.
3. Outbreak.
4. Pandemic.

Answer: 2

Rationale: An endemic disease is one that demonstrates a consistent chain of transmission from person to person for 12 months or more in a particular geographic area. An epidemic involves the occurrence of a great number of cases of a disease far beyond what would ordinarily be expected in a given population. An outbreak is an increased number of cases in the population that does not approach epidemic proportions. A pandemic is the simultaneous, extensive outbreak of disease or epidemics in several parts of the world.

Step in the Nursing Process: Assessment

Category of Client Need: Health Promotion and Maintenance

Cognitive Level: Application

Learning Objective 28-1: Analyze major trends in the incidence of communicable diseases.

Test Taking Tip: Understand the differences among the terms endemic, epidemic, outbreak, and pandemic.

28.3 The nurse is making a graph to show some of the common diseases that are transmitted through sexual contact. The diseases that should be on the graph are:
1. Chlamydia, hepatitis A, and human immunodeficiency virus.
2. Gonorrhea, hepatitis C, and hepatitis A.
3. Herpes simplex, hepatitis B, and syphilis.
4. Syphilis, haemophilus influenzae type B, and gonorrhea.

Answer: 3

Rationale: Diseases transmitted by sexual contact include chlamydia; gonorrhea; hepatitis B, C, and D; HIV infection; herpes simplex virus infection; and syphilis. Hepatitis A is transmitted by fecal-oral/infection and haemophilus influenzae is transmitted by the airborne mode.

Step in the Nursing Process: Implementation

Category of Client Need: Health Promotion and Maintenance

Cognitive Level: Application

Learning Objective 28-2: Identify the modes of transmission for communicable diseases.

Test Taking Tip: Distinguish among the modes of transmission for common diseases.

28.4 The client had an open wound and was splashed with contaminated body fluid. The diseases the client is most at risk for include:
1. All of the hepatitis diseases.
2. Human immunodeficiency virus and only hepatitis C.
3. Salmonellosis, typhoid, and HIV.
4. HIV, and hepatitis B, C, and D.

Answer: 4
Rationale: Diseases commonly spread by direct inoculation include HIV and hepatitis B, C, and D. Hepatitis A and E are transmitted by fecal-oral/ingestion. Salmonellosis is also spread by fecal-oral/ingestion. Typhoid is most often ingested in contaminated food or drink.
Step in the Nursing Process: Planning
Category of Client Need: Health Promotion and Maintenance
Cognitive Level: Application
Learning Objective 28-2: Identify the modes of transmission for communicable diseases.
Test Taking Tip: Understand the modes of transmission for common diseases.

28.5 The mother brought her four-year-old into the emergency room. The child had multiple tick bites over the abdomen and lower extremities. The child is most at risk for:
1. Plague.
2. Malaria.
3. Rocky Mountain spotted fever.
4. Rabies.

Answer: 3
Rationale: All of the diseases listed are transmitted by insect or animal bites, but Rocky Mountain spotted fever is transmitted by the bite of infected ticks. Plague can be transmitted by fleas on infected rodents. Malaria is transmitted by the Anopheles mosquito. Rabies is usually transmitted by a non-immunized pet or by a bat.
Step in the Nursing Process: Assessment
Category of Client Need: Health Promotion and Maintenance
Cognitive Level: Application
Learning Objective 28-2: Identify the modes of transmission for communicable diseases.
Test Taking Tip: Know which diseases are transmitted by insect or animal bites.

28.6 A client and the client's caretaker are talking with the nurse in the community chronic disease clinic. The caretaker is complaining that the client is more difficult to care for and is having altered behavior. The nurse suspects dementia. What disease does this scenario most likely describe?
1. Tuberculosis.
2. HIV/AIDS.
3. Hepatitis C.
4. Hepatitis A.

Answer: 2
Rationale: Clients with HIV/AIDS may develop dementia, which alters behavior and makes caring for them difficult. Clients with tuberculosis and hepatitis C and A are not prone to developing dementia.
Step in the Nursing Process: Implementation
Category of Client Need: Health Promotion and Maintenance
Cognitive Level: Analysis
Learning Objective 28-3: Describe the influence of biophysical, psychological, physical environmental, sociocultural, behavioral, and health system factors on communicable diseases.
Test Taking Tip: Understand the psychological considerations of communicable diseases.

28.7 The nurse is working in a community that has significant problems with sanitation and disposal of both human and animal feces. Which communicable diseases is the community most at risk for developing?
1. Hepatitis A, tetanus, and polio.
2. Hepatitis A, botulism, and tuberculosis.
3. Plague, malaria, and hepatitis E.
4. Diphtheria, varicella, and tetanus.

Answer: 1
Rationale: Sanitation and disposal of both human and animal feces are other factors in the physical environmental dimension that affect the development of communicable diseases, particularly hepatitis A, tetanus, and polio. Crowded living conditions enhance the spread of tuberculosis. Poor environmental sanitation contributes to the incidence of poliomyelitis and hepatitis E. Overcrowded conditions contribute to the incidence of polio and diphtheria and varicella. Plague is spread by insect or animal bites. Botulism is spread by contaminated food and water.
Step in the Nursing Process: Assessment
Category of Client Need: Health Promotion and Maintenance
Cognitive Level: Application
Learning Objective 28-3: Describe the influence of biophysical, psychological, physical environmental, sociocultural, behavioral, and health system considerations on communicable diseases.
Test Taking Tip: Understand physical environmental considerations and communicable diseases.

28.8 The student nurse needs to administer an injection to a client with human immuno-deficiency virus infection. The student is extremely fearful of administering the injection. The instructor informs the student that the average risk of human immunodeficiency virus infection after

Answer: 2
Rationale: The average risk of HIV infection after percutaneous exposure among health care workers is estimated at 0.3%, not at 0%, 1.5% or 5.0%.
Step in the Nursing Process: Implementation
Category of Client Need: Health Promotion and Maintenance
Cognitive Level: Application
Learning Objective 28-3: Describe the influence of biophysical, psychological, physical environmental, sociocultural, behavioral, and health system factors on communicable diseases.

percutaneous exposure is estimated at:

1. 0%.
2. 0.3%.
3. 1.5%.
4. 5.0%.

Test Taking Tip: Understand sociocultural considerations related to communicable diseases.

28.9 Botulism is a disease in which the causative organism is ingested with contaminated food or water. Contamination usually occurs by accident through inadequate canning and preserving processes, but it also could occur as a result of:

1. Preservatives used on the food.
2. Environmental contamination.
3. Bioterrorist activity.
4. Insecticides used on crops.

Answer: 3
Rationale: Botulism can be caused by contamination by accident through inadequate canning and preserving processes, but could potentially occur as a result of bioterrorist activity. Insecticides used on crops are not a cause of botulism. Food preservatives are not a source of botulism.
Step in the Nursing Process: Assessment
Category of Client Need: PromotionHealth Promotion and Maintenance
Cognitive Level: Application
Learning Objective 28-4: Analyze the potential effects of epidemics due to bioterrorist activity.
Test Taking Tip: Understand the health effects of bioterrorist activity.

28.10 The nurse came to work in the nursery after being sick for 24 hours with an elevated temperature and diarrhea. After working the 12-hour shift, several of the newborns showed the same symptoms. This best describes a/an:

1. Communicable disease.
2. Epidemic.
3. Outbreak.
4. Nosocomial infection.

Answer: 4
Rationale: Nosocomial infections are spread as a result of exposure in a health care setting, in hospitals and physicians' offices. Even though this is also a communicable disease or an outbreak, the best description is nosocomial infection. An epidemic involves the occurrence of a great number of cases of a disease far beyond what would ordinarily be expected in a given population.
Step in the Nursing Process: Implementation
Category of Client Need: Health Promotion and Maintenance
Cognitive Level: Analysis
Learning Objective 28-5: Analyze the role of community health nurses in controlling communicable diseases as it interfaces with those of other health professionals.
Test Taking Tip: Understand that characterizing infection types changes according to the setting in which the infection occurred.

28.11 Some of the major areas of emphasis in preventing communicable diseases include: (Select all that apply.)

1. Post-exposure prophylaxis.
2. Immunizations.
3. Screening.
4. Surveillance.
5. Monitoring

Answer: 1, 2
Rationale: Primary prevention of communicable diseases is directed toward preventing the occurrence of disease. Major emphases in preventing communicable diseases include immunization and post-exposure prophylaxis. Screening, monitoring and surveillance are secondary prevention measures.
Step in the Nursing Process: Implementation
Category of Client Need: Physiological Integrity
Cognitive Level: Application
Learning Objective 28-6: Provide examples of approaches to primary prevention of communicable diseases.
Test Taking Tip: Review primary prevention.

28.12 Secondary prevention activities in relation to communicable diseases include reporting. Five categories are generally recognized for reporting of communicable diseases. In what class does the common cold belong?

1. 1.
2. 2.
3. 4.
4. 5.

Answer: 4
Rationale: Class 5 diseases are not ordinarily reportable because they are uncommon, not directly transmissible from person to person, or because reporting does not enhance the potential for controlling the spread of disease, such as with the common cold. Class 1 diseases are reportable internationally to the World Health Organization (examples include cholera, plague, and yellow fever). With class 2 diseases, a case report is required wherever the disease is diagnosed and includes all of the officially reportable diseases in a given jurisdiction. Class 4 diseases are required to be reported in the instance of outbreaks only and reporting of individual sporadic diagnoses is not required.
Step in the Nursing Process: Implementation
Category of Client Need: Health Promotion and Maintenance
Cognitive Level: Application
Learning Objective 28-7: Describe major considerations in secondary prevention for communicable diseases.
Test Taking Tip: Know reporting requirements for communicable diseases.

28.13 The nurse works in a human immunodeficiency virus (HIV) screening clinic. Two priority concerns for the nurse are:
1. Confidentiality and final results.
2. Results and gender.
3. Confidentiality and length of time to obtain results.
4. Age and race.

Answer: 3
Rationale: Two concerns with respect to human immunodeficiency virus screening are confidentiality and the length of time before results are known.
Step in the Nursing Process: Implementation
Category of Client Need: Safe, Effective Care Environment
Cognitive Level: Application
Learning Objective 28-6: Provide examples of approaches to primary prevention of communicable diseases.
Test Taking Tip: Know the elements of a comprehensive disaster plan.

28.14 There is an epidemic of influenza in a small, rural community. The leaders of the community are so concerned about the epidemic that they canceled all planned public events. This is an example of:
1. Social distancing.
2. Quarantine.
3. Isolation.
4. Restricting.

Answer: 1
Rationale: Social distancing involves voluntarily limiting one's interactions with others in order to prevent potential exposure to pathogenic microorganisms. Social distancing measures taken at the population level would be tertiary prevention interventions aimed at preventing the spread of existing disease in the community, such as canceling public events. Quarantine restricts the movements of healthy people who have been exposed to a particular disease. Isolation is the process of limiting the movement and interactions of people who have a communicable disease to prevent the spread of the disease to others. Restricting is not an approach used to prevent the spread of communicable diseases within the population.
Step in the Nursing Process: Implementation
Category of Client Need: Health Promotion and Maintenance
Cognitive Level: Analysis
Learning Objective 28-8: Discuss tertiary prevention of communicable diseases.
Test Taking Tip: Understand approaches used to prevent the spread of communicable diseases

28.15 A diabetic client is being screened for tuberculosis. The nurse administers the tuberculin skin test. Instructions related to the skin test include:
1. The client must return within 24 to 36 hours to have the test assessed.
2. A positive reaction to the skin test is based upon redness around the injection site.
3. An induration area of 15 mm or greater is significant in this client.
4. An induration area of 10 mm or more is considered positive in this client.

Answer: 4
Rationale: For persons with diabetes, 10 mm or more induration is considered positive. The skin test is read within 48 to 72 hours of administration. A positive or significant reaction is based on the degree of induration, not the redness around the site. In a person with normal immune function an area of induration of 15 mm or greater is considered significant.
Step in the Nursing Process: Implementation
Category of Client Need: Health Promotion and Maintenance
Cognitive Level: Analysis
Learning Objective 28-7: Describe major considerations in secondary prevention for communicable diseases.
Test Taking Tip: Understand tuberculosis screening.

CHAPTER 29

29.1 The student is preparing a presentation on common chronic diseases. The best definition of a chronic disease is:
1. A condition that requires ongoing medical care, limits what one can do, and is likely to last longer than one year.
2. Problems in body function and structure such as significant deviation or loss.
3. A multidimensional phenomenon that results from the interaction between people and their physical and social environment.

Answer: 1
Rationale: A chronic disease is defined as a condition that requires ongoing medical care, limits what one can do, and is likely to last longer than one year (Partnership for Solutions, 2002). Impairment refers to problems in body function and structure such as significant deviation or loss (WHO as quoted in Kearney & Pryor, 2004). Activity limitations are defined as difficulties an individual may have in executing activities (Kearney & Pryor, 2004). Disability is a multidimensional phenomenon resulting from the interaction between people and their physical and social environment (WHO, as quoted in Kearney & Pryor, 2004). Participation restrictions are problems an individual may experience in life situations.
Step in the Nursing Process: Assessment
Category of Client Need: Psychological Integrity
Cognitive Level: Comprehension
Learning Objective 29-1: Describe personal and population effects of chronic physical health problems.

4. Problems an individual may experience in life situations.	Test Taking Tip: Understand chronic diseases.
29.2 The nurse is preparing a class about pain. The percentage the nurse cites for how many adults in the United States experience daily pain is: 1. 27%. 2. 42%. 3. 55%. 4. 63%.	Answer: 2 Rationale: It is estimated that 42% of US adults experience daily pain, not 27%, 55%, or 63%. Step in the Nursing Process: Assessment Category of Client Need: Psychosocial Integrity Cognitive Level: Comprehension Learning Objective 29-1: Describe personal and population effects of chronic physical health problems. Test Taking Tip: Recognize how often pain accompanies chronic conditions.
29.3 The community is conducting a seminar to encourage health promotion. A portion of the seminar will discuss the cost of chronic health conditions. The most relevant information that should be included in the seminar is that: 1. Heart disease accounted for 5% of United States hospitalizations in 2003. 2. Direct and indirect costs for diabetes amounted to $50 million in 2002. 3. Chronic diseases account for 75% of health care expenditures in the United States. 4. Overall costs of epilepsy are as much as $5 billion each year.	Answer: 3 Rationale: Chronic diseases account for 75% of health care expenditures in the United States. Heart disease accounted for 13% of United States hospitalizations in 2003. Direct and indirect costs for diabetes amounted to $132 million in 2002. Overall costs of epilepsy are as much as $12.5 billion each year. Step in the Nursing Process: Assessment Category of Client Need: Health Promotion and Maintenance Cognitive Level: Application Learning Objective 29-1: Describe personal and population effects of chronic physical health problems. Test Taking Tip: Understand the costs related to chronic physical health problems.
29.4 The nurse is preparing a presentation about pediatric health care. Since most people believe that chronic health problems occur primarily among the elderly, the nurse should include which of the following information in the presentation? 1. In the United States, 7.8% of children experience some form of disability related to a variety of chronic conditions. 2. Disabilities are rarely seen in the pediatric population. 3. Diabetes is more common in the pediatric population than in the adult population. 4. Young children are the only high-risk age group for epilepsy.	Answer: 1 Rationale: It is a fact that 7.8% of United States children experience some form of disability related to chronic health conditions. Diabetes prevalence is more than two times higher in people over age 60 than in younger people. Young children and the elderly are at higher risk for epilepsy than other age groups. Step in the Nursing Process: Assessment Category of Client Need: Health Promotion and Maintenance Cognitive Level: Application Learning Objective 29-2: Identify biophysical, psychological, physical environmental, sociocultural, behavioral, and health system factors that influence the development of chronic physical health problems. Test Taking Tip: Recognize how maturation and aging is related to chronic physical health problems.
29.5 The nurse is preparing a community health program about women's health care issues. Which of the following statements should the nurse include in the program? 1. Women have higher incidence rates for hypertension. 2. Women are more likely than men to die of chronic liver disease.	Answer: 4 Rationale: Arthritis prevalence for women exceeds that for men at all ages. Women have a lower incidence for hypertension. Men are more likely to die of chronic liver disease and from stroke. Step in the Nursing Process: Assessment Category of Client Need: Health Promotion and Maintenance Cognitive Level: Application Learning Objective 29-2: Identify biophysical, psychological, physical environmental, sociocultural, behavioral, and health system factors that influence the development of chronic physical health problems.

3. Women have a higher risk of death from stroke.
4. Women have a higher risk for arthritis than men.

Test Taking Tip: Understand the chronic physical health problems that women experience.

29.6 Factors that help to identify persons who may have an elevated chance of developing a specific condition, but do not contribute to its development, are called:
1. Tendencies.
2. Risk markers.
3. Predispositions.
4. Familial.

Answer: 2
Rationale: Risk markers are factors that help to identify persons who may have an elevated risk of developing a specific condition, but do not contribute to its development. Familial refers to factors that are found in families. A predisposition refers to a tendency to develop a disease.
Step in the Nursing Process: Assessment
Category of Client Need: Health Promotion and Maintenance
Cognitive Level: Comprehension
Learning Objective 29-2: Identify biophysical, psychological, physical environmental, sociocultural, behavioral, and health system factors that influence the development of chronic physical health problems.
Test Taking Tip: Review biophysical considerations and chronic health problems.

29.7 The nurse wants to work with the group that is most at-risk for hypertension. Which group is this?
1. Hispanics.
2. Caucasians.
3. African-Americans.
4. Latinos.

Answer: 3
Rationale: African-Americans are more likely than Caucasians, Hispanics, and Latinos to have hypertension.
Step in the Nursing Process: Assessment
Category of Client Need: Health Promotion and Maintenance
Cognitive Level: Application
Learning Objective 29-2: Identify biophysical, psychological, physical environmental, sociocultural, behavioral, and health system factors that influence the development of chronic physical health problems.
Test Taking Tip: Know which group is most at-risk for hypertension.

29.8 The client explains to the nurse that his father died from malignant melanoma. The nurse knows that this client has:
1. An eightfold increase in risk for malignant melanoma.
2. The same risk for malignant melanoma as the general population.
3. A lower risk of developing malignant melanoma.
4. The same risk for malignant melanoma as the father had.

Answer: 1
Rationale: A family history of malignant melanoma in a first-degree relative has been associated with an eightfold increase in risk for developing that disease. The client whose father died from malignant melanoma does not have the same risk for developing the disease as the general population, does not have a lower risk of developing malignant melanoma, nor the same risk for malignant melanoma as the father had; the client has an eightfold increase in risk for malignant melanoma.
Step in the Nursing Process: Assessment
Category of Client Need: Health Promotion and Maintenance
Cognitive Level: Application
Learning Objective 29-2: Identify biophysical, psychological, physical environmental, sociocultural, behavioral, and health system factors that influence the development of chronic physical health problems.
Test Taking Tip: Understand genetic inheritance factors in chronic physical health problems.

29.9 The nurse is discussing the effects of obesity with a group of adolescents. Information the nurse should share with the group includes: (Select all that apply.)
1. Obesity may exacerbate the effects of arthritis.
2. Obesity can contribute to heart disease.
3. Obesity is associated with increased disability among people with chronic illnesses.
4. Obesity is decreasing among the younger population.
5. Obesity decreases with age.

Answer: 1, 2, 3
Rationale: Obesity places a greater strain on joints and may exacerbate the effects of arthritis on affected joints. Obesity is a physiological factor that can contribute to heart disease. Obesity is associated with increased disability among people with chronic illnesses. Obesity is not decreasing among the younger population. Increase in age does not decrease the incidence of obesity.
Step in the Nursing Process: Assessment
Category of Client Need: Health Promotion and Maintenance
Cognitive Level: Comprehension
Learning Objective 29-2: Identify biophysical, psychological, physical environmental, sociocultural, behavioral, and health system factors that influence the development of chronic physical health problems.
Test Taking Tip: Understand the relationship of obesity to chronic physical health problems.

29.10 The major psychological factor that contributes to chronic health problems is:
1. Depression.
2. Anxiety.
3. Stress.
4. Social isolation.

Answer: 3
Rationale: The major psychological factor that contributes to chronic health problems is stress. Depression, anxiety and social isolation are not the major psychological factor contributing to chronic health problems.
Step in the Nursing Process: Assessment
Category of Client Need: Psychosocial Integrity
Cognitive Level: Comprehension
Learning Objective 29-2: Identify biophysical, psychological, physical environmental, sociocultural, behavioral, and health system factors that influence the development of chronic physical health problems.
Test Taking Tip: Review the psychological considerations in chronic physical health problems.

29.11 The nurse is planning a month-long series related to healthy lifestyles. Some of the most relevant topics should include: (Select all that apply.)
1. Diet.
2. Exercise.
3. Pharmacotherapy.
4. End-of-life care.
5. Immunization for selected conditions.

Answer: 1, 2, 5
Rationale: Strategies to promote healthy lifestyles should focus on diet, exercise, and immunizations for selected conditions. Pharmacotherapy is secondary prevention, and end-of-life care is tertiary prevention.
Step in the Nursing Process: Planning
Category of Client Need: Physiological Integrity
Cognitive Level: Application
Learning Objective 29-3: Describe strategies for primary prevention of chronic physical health problems and analyze the role of the community health nurse related to each.
Test Taking Tip: Know the strategies that promote health lifestyles.

29.12 The nurse is working in a clinic whose clientele has existing liver disease. The nurse knows that these clients need which of the following immunizations?
1. Pneumococcal.
2. Meningococcal.
3. Varicella.
4. Rubella.

Answer: 1
Rationale: Clients with existing liver disease should receive pneumococcal vaccine. Clients with existing liver disease do not have a need for meningococcal, varicella or rubella immunizations.
Step in the Nursing Process: Planning
Category of Client Need: Physiological Integrity
Cognitive Level: Application
Learning Objective 29-3: Describe strategies for primary prevention of chronic physical health problems and analyze the role of the community health nurse related to each.
Test Taking Tip: Understand the immunizations needed by the client with chronic physical health problems.

29.13 One of the three major foci of secondary prevention includes:
1. Assisting the client to adjust to a chronic condition.
2. Providing end-of-life care.
3. Screening for existing chronic conditions.
4. Monitoring health status.

Answer: 3
Rationale: One of the three major foci of secondary prevention includes screening for existing chronic conditions. Tertiary prevention includes assisting the client to adjust to a chronic condition, providing end-of-life care, and monitoring health status.
Step in the Nursing Process: Planning
Category of Client Need: Health Promotion and Maintenance
Cognitive Level: Comprehension
Learning Objective 29-4: Identify the major aspects of secondary prevention of chronic physical health problems and analyze community health nursing roles with respect to each.
Test Taking Tip: Review secondary prevention strategies for chronic physical health problems.

29.14 The nurse is working with a program to encourage clients with cardiovascular disease to participate in cardiac rehabilitation. The nurse knows that the percentage of people with cardiovascular disease that do participate in such rehabilitation is:
1. 5%.
2. 10%.
3. 15%.
4. 20%.

Answer: 4
Rationale: Only about 20% of people with cardiovascular disease begin and maintain a cardiac rehabilitation program.
Step in the Nursing Process: Assessment
Category of Client Need: Health Promotion and Maintenance
Cognitive Level: Comprehension
Learning Objective 29-5: Analyze community health nursing roles in tertiary prevention of chronic physical health problems.
Test Taking Tip: Review tertiary prevention strategies for chronic physical health problems.

29.15 The nurse is working with a client who is recovering from a debilitating stroke. The nurse is encouraging the client to continue to feed himself and to continue taking care of his toileting needs. What is the most important reason that the nurse is encouraging the client?
  1. Because it was a physician's order.
  2. To promote a positive self-image.
  3. To prevent joint involvement.
  4. To prevent depression.

Answer: 2
Rationale: A chronic disease may make a client more dependent on others and less able to engage in activities of daily living. Being able to engage in those activities promotes a positive self-image. Dependence is often demeaning to one who has been self-reliant. The physician would not have to write an order to encourage the client to feed himself and to continue taking care of his toileting needs. Even if there was a physician order, the most important reason that the client needs to continue feeding himself and to continue taking care of toileting needs is because it will promote self-image. Even though assisting with feeding and toileting needs would encourage the use of some joints the best answer is participating in these activities will promote positive self-image. Participating in these activities will not prevent depression.
Step in the Nursing Process: Implementation
Category of Client Need: Physiological Integrity
Cognitive Level: Analysis
Learning Objective 29-5: Analyze community health nursing roles in tertiary prevention of chronic physical health problems.
Test Taking Tip: Review tertiary prevention strategies for chronic physical health problems.

CHAPTER 30

30.1 A student is teaching a class on the impact of mental health on the community. The student would include which of the following information in the presentation?
  1. An estimated 20-29% of the population of the United States will experience some level of mental health problems this year.
  2. The incidence of depression is expected to decrease within the next ten years.
  3. Mental illness is an increasing problem only in the more populated areas of the world.
  4. Post-traumatic stress disorder is the most common of the anxiety disorders.

Answer: 1
Rationale: An estimated 20-29% of the United States population will experience some level of mental health problems this year. In the next ten years, depression is expected to become the second greatest cause of disability in the world. Mental illness is a growing problem throughout the world. Phobias, not post-traumatic stress disorder, are the most common anxiety disorder.
Step in the Nursing Process: Assessment
Category of Client Need: Psychosocial Integrity
Cognitive Level: Comprehension
Learning Objective 30-1: Analyze the personal, family, and societal impact of mental illness and mental health problems.
Test Taking Tip: Recognize the impact of mental health problems.

30.2 The reason that mental illness often results in worsening of physical health problems is because of the:
  1. Inability or lack of motivation for effective self-care.
  2. Side effects of the mental health medications.
  3. Loss of cognitive function.
  4. Feelings of inadequacy.

Answer: 1
Rationale: Mental illness may result in worsening of physical health problems due to inability or lack of motivation for effective self-care. In general, side effects of the mental health medications do not result in worsening of physical health problems. Loss of cognitive function is not a reason that mental illness results in worsening of physical health problems. Feelings of inadequacy are not a reason mental illness results in worsening of physical health problems.
Step in the Nursing Process: Assessment
Category of Client Need: Psychosocial Integrity
Cognitive Level: Application
Learning Objective 30-1: Analyze the personal, family, and societal impact of mental illness and mental health problems.
Test Taking Tip: Recognize the impact of mental illness on physical health.

30.3 The nurse is working in a mental health clinic. A client has just been diagnosed with schizophrenia. The client asks the nurse if his son has a

Answer: 3
Rationale: The lifetime risk of developing schizophrenia for someone with one or more family members with schizophrenia is ten times greater than for those with no family history of the disease. The son does have a greater risk of developing

greater risk for schizophrenia. The nurse knows that:

1. The client's son does not have a greater risk of developing schizophrenia.
2. Schizophrenia skips a generation so the client's son will not have a greater risk of developing schizophrenia.
3. The son has a ten times greater risk for developing schizophrenia.
4. Only the client's daughters have a greater risk for developing schizophrenia.

schizophrenia. Schizophrenia does not skip a generation so the son does have a greater risk of developing schizophrenia. All children have a greater risk for developing schizophrenia.
Step in the Nursing Process: Assessment
Category of Client Need: Psychosocial Integrity
Cognitive Level: Analysis
Learning Objective 30-2: Analyze factors influencing the development of mental health problems.
Test Taking Tip: Understand the genetic impact on mental illness.

30.4 The increasing number of mental health problems in the pediatric population is related to: (Select all that apply.)

1. Family unemployment.
2. Poverty.
3. Loss of community environment support.
4. Changes in family structure.
5. Age of the parents.

Answer: 1, 2, 3, 4
Rationale: Increasing mental health problems in the pediatric age group are related to changes in family structure, family unemployment, loss of traditional community environment supports, and poverty. Age of the parents is not a factor in the increasing mental health problems among the pediatric age group.
Step in the Nursing Process: Assessment
Category of Client Need: Psychosocial Integrity
Cognitive Level: Application
Learning Objective 30-2: Analyze factors influencing the development of mental health problems.
Test Taking Tip: Recognize how mental health problems affect the pediatric population.

30.5 The nurse wants to work with the group that is most prone to depression. That group would be:

1. African-Americans.
2. Caucasians.
3. Mexican-Americans.
4. Asian-Americans.

Answer: 2
Rationale: Based on data from the National Health and Nutrition Examination Survey III, major depression is more common among Caucasians than African-Americans, Asian-Americans, or Mexican-Americans.
Step in the Nursing Process: Planning
Category of Client Need: Health Promotion and Maintenance
Cognitive Level: Application
Learning Objective 30-2: Analyze factors influencing the development of mental health problems.
Test Taking Tip: Understand the connections between race, ethnicity, and mental health illness.

30.6 The client is seen in the postpartum clinic. She is complaining of tearfulness, mood swings, feelings of guilt, and inability to cope. The nurse suspects that the client is suffering from which condition?

1. Substance abuse.
2. Postpartum psychosis.
3. Seasonal affective disorder.
4. Postpartum depression.

Answer: 4
Rationale: Symptoms of postpartum depression are similar to those of other major depressive episodes but may also include tearfulness, mood swings, feelings of guilt and inadequacy as a mother, and inability to cope with the demands of an infant. Substance abuse would not be suspected in this scenario. Postpartum psychosis is characterized by mood fluctuations, disorganized behavior, and possible delusions or hallucinations. Seasonal affective disorder is a form of depression that varies with the seasons, and results in depression in the fall and winter when exposure to natural light is diminished and positive mood in spring and summer when natural light is more abundant.
Step in the Nursing Process: Assessment
Category of Client Need: Psychosocial Integrity
Cognitive Level: Application
Learning Objective 30-2: Analyze factors influencing the development of mental health problems.
Test Taking Tip: Recognize the relationship of physiologic function and mental health.

30.7 The client is complaining of episodes of intense fear without any identifiable basis. During the episodes the client says he experiences shortness of breath and palpitations.

Answer: 1
Rationale: Panic disorder is characterized by episodes of intense fear without any identifiable basis. Panic is manifested in cardiac, respiratory, and gastrointestinal symptoms. Bipolar disorder is characterized by unusual shifts in mood, energy, and functional ability. Schizophrenia is characterized by three types of symptoms: positive

The nurse suspects that this client has which disorder?
1. Panic disorder.
2. Bipolar disorder.
3. Schizophrenia.
4. Borderline personality disorder.

symptoms (unusual thought or perceptions that are not present in normal people); negative symptoms (absence of normal behaviors and emotional states); and cognitive symptoms that reflect deficits in attention, memory, and executive functions that permit planning and organizing thoughts and behaviors. Borderline personality disorder is characterized by rapidly changing moods and and results in difficulty with interpersonal relationships and an inability to function effectively in society.
Step in the Nursing Process: Planning
Category of Client Need: Psychosocial Integrity
Cognitive Level: Analysis
Learning Objective 30-3: Identify symptoms characteristic of common mental health problems.
Test Taking Tip: Recognize symptoms of the most common mental health problems.

30.8 The client has been diagnosed with bulimia nervosa. The signs and symptoms the nurse knows are most characteristic of this disease include;
1. Intense fear of gaining weight.
2. Uncontrollable eating followed by purging.
3. Excessive overeating without compensatory purging.
4. Not eating for days at a time.

Answer: 2
Rationale: Bulimia nervosa is characterized by uncontrollable eating followed by compensatory purging. The client with anorexia nervosa has an intense fear of gaining weight. Excessive overeating without compensatory purging and other behaviors is referred to as binge eating. Not eating for days at a time is not a characteristic of one of the major eating disorders.
Step in the Nursing Process: Assessment
Category of Client Need: Psychosocial Integrity
Cognitive Level: Analysis
Learning Objective 30-3: Identify symptoms characteristic of common mental health problems.
Test Taking Tip: Understand the symptoms of the major eating disorders.

30.9 A group of middle-aged women asks the nurse to prepare a presentation on the relationship of menopause and depression. The nurse researches the topic and includes the following information in the presentation:
1. Progression through natural menopause is not a risk for major depression.
2. Depression prior to menopause actually delays menopause.
3. Menopause is a risk for major depression.
4. Postpartum depression leads to a lower risk for depression during perimenopause.

Answer: 1
Rationale: Progression through natural menopause is not a risk for major depression, but women who have a history of postpartum depression may be at higher risk for depression during perimenopause than other women. Depression prior to menopause may lead to earlier onset of menopause. Menopause is not a risk for major depression.
Step in the Nursing Process: Planning
Category of Client Need: Health Promotion and Maintenance
Cognitive Level: Application
Learning Objective 30-2: Analyze factors influencing the development of mental health problems.
Test Taking Tip: Recognize how menopause affects mental health.

30.10 The client has taken an overdose of lithium. Which of the following signs and symptoms should the nurse assess for?
1. Seizures and hyperactive reflexes.
2. Inability to sleep and vomiting.
3. Diarrhea and vomiting.
4. Purpura and incontinence.

Answer: 1
Rationale: Signs of lithium toxicity include confusion, dizziness, hyperactive reflexes, incontinence, nausea, polyuria, restlessness, seizures, slurred speech, somnolence, stupor, thirst, tremor, and vertigo. Vomiting is not a sign of lithium overdose. Diarrhea is not a sign of lithium overdose. Purpura and incontinence are not seen with lithium overdoses.
Step in the Nursing Process: Assessment
Category of Client Need: Physiological Integrity
Cognitive Level: Application
Learning Objective 30-4: Analyze the role of the community health nurse in strategies to prevent mental health problems.
Test Taking Tip: Review the signs and symptoms of lithium toxicity.

30.11 The client is taking second-generation antipsychotic medications for schizophrenia. The most appropriate teaching topic for this client is:
1. Diet and physical activity.
2. The need for regular blood work.

Answer: 1
Rationale: Second generation antipsychotic medications increase the risk of weight gain and metabolic disorder, so people taking these drugs need primary prevention interventions to control weight, such as diet instruction and encouraging physical activity. The most appropriate teaching topic for this client would be diet and physical activity and not the need for blood work. Hair loss is not a probability with

3. The probability of hair loss.
4. The need to take the medications on an empty stomach.

second-generation antipsychotic medications. All second-generation antipsychotic medications do not need to be taken on an empty stomach.
Step in the Nursing Process: Implementation
Category of Client Need: Physiological Integrity
Cognitive Level: Analysis
Learning Objective 30-4: Analyze the role of the community health nurse in strategies to prevent mental health problems.
Test Taking Tip: Review the side effects of the major antipsychotic medications.

30.12 The nurse is working with a group of elderly clients who are being treated for major depression. The nurse's first goal is to:
1. Increase compliance with medications.
2. Improve level of function.
3. Improve quality of life.
4. Reduce suicide risk.

Answer: 4
Rationale: Treatment goals have been developed for treatment of depression in the elderly. The first goal is to reduce suicide risk. The second goal is to improve the client's level of function and the third goal is to improve the client's quality of life.
Step in the Nursing Process: Planning
Category of Client Need: Psychosocial Integrity
Cognitive Level: Analysis
Learning Objective 30-5: Discuss approaches to community treatment of mental health problems and analyze the community health nurse's role in each.
Test Taking Tip: Understand treatment goals for depression in the elderly.

30.13 Most pharmacologic agents that are used in the treatment of mental disorders act by: (Select all that apply.)
1. Increasing the action of neurotransmitters in the brain.
2. Decreasing the action of neurotransmitters in the brain.
3. Slowing activity in the beta cells.
4. Decreasing metabolic activity.
5. Decreasing protein binding.

Answer: 1, 2
Rationale: Most pharmacologic agents used in the treatment of mental disorders alter the action of neurotransmitters in the brain by either increasing or decreasing their activity. Most mental disorder pharmacologic agents do not act by slowing activity in the beta cells. Mental disorder pharmacologic agents do not act by decreasing metabolic activity. Mental disorder pharmacologic agents do not affect protein binding.
Step in the Nursing Process: Assessment
Category of Client Need: Physiological Integrity
Cognitive Level: Application
Learning Objective 30-5: Discuss approaches to community treatment of mental health problems and analyze the community health nurse's role in each.
Test Taking Tip: Understand the action of pharmacologic agents that are used in the treatment of mental disorders.

30.14 The intent of psychotherapy is to:
1. Control one's behavior.
2. Develop an understanding of one's problems.
3. Promote medication compliance.
4. Promote normal behaviors.

Answer: 2
Rationale: The intent of psychotherapy is to develop an understanding of one's problems and ways of dealing with them. The intent of psychotherapy is not to control behavior but to understand and deal with one's problems. The intent of psychotherapy is not to promote medication compliance. Psychotherapy's intent is not to promote normal behaviors but is to help individuals or groups develop an understanding of problems and find ways to deal with them.
Step in the Nursing Process: Assessment
Category of Client Need: Psychosocial Integrity
Cognitive Level: Comprehension
Learning Objective 30-6: Describe areas of emphasis in maintenance therapy for mental health problems and analyze the role of the community health nurse in maintenance.
Test Taking Tip: Know the intent of psychotherapy.

30.15 The nurse is working with a client who has a chronic mental illness. Which goal should be the nurse's priority?
1. Assess for circumstances that may contribute to mental health difficulties.
2. Maintain the client's level of function and prevent frequent hospitalizations.
3. Increase the client's ability to deal with challenges.
4. Assist the client to develop coping skills.

Answer: 2
Rationale: The goal of maintenance in chronic mental illness is to maintain the client's level of function and to prevent frequent hospitalizations. Even though the other answers may be goals that could be included on a care plan, the goal of maintaining function and preventing frequent hospitalizations is the priority and therefore the best answer.
Step in the Nursing Process: Implementation
Category of Client Need: Health Promotion and Maintenance
Cognitive Level: Analysis
Learning Objective 30-6: Describe areas of emphasis in maintenance therapy for mental health problems and analyze the role of the community health nurse in maintenance.
Test Taking Tip: Understand the priority nursing goals for chronic mental illness.

31.1 The nurse is completing a history on a client who has been referred to a substance abuse clinic. Which of the following statements by the client would most indicate a problem with abuse of a psychoactive substance?
1. "I do not have a job."
2. "I cannot get along with people at work."
3. "I have never had a positive drug test."
4. "I am not married."
5. "I have been arrested several times in the last two months."

Answer: 2, 5
Rationale: General indicators that a person has a problem with abuse of psychoactive substance include frequent intoxication, preoccupation with obtaining and using the substance, binge use, change in personality or mood, withdrawal, problems with family members related to use of the substance, problems with friends or neighbors, problems on the job, and conflicts with law enforcement officials. The best answers include the response that the client cannot get along with people at work and that he has had conflict with law enforcement officials. Unemployment, negative drug testing and not marrying are not indicators that a person has a problem with abuse of psychoactive substances.
Step in the Nursing Process: Assessment
Category of Client Need: Psychosocial Integrity
Cognitive Level: Analysis
Learning Objective 31-1: Identify signs and symptoms of psychoactive substance dependence.
Test Taking Tip: Know the signs of psychoactive substance abuse.

31.2 The nurse suspects that the client has psychoactive substance dependence. Which of the following assessments made the nurse most suspicious?
1. Decreased tolerance to the substance.
2. Lack of the characteristic withdrawal symptoms.
3. Decreased substance use to decrease withdrawal symptoms.
4. Increased time spent recovering from the effects.

Answer: 4
Rationale: Diagnosis of psychoactive substance dependence is based on increased tolerance to the substance, experience of characteristic withdrawal symptoms, increased substance use to decrease withdrawal symptoms, and increased time spent recovering from the effects.
Step in the Nursing Process: Assessment
Category of Client Need: Physiological Integrity
Cognitive Level: Application
Learning Objective 31-2: Distinguish between psychoactive substance dependence and abuse.
Test Taking Tip: Know the signs and symptoms of psychoactive substance dependence.

31.3 The community is conducting a series of forums about alcoholism. What information should the forum include?
1. Alcohol use is the tenth leading cause of death in the United States.
2. Ten percent of high school students engage in periodic heavy drinking.
3. Almost 5% of the United States population meets diagnostic criteria for alcohol dependence.
4. Alcohol use contributes to more than 100,000 deaths per year in the United States.

Answer: 4
Rationale: Alcohol use is the third leading cause of death in the United States, and contributes to more than 100,000 deaths per year. The Youth 2005 Risk Behavior Surveillance indicated that 25.5% of high school students engage in periodic heavy drinking. Nearly 8% of the United States population meets diagnostic criteria for alcohol dependence or abuse.
Step in the Nursing Process: Assessment
Category of Client Need: Psychosocial Integrity
Cognitive Level: Application
Learning Objective 31-3: Identify substances that led to dependence and abuse.
Test Taking Tip: Understand alcohol dependence.

31.4 The nurse is teaching a class about substance abuse. A portion of the class discusses the desirable initial effects of some of the substances. Which substances should be cited as producing a euphoricinitial effect? (Select all that apply.)
1. Phencyclidine (PCP).
2. Cocaine.
3. Nicotine.
4. Amphetamines.
5. Inhalants.

Answer: 1, 2, 3, 4, 5
Rationale: Phencyclidine (PCP) causes heightened sensitivity to stimuli, mood elevation, a sense of omnipotence, and relaxation. Cocaine produces euphoria, a sense of competence, increased energy, and clarity of thought. Nicotine produces feelings of well-being, increases mental acuity and ability to concentrate, and heightens one's sense of purpose. Amphetamines produce feelings of euphoria, energy, confidence, increased ability to concentrate, and improved physical performance. Inhalants usually produce a sense of euphoria, loss of inhibition, and excitement.
Step in the Nursing Process: Assessment
Category of Client Need: Physiological Integrity
Cognitive Level: Application
Learning Objective 31-3: Identify substances that lead to dependence and abuse.
Test Taking Tip: Review initial desired effects among the commonly-abused substances.

31.5 The nurse is interviewing the spouse of a client who is being treated for substance abuse. The nurse suspects co-dependence exists between the client and the spouse. Characteristics of co-dependence include:
1. Evidence of high self-esteem.
2. The ability to freely express feelings.
3. Control of others.
4. The ability to stand up for one's own desires.

Answer: 3
Rationale: Characteristics of co-dependence center on patterns of denial of feelings, low self-esteem, and compliance with others' desires over personal interests, and control of others.
Step in the Nursing Process: Assessment
Category of Client Need: Psychosocial Integrity
Cognitive Level: Application
Learning Objective 31-4: Analyze personal, family, and societal effects of substance abuse.
Test Taking Tip: Understand the phenomenon of co-dependence.

31.6 The community is experiencing an unusual increase in crime. A summit is being planned to discuss the effects of substance abuse on crime in the community. Information that should be discussed in the summit includes:
1. In 2004, there were 100,000 drug-related arrests among adults and another 194,000 among juveniles in the United States.
2. In 2003 the majority of juvenile arrests (84%) involved illegal possession of drugs.
3. The majority of drug arrests by adolescents involved cocaine.
4. Twenty percent of state prison inmates were using drugs or alcohol at the time they committed the crime for which they were incarcerated.

Answer: 2
Rationale: In 2003 the majority of juvenile arrests (84%) involved illegal possession of drugs. In 2004 there were 1.5 million drug-related arrests among adults and another 194,000 among juveniles in the United States. The majority of drug arrests by adolescents involved marijuana. Forty percent of state prison inmates were using drugs or alcohol at the time they committed the crime for which they were incarcerated.
Step in the Nursing Process: Planning
Category of Client Need: Health Promotion and Maintenance
Cognitive Level: Application
Learning Objective 31-4: Analyze personal, family, and societal effects of substance abuse.
Test Taking Tip: Understand the effects of substance abuse on crime.

31.7 A mother visits the clinic to talk with the nurse. The mother states she is fearful that her son is demonstrating some behaviors that place him at risk for substance abuse. Which behaviors most contribute to problems of substance abuse?
1. Conformity.
2. Patience with failure.
3. Easily acknowledging feelings.
4. Tolerance of deviant behavior.

Answer: 4
Rationale: Personality traits that may place one at risk for substance abuse include rebelliousness and nonconformity, poor tolerance for failure, difficulty acknowledging feelings, and greater tolerance of deviant behavior.
Step in the Nursing Process: Assessment
Category of Client Need: Psychosocial Integrity
Cognitive Level: Application
Learning Objective 31-5: Analyze biophysical, psychological, sociocultural, behavioral, and health systems factors that influence substance abuse.
Test Taking Tip: Understand personality traits that contribute to problems of substance abuse.

31.8 The nurse is assisting the community by performing a comprehensive assessment of substance abuse within the community and by identifying existing resources and opportunities for substance abuse intervention. The nurse plans to then assist the community by developing and implementing some new resources to deal with the abuse. What is the nurse performing?
1. Community assessment.
2. Risk appraisal.
3. Rapid assessment and response.
4. Community surveillance.

Answer: 3
Rationale: Rapid assessment and response is the best answer, because it is a means of undertaking comprehensive assessment of an issue as substance abuse. It identifies existing resources and opportunities for intervention and helps plan, develop, and implement interventions.
Step in the Nursing Process: Assessment
Category of Client Need: Psychosocial Integrity
Cognitive Level: Application
Learning Objective 31-6: Discuss aspects of community health assessment in relation to substance abuse.
Test Taking Tip: Understand aspects of community health assessment in relation to substance abuse.

31.9 The nurse is working with a group of adolescents every Saturday at a local community clinic, and is trying to discourage them from trying alcohol. Which of the following is the best description of this nursing action?
1. Primary prevention.
2. Secondary prevention.
3. Tertiary prevention.
4. Education.

Answer: 1
Rationale: Primary prevention involves trying to prevent nonusers from initiating use of substances. Secondary prevention is employed when there is an existing problem with substance abuse. Tertiary prevention involves rehabilitation. Education would involve providing information to the adolescents as to why substance abuse should be avoided.
Step in the Nursing Process: Implementation
Category of Client Need: Psychosocial Integrity
Cognitive Level: Application
Learning Objective 31-7: Identify major approaches to primary prevention of substance abuse and analyze the role of the community health nurse with respect to each.
Test Taking Tip: Review prevention and substance abuse.

31.10 Which is the best example of secondary prevention?
1. The nurse who works in an alcohol use screening program.
2. The nurse who participates in a school-based education program to prevent drug-related motor vehicle facilities.
3. The nurse who assists clients experiencing stress to eliminate or modify sources of stress in their lives.
4. The nurse who engages in political activity to control availability of psychoactive substances.

Answer: 1
Rationale: Secondary prevention is employed when there is an existing problem with substance abuse. Secondary prevention begins with screening for inappropriate use of psychoactive substances, as an alcohol use screening program. Primary prevention involves education programs, as with the nurse who participates in the school-based program. Primary prevention also involves risk factor modification, as with the nurse who assists the clients experiencing stress. Primary prevention includes the community health nurses who engage in political activity to control access to the availability of psychoactive substances.
Step in the Nursing Process: Implementation
Category of Client Need: Psychosocial Integrity
Cognitive Level: Analysis
Learning Objective 31-8: Describe the components of the intervention process in secondary prevention of substance abuse.
Test Taking Tip: Review secondary prevention and substance abuse.

31.11 An adolescent who has been treated twice in the last three years for substance abuse is in the clinic today with his mother. The adolescent has been warned by the court that further problems with the law will result in his incarceration. The mother is in total denial of the adolescent's problem. The nurse is trying to convince the mother to have the adolescent admitted to a local rehabilitative program. What substance abuse treatment principle does this best represent?
1. Multiple episodes of treatment may be necessary.
2. Medications in conjunction with other behavioral therapies are important to treatment.
3. No single treatment is appropriate for all individuals.
4. Treatment does not need to be voluntary to be effective.

Answer: 4
Rationale: Even though each possible answer is a principle of treatment for substance abuse, the principle the nurse is working with is that treatment does not need to be voluntary to be effective. The nurse is not addressing that multiple episodes of treatment may be necessary. The nurse is not discussing medications that may be used in conjunction with other therapies. The nurse is not emphasizing that no single treatment is appropriate for all individuals.
Step in the Nursing Process: Implementation
Category of Client Need: Psychosocial Integrity
Cognitive Level: Analysis
Learning Objective 31-9: Identify general principles in the treatment of substance abuse.
Test Taking Tip: Understand the general principles in the treatment of substance abuse.

31.12 The client explains to the nurse that he has been treated with aversive conditioning, hypnotherapy, abrupt abstinence, and desensitization. The nurse is aware that the client has been treated for substance abuse of:
1. Amphetamines.
2. Opioids.

Answers: 3
Rationale: Treatment for nicotine abuse includes aversive conditioning, desensitization, substitution, hypnotherapy, group therapy, relaxation training, supportive therapy, and abrupt abstinence. Treatment for amphetamines has no established treatment guidelines but treatment is similar to cocaine abuse, which includes: hospitalization, mutual-help groups, contingency contracting, and tricyclic antidepressants. Treatment for opioids includes therapy with methadone, opioid antagonists, group therapy, assistance with social skills, vocational training, family

3. Nicotine.
4. Hypnotics.

therapy, mutual-help groups, and psychotherapy. Treatment for hypnotics includes detoxification, psychotherapy, and group therapy.
Step in the Nursing Process: Implementation
Category of Client Need: Psychosocial Integrity
Cognitive Level: Analysis
Learning Objective 31-10: Describe treatment modalities in substance abuse control and analyze the role of the community health nurse in their implementation.
Test Taking Tip: Review treatment modalities for the most commonly abused substances.

31.13 The nurse is working in a program whose clients are substance abusers who are trying to avoid relapse. The nurse is assisting one client to recognize personal warning signs of relapse. Which principle of relapse prevention does this best represent?
1. Self-regulation.
2. Integration.
3. Self-knowledge.
4. Awareness.

Answer: 3
Rationale: Self-knowledge is when clients are able to recognize personal warning signs of relapse. Self-regulation is the client's ability to self-regulate thoughts, emotions, memory, and judgment. Integration involves conscious understanding and acceptance of situations including previous relapses. Awareness reflects use of a daily inventory to check for the presence of warning signs.
Step in the Nursing Process: Implementation
Category of Client Need: Health Promotion and Maintenance
Cognitive Level: Analysis
Learning Objective 31-11: Analyze the role of the community health nurse in tertiary prevention of substance abuse.
Test Taking Tip: Know the principles that guide relapse prevention.

31.14 The nurse is working in a methadone clinic. What type of intervention does this best describe?
1. Health promotion.
2. Harm reduction.
3. Tertiary prevention.
4. Pharmacological intervention therapy.

Answer: 2
Rationale: Harm reduction is an alternative approach to the control of substance abuse. It is an approach to drug use that focuses on moderation of substance use and minimization of its harmful effects. One such approach is administering methadone to heroin users.
Step in the Nursing Process: Implementation
Category of Client Need: Health Promotion and Maintenance
Cognitive Level: Analysis
Learning Objective 31-12: Discuss harm reduction and its role in control of substance abuse.
Test Taking Tip: Understand the different interventions in the control of substance abuse.

31.15 The client tells the nurse he is using blue velvet. The nurse knows that he is using:
1. Codeine.
2. Demerol.
3. Opium.
4. Cocaine.

Answer: 3
Rationale: The street name(s) for codeine is schoolboy; for demerol it is demies, dolls, or dollies; for opium it is blue velvet, black stuff, or dover's powder; and for cocaine it is coke, snow, uptown, flake, crack, bump, toot, c, or candy.
Step in the Nursing Process: Assessment
Category of Client Need: Physiological Integrity
Cognitive Level: Comprehension
Learning Objective 31-3: Identify substances that lead to dependence and abuse.
Test Taking Tip: Know street names of commonly-abused substances.

CHAPTER 32

32.1 The nurse is discussing child abuse with a group of new elementary teachers. One of the teachers asks who is most likely to be the perpetrator of child abuse. The correct answer would be:
1. Strangers.
2. Baby-sitters.
3. Parents.
4. Siblings.

Answer: 3
Rationale: Perpetrators of child abuse tend to be family members, typically parents. More parents are involved in child abuse than are strangers, baby-sitters or siblings.
Step in the Nursing Process: Assessment
Category of Client Need: Psychosocial Integrity
Cognitive Level: Comprehension
Learning Objective 32-1: Compare types of societal violence.
Test Taking Tip: Understand child abuse.

32.2 The nurse is working in a rural community health clinic. A new client comes in complaining of nightmares and feelings of anxiety. The client is twenty pounds below normal weight without any physical complaints at this time. The client admits to a recent suicide attempt but is very casual in talking about the attempt. The client is married but states that she does not want to be questioned about her immediate family. The nurse suspects which of the following issues or disorders?

1. Anorexia.
2. Intimate partner violence.
3. Substance abuse.
4. Child abuse.

Answer: 2

Rationale: Intimate partner violence refers to any behavior within an intimate relationship that causes physical, psychological, or sexual harm to those in the relationship. Psychological indications of intimate partner violence include casual response to an injury, nightmares, anxiety, anorexia, and suicide attempts. Even though a psychological indication of intimate partner violence may include anorexia, anorexia would not be the best answer as the scenario describes a much greater problem than just anorexia. The scenario does not describe the typical picture of one who is a substance abuser or one who was abused as a child.

Step in the Nursing Process: Planning
Category of Client Need: Physiological Integrity
Cognitive Level: Analysis
Learning Objective 32-1: Compare types of societal violence.
Test Taking Tip: Review the symptoms of societal violence.

32.3 The community is conducting a series of panel discussions about suicide. Information that should be discussed includes:

1. An estimated 2% of Americans attempt suicide at some point in their life.
2. Suicide is the third leading cause of death for men between the ages of 15 to 24 years.
3. In 2002, more than 50,000 people were hospitalized in the United States as a result of attempted suicide.
4. The suicide rate is highest among the middle-age population.

Answer: 2

Rationale: Suicide is the third leading cause of death for men between the ages of 15 to 24 years. An estimated 4.5% of Americans attempt suicide at some point in their lifetime. In 2002 more than 132,000 people were hospitalized in the United States as a result of attempted suicide. Suicide is highest among elderly members of the population.

Step in the Nursing Process: Planning
Category of Client Need: Psychosocial Integrity
Cognitive Level: Application
Learning Objective 32-1: Compare types of societal violence.
Test Taking Tip: Know suicide statistics.

32.4 The nurse is working with a young adult female who admits to being severely abused as a child. The teaching that would be most appropriate initially is about:

1. The results of risky sexual behavior.
2. The possibility of her becoming a child abuser.
3. General hygiene needs.
4. General coping skills.

Answer: 1

Rationale: Experience of abuse as a child has been shown to lead to risky sexual behavior and early pregnancy. Since the young adult admits to being severely abused, the most appropriate initial teaching should be the results of risky behavior. A later teaching topic might include the possibility of her becoming a child abuser. General hygiene needs would not be an appropriate initial teaching as compared to the results of risky sexual behavior. Even though she might need some general coping skills that would not be the initial most appropriate teaching topic.

Step in the Nursing Process: Assessment
Category of Client Need: Physiological Integrity
Cognitive Level: Analysis
Learning Objective 32-2: Analyze the influence of biophysical, psychological, physical environmental, sociocultural, behavioral, and health system factors on societal violence.
Test Taking Tip: Review how age and physiological status interact in terms of their influence on family violence.

32.5 A nurse is teaching a class on suicide prevention to a group of elderly adults. The nurse is trying to emphasize that methods of suicide vary with different age groups. The example the nurse uses is the preferred method of suicide among the elderly in New York City, which is:

1. Firearms.
2. Overdose of prescribed medications.

Answer: 3

Rationale: Among elderly suicide victims in New York City, falling from a height was the preferred method of suicide. Even though firearms may be used in some suicides in New York City, the preferred method of suicide by elderly victims is falling from a height. Even though overdosing on prescribed medications may be the cause of some suicides in New York City, the preferred method of suicide by elderly victims is falling from a height. Hanging is not the preferred method of suicide in elderly victims in New York City.

Step in the Nursing Process: Assessment
Category of Client Need: Psychosocial Integrity
Cognitive Level: Comprehension

3. Falling from a height. 4. Hanging.	Learning Objective 32-2: Analyze the influence of biophysical, psychological, physical environmental, sociocultural, behavioral and health system factors on societal violence. Test Taking Tip: Understand the impact of age on suicide.
32.6 The nurse is discussing societal violence with a group of community leaders. The nurse is trying to show that traditionally there has not been enough attention given to the problem. The example the nurse could use to make this point is that traditionally, the most attention given to societal violence has been related to: 1. Identification and treatment of abuse. 2. Prevention strategies. 3. Ways to increase personal abilities to deal with stress. 4. Ways to increase personal aversion to violence.	Answer: 1 Rationale: Identification and treatment of abuse are secondary prevention and have received more attention than primary prevention. Less attention has been given to primary prevention of societal violence in the United States. Primary prevention includes prevention strategies, increasing personal abilities to deal with stress, and increasing personal aversion to violence. Step in the Nursing Process: Planning Category of Client Need: Psychosocial Integrity Cognitive Level: Comprehension Learning Objective 32-3: Identify major foci in primary prevention of societal violence. Test Taking Tip: Understand the area of prevention related to societal violence that has not received as much attention in the United States.
32.7 A series of recommendations for decreasing the incidence of violence against women was developed at the international level. Included in the recommendations were: (Select all that apply.) 1. Segregating girls from boys during high school. 2. Promoting gender equality. 3. Sensitizing legal systems to the needs of abused women. 4. Increasing funding to certain programs. 5. Supporting research on factors that contribute to violence.	Answer: 2, 3, 4, 5 Rationale: At the international level, the World Health Organization (WHO) developed a series of recommendations for decreasing the incidence of domestic violence against women. Included in the recommendations were making schools safe for girls, promoting gender equality, sensitizing legal systems to the needs of abused women, increasing funding to certain programs, and supporting research on factors contributing to violence. A recommendation was to make schools safer for girls, not to segregate girls and boys during high school. Step in the Nursing Process: Implementation Category of Client Need: Psychosocial Integrity Cognitive Level: Application Learning Objective 32-3: Identify major foci in primary prevention of societal violence. Test Taking Tip: Understand the World Health Organization (WHO) recommendations for decreasing the incidence of domestic violence against women.
32.8 The most appropriate intervention when screening to identify persons at risk for violence is to: 1. Report instances of violence. 2. Refer these persons for counseling. 3. Engage in case finding to teach others how to recognize signs of abuse or potential violence. 4. Engage in political activity to advocate for adequate treatment facilities for persons at risk.	Answer: 3 Rationale: The best approach in screening to identify persons at risk for violence is to engage in case finding. Teachers and counselors are in a good position to recognize signs of potential abuse and violence, and should be taught how to recognize abuse or potential for violence. Reporting instances of violence is an intervention, but does not address how to identify persons at risk. Referring for counseling is an intervention done after the identification of violence risk has been made. Advocating for shelters is an intervention that addresses provisions for persons at risk for violence, but does not address identifying the at-risk person. Step in the Nursing Process: Implementation Category of Client Need: Safe, Effective Care Environment Cognitive Level: Application Learning Objective 32-4: Describe approaches to the secondary prevention of societal violence. Test Taking Tip: Understand how identification needs precede other approaches.
32.9 What should a community approach to provide treatment for violent persons include? 1. Advocate for availability of treatment services and facilities. 2. Referral for necessary services. 3. Educate the public about factors that contribute to the risk of violence.	Answer: 1 Rationale: Advocating for treatment services and facilities addresses the goal of providing treatment for violent persons with a community approach. Referral to necessary services and removing victims of abuse addresses approaches on an individual level. Educating the public about factors that contribute to the risk of violence is a community approach that addresses identifying persons at risk for violence, not providing treatment for violent persons. Step in the Nursing Process: Implementation Category of Client Need: Safe, Effective Care Environment

4. Remove victims of abuse to safe environments as needed.	Cognitive Level: Application Learning Objective 32-4: Describe approaches to the secondary prevention of societal violence. Test Taking Tip: Understand the differences between individual and community approaches.
32.10 Advocating for available shelter and other resources and having a safety plan addresses which prevention goal? 1. Provide treatment for victims of violence. 2. Identify persons at risk for violence. 3. Identify episodes of violence. 4. Provide safe environments.	Answer: 4 Rationale: Having a safety plan and advocating for available shelters address the goal of providing a safe environment for victims of abuse when they decide to leave. A safety plan is an individual approach and the advocacy is a community approach. Providing treatment, identifying episodes of violence and identifying persons at risk do not address the goal of providing a safe environment. Step in the Nursing Process: Implementation Category of Client Need: Safe, Effective Care Environment Cognitive Level: Application Learning Objective 32-4: Describe approaches to the secondary prevention of societal violence. Test Taking Tip: Understand how each goal has different approaches at the individual and community level.
32.11 A consideration for preventing suicide clusters and copycat murders on a community level would be to: 1. Assist family members who are affected work through feelings of guilt and grief. 2. Advocate for services to address victims and perpetrators of violence. 3. Assist in developing community response plans to these events. 4. Reduce the sources that contribute to suicide or homicide.	Answer: 3 Rationale: A community consideration for preventing suicide clusters and copycat murders is to have a community response plan. In addition, media exposure to these events can be controlled. Assisting family members and reducing sources that contribute to suicide and homicide address other tertiary prevention goals. Advocating for available services for victims and perpetrators of violence is not considered preventing suicide clusters and copycat murders, but a treatment of the consequences of violence. Step in the Nursing Process: Implementation Category of Client Need: Safe, Effective Care Environment Cognitive Level: Application Learning Objective 32-5: Discuss considerations in tertiary prevention of societal violence. Test Taking Tip: Understand a community approach to preventing suicide and homicide.
32.12 What do individual approaches to reduce sources of stress that could lead to violence include? (Select all that apply.) 1. Referral to sources of assistance. 2. Develop or expand social support networks. 3. Assist with employment and other social needs. 4. Arrange for respite care as needed. 5. Assist in developing a community response plan to stress.	Answer: 1, 2, 3, 4 Rationale: On the individual level, addressing approaches to reduce sources of stress are referral to sources of assistance, developing or expanding social support networks, assisting with employment and other social needs, and arranging for respite care as needed. These approaches address potential sources of abuse: elder, child, and self. Assisting in developing a community response plan to stress addresses a community response and not an individual one. Step in the Nursing Process: Implementation Category of Client Need: Psychosocial Integrity Cognitive Level: Application Learning Objective 32-5: Discuss considerations in tertiary prevention of societal violence. Test Taking Tip: Understand how reducing stress can decrease or prevent violence.
32.13 How would providing care to families of homicide and suicide victims best be addressed on the community level? 1. Assist family members to work through feelings of grief and guilt. 2. Advocate for support services for families of victims. 3. Referral to assistance with legal and other tasks as needed. 4. Assist families to find positive ways to cope with loss.	Answer: 2 Rationale: Advocating for support services for families of victims is a community consideration in providing care to homicide and suicide victims. Assisting family members to work through their feelings and finding positive ways to cope addresses individual considerations, as does referral to assistance in legal matters and other tasks. Step in the Nursing Process: Implementation Category of Client Need: Psychosocial Integrity Cognitive Level: Application Learning Objective 32-5: Discuss considerations in tertiary prevention of societal violence. Test Taking Tip: Understand the difference between individual and community approaches.

32.14 An important consideration for the community health nurse to address societal violence is to:

1. Assess for environmental factors that could lead to violence.
2. Ask all female members of the community if they have been abused.
3. Ensure that adolescent males in the community are aware of suicide risks.
4. Advocate for gun control in the community.

Answer: 1

Rationale: Before acting on the other aspects of societal violence, the nurse needs to first assess the community for risk factors that could lead to violence. Asking all female members of the community if they have been abused is unrealistic and may generate false answers. While adolescent males have higher suicide risk potential, targeting them will not decrease suicide. Advocating for gun control may decrease violence, but is controversial given constitutional considerations.

Step in the Nursing Process: Assessment

Category of Client Need: Safe, Effective Care Environment

Cognitive Level: Application

Learning Objective 32-6: Analyze the role of community health nurses with respect to societal violence.

Test Taking Tip: Understand how assessment is an important component in the community health nurse's role in societal violence.

32.15 The unemployment rate has increased in the community. The nurse should:

1. Monitor whether more community members receive food assistance.
2. Monitor whether more community residents receive health services at the local health clinic.
3. Monitor for an increase in domestic violence and child abuse as frustrations rise over loss of income.
4. Monitor for an increase in liquor sales in the community.

Answer: 3

Rationale: As unemployment rises, frustrations may increase as income loss creates hardships in families and may manifest in domestic violence and child abuse. The nurse will need to be alert to this potential. Increased liquor sales, increased numbers of residents using the local health clinic, and requiring food assistance can create health concerns for the community, but not necessarily result in a potential for violence.

Step in the Nursing Process: Planning

Category of Client Need: Psychosocial Integrity

Cognitive Level: Application

Learning Objective 32-6: Analyze the role of community health nurses with respect to societal violence.

Test Taking Tip: Understand how community events can lead to violence and what the community health nurse must be attuned to.

TRANSITION GUIDE

COMPANION WEBSITE ADVOCACY INTERVIEWS

Rita Lourie of Temple University interviews four people who have been influential in advocating for community health throughout their careers in nursing. Biographies of these four outstanding women are below.

TINE HANSEN-TURTON, *EXECUTIVE DIRECTOR OF THE NATIONAL NURSING CENTERS CONSORTIUM*

As the head of the National Nursing Centers Consortium (NNCC), Tine Hanson-Turton oversees 150 nurse-managed health centers in the U.S. that provide quality primary health care, health promotion, and disease prevention to over two million families. She has a strong policy development background and has been instrumental in changing health policies and regulations at the state and national level. She is the author of *Community and Nurse-Managed Health Centers: Getting Them Started and Keeping Them Going*.

CONGRESSWOMAN EDDIE BERNICE JOHNSON, *REPRESENTING THE 30TH DISTRICT OF TEXAS*

Congresswoman Eddie Bernice Johnson is widely recognized as one of the most effective legislators in Congress. She is credited with originally authoring and co-authoring more than 120 bills that were passed by the House and Senate and signed into law by the president. Congresswoman Johnson studied nursing at St. Mary's College at the University of Notre Dame and earned a bachelor's degree in nursing from Texas Christian University in 1967. She received a master's degree in public administration from Southern Methodist University in 1976 and subsequently served as the chief psychiatric nurse at the Veterans Administration Hospital in Dallas. Congresswoman Johnson was elected to the Texas House of Representatives in 1972 and became the first woman in Texas history to lead a major Texas House committee, the Labor Committee.

Congresswoman Johnson has a long-standing reputation for providing excellent constituent services. As an advocate for workers, children, and families, she was recognized and appointed by President Jimmy Carter to serve as regional director of the Department of Health, Education, and Welfare in 1977. Her district offices in downtown Dallas specialize in working with all federal departments and agencies to assist citizens in solving a wide range of individual problems.

VERNICE FERGUSON, *SENIOR FELLOW EMERITUS, UNIVERSITY OF PENNSYLVANIA, AND AMERICAN ACADEMY OF NURSING "LIVING LEGEND"*

Ms. Vernice Ferguson RN, MA, FAAN, FRCN was Senior Fellow in the School of Nursing at the University of Pennsylvania and held the Fagin Family Chair in Cultural Diversity from 1993–1996. Prior to this, Ms. Ferguson served for 12 years as the Assistant Chief Medical Director for Nursing Programs in the Department of Veteran Affairs. She is the recipient of eight honorary doctorates and two fellowships; one in physics, the others in alcohol studies. She is an Honorary Fellow in the Royal College of Nursing of the United Kingdom. She has devoted her life and talent to the field of nursing, shaping with her professional leadership hundreds of nurses.

SISTER ROSEMARY DONNELLY, FORMER EXECUTIVE VICE PRESIDENT OF CATHOLIC UNIVERSITY AND FORMER DEAN OF THE SCHOOL OF NURSING, AND FORMER PRESIDENT OF SIGMA THETA TAU INTERNATIONAL HONOR SOCIETY

Sister Donley has a long history of academic pursuits and influencing policy at many institutional and government levels. After her years as executive vice president of Catholic University, she continued her education to become a certified nurse practitioner and to study administration. She is a former Robert Wood Johnson health policy fellow, and has been awarded many other honors. Currently, she teaches at Catholic University and is the director of its Community Public Health Care of the Vulnerable programs. Her current interest is in studying the link between ethics and policy.

THINKING ADVOCACY QUESTIONS AND RESPONSES

What follows are the questions and suggested guidelines for evaluating answers to the "Think Advocacy" boxes that appear in each chapter. After some answers are additional questions for use in classroom discussions or as assignments.

CHAPTER 1

Page 8
1.1 Talk with your classmates. What needs for advocacy with individual clients and families have arisen in your community health nursing clinical practice? Who were the participants in the advocacy situation? What actions were undertaken by the advocate? What were the consequences of those actions?

Evaluating Student Responses: Advocacy as it relates to community health nursing involves actions that create or support healthy environment. Most students will be familiar with situations that involve participants in the WIC program, which promotes proper nutrition for pregnant women and young children. The student may also be familiar with TB screenings and treatment of infected individuals. Many communities have programs that deal with preventing sexually transmitted diseases. There are also programs aimed at providing Pap smears and mammograms to women who do not have health insurance. The student will relate advocacy actions such as immunization clinics, TB testing and WIC clinics. They may relate that their limited clinical times keeps them from seeing the results of these actions. They may also realize that the results may not be seen in a community for months or years.

1.2 Based on the overall needs of the population you have witnessed in your community health nursing clinic rotation, where is advocacy needed at the population level? What risks might community health nurses experience in advocating in these areas?

Evaluating Student Responses: The overall needs of the population will depend upon the specific community that the student is involved in. It will also depend upon whether it is an urban or a rural community. Some urban populations have large communities of people dealing with HIV/AIDS. This may also be true in a rural community. Smaller communities may have higher concentrations of lung cancer especially if the community is tobacco producing. The urban community health nurse must deal with the inherent dangers of working alone and visiting in areas that are not considered "safe."

CHAPTER 2

Page 27
2.1 How might community health nurses in your area promote a population-health focus for local health services? What segments of the population are not currently being effectively served by existing services? How might these subpopulations be better served using a population-health approach?

Evaluating Student Responses: Community health nurses would begin a population health focus with an assessment of the health needs of the dominant populations. The nurse may do this informally by observing which conditions appear to predominate in the community and if these conditions are associated with specific population groups or the nurse could work through the local public health department or other government agency to formally assess the community.

Possible segments that are not being served are the "anonymous" members of the community such as undocumented workers or transients and homeless persons.

The population health approach requires community ownership to be effective. Therefore community health nurses should focus attention on educating the community about meeting the needs of the underserved subpopulations and how that will aid the health of the community as a whole.

Additional Discussion: You have discovered an underserved subpopulation in your community and feel that treating that subpopulation will have a significant impact on your community. Who would you seek out first to present this need? What would you use as the "selling points" of your argument for resources to meet these needs?

CHAPTER 3

Page 47

3.1 Kalisch and Kalisch (2004) described the role of Margaret Sanger in promoting women's access to contraceptive services at the beginning of the 20th century. According to the authors, in 1912, Sanger cared for a 28-year-old mother of three who attempted a self-induced abortion of an unwanted pregnancy. The woman pleaded with Sanger to give her information to prevent subsequent pregnancies. Sanger, constrained by the 1873 Comstock Act, which classified contraceptive information as obscene, could not accede to her request and was later called by the woman's husband to attend her deathbed. This event was a catalyst for Sanger's activities to make contraceptive services available to women. She studied contraceptive technology in France and educated women by means of a journal she published entitled *The Woman Rebel*. In 1916, she opened a birth control clinic, which saw 150 women in its first day of operation. Arrested by an undercover policewoman posing as a client, Sanger was jailed. She publicly refused to abide by the law and was sentenced to 30 days in the workhouse. In spite of these sanctions, Sanger continued to promote access to contraceptive services for women and educate women in their use. She solicited the support of wealthy and influential women who were able to influence the policy makers of the day, and in 1921 instituted the American Birth Control League, the forerunner of the Planned Parenthood Federation.

- What community health issues in your community will require the level of commitment displayed by Margaret Sanger?
- How might you go about influencing those issues? What influential individuals and groups would you approach for support of your initiative?

Evaluating Student Responses: It is difficult to imagine a situation today where a nurse would have to go to jail for a public health issue. Some highly charged issues today still relate to reproductive issues. Just as Margaret Sanger went to jail for the right of a woman to take a contraceptive, other nurses may be willing to go to jail to prevent a woman from obtaining an abortion, even though abortion is legal.

CHAPTER 4

Page 75

4.1 Does the agency in which you are obtaining your clinical experience in community health nursing expect

Evaluating Student Responses: Many communities use the Dimensions Model of Community Health or a variant that resembles this model. This allows a community health agency to look at the dimensions of health, health care and the nursing process. The advantage of the dimensions model is that it looks at all facets of

employees to base their practice on a particular community health nursing model? If so, which model is being used? If not, how might you advocate for the use of the dimensions model as a foundation for community health nursing practice in the agency? What advantages to the use of the model could you point out to agency staff? What disadvantages might there be to adopting a specific model for community health nursing practice in the agency?

community health and all of the factors that can influence it. It also incorporates the nursing process upon which all nursing actions and interventions should be based. The community health nurse employed by an agency that did not use a dimensions model could show how this model would more effectively identify factors that influence community health and the money that could be saved by utilizing the dimensions model.

Additional Discussion: What are the major causes of morbidity and mortality in your community? How could the model that your public health agency uses influence the morbidity and mortality?

CHAPTER 5

Page 88
5.1 Your community includes a number of relatively large refugee populations from different war-torn areas of the world. Some members of these populations have been in the United States for 2 to 3 years and some have recently arrived. All of them have difficulty obtaining services to address health care needs they are currently experiencing. What might you do to address their lack of care? What other groups or agencies might you attempt to bring into a coalition to address the health needs of this population?

Evaluating Student Responses: The nurse could begin by assessing the general areas in which the refugees live. Many people will live in an area where they will find people of a common culture and language. It would also be important to know the value of health care in these cultures. A nurse could visit the leader of these cultural groups to give information about services that are available in that community.

Other groups that could possibly be approached would be the faith-based communities where the refugee groups worship or gather. It might be possible to arrange meetings with the refugees in a comfortable place as well as set up clinics for basic things such as immunizations or health screenings.

Additional Discussion: A large group of refugees from Africa have arrived in your community. In this group are 12 women who are pregnant. None have had any prenatal care up to this point. This group is from an area where HIV infection is prevalent. You are able to organize a prenatal clinic for these women but cannot find a female physician or ARNP to staff it. What first steps would you take? What resources might you draw upon?

CHAPTER 6

Page 116
6.1 Many Mexican citizens are legally employed to work in the United States. They are sometimes employed in positions that provide health care benefits. Many of those who are eligible for health insurance prefer to obtain medical care from familiar providers in Mexico rather than from U.S. providers. Their insurance benefits, however, do not cover services provided in Mexico. What kind of advocacy would be required to encourage insurance companies to cover services on both sides of the border? What groups or coalitions might be able to engage in such advocacy? What might be the role of community health nurses in this kind of advocacy?

Evaluating Student Responses: To help Mexican citizens obtain medical care on both sides of the border would be to prove to the insurance companies that it is more cost effective to do it that way. Possible groups that might advocate for this change might be the governments of the communities involved because it would bring increased revenue. The community health nurse might obtain the needed statistics and also might show the increase in compliance as well as improved health of this Mexican population.

Additional Discussion: What healthcare services would be available to Mexican workers who are undocumented? How do community health nurses attempt to meet the needs of these people?

CHAPTER 7

Page 150
Tsoukalas and Glantz (2003) described the efforts of health advocacy groups to promote clean air legislation in

Evaluating Student Responses: The tobacco industry formed coalitions, networked and lobbied those that supported them.

Duluth, Minnesota. After passage of an initial weak ordinance, the advocacy group analyzed strategies used by the tobacco industry to oppose the ordinance. Strategies that led to initial tobacco industry success included framing the issue as one of individual rights, recruiting support from third-party groups such as the National Smokers Alliance and manufacturers of ventilation equipment, and promulgating claims of lost revenue among members of the Minnesota Licensed Beverage Association and the Duluth Hospitality Association. Knowledge of these tactics allowed the health advocacy coalition to mount a successful campaign for a stronger ordinance.

7.1 What principles of political activism described in the chapter did the tobacco industry successfully employ?

7.2 How might community health nurses have been involved in the health coalition's advocacy effort?

Evaluating Student Responses: Community health nurses would have been helpful in gathering the statistics of the incidence of tobacco related diseases in the community. The nurses would also have been helpful in showing the economic benefit to the community of clean air legislation.

CHAPTER 8

Page. 171

8.1 National studies have found that immigrants, both legal and undocumented, have lower rates of insurance coverage than native-born Americans and that immigrants who are noncitizens are less likely to have health insurance than those who are citizens (Prentice, Pebley, & Sastry, 2005). Yet immigrants, particularly those who are refugees, may have significant health care needs that go unmet because of their lack of health insurance. What programs exist in your local area to address these needs? How adequate are these programs? How might community health nurses engage in initiatives to better address the health needs of these groups?

Evaluating Student Responses: Local programs will depend upon whether it is a rural or urban area. Urban areas may have large-scale clinics set up on a daily basis to meet health care needs of non-citizens. Large cities may have clinics that exist within the school systems that meet the health care needs of the students. Rural areas may have local free clinics that meet once or twice a week with volunteer help. Other sources may be through faith-based communities where clinics may be set up.

It is difficult to assess the adequacy of these programs because so many of the non-citizens are "invisible." Very few of these programs are able to meet all of the needs. They function more as a "fire extinguisher" to handle health crises. There aren't enough funds to meet the needs.

Community health nurses could investigate grants that would help to meet these health care needs. They could also discover where the most pressing health care needs are for the non-citizens in the area. Using this information, the community health nurses could then seek funding for the most common or important health care needs.

CHAPTER 9

Page 206

9.1 There is significant evidence that tobacco companies specifically target U.S. immigrants as potential markets, using culture-based marketing strategies. This evidence is based on a review of tobacco company documents that put forth specific recommendations for

Evaluating Student Responses: Community health nurses need to use the same strategies that successful marketing groups use to sell tobacco. The nurses must use techniques that sell their product, which is anything anti-tobacco. Some examples would be posters and slogans that are colorful and flashy. Some techniques also might include peer pressure not to use tobacco, especially if marketing to the teen population. The problem for the community health nurse is the lack of resources to produce the flashy products. Community health nurses may try to work with local high schools or college art departments to develop and produce products at a lower cost.

marketing to selected immigrant groups (Acevedo-Garcia, Barbeau, Bishop, Pan, & Emmons, 2004). What strategies might be used by community health professionals to counteract these highly successful marketing approaches?

Additional Discussion: A local health department would like to decrease the number of pregnant women who smoke. What type of slogan or product might produce the effect they are looking for?

CHAPTER 10

Page 239

10.1 If access to water is a basic human right, how should community health nurses deal with the practice of cutting off access to water sources when clients are not able to pay their water bills or purchase bottled water for family members who are immunocompromised?

Evaluating Student Responses: Community health nurses must work with the utility companies and non-governmental organizations to work on funding for people who legitimately cannot pay their water bill. The community health nurse might also work on a grant to provide bottled water for the immunocompromised patient or the bottled water company may be willing to provide it free or at very reduced cost up to a certain amount of water.

Additional Discussion: A family of 5 is living in a home where a home health nurse visits every week. At the weekly visit the nurse discovers that there is no running water in the home. The family is obtaining water from a creek behind their home. What would be the most appropriate action for this community health nurse?

CHAPTER 11

Page 263

11.1 The Healthy People Curriculum Task Force has recommended incorporation of a common curriculum framework related to health promotion and illness prevention in clinical practice for the education of all health professionals (Allan et al., 2004). Suggested curricular elements include the following:

- Evidence base of practice
  Epidermiology and biostatistics
  Evaluation of health-related literature
  Outcome of measurement
  Health surveillance measures
  Determinants of health
- Clinical preventive and health promotion services
  Screening
  Counseling
  Immunization
  Chemoprevention
- Health systems and health policy
  Health system organization
  Health services financing
  Health workforce
  Health policy formation
- Community aspects of practice
  Communicating with the public
  Environmental health
  Occupational health
  Global health issues
  Cultural dimensions of practice
  Community services

To what extent are these areas reflected in your nursing curriculum? What might you do to advocate adoption of this common curriculum framework in your nursing program?

Evaluating Student Responses: In most nursing curriculum, the elements of the framework can be found. The topics of screenings and immunizations are usually emphasized more than others. Most nursing schools are beginning to emphasize evidenced-based practice. When advocating for anything, it is important to demonstrate the reason the framework should be completely instituted into the curriculum and why it would improve the effectiveness of the nursing school program.

Additional Discussion: You believe it would be important to integrate community health principles into the nursing curriculum. What type of activities could be instituted to assist in this?

CHAPTER 12

Page 284

12.1 There is a high rate of adolescent pregnancy in your community. The large majority of pregnant teenagers choose to keep their babies. Most of them end up dropping out of school, and approximately half become pregnant again within a year. You think case management services might help improve outcomes for these girls and their children, but no such services are available in the community. How would you go about initiating such services? What community partners should be involved in advocating for and developing case management services for pregnant adolescents? How would you get the community partners involved?

Evaluating Student Responses: The community health nurse should begin by reviewing the process already in place for dealing with pregnant teenagers. The nurse could see if case management could be implemented by revising the present process. If this is not possible, case management could be best handled through an agency such as the local schools. The community partners would include the school districts, local medical clinics, public health agencies and local hospitals. There may also be a need to include day care facilities that receive federal funds. The nurse could begin by visiting each community partner to discuss the vision for case management. It would be important to emphasize the benefit of case management to the community partner. Then the nurse could hold a planning meeting to determine the responsibilities of each partner.

Additional Discussion: What population-based case management exists in your community? If there are none, what programs would be best implemented?

CHAPTER 13

Page 310

13.1 Gunther (2005) described 10 principles for effective advocacy campaigns. These principles are:

- Communicate values underlying the advocacy initiative.
- Frame discourse in an oppositional framework in which people can be *against* something.
- Focus on winning over those who are undecided regarding an issue.
- Project confidence and take the high moral ground to persuade the undecided.
- Aggressively confront opposition. Identify them and attack their motives.
- Convince target audiences that they, as individuals, can make a difference.
- Minimize campaign costs by focusing on opinion leaders who will further disseminate your position to others.
- Project responsible extremism, rather than reasonable moderation, to influence the media.
- Don't stop with passage of the law or problem resolution; your position will likely need to be reiterated and defended on an ongoing basis.
- Strategic diversity in approaches is critical to successful advocacy, with multiple independent advocacy campaigns focused on

Evaluating Student Responses: Many communities in this country are struggling with the issue of smoking in restaurants. One of the ways communities have been successful is by looking at the health value to the employees of the restaurant or indoor areas. This takes the personal aspect of smoking away and turns it to the "secondhand smoke" issue.

Additional Discussion: Your community would like to ban smoking at all community events whether indoors or outdoors. How can the community health nurses assist in this endeavor?

the same issue (e.g., within different cultural or ethnic groups or other target audiences). Examine a community organization issue in your area. How might these principles of effective advocacy be implemented in the process?

CHAPTER 14

Page 336

14.1 In conducting an assessment of families in your community, you find that there are a number of families with older members in which all other adult members are employed. Many of these older family members feel socially isolated because their children are not available to take them to participate in local activities designed for senior citizens. There is a local senior citizens center that has a variety of activities these individuals might enjoy, but there is no public transportation to allow them to reach the center. How might you begin to address this problem within the community?

Evaluating Student Responses: The community health nurse might begin by assessing what government grants are available for transportation in the area. The local churches might be useful in taking turns at providing transportation. (With enough churches, one church might only have to provide transportation once a month). Lastly, local bus and taxi companies might be contacted to see how to lower the cost of meeting this need.

Additional Discussion: A family is dealing with a 32-year-old severely developmentally delayed child and a 78-year-old grandparent with Alzheimer's disease. What would be the best ways to assist this family?

CHAPTER 15

Page 365

15.1 Policy makers in your community have decided to conduct a comprehensive community assessment to determine what public health services should be expanded, what services can be eliminated, and what additional services are needed. You have been appointed to the committee planning the assessment. At the first meeting you notice that there are no community residents represented on the committee. How would you go about advocating for community participation in all facets of the assessment and subsequent decision making?

Evaluating Student Responses: At the first meeting, the community health nurse might suggest that each committee member introduce themselves and tell who they are representing (agency, etc.). This might be a perfect opportunity to point out that no individual community members are on the committee. If the committee as a whole will not agree to adding an individual community member, the community health nurse might suggest the formation of an ad hoc committee made up of individual community members who could bring a consensus to the committee.

Additional Discussion: Has your community had a recent community assessment? What were the results? What matters of public health were identified?

CHAPTER 16

Page 407

16.1 Rowe, Onikpo, Lama, and Deming (2001) conducted a study to examine the extent to which community health workers (CHWs) implemented WHO strategies for Integrated Management of Childhood Illness for children under the age of 5 years. They found that a significant portion of the community health workers failed to correctly implement the guidelines. Major areas

Evaluating Student Responses: The CHW should begin by assessing which factor contributes the most to the lack of implementation of guidelines. The CHW would then see if it is feasible to address that factor. For example, poor staffing may be the primary reason for lack of implementation, yet it is an area a CHW would not have the authority to rectify. The CHW should begin by choosing a factor that is easily rectified. This would be the springboard to improving the quality of the entire process.

Additional Discussion: How well does your local health department implement the guidelines? Where would you start to increase the implementation?

of deficit included incomplete assessment, incorrect diagnosis and treatment, inappropriate drug therapy, missed opportunities for immunizations, and failure to refer children for professional care when needed. Qualitative data obtained from CHWs indicated reasons for these deficits included conflicts among health workers, overload, failure to use knowledge acquired in training, low morale and motivation, poor time management, lack of equipment, and lack of fluency in the local language. Other reasons given for poor implementation of guidelines were impatient parents or other caregivers, caregiver demands for medications, CHW perceptions that caregivers would report all of a child's symptoms without questioning or prompting or would be alarmed if told of a child's diagnosis, and CHW unwillingness to use charts or other diagnostic and treatment aids for fear of being thought incompetent. How might you address the factors contributing to poor implementation of guidelines by CHWs so that all the children seen receive adequate treatment for their illness?

CHAPTER 17

Page 441

17.1 How would you go about advocating for rights for LGBT couples equal to those afforded to heterosexual married couples in your state? What activities, if any, are already underway in this effort? Who is engaged in these advocacy activities? What sources of resistance would this kind of policy change encounter? How would you counteract that resistance? What groups or agencies might support your advocacy efforts?

Evaluating Student Responses: The community health nurse would begin by assessing what rights heterosexual couples are afforded that are not available to LGBT couples. Most states are looking at providing employer-provided medical coverage for same sex couples just as it is available to heterosexual couples. Some states are looking at allowing marriage to be more than a heterosexual relationship. Not all areas of the country will approach this in the same way. It appears that most of the changes have occurred in states in the west and the northeast. Traditionally, these areas of the country have a more liberal point of view both socially and politically. It appears most of this is found in the political arena at this time. One of the problems is that the agencies that stand strongly for these issues are often felt to be at odds with traditional moral values.

Resistance is found in groups that feel that the traditional moral values are assaulted by changes that would give rights to LGBT couples. This resistance is found in fundamental Christian churches and other groups that espouse these values. Resistance may be counteracted by demonstrating the benefit to the community by giving more rights to the LGBT couples. A group that might be helpful would be P-FLAG, which is made up of parents and family members who have a gay family member.

Additional Discussion: How would you go about setting up a P-FLAG group in your community? What issues would be most important to this group?

CHAPTER 18

Page 485

18.1 Howard, Davis, Evans-Ray, Mitchell, and Ampomah (2204) described the establishment of a "teen-friendly" clinic

Evaluating Student Responses: Different communities may view this service differently. Urban schools with large populations of teen pregnancies may see this as a service to both the teen and the community. Resistance to these programs usually originates with the parents who want to believe that their children do not engage in

for both male and female adolescents to meet the need for sexual clinical and education services for this age group. The clinic was established based on the evaluation of an educational program in which adolescent boys achieved gains in knowledge about and changes in attitude toward sexual activity and indicated that they would use protection during sexual intercourse if available. Provision of such services is often resisted in many communities in the belief that it promotes sexual activity among adolescents. How would such a service be viewed in your community? Where might resistance to the program originate? How would you go about advocating for such a program?

sexual activity. Advocating for the program should include a focus on a benefit that is not involved with the provision of sexual protection.

Additional Discussion: The local high school wants to hire a school nurse who is a nurse practitioner. The purpose will be to provide reproductive services to all high school students. No parental permission will be sought and parents will not be given any access to these health records. How could this community health nurse get parents to understand the necessity for this service?

CHAPTER 19

Page 508

19.1 What groups might be approached to form a coalition to advocate for support services for caregivers of older clients with Alzheimer's disease? Why would you include these specific groups in your coalition?

Evaluating Student Responses: The community health nurse could approach the largest employer in the area, the local hospitals, the churches and the local colleges. The largest employer needs to see how many employees are dealing with a family member with Alzheimer's and how support services could decrease lost work days. Local hospitals might already have services in place that could be expanded to meet the needs of these caregivers. Churches often have a large population of caregivers. Many churches could provide facilities for things such as adult day care and also could provide spiritual support to the caregiver. Lastly, local colleges have programs offered free to people over age 65. The college might also be willing to begin programs especially suited to the caregiver and also see the need to provide care for the family member while the class is going on.

Additional Discussion: A local church has expressed an interest in starting an adult day care 2 days a week. The church would like it to be for adults with Alzheimer's disease or other forms of dementia but some members of the community would like the day care to also care for some severely developmentally delayed adults. Would this be feasible? If the church agrees to do this, what specific facilities will need to be available to meet the needs of these diverse groups?

CHAPTER 20

Page 559

20.1 The Bringing America Home Act (Bringing America Home, 2005a) is an ambitious piece of legislation aimed at addressing the multiple factors that contribute to homelessness in the Unites States. Access the Web site at http://bringingamericahome.org to see what organizations in your area have endorsed this legislation. What organizations in your area might endorse this Act? How might you organize a campaign to support this piece of legislation?

Evaluating Student Responses: Students could begin by assessing where the homeless populations in their community go for help, such as a mission. The students would also need to determine the size of the homeless population. The students could begin to establish services by going where the homeless already are. Some of the most common services are treatment for chronic illnesses such as HTN and diabetes. There are also possible underlying conditions such as alcoholism, TB and HIV infection. The students could provide screenings such as blood pressure and blood sugar monitoring. The students could also see what immediate needs the person has such as need of food or shelter. The provision of medical care and medications, as well as the arrangement for monetary benefits, are best handled by others. Students could contact local ARNPs and physicians to determine the willingness to provide medical services. Students could contact pharmaceutical representatives to determine what drugs could be obtained free or at a very reduced cost. Students should look closely at retired health care professionals to provide the care needed.

Most communities are represented by at least one organization on this list. The organizations that would support the act are those that represent the needs of people who are dealing with homelessness. It is important to emphasize the benefit to the entire community of supporting this legislation.

Additional Discussion: A large manufacturing company in your town has just closed. It employed 1500 people. There is not enough industry in your town to absorb the loss. What type of plans should this community have in place to deal with the potential increase in homelessness related to the closing of the industry?

CHAPTER 21

Page 581

21.1 Berg, Hines, and Allen (2002) found that only 4% of homes of clients who used wheelchairs had received all five recommended structural modification designed to address clients' functional limitations. Lack of modifications led to a higher incidence of falls with injuries. In part, modifications were not made because they were not covered by either private or governmental insurance programs. The authors suggested that "home environments that facilitate independence and that make it easier to move around should be considered a basic need for disabled persons" (p. 48). How might community health nurses advocate for this basic right? What might nurses and others do to get home modifications covered by health insurance plans?

Evaluating Student Responses: A community health nurse might ask community leaders to gather in a home and spend some time attempting to get around in a wheelchair. Ask them to go to the bathroom and then ask them to get out of the house into the car. This often opens eyes, especially if the local media is contacted. The community health nurse might also ask the media to spotlight a person who is struggling with these issues.

The community health nurse needs to have home modifications designated as durable medical equipment, which is usually covered at 50–80% by most health insurance plans. It is also important to prove to the insurance companies that providing these modifications will ultimately cost them less over the lifetime of the individual.

Additional Discussion: How has your community complied with ADA regulations? Are all public buildings able to be accessed by a disabled person? Are all restaurants and stores easily accessed? If not, how could you encourage these places to become compliant?

CHAPTER 22

Page 613

22.1 Esperanza Gutierrez is a public health nurse working for the Jackson County Health Department. She is responsible for a low-income area in which many Latino clients live. Many of her clients live in apartment complexes owned by a few absentee Caucasian landlords. On several of her visits, Esperanza has noticed that the apartments are in need of repair and many are lacking smoke detectors, although they are required in rental units by state law. Others have bars on the windows that would prevent escape in the case of fire. Her clients tell her that they have spoken to their landlords about repairs, but have received no response or are told to call a repairman and pay for the repairs themselves. Many of her clients speak no English and are afraid to report the safety hazards to the local housing authority for fear they will be evicted in retaliation. There are not enough rental units to meet the housing demand in the area, and apartments are often rented within a day of vacancy.

Evaluating Student Responses: Some of the factors would be language, poverty and fear. Also, the cultural problems with dealing with an authority figure by people who consider themselves subservient to that person.

This public health nurse should bring this issue to the attention of the entire public health department. If her employer will not allow her to do it, she should encourage the residents to contact the media about the problems.

The nurse should contact the county government to determine if the landlord can be forced to provide the services. The fire department often provides smoke detectors for free or at a very low cost to those who can't afford them. The nurse could continually bring individual cases to the attention of authorities so eventually it couldn't be ignored. The nurse should also emphasize that intervening now might prevent a serious incident that could result in death.

The residents could form a renters organization. There are specific rights for renters and as a group they could advocate for these rights. It is more difficult to get rid of a group than an individual.

Additional Discussion: Does your community have specific regulations for landlords? Which of these regulations pertain to the health of the renters? How could you ensure that your community has the needed health regulations?

- What factors are influencing this situation?
- What action might Esperanza take to remedy the situation?
- What other segments of the county government might she involve in her efforts? What other community agencies might she involve? How might she go about obtaining their involvement?
- How might residents of the apartment complexes become involved?

CHAPTER 23

23.1 The local elementary school where you work has a policy that students may not self-medicate, including the use of inhalers by students with asthma. The reasoning of the administration is that students may overuse medications or share medications with classmates. According to school policy, students are to give their inhalers to the school nurse and come to the nursing office when they need to use them. You are present at this school only two and a half days a week. In your absence, the principal's secretary is supposed to unlock the nursing office and provide students with access to their inhalers. Each week, you have 10 to 12 students visiting the nursing office during the hours you are there to use inhalers. Because the campus is quite large, students may be coming from quite a distance and their asthma symptoms may be quite pronounced before they reach the nursing office. How would you go about advocating for a change in this policy? Would you advocate a change in policy for all children (K-6) or only for selected students? Why? What support might you try to draw on from other elements of the school population or from the outside community?

Evaluating Student Responses: The nurse could begin by gathering the data about the number of students, the disorders and the ages of the children involved. It would also be necessary to know at which schools these children are located. Then the nurse could gather data on problems that have been encountered and which problems occurred because of the length of time it took the child to reach the nurse. After gathering the data the nurse could decide if the policy should be applicable for all students. It rarely can be. Certainly, self-medication may not be appropriate for all children (such as special needs or very young children). The nurse should look to the teachers of the children and the parents of the children to assist in advocating for the self-medication.

CHAPTER 24

Page 694

24.1 The work setting where you are employed as an occupational health nurse has recently developed a policy that employees are no longer allowed to eat on the premises except in a designated dining area. In addition, employees will not be allowed to keep

Evaluating Student Responses: The nurse should document the number of persons with diabetes in the work environment and the number of cases of hypoglycemia that have occurred since the implementation of the policy. The nurse could suggest an easy situation. The first would be that diabetic employees could keep glucose tablets in their pockets. The nurse could also suggest that an additional dining room be added in the work environment.

Additional Discussion: A company decided to limit the number of bathroom breaks an employee could take to decrease lost time. Many employees are very upset

any kind of food or beverages in their work areas, even if they are sealed in air-tight containers. The intent of the policy is to deal with insect infestations that have been getting worse in the last few months. As the nurse in the setting, you realize that there are several employees with diabetes. The distance from some worksites to the dining area is quite long, and a couple of employees have come to see you about their concerns if they should experience hypoglycemia during the workday. What will you do in this situation?

by this new rule. In fact, many employees are planning an action such as a "sit in" in the bathroom. How would the occupational health nurse advocate for the employees in this situation?

CHAPTER 25

Page 709

25.1 Millersville is a small town of 3,000 people in rural Arizone, The main street of town is part of a four-lane undivided highway to Phoenix. The part of town traversed by the highway comprises about 20 blocks, four of which are lined by local stores and diagonal parking on either side. Except when it's raining, which is infrequent, most of the town's children ride their bicycles to the local elementary school, which is located on the highway three blocks south of the main shopping area. In the past 2 years, three children have been killed and seven other injured by cars speeding through town on the highway. There is a stop sign in the middle of town, but it does not seem to have reduced speeds or accidents. Research suggests that bicycle lanes divided from motor vehicle traffic by concrete barriers reduce child bicycle injuries. Although you have suggested creation of bicycle lanes on the section of the highway that bisects the town, the idea has been resisted by local merchants who do not want to give up the parking in front of their stores. They are afraid that if people from the outlying ranches have to park elsewhere and walk to the stores, they will take their business to the city 40 miles away. How would you go about advocating for a bicycle lane in town?

Evaluating Student Answers: The nurse in this situation will have to look beyond the economics of adding the bicycle lane. The nurse could gather the merchants together and ask them to help devise a way to improve the safety of children who ride bicycles. The nurse would present the data that showed the number of injuries (both fatal and nonfatal) and share that a bicycle lane has been considered. The nurse could then turn it over to the merchants and ask them to brainstorm ways to improve safety and still maintain the parking spaces. The merchants could then market the idea as their own.

Additional Discussion: It has been proven that wearing a bicycle helmet decreases the number of head injuries in children. How could you improve the number of children who regularly wear helmets while riding a bicycle?

CHAPTER 26

Page 746

26.1 In October 2004, the *San Diego Union Tribune*, the major newspaper in the San Diego area, published an Associated Press story on citizens who

Evaluating Student Responses: Any person who lives in a community where there is close contact should be immunized against the flu, even when vaccine is short. The cost of providing the vaccine is much less than the cost to care of those who get the flu and then spread it to others. It also cuts down on cases being spread to those who work at the prison and their family members. The nurse should begin by

were irate that prisoners were being given influenza immunizations when vaccine shortages prevented community members from obtaining protective immunization (Flu shots for inmates, 2004). Who do you think should receive priority access to a limited supply of vaccine? Why? What actions might you take to advocate for access to vaccines for the group you think should receive priority?

gathering data that reflect the number of inmates, along with their age and the number who also are at increased risk for viral illness. The nurse should see how many people (besides the inmates) the flu would impact if the flu began to appear in the prison population.

Additional Discussion: A federal prison is on 23-hour lock-down. What type of problems will a nurse see as a result of this? What nurses' actions would be appropriate in this situation?

CHAPTER 27

Page 781

27.1 Many segments of society do not have the financial resources to comply with recommendations for disaster preparedness. This is particularly true of homeless individuals. How might you go about assuring that the disaster response plans address the special needs of homeless populations in your area?

Evaluating Student Responses: The nurse would begin by gathering data about how many people usually experience homelessness in the community and where most of these people can be found. This will give the disaster planners an idea of who and where this population is and how at risk they are depending upon the situation. Because many of these people will not have personal transportation to leave the area, the disaster plan must include some way for transportation to be made available for them.

Additional Discussion: You have been asked to serve on a disaster planning team. What areas in your community are especially vulnerable to disaster? What industries in your community could cause a disaster? What could you do now to mitigate the possibility of a disaster occurring?

CHAPTER 28

Page 827

28.1 A local university does not require proof of immunization from incoming students. The university administration is afraid that requiring evidence of immunization will deter students from registering for courses. How might you go about convincing the administration that immunization status should be validated before students are allowed to register?

Evaluating Student Responses: The nurse could begin by showing the cost to the university of an epidemic of a disease as opposed to the cost of lost students. This might be very enlightening. The nurse could also show the statistics that show the risk of disease in the university population. The nurse could emphasize the fact that university students live in dorms, which increases the probability of spreading communicable diseases.

Additional Discussion: You believe that all college students should receive a meningitis vaccination prior to enrolling. What do you believe would work better—requiring the immunization before the student arrives at the college, or providing the vaccination upon the student's arrival at college?

CHAPTER 29

Page 865

29.1 Exposure to pesticides and other chemicals used in agriculture increases the risk of chronic health problems for agriculture workers. Although OSHA regulations control use of such chemicals in large farming operations, they are not applicable to farms with only a few employees. In working in an area with many small family-operated farms that may employ two or three nonfamily members, you become aware of an increase in pesticide-related neurological conditions. How would you go about advocating for more effective control measures for pesticide use in the area? Who else would you involve in your advocacy efforts?

Evaluating Student Responses: As with any effort to change something, the nurse would begin by gathering data that shows the incidence of the neurological problems that are associated with small farm operations. The nurse could present this to the local health department to see if there are any rules or regulations already in place that address this issue. The problem is reaching the small farm owners to share the danger of the chemicals being used. The nurse could attend local government meetings and share the results of the data and see if local government would be willing to address this issue. The nurse should look to the local small farm association, the local agricultural department representative and the state farm bureau for help in addressing this issue.

Additional Discussion: In your local community, how does an individual obtain a handicapped parking permit? What are the laws that mandate how many handicapped parking places are available in each parking lot? What can the community health nurse do to improve the ability of the disabled to get around in the community?

© 2008 Pearson Education, Inc.

CHAPTER 30

Page 914

30.1 Your educational institution has determined that it needs to have a policy in place for the involuntary withdrawal of students from the institution who have not violated any specific regulation, policy, or law, but who engage in behaviors that disrupt the learning environment or create potentially dangerous situations. One of the behaviors specifically listed in the policy that would prompt involuntary withdrawal is attempted suicide. How would you go about getting this provision removed from the policy? What other type of policy might be needed instead of involuntary withdrawal to address the issue of attempted suicide?

Evaluating Student Responses: The nurse would begin by showing that removing the student from school may increase the student's chance of trying suicide again because it might increase the student's sense of isolation. This student should be treated as any student who has a physical illness during the semester. Each individual teacher would make a decision about whether the student can make up the work during the semester or give the student an incomplete and allow him to finish the work when mental health returns.

Additional Discussion: The local vocational rehabilitation department in your community would like to place an individual with schizophrenia in the office of your local health department. The office where this individual is to be placed is very against this placement. How would you go about advocating for this individual with the persons in your office?

CHAPTER 31

Page 961

31.1 Most State Board of Nursing disciplinary actions involve substance abuse by nurses. State Boards of Nursing and Medicine often have different perspectives on substance abuse by members of the two professions. Among physicians, problems of abuse are often handled by physician addiction specialists outside of the licensing board, and cases often are not referred to the board if they can be handled at this peer counseling level (Haack & Yocom, 2002). What are the policies for dealing with substance abuse by nurses and physicians in your state? Are they the same? If there are differences, how might you go about advocating for equitable treatment for substance abuse problems between the two professions?

Evaluating Student Responses: Most states have some program for dealing with impaired nurses. Some states do not automatically suspend the license of the impaired nurse while others do. Most states require a nurse to participate in random drug screenings as proof that the nurse is staying "clean." Many times a nurse's license is probated upon return to work. The nurse may be limited in the scope of practice (administering narcotics) for a period of time upon return to work. States differ in their treatment of physicians but most require physicians to seek treatment and limit their ability to prescribe Schedule 3 drugs for a period of time.

If the treatment was inequitable, the nurse should gather data that shows the inequities and the effects upon the individuals' careers. It would also be important to bring it to the attention of the local and state legislators who have the authority to correct the situation.

Additional Discussion: You are visiting an older woman with cancer. She is receiving treatment (chemo and radiation) and has been given a positive prognosis. On one of your visits you notice evidence of marijuana use in the home. The woman states that she has used it occasionally for years but is using it a few times every day to take away the nausea from the treatments. How would you advise this woman?

CHAPTER 32

Page 981

32.1 Several of the references cited in this chapter suggest that little attention has been given to intimate partner violence directed against men. Social stigma, legal system biases, and lack of support services are some of the factors that have been identified as mitigating against equitable treatment of male victims of IPV. How might you go about changing societal awareness of and attitudes toward IPV directed against men?

Evaluating Student Answers: Men often do not report IPV if the abuser is a woman. This may be because of shame that the abuse occurred in the first place. The community health nurse can begin by contacting abuse services and see what services could be adapted for male victims. One of the problems is that there is little if any housing for male victims of abuse. Local abuse services are at a disadvantage because housing for victims is kept secret from the general public. It is difficult to find this type of housing for the male victim. The nurse could advocate for money to be set aside for motel rooms for short-term use. Male victims are hidden victims. The nurse can include information about male abuse in any information presented about abuse in general.

Additional Discussion: A local LGBT group is concerned because of an increase in abuse among individuals with HIV. This group feels there is prejudice among the justice and medical community that keeps the victims from receiving adequate care. How can the local community health nurse help these victims?

THINKING CRITICALLY QUESTIONS AND RESPONSES

The questions that follow are provided for classroom discussion or to be assigned as homework. They do not appear in the textbook or on the Companion Website. Students responses will vary, and the "Evaluating Student Responses" comment will point to common areas that students may address.

CHAPTER 1

1.1 What are the specific community health focuses for your community?

Evaluating Student Responses: Many states and communities are using Tobacco Settlement money to conduct smoking cessation for adults and antismoking campaigns for teens. Many community health nurses conduct diabetic care classes. There is also an outreach to at-risk teens and adults to be tested for HIV.

1.2 The community health nurse serves many roles. Which of these roles do you believe has the most impact on the community itself?

Evaluating Student Responses: The nurse as educator may be the role that is a part of every aspect of community health nursing. The community health nurse is always educating community members, whether it is about disease prevention, disease detection, or disease maintenance.

CHAPTER 2

2.1 Who is the lead agency in your community that monitors the objectives for Healthy People 2010?

Evaluating Student Responses: Local communities may have a city or county health department that monitors these objectives or it may be an agency that covers multiple counties or areas. It may depend upon whether you live in an urban or rural area.

2.2 What activities would be considered primary prevention when dealing with population-based health concerns?

Evaluating Student Responses: An example of primary prevention would be classes aimed at preventing diabetes, especially in persons who are already identified as being at high risk.

CHAPTER 3

3.1 Community health nurses may be utilized in local public health agencies providing services such as immunization and family planning clinics or they may function as home health nurses. How do you think the community's resources are best used, in clinic-type activities or in home health activities?

Evaluating Student Responses: Many local community health departments are dropping home health services because of the amount of resources that are required and that the clients served are often those that cannot pay at all. Though it meets the needs of this population, most health departments will not bear this cost so they focus on traditional public health services such as TB prevention and immunizations for children.

3.2 What local community activities would be most appropriate to combat terrorism?

Evaluating Student Responses: Possible local community activities that combat terrorism include educating the community about preparing for emergency situations and developing plans for mass immunizations in the case of bacterial terrorism.

CHAPTER 4

4.1 What dimension (psychological, biological, social, etc.) affects your community the most?

Evaluating Student Responses: The dimension will depend upon the particular community. The student will usually find that different dimensions have differing impacts, depending upon the situation.

4.2 Which dimension of nursing do you believe has the greatest impact on your community nursing career?

Evaluating Student Responses: Many nurses believe that the interpersonal dimension has the greatest impact because it affects all of a nurse's interactions with others, both peers and clients.

CHAPTER 5

5.1 Most public health systems are supported by taxes. How is your local public health system supported?

Evaluating Student Responses: Most will find that the local public health system is supported through a portion of property taxes, though there may be other formulas.

5.2 Who makes the decision in your community about the taxes or other monies that fund the local public health system?

Evaluating Student Responses: Each community handles it differently. It may be a county or city commission decision or there may be a board that oversees this and sets the tax rate.

CHAPTER 6

6.1 Fear of terrorism is in the minds and on the hearts of many people in both the United States and in the world at large. What impact has the increase in terrorism had on the health of both U.S. and world citizens?

Evaluating Student Responses: Terrorism has gravely impacted the mental health of people all over the world. It has also increased the number of injuries and deaths worldwide from explosives and firearms, therefore there are more people dealing with large traumatic injuries as well as the disruption of the family.

6.2 Compare the policy of Homeland Security and HIPPA. Which is more important?

Evaluating Student Responses: Most people would answer this question by saying that it depended upon the situation. In reality, though, as nurses we are bound by law to abide by HIPPA. The reporting of someone suspicious is not yet law so nurses must abide by the law first.

CHAPTER 7

7.1 Professional organizations such as ANA (American Nurses Association) are often called upon to speak for the nursing profession as a whole. What are some reasons that registered nurses do not join a professional organization?

Evaluating Student Responses: Many nurses point to the cost of joining the organization. Many also say they don't have time to belong to an organization. Other object to the political action committees that arise from these professional organizations.

7.2 What is an example of a professional nursing organization making a difference in policy development?

Evaluating Student Responses: The American Nurses Association spoke loudly in states that were considering limiting mandatory overtime. They have also been effective in lobbying for whistleblower laws.

CHAPTER 8

8.1 At your local health department, how are the major programs funded?

Evaluating Student Responses: Most of the major programs will be funded differently. The immunization program will receive a lot of the vaccines from the Vaccines for Children program. These vaccines can only be given to children, though. Most health departments also provide WIC services. These monies come from both federal and state funds. Most major programs will be funded with a combination of funds.

8.2 Who receives the majority of services at your local health department? How are they funded?

Evaluating Student Responses: Most local health departments will see children as one of the largest consumers of service. This is because of the number of immunizations children need and the availability of these immunizations at the local health departments. The same may be said about other services such as WIC.

CHAPTER 9

9.1 The Hispanic population is growing in the United States and will soon be the largest minority group in the United States. In your community, what are the most common health care needs that occur within the Hispanic population?

Evaluating Student Responses: In most communities, community health nurses will see hypertension, obesity, diabetes and lack of adequate care.

9.2 How does the value of male dominance influence the provision of health care services?

Evaluating Student Responses: It may be necessary for the community health nurse to speak to the male, even if the patient is female. In situations dealing with childbearing, the patient's mother is usually the person that receives all information.

9.3 How does the economic status of the Hispanic population in your community affect health care?

Evaluating Student Responses: Though not all Hispanics have low paying jobs, many of them do, therefore there is little money for medicine or regular visits to a physician.

CHAPTER 10

10.1 In your community, what environmental issues may cause health problems?

Evaluating Student Responses: Most urban areas deal with clean air problems that impact individuals with underlying respiratory conditions such as asthma and COPD. Other communities have difficulties with clean water. Manufacturers may put waste into the local water supply. Waste from septic tanks can also get into the ground water and cause problems for individuals who are immunocompromised. Other communities have environmental issues that are specific to their geographic area such as areas that are near nuclear and chemical plants.

10.2 How is your local health department handling these issues?

Evaluating Student Responses: Most local health departments have environmental specialists on staff or share one with other local health departments.

CHAPTER 11

11.1 How can the community health nurse utilize the Internet to promote empowerment to improve the health of the community?

Evaluating Student Responses: The community health nurse can develop (or have developed) a website that is attractive and invites visitors. This website could be used to promote health related activities that are important to those people who are most comfortable surfing the web.

11.2 How can the community health nurse use social marketing to reach the increasing number of older adults in the community?

Evaluating Student Responses: The community health nurse begins the process by describing the problem (for example, a significant increase in alcoholism in recently widowed persons). The characteristics of this audience would be determined and then a strategy would be developed (finding participants through the local funeral homes) and an intervention would be designed. A plan to monitor the program would be developed and then the program would be implemented.

CHAPTER 12

12.1 The community health nurse often sees a client after the acute phase of an illness or injury has passed. The client has returned home and arrangements for visits by a home health nurse have been made while the client was hospitalized. The community health nurse is now expected to handle the case management of this client. How could the community health nurse be a part of the client's entire illness or injury?

Evaluating Student Responses: The community health nurse may or may not be asked to attend the discharge planning conference to set up long term plans for the client. The community health nurse could begin by setting up a system to include the community health nurse if needs are anticipated early in the admission process.

CHAPTER 13

13.1 How could the community health nurse encourage empowerment in the developmentally delayed population within the community?

Evaluating Student Responses: Fostering independence is always the goal in working with individuals who are developmentally delayed. The community health nurse may work with groups of DD individuals on certain skills needed to function more independently in the community. The community health nurse could also determine if there are agencies that could be adapted to assist with rather than take over certain skills. The community health nurse could also work with the families or guardians of DD individuals to encourage them to allow these individuals to be responsible for certain things.

CHAPTER 14

14.1 When a family is in crisis, they often use defense mechanisms to cope with the stress. How might the community health nurse help a family to turn these defense mechanisms into strengths?

Evaluating Student Responses: The community health nurse may be able to use intellectualization and rationalization as ways to promote resiliency. As the family rationalizes the event, the community health nurse can move the conversation to ways that demonstrate the already present strength of the family. As the family intellectualizes, the nurse can help the family see the knowledge they already have and build on it.

CHAPTER 15

15.1 What type of programs would be appropriate for a community that has chemical and nuclear waste industries?

Evaluating Student Responses: The assessment team would first assess if there has been any type of illness or injury related to these industries that are seen in the population, both those that work at the facilities and those that live in the proximity of these industries. The assessment team would then prioritize the problems found. The program would depend upon what type of problem was the priority. For example, is there a specific illness found in persons who worked in the nuclear waste industry that has caused death above the national average? Or is it a problem that has a wider population base, such as increased level of miscarriage in the community? The program developed would depend upon the problem. It may ultimately end in the closure of one or more of the products made or of the industry itself.

CHAPTER 16

16.1 Women who receive prenatal care through the local health department receive an alpha fetaprotein test during the pregnancy. Women who have positive results are referred for a diagnostic ultrasound. In some cases, Down's syndrome is diagnosed. For those women who decide to continue the pregnancy, how could the community health nurse intervene to begin assisting the parent in the unique developmental needs of this unborn child?

Evaluating Student Responses: It is well known that early stimulation is effective in increasing the developmental abilities of a child with known developmental delays. The community health nurse could begin to educate the woman (parents if applicable) about the condition. The community health nurse could inform the early childhood specialists who could then meet the mother prior to the birth. The community health nurse could also begin the case management process by helping the mother to know the services that will possibly be needed at the birth and after.

CHAPTER 17

17.1 How can the community health nurse best educate women concerning hysterectomy surgery and any sexual implications involved in this surgery?

Evaluating Student Responses: The community health nurse can help women to understand that in most cases a hysterectomy only removes the uterus itself, which will not change anything except the ability to become pregnant. Women who also have their ovaries removed will experience immediate menopause and will then use synthetic hormones, which may affect sex drive in the short term. Women should inform their health care practitioners if sex drive doesn't return to normal.

CHAPTER 18

18.1 Drugs for erectile dysfunction have become popular with men, especially older men. The marketing leads men to believe that erectile dysfunction is a common occurrence. How can the community health nurse use these same marketing tools to increase men's compliance with regular screening activities?

Evaluating Student Responses: The community health nurse can connect the fact that if someone feels they have erectile dysfunction, their health care provider is the best one to talk to. While they are there at the health care provider, encourage men to get regular screening tests done such as a PSA, stool for occult blood and a manual exam of the prostate.

CHAPTER 19

19.1 Recently, a local newspaper in your community featured an article about a 78-year-old man who had written a living will. He stated that he desired no heroic measures taken if he fell ill. The man had fallen off of his porch and was taken to the hospital. His wife brought his living will to the hospital but the physician did not follow the man's wishes because he felt the man had a good chance to survive the accident if heroic measures were taken. How can the community health nurse best educate the public about living wills and other measures that can be taken to assure that a person's wishes are granted?

Evaluating Student Responses: The community health nurse can have living will forms already printed and ready to be handed out when someone asks about them. The community health nurse could give it to a person and explain it on one visit and then help him or her complete it at the next visit so the person can make the necessary decisions. It is also important for persons to understand that it is all right to want to have all measures taken, no matter what the circumstances. Older persons should also know that a copy of the living will should be kept on their person at all times and also a copy given to their medical surrogate or their significant other.

CHAPTER 20

20.1 Most communities in the United States have some type of temporary housing for the homeless. Many of these are run by religious agencies and are for men only. How can the community health nurse advocate for homeless women?

Evaluating Student Responses: This is a difficult situation. The nurse can begin by visiting the agencies in the community that provide housing for the homeless and see if modifications could be made to make some of the housing for women and children. In the agencies that require a person to work for housing, the nurse could see if daycare is available for the women with children. It is important that agencies that provide housing understand the importance of providing it to all people.

CHAPTER 21

21.1 What types of interventions would be appropriate for the home health nurse who is visiting an 80-year-old man who now requires home oxygen due to an exacerbation of COPD? This client also has Type II diabetes and severe arthritis.

Evaluating Student Responses: After assessing all the body systems of this client, the home health nurse would assess the environment. Does this client still smoke? Who is available to help this client on a daily basis? Is there enough oxygen tubing to allow the client to get to the bathroom? If not, can this client safely go to the bathroom without oxygen? The nurse should also assess the client's ability to handle his diabetes. Because of the arthritis, is this client able to bathe properly and therefore able to wash and dry his feet carefully? Can he even view his feet properly?

CHAPTER 22

22.1 How would a nurse begin a faith-based community nursing program?

Evaluating Student Responses: Prior to beginning a program, the nurse must have the support of the church. Then the nurse must complete a Basic Preparation for Parish Nurse course. This course may be available locally or can be obtained from a college via the Internet. The nurse then forms a committee to meet the health needs of the congregation. The committee assesses the congregation to see what needs are the most important and then prioritizes them and begin to meet those needs.

CHAPTER 23

23.1 Your local school district does not have a nurse in every school. Regularly scheduled medications (such as ADHD meds) are administered by the school secretary. How would you go about changing this policy so that a nurse administers all medications?

Evaluating Student Responses: Most of the time, districts do not want to hire a licensed person for each school and site the lack of money. The community nurse could begin by showing how much money the school could lose if a child were injured due to a medication error. The nurse could also point out the benefits of having someone knowledgeable about medication side effects. The nurse should also share the dangers of unlicensed persons administering medications with the entire school district. This will often help to change policy.

CHAPTER 24

24.1 Short and long term disability caused by back injury happens in many work environments. What can the nurse do to decrease the incidence of back injuries?

Evaluating Student Responses: The nurse should begin by gathering data on the persons who have experienced back injuries and if there are any commonalities in their jobs, or if there are other commonalities such as age, sex and weight. Once the data are gathered, the nurse should begin a back injury prevention program aimed at those who have experienced the most problems and then expand the program to the entire work place.

CHAPTER 25

25.1 Individuals in rural communities may have to travel great distances to access health care. Public transportation is usually not available to these people. What could the community health nurse do to assist these individuals?

Evaluating Student Responses: The nurse could advocate for 2 different things. In one case, the nurse could advocate for the health care to go to the people. Many practices that have a large rural population will travel to different communities from time to time (such as a monthly basis). The nurse could also look at ways to provide affordable transportation to individuals in rural communities. One way would be for local churches to provide transportation on a weekly basis. The nurse could coordinate with health care offices to try and schedule appointments for individuals on the same day.

CHAPTER 26

26.1 The local correctional institution often has pregnant women who are incarcerated for short-term sentences. How would you advocate for instituting a program where the infants live in the jail for the first 6 months of their lives?

Evaluating Student Responses: The nurse could first look at the average sentence of the women at the prison. The nurse could then see how much it would cost to implement the program and then compare it to the cost of providing foster care for the children until the mother is released. The nurse could also point out the advantage of letting the women assume responsibility while still in prison.

CHAPTER 27

27.1 Your community is home to four chemical plants. One plant experienced a dangerous release of chemicals that could have injured many people if the chemical had escaped into the community. What safety features should be present in the community to alert the population to dangers from the industries?

Evaluating Student Responses: Each chemical plant should be equipped with telephone and computer alert systems that automatically contact the police and fire departments of the community when a dangerous chemical is released. The area should be assessed to see what other communities could be impacted by the plants, depending upon wind conditions. The communities should have action plans for alerting the community members such as alert sirens and automatic telephone calls as well as roadblocks to prevent people from entering the community.

CHAPTER 28

28.1 Many schools no longer require TB tests prior to entering an elementary or secondary school. How can the community health nurse prevent the spread of TB without this useful screening tool?

Evaluating Student Responses: The community health nurse must educate those that interact with the children and their families the most, which is the school. Teachers should be instructed in the S/S of TB and how to refer possible cases. The nurse can also prepare handouts that can be sent home describing TB and its spread as well as the symptoms and how it is treated. The nurse can also gather data on the cases already diagnosed in the community and focus attention on those areas and populations (such as migrant workers and the homeless).

CHAPTER 29

29.1 Chronic illness is often thought of as natural progression of the aging process. How can the community health nurse change this perception and what can be done to decrease the incidence of chronic illness in the older population?

Evaluating Student Responses: This is a very difficult perception to change. One way is to meet with older individuals who do not have chronic illness or disability. It might be possible to get some case studies that show how prompt attention to a problem can prevent it from progressing. The nurse might also meet with groups of older individuals who are presently dealing with a disability but have maintained independence through it. Some things to consider may be newspaper articles and television interviews and then some type of program that deals with the myth of aging and encourages people who are aging to stay active and to keep regular medical checkups.